PATHOPHYSIOLOGY OF SEVERE ISCHEMIC MYOCARDIAL INJURY

Developments in Cardiovascular Medicine

VOLUME 104

PATHOPHYSIOLOGY OF SEVERE ISCHEMIC MYOCARDIAL INJURY

edited by

Hans Michael Piper

Institute of Physiology
University of Düsseldorf
Düsseldorf, FRG

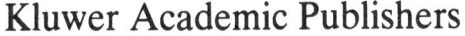

Kluwer Academic Publishers

Dordrecht / Boston / London

Library of Congress Cataloging-in-Publication Data

Pathophysiology of severe ischemic myocardial injury / edited by Hans
  Michael Piper.
       p.   cm. -- (Developments in cardiovascular medicine ; 104)

    1. Heart--Infarction--Pathophysiology. 2. Coronary heart disease-
  -Pathophysiology.   I. Piper, Hans Michael. II. Series:
  Developments in cardiovascular medicine ; v. 104.
    [DNLM: 1. Myocardial Reperfusion Injury--etiology. 2. Myocardial
  Reperfusion Injury--physiopathology.   W1 DE997VME v. 104 / WG 300
  P2977]
  RC685.I6P39   1990
  616.1'2307--dc20
  DNLM/DLC
  for Library of Congress   89-19985

ISBN-13: 978-94-010-6699-0   e-ISBN-13: 978-94-009-0475-0
DOI: 10.1007/978-94-009-0475-0

Published by Kluwer Academic Publishers,
P.O. Box 17, 3300 AA Dordrecht, The Netherlands.

Kluwer Academic Publishers incorporates
the publishing programmes of
D. Reidel, Martinus Nijhoff, Dr W. Junk and MTP Press.

Sold and distributed in the U.S.A. and Canada
by Kluwer Academic Publishers,
101 Philip Drive, Norwell, MA 02061, U.S.A.

In all other countries, sold and distributed
by Kluwer Academic Publishers Group,
P.O. Box 322, 3300 AH Dordrecht, The Netherlands.

Printed on acid-free paper

Table of Contents

vi

PART IX: CONCLUSIONS

Foreword

In industrialized countries, ischemic heart disease is by far the most common organ-specific cause of death. The thrombotic occlusion of a coronary artery which had previously been severely altered by atherosclerosis, is the most frequent cause of ischemic deterioration of myocardial tissue, i.e. myocardial infarction. Death of the human individual occurs when myocardial ischemia causes a critical impairment of cardiac pump function. The failure of a heart with an ischemic area may be due to the amount and location of contractile tissue becoming paralyzed or even necrotic, or to arrhythmias provoked by the ischemic condition, or by a combination of both factors.

Considerable progress has been made in the development of antiarrythmic therapy. Effective tools have been developed to reperfuse ischemic myocardial tissue as soon as the patient reaches hospital. However, therapeutical principles for the ischemic-reperfused myocardium which would specifically interfere with the state of injury of the ischemic tissue at the onset of reperfusion, and avoid the apparent hazards of the reperfusion process itself, have yet to be established. But not only approved therapeutical concepts are lacking, the pathophysiology of myocardial cell injury in progressive ischemia and under reperfusion is in itself only partly understood. In this book, an attempt has been made to give a critical overview of current factual knowledge and the prevailing ideas about the causes of severe ischemic myocardial injury and the possible outcomes of reperfusion which are either myocardial recovery or aggravation of the state of injury ('reperfusion injury'). It is the hope of the authors that a better understanding of the pathophysiology stimulates the development of new therapeutic approaches to the ischemic-reperfused myocardium.

Hans Michael Piper

List of Contributors

A.P. Allshire, Department of Human Anatomy and Cell Biology, The University of Liverpool, P.O. Box 147, Liverpool L69 3BX, UK
Co-author: P.H. Cobbold

M. Borgers, Laboratory for Cell Biology, Department of Life Sciences, Janssen Research Foundation, B-2340 Beerse, Belgium

R.S. Decker, Department of Medicine, Cardiology Division, Northwestern University, Medical School, 303 East Chicago Avenue, Chicago, IL 60611, USA
Co-author: M.L. Decker

C.E. Ganote, Department of Pathology, Northwestern University, Medical School, 303 East Chicago Avenue, Chicago, IL 60611, USA
Co-author: R.S. Vander Heide

R. Ferrari, Cattedra di Cardiologia, University of Brescia, Civil Hospital, I-25100 Brescia, Italy
Co-authors: S. Curello, A. Cargnoni, E. Condorelli, L. Comini, S. Ghielmi, C. Ceconi

H.K. Hagler, Department of Pathology, University of Texas, Southwestern Medical Center, 5323 Harry Hines Blvd., Dallas, TX 75235–9072, USA
Co-author: L.M. Buja

A.J. Liedtke, Cardiology Section, Department of Medicine, University of Wisconsin Hospital, 600 Highland Avenue, H6/339, Madison, WI 53792, USA
Co-author: E. Shrago

L.H. Opie, Heart Research Unit, University of Cape Town, Medical School, Cape Town 7925, South Africa

K.M. Mullane, Gensia Pharmaceuticals, Inc., 11075 Roselle Street, San Diego, CA 92121-1207, USA
Co-author: C.W. Smith

H.M. Piper, Institute of Physiology, University of Düsseldorf, Moorenstr. 5, D-4000 Düsseldorf 1, FRG
Co-authors: S. Buderus, A. Krützfeldt, T. Noll, S. Mertens, R. Spahr

P.A. Poole-Wilson, Department of Cardiac Medicine, National Heart and Lung Institute, Dovehouse Street, London SW3 6LY, UK

W. Schaper, Max-Planck-Institute, Department of Experimental Cardiology, Benekestrasse 2, D-6350 Bad Nauheim, FRG
Co-author: J. Schaper

A. Schömig, Department of Cardiology, University of Heidelberg, Bergheimerstr. 58, D-6900 Heidelberg, FRG
Co-authors: R. Strasser, G. Richardt

K. Schrör, Institute of Pharmacology, University of Düsseldorf, Moorenstr. 5, D-4000 Düsseldorf 1, FRG
Co-author: Th. Hohlfeld

P.G. Spieckermann, Institute of Medical Physiology, University of Vienna, Schwarzspanierstr. 17, A-1090 Vienna, Austria

G.J.M. Stienen, Laboratory of Physiology, Free University, Van der Boechorststraat 7, 1081 BT Amsterdam, The Netherlands
Co-author: G. Elzinga

G.J. van der Vusse, Department of Physiology, University of Limburg, Biomedical Center, P.O. Box 616, 6200 MD Maastricht, The Netherlands
Co-authors: M. van Bilsen, T. Sonderkamp, R.S. Reneman

PART I

Introduction

Irreversible ischemic injury – definition of the problem

HANS MICHAEL PIPER

Institut für Physiologie I der Universität Düsseldorf, Moorenstr. 5, D-4000 Düsseldorf, FRG

Introduction

In spite of tremendous strides forward in cardiac pathophysiology over the past 30 years, knowledge of the genesis of irreversible ischemic myocardial injury is still limited. Ischemic myocardial heart disease is predominantly caused by the thrombotic occlusion of coronary arteries. After an initial period of ischemia during which restoration of supply conditions still allows structural and functional recovery of the myocardial cell, ischemic injury becomes irreversible or, in other words, reversible ischemia turns into infarction.

In recent years, three theories have been discussed most thoroughly which relate the onset of irreversibility to either: a critical energy loss; a critical accumulation of cellular calcium; or to the deleterious effects of free radical formation. But other concepts have also been proposed, relating irreversible injury to the functional failure or structural deterioration of a certain cell structure, such as the sarcolemmal barrier; a critical disturbance of cellular lipid metabolism; or to the dysfunction of a particular non-muscular cell type, e.g. the endothelial cell. Together, these theories do not represent mutually exclusive alternatives; rather each of them accentuates a certain aspect of the pathophysiological process leading to irreversible myocardial injury. In certain experimental models, favourable results for each of these theories have been obtained.

During the past ten years, techniques to re-open a fresh thrombotic occlusion of a coronary vessel have come widely into use (percutaneous transluminal coronary angioplasty, intracoronary thrombolysis). But since a considerable time delay is usually unavoidable before the patient arrives at hospital, progressed stages of ischemic myocardial injury prevail in the clinical situation. It is therefore of great therapeutic value to better understand the causal key events in the process which leads to irreversible injury in ischemic-reperfused myocardium. In clinical practice, a very pragmatic definition of irreversible injury is generally applied; that is that all available techniques have failed to resuscitate the tissue. This operational definition, however, does not differentiate between the various possible causes of fail-

H.M. Piper (ed.) Pathophysiology of severe ischemic myocardial injury, 3–14.
© *1990 Kluwer Academic Publishers, Dordrecht –*

ure. Additionally, present practical limitations of resuscitation of ischemic myocardium may soon be overcome with the development of new therapeutic principles.

After prolonged ischemia, myocardial injury is not reversed but exacerbated as the tissue is re-supplied with oxygen and substrates. It has been debated whether this 'reperfusion injury' is actually caused by the process of reperfusion/reoxygenation or merely exposes pre-existing irreversible injury. If reperfusion injury is a genuine phenomenon, then a problem arises for the verification of irreversible ischemic injury. This is because it remains an important test for the reversible or irreversible character of ischemic injury to see whether the restoration of normal supply conditions leads to functional and structural recovery of the myocardium.

In summary, therapeutic principles are needed which can salvage myocardium at the point of irreversible injury. But in order to develop more effective treatment, a sound basis of pathophysiological knowledge is required. The hypotheses most adhered to currently about the pathogenesis of irreversible ischemia-reperfusion injury are discussed in this book.

Key events and secondary effects in the development of irreversible ischemic injury

Conceptual distinctions

In the analysis of the pathogenesis of irreversible myocardial injury under ischemia-reperfusion or hypoxia-reoxygenation, some conceptual distinctions should first be made (Table 1), since they are helpful in the analysis of the pathogenesis of irreversible myocardial injury. They serve to distinguish between key events and secondary effects in the development of injury. Key events are the basic steps in the process leading to cell deterioration, found in all models of the oxygen depleted and reoxygenated cardiomyocyte. Secondary effects may differ among the various models; they are either effects the energy depleted cardiomyocyte exerts on its environment or effects by which the injured cardiomyocyte is affected by its environment.

Regionality

When investigating the performance of the whole heart with an ischemic area of limited size, malfunctions may have their origin within the ischemic area or they may be caused by something, for example catecholamines, which is released by the ischemic tissue and influences the performance of the surrounding tissue. In the clinical situation, such an effect can be of primary importance since it might provoke unmanageable arrhythmias; but for the analysis of the process of ischemic injury it represents a secondary effect.

Table 1. Necessary distinctions in the analysis of irreversible ischemic myocardial cell injury.

1. Regionality
   * Condition of the ischemic area
     vs. secondary effects on the surrounding tissue
2. Injured cell type
   * Injury of the myocardial cell
     vs. injury of the vasculature
3. Cellular interactions
   * Injury of a cell caused by its own condition
     vs. injury by interference of adjacent cells
4. Course of injury development
   * Factors influencing the velocity of changes
     vs. factors interfering with key events
5. Effects of reperfusion/reoxygenation
   * Injury becoming apparent on reperfusion/reoxygenation
     vs. injury caused by reperfusion/reoxygenation
6. Indicators of irreversible cell injury
   * Indicators of manifest irreversible cell injury
     vs. indicators of the onset of irreversible injury

Injured cell type

A biological definition of irreversible myocardial injury should differentiate between irreversibility primarily due to cardiomyocyte damage, and irreversibility due to circulatory malfunction which prevents a re-supply of the ischemic cardiomyocyte with oxygen and substrates.

Cellular interactions

In contractile tissue, many cells may suffer from mechanical forces imposed on them by severely injured neighbouring cells. There should be further investigation into how well the individual cardiomyocyte could by itself recover from hypoxic injury at various stages of severity; and which external factors could prevent the cell's survival up to its own ultimate limit of reversibility.

Course of injury development

The various conditions and experimental models in which the myocardial cell is submitted to oxygen deficiency differ in the time needed for manifestation of irreversible injury. But do they also differ in the succession of the basic key events in the process of progressive injury? Which of the factors, known to influence the development of cell injury, change only the velocity of this development and which, by specific interference with such key events, are able to alter the direction of the development? It seems particularly important to make such distinctions when searching for new therapeutic principles.

Effects of reperfusion/reoxygenation

The most important test as to whether a certain state of ischemic or hypoxic myocardial cell injury is still reversible, is the re-supply with oxygen and substrates and washout of waste products. If this is done during the early phase of injury, aerobic energy metabolism will start working again, the ultrastructure will recover, and to a variable extent contractile function will be restored. But re-establishment of normal aerobic supply conditions does not always improve the condition of the tissue. After extended periods of ischemia or hypoxia, myocardial cell injury seems to become exacerbated rather than diminished, a phenomenon termed 'oxygen paradox' [1]. (Here, the terms 'reperfusion injury' for ischemically damaged myocardium and 'reoxygenation injury' for myocardium damaged by hypoxia are used as synonyms for 'oxygen paradox'.) The oxygen paradox is characterized by an abrupt release of intracellular constituents due to the sudden rupture of cell membranes and the unique phenomenon of contraction band formation [2]. Whether this reperfusion- or reoxygenation-induced injury is a manifestation of cell damage which was already present in the hypoxic cell, or is immediately caused by the re-introduction of oxygen, is still a matter of debate.

Indicators of irreversible heart cell injury

Macromolecule release or certain histological indicator reactions are frequently used as criteria for irreversible myocardial cell injury. But the logical status of these criteria is often unclear. First, they may indicate the onset of irreversible injury or the already manifest cell necrosis. For the causal analysis of the pathogenesis of irreversible injury only those criteria which identify its onset are useful (the point of no-return). Second, these criteria are often believed to be sufficient and necessary, that is, indicators which are always and only found to be positive when cell injury is irreversible. If the criteria in fact used are carefully examined, however, none of them represents such a reliable tool to detect the starting point of irreversible injury in ischemia-reperfusion of hypoxia-reoxygenation.

The release of enzymes is often regarded as an indicator of irreversible cell injury [3]. Enzyme release, however, is not always caused by irreversible cell disruption, since at moderate energetic stress, myocardial tissue can release small amounts of macromolecules from the cytosolic compartment by mechanisms other than persistent membrane perforation [4–6]. Histological techniques are applied in many studies to evaluate the 'viability' of injured myocardial tissue. On the light microscopic level, tetrazolium salt stain is used most frequently for tissue samples, and trypan blue for isolated cells. Both methods, however, have also been shown to produce false results [7, 8]. But also on the ultrastructural level, morphology alone has not been able to define the point of no-return. It might be a certain degree of metabolic failure which marks the onset of irreversible injury, rather than structural damage. But which metabolic function has to fail, and to what extent?

The search for causal key events

A number of conceptual distinctions are needed to analyze the process leading to irreversible injury of the cells contained in myocardial tissue. One possible approach to examining the causal connections of this process in greater detail is the reduction of variables of the pathophysiological situation. For this purpose, model studies using isolated cardiomyocytes under hypoxic conditions have been introduced in experimental research [8]. In such studies, one may find the ultimate biological borderline up to which functional and structural recovery of the energy depleted cardiomyocyte is possible. When the causal key events in this process become known, it might also be understood how far cell survival in the natural course of ischemic injury is limited by secondary factors, such as mutual mechanical cell interaction.

Determinants of severe ischemic and hypoxic injury

The role of energy deficiency

Since extensive energy depletion leads to severe cellular injury, it is tempting to search for a critical energetic threshold defining the point of no-return. An apparent ATP threshold (1–2 μmol/g wet weight) for resuscitability has been described for ischemic dog myocardium [9, 10], ischemic rat hearts [11] and anoxic cultured rat cardiomyocytes [12].

Coincidence of the practical limit of reversibility of injury with a certain tissue content of ATP may indicate a causal connection. Kübler and Spieckermann hypothesized that the decrease of tissue ATP below a threshold level leads to the irreversible cessation of glycolysis [9]. According to this hypothesis, the critical threshold must be found in all heart cell models. Alternatively, the relationship between the loss of tissue ATP and reversibility of injury may be indirect and accidental, in that a depressed energetic state severely disturbs crucial cell functions and crucial cell structures, like the homeostasis of the cystosolic cation content and the stability of phospholipid membranes. Since for the development of these defects the available energy is only one determinant among others, a single fixed ATP threshold for all models in which cardiomyocytes are made hypoxic is not to be expected.

Critical cellular structures

Irreversibility of myocardial cell injury may be due to functional failure or physical destruction of a certain cell structure. The sarcolemma could be the structure whose deterioration limits the survival of the whole cell. But sarcolemmal perforations, if not long-lived, can obviously be survived by cardiomyocytes. Transient sarcolemmal perforations occur, for example, when single cells are impaled by microelectrodes. Therefore, the question arises whether persistent holes have to be regarded as a phenomenon secondary to other crucial physicochemical changes of the sarcolemma, such as alterations in their phospholipid composition [13]. Sarcolemmal discontinuities may therefore represent only the inevitable consequence of previous crucial changes in the cell's metabolic state.

Damage to the mitochondria may be of crucial importance for the recovery from ischemic or hypoxic injury. Recovery of the myocardial cell after a period of oxygen depletion requires sufficient preservation of mitochondrial function. Apart from their central role in energy metabolism, mitochondria perform a vital function in cellular Ca^{2+} homeostasis, since they represent the largest intracellular compartment for the sequestration of cytosolic Ca^{2+}.

The role of lipids

In ischemic myocardial tissue, long-chain fatty acyl CoA and carnitine esters were found to accumulate quickly even in the absence of exogenous fatty acids [14]. Most of the accumulating long-chain acyl derivatives are hydrolysed from triglycerides and from membrane phospolipids [15]. Exogenous fatty acids, being the main fuel for the myocardium under aerobic conditions, are disadvantageous under oxygen deprivation since their presence further augments the accumulation of long-chain acyl esters in the myocardial cell [16, 17].

The accumulation of lipids as free amphiphiles and the degradation of lipids from cellular membranes may contribute to the progression of injury [18]. Both the detergent effect of long-chain acyl compounds and the loss of constituent phospolipids can alter the barrier and transport functions of cellular membranes and lead, ultimately, to their physical destruction. Such deleterious effects have been demonstrated with isolated membranes in the test tube. But it has not yet been clearly demonstrated that these compounds reach a free concentration in the ischemic cell, which is as harmful as in the cell-free system.

The role of oxygen radicals

The role of free radicals in severe myocardial injury has been extensively discussed during recent years. The term 'free radicals' refers to molecules with an unpaired electron, most of which are chemically highly reactive. Chemical radicals are intermediates of a number of biochemical reactions, and usually the cell is protected from their potentially deleterious effects [19, 20]. A crucial role of free radicals in myocardial injury could relate to an increase in free radical formation, greater toxicity of the species formed, and defects in the defence system. According to the most likely theory, oxygen radicals represent a crucial factor in reperfusion/reoxygenation injury [21] due to both their enhanced formation and to a weakening of the normal cellular defence mechanisms during ischemic or hypoxic stress. Toxicity of free radicals seems to enhance injury in certain experimental models as suggested by the beneficial effect of anti-free radical-directed interventions in these models.

The generation of oxygen radicals during reperfusion of ischemic myocardium has been clearly demonstrated [22–25]. It has, however, not yet been proven that these compounds are indeed of critical causal importance. Nor is the major source of oxygen radical formation known with any degree of certainty. This is partly due to the fact that current methodology is unable to determine precisely the quantity and molecular nature of the generated free radicals [25].

Oxygen free radical toxicity also represents one of the major ways in which white blood cells can augment tissue injury [26, 27]. But activated neutrophils are not of decisive importance for either the primary process of ischemic injury or for the rapidly developing reperfusion injury. The effect of activated neutrophils on ischemic-reperfused myocardium peaks after several hours of reperfusion [26, 27].

The role of calcium

Ultimately, irreversibly injured myocardial cells lose their ability to maintain the transsarcolemmal gradient of Ca^{2+} which comprises 4 orders of magnitude under resting conditions. High cytosolic Ca^{2+} concentrations cause hypercontracture when a sufficient amount of ATP is still or again available at myofibrillar sites [28]. Hypercontracture leads to massive disruptions of cytoskeletal cell structures.

Reoxygenation of myocardial cells which have accumulated high cytosolic Ca^{2+} levels causes problems not only for the myofibrils but also for the mitochondria. At elevated Ca^{2+} concentrations, mitochondria start to accumulate Ca^{2+} when respiratory energy is generated. Expenditure of respiratory energy for the accumulation of Ca^{2+} reduces the energy available for the formation of ATP [29]. It therefore prevents the mitochondria from rapidly providing energy for the sarcolemmal pump mechanisms which could reestablish a normal cytosolic cation homeostasis. Massive Ca^{2+} overload causes irreversible injury of the mitochondria [30].

An energy depleted myocardial cell seems better able to tolerate Ca^{2+} overload than the cell resupplied with oxygen [31]. But Ca^{2+} overload may also cause injury under such conditions, for instance, by the activation of phospholipases [32], so that eventually high cytosolic Ca^{2+} concentrations invariably lead to cell deterioration. It is not yet known for precisely how long Ca^{2+} overload can be tolerated by an energy depleted cardiomyocyte.

Mechanical factors

The oxygen paradox is characterized by a sudden onset of contracture and sarcolemmal disruption of myocardial cells when the myocardium is reoxygenated after a prolonged period of oxygen deficiency. Contracture could be the immediate cause of sarcolemmal disruptions, but it is also conceivable that sarcolemmal integrity is lost first of all with contracture developing thereafter. Experiments with isolated cardiomyocytes, exposed to anoxia-reoxygenation, seem to permit a decision between these alternatives. When isolated cardiomyocytes are reoxygenated after a prolonged period of hypoxia, they develop hypercontracture, but retain sarcolemmal integrity. Even after the development of hypercontracture, they are able to re-establish a normal phosphorylation potential [33] and to renormalize their cytosolic Ca^{2+} homeostasis [31, 33]. These results suggest that this cell type could, in principle, survive the conditions that elicit hypercontracture upon reoxygenation. In tissue where the cells are mutually mechanically coupled, contracture causes mechanical cell disruption. It is possible that only a minority of the myocardial cells in reoxygenated tissue needs to be prone to hypercontracture in order to trigger the deterioration of the whole. Increased fragility of the cardiomyocytes [34] after ischemia can increase this snowball effect.

The role of endothelial cells and neurons

When the metabolic function of endothelial cells in ischemic tissue becomes seriously altered, this may render successful reperfusion impossible. Energy depleted endothelial cells can swell so extensively that the capillary bed becomes completely occluded. This in turn creates a situation which is almost irreversible for the affected area of tissue, a phenomenon termed 'no-reflow' [35]. But in successfully reperfused myocardium, endothelial dysfunction can also influence the recovery of myocardial tissue. Increased permeability of the endothelial lining to water and solutes contributes to the development of edema [36]. It has been discussed whether endothelial dysfunction during reperfusion also clearly exacerbates tissue injury in that it becomes the primary cause of reperfusion injury [37]. Endothelial cells might be the source of oxygen radicals generated by xanthine oxidase [21], an enzyme localized in the heart only in the endothelial cell compartment [38].

The mass of neuronal cells in the myocardium is negligibly small. Therefore, their direct metabolic contribution to the metabolism of the whole tissue is minimal. A metabolic dysfunction of cardiac neurons can, nevertheless, have serious consequences for the ischemic and the adjacent myocardial tissue if release and re-uptake of transmitter hormones is altered. The loss of noradrenaline from adrenergic nerve endings in ischemic myocardium is best investigated. The effects of increased interstitial concentrations of catecholamine are multifold. The stimulation of β-adrenoreceptors on the cardiomyocytes may directly increase their metabolic demand, thereby shortening their lifespan. Possibly of greater pathophysiological significance are the actions of catecholamines which leak from the ischemic into the adjacent tissue. There, they can cause life threatening arrhythmias [39]. The α-adrenoreceptor mediated vasoconstrictory effect can further enhance the underperfusion [40]. *In vivo*, the pain reaction to myocardial ischemia stimulates additional catecholamine release in the injured heart [41].

Neurons in myocardial tissue also contain transmitters other than catecholamines. Neuropeptide Y, which is contained both in the adrenergic nerve endings and in intrinsic myocardial neurons [42, 43], has a pronounced vasoconstrictory effect [44]. It is conceivable that its release into ischemic tissue aggravates the degree of underperfusion of the ischemic area. Neuropeptide Y also exerts, however, a direct anti-adrenergic effect on the cardiomyocyte [45, 46] and has an inhibitory effect on the release of noradrenaline from adrenergic nerve endings [44]. In general, then, its role in ischemic myocardium could be beneficial.

Conclusions

Any discussion of the pathophysiology of severe ischemic myocardial injury has to encounter the problem that the immediate determinants which at some stage render progressive cell injury irreversible, are not yet clearly identified. The usual ways of reperfusing ischemic tissue may not be delicate enough to allow recovery, and therefore failure to restore myocardial function after a short period of reperfusion cannot be accepted as proof of the irreversibility of cell injury.

The analysis of the pathogenesis of severe ischemia-reperfusion injury in the heart *in situ* is hampered by the great complexity of this process. From studies on the ischemic heart in situ many factors have become known which influence the natural course of injury development. While such studies have elucidated many details of the pathophysiological process, they have also led to a great number of divergent opinions concerning the basic causal mechanisms. The basic mechanisms are more likely to be identified by searching for key events common to the development of cell injury in models of reduced complexity. In combining both approaches, it may be possible to identify events of primary and secondary causal importance for the manifestation of irreversible myocardial injury.

12

Acknowledgements

This study was supported by the Deutsche Forschungsgemeinschaft, grants Pi 162/2-1 and A6 of SFB 242.

References

1. Hearse DJ, Humphrey SM, Chain EB (1973) Abrupt reoxygenation of the anoxic potassium-arrested perfused rat heart: A study of myocardial enzyme release. J Mol Cell Cardiol 5: 395–407
2. Ganote CE (1983) Contraction band necrosis and irreversible myocardial injury. J Mol Cell Cardiol 15: 67–73
3. Ahmed SA, Williamson JR, Roberts E, Clark RE, Sobel BE (1976) The association of increased plasma MB CPK activity and irreversible ischemic myocardial injury in the dog. Circulation 54: 187–193
4. Spieckermann PG, Nordbeck H, Preusse CJ (1979) From heart to plasma. In: Hearse DJ, De Leiris J (eds) Enzymes in Cardiology: Diagnosis and Research. New York, John Wiley, pp 59–79
5. Piper HM, Schwartz P, Hütter JF, Spieckermann PG (1984) Energy metabolism and enzyme release of cultured adult rat heart muscle cells during anoxia. J Mol Cell Cardiol 16: 995–1007
6. Wienen W, Kammermeier H (1988) Intra- and extracellular markers in interstitial transsudate of perfused rat hearts. Am J Physiol 254: H785–H794
7. Barnard RJ, Okamoto F, Buckberg GD, Sjostrand F, Rosenkranz ER, Vinten-Johansen J, Allen BS, Leaf J (1986) Studies of controlled reperfusion after ischemia. III. Histochemical studies: Inability of triphenyltetrazolium chloride nonstaining to define tissue necrosis. J Thorac Cardiovasc Surg 92: 5002–5012
8. Piper HM (1988) Evaluation of anoxic injury in isolated adult cardiomycytes. In: Clark WA, Decker RS, Borg TK (eds) Biology of Isolated Adult Cardiac Myocytes. New York, Elsevier, pp 68–81
9. Kübler W, Spieckermann PG (1970) Regulation of glycolysis in the ischemic and the anoxic myocardium. J Mol Cell Cardiol 1: 351–377
10. Jennings RB, Hawkins HK, Lowe JE, Hill ML, Klotman S, Reimer KA (1978) Relation between high energy phosphate and lethal injury in myocardial injury in the dog. Am J Pathol 92: 187–241
11. Taegtmeyer H, Roberts AFC, Raine AEG (1985) Energy metabolism in reperfused heart muscle: metabolic correlates to return of function. J Am Coll Cardiol 6: 864–870
12. Schwartz P, Piper HM, Spahr R, Spieckermann PG (1984) Ultrastructure of adult myocardial cells during anoxia and reoxygenation. Am J Pathol 115: 349–361
13. Chien KR, Han A, Sen A, Buja LM, Willerson JT (1984) Accumulation of unesterified arachidonic acid in ischemic canine myocardium: Relation to a phosphatidylcholine deacylation-reacylation cycle and the depletion of membrane lipids. Circ Res 54: 313–322
14. Idell-Wenger JA, Grotyohann LW, Neely JR (1978) Coenzyme A and carnitine distribution in normal and ischemic hearts. J Biol Chem 253: 4310–4318
15. Van der Vusse GJ, Stam H (1987) Accumulation of lipids and lipid-intermediates in the heart during ischaemia. Basic Res Cardiol 82, suppl 1: 157–167
16. Piper HM, Das A (1987) Detrimental actions of endogenous fatty acids and their derivatives. A study of ischaemic mitochondrial injury. Basic Res Cardiol 82, suppl 1: 187–196
17. Piper HM, Das A (1986) The role of fatty acids in ischemic tissue injury: difference between oleic and palmitic acid. Basic Res Cardiol 81: 373–383
18. Katz AM, Messineo FC (1981) Lipid-membrane interactions and the pathogenesis of ischemic damage in the myocardium. Circ Res 48: 1–16

19. Slater TF (1984) Free radical mechanisms in tissue injury. Biochem J 222: 1–15
20. Sies H, Cadenas E (1985) Oxidative stress: damage to intact cells and organs. Phil Trans R Soc Lond B 311: 617–631
21. McCord JM (1988) Free radicals and myocardial ischemia: Overview and outlook. Free Rad Biol Med 4: 9–14
22. Arroyo CM, Kramer JH, Dickens BF, Weglicki WB (1987) Identification of free radicals in myocardial ischemia reperfusion by spin trapping with nitrone DMPO. FEBS Lett 211: 101–104
23. Garlick PB, Davies MJ, Slater TS, Hearse DJ (1987) Detection of free radical production in the isolated rat heart using a spin trap agent and electron spin resonance. Circ Res 61: 757–760
24. Zweier JL, Flaherty JT, Weisfeldt ML (1987) Direct measurement of free radical generation following reperfusion of ischemic myocardium. Proc Natl Acad Sci USA 84: 1404–1407
25. Baker JE, Felix CC, Olinger GN, Kalyanaraman B (1988) Myocardial ischemia and reperfusion: Direct evidence for free radical generation by electron spin resonance spectroscopy. Proc Natl Acad Sci USA 85: 2786–2789
26. Mullane KM, Salmon JA, Kraemer R (1987) Leukocyte-derived metabolites of arachidonic acid in ischemia-induced myocardial injury. Fed Proc 46: 2422–2433
27. Werns SW, Lucchesi BR (1988) Leukocytes, oxygen radicals, and myocardial injury due to ischemia and reperfusion. Free Rad Biol Med 4: 31–37
28. Piper HM (1989) Energy deficiency, calcium overload or oxidative stress: possible causes of irreversible ischemic myocardial injury. Klin Wschr 67: 465–476
29. Carafoli E (1985) The homeostasis of calcium in heart cells. J Mol Cell Cardiol 17: 203–212
30. Nicholls DG, Crompton M (1980) Mitochondrial calcium transport. FEBS Lett 111: 261–268
31. Piper HM, Jacobson SL, Schwartz JL, Mealing GAR, Whitfield JF (1988) Disturbance of Ca^{2+} homeostasis in restrained cardiomyocytes under anoxia and reoxygenation. J Mol Cell Cardiol 20, suppl V: 35
32. Weglicki WB, Low MG (1987) Phospholipases of the myocardium. Basic Res Cardiol 82, suppl 1: 107–119
33. Siegmund B, Koop A, Klietz T, Schwartz P, Piper HM (1989) Sarcolemmal integrity and metabolic competence of cardiomyocytes under anoxia-reoxygenation. Am J Physiol: in press
34. Ganote CE, Vander Heide RS (1988) Irreversible injury of isolated adult rat myocytes. Osmotic fragility during metabolic inhibition. Am J Pathol 132: 212–222
35. Kloner RA, Ganote CE, Jennings RB (1974) The 'no-reflow' phenomenon after temporary coronary occlusion in the dog. J Clin Invest 54: 1496–1508
36. Sunnergren KP, Rovetto MJ (1987) Myocyte and endothelial injury with ischemia reperfusion in isolated rat hearts. Am J Physiol 252: H1211–H1217
37. Buderus S, Siegmund B, Spahr R, Krützfeldt A, Piper HM (1989) Resistance of endothelial cells to anoxia-reoxygenation in isolated guinea pig hearts. Am J Physiol 257: 488–493
38. Jarasch ED, Grund C, Bruder G, Heid HW, Keenan TW, Franke WW (1981) Localization of xanthine oxidase in mammary gland epithelium and capillary endothelium. Cell 25: 67–82
39. Penny WJ (1984) The deleterious effects of myocardial catecholamines on cellular electrophysiology and arrhythmias during ischemia and reperfusion. Eur Heart J 5: 960–973
40. Heusch G, Deussen A (1983) The effects of cardiac sympathetic nerve stimulation on the perfusion of stenotic coronary arteries in the dog. Circ Res 53: 8–15
41. Kröger K, Schipke J, Heusch G, Thämer V (1989) Myocardial dysfunction induced by peripheral nociceptive stimulation. Europ Heart J : in press
42. Gu J, Polak JM, Allen JM, Huang WM, Sheppard MN, Tatemoto K, Bloom SR (1984) High concentrations of a novel peptide, neuropeptide Y, in the innervation of mouse and rat heart. J Histochem Cytochem 32: 467–472
43. Hassall CJS, Burnstock G (1984) Neuropeptide Y-like immunoreactivity in cultured intrinsic neurones of the heart. Neuroscience Lett 52: 111–115
44. Edvinsson L, Hakanson R, Wahlestedt C, Uddman R (1987) Effects of neuropeptide Y on the cardiovascular system. Trends Pharmacol Sci 8: 231–235

45. Millar BC, Piper HM, McDermott BJ (1988) The antiadrenergic effect of neuropeptide Y on the ventricular cardiomyocyte. Naunyn Schmiedeberg's Arch Pharmacol 338: 426–429
46. Piper HM, Millar BC, McDermott BJ (1989) The negative inotropic effect of neuropeptide Y on the ventricular cardiomyocyte. Naunyn Schmiedeberg's Arch Pharmacol 340: 333–337

Recovery of severely ischemic myocardium – a challenge for the clinical cardiologist

PHILIP A. POOLE-WILSON

Department of Cardiac Medicine, National Heart and Lung Institute, Dovehouse Street, London SW3 6LY, UK

Introduction

The presence of atheroma in the coronary arteries of humans can lead to many clinical syndromes including angina, sudden death and myocardial infarction. These entities, collectively referred to as coronary or ischemic heart disease, cause substantial morbidity and mortality in many countries and particularly in men in the age range 45–65 years. Expenditure on the prevention and treatment of coronary artery disease is massive. The consequences of coronary artery disease for health care in the community represent a major challenge to doctors, scientists, epidemiologists and public health workers.

The initiating cause of coronary events

Several early descriptions exist of what were probably heart attacks or angina. The best modern description of angina is attributed to Heberden [1] and the diagnosis of myocardial infarction in the living to Obrastzow and Straschenko [2] and Herrick [3]. Controversy used to exist with regard to the pathology of myocardial infarction and in particular whether infarction was initiated by coronary vasoconstriction or by thrombosis in the coronary artery. Only recently has this controversy been resolved. Coronary angiography undertaken soon after myocardial infarction [4] has shown that thrombosis occurs in 80% of full thickness infarcts and the frequency of observing an obstruction decreases subsequently. This is interpreted as suggesting that thrombosis is an early event and that the thrombosis can spontaneously resolve. In non-Q wave infarcts the opposite is found [5]. Total occlusion of a coronary artery by a thrombus is rare and the incidence increases with time. Thus thrombosis in this clinical context is a late event. This apparent contradiction is explained by current ideas on the earliest pathological events in the development of myocardial infarction.

The initial event seems to be rupture or a bleed in the wall of the coronary

H.M. Piper (ed.) Pathophysiology of severe ischemic myocardial injury, 15–24.
© *1990 Kluwer Academic Publishers, Dordrecht –*

artery in the immediate vicinity of an atheromatous plaque. The raw surface of the artery initiates a series of biochemical processes involving an interaction between the components of the blood stream and the vessel wall which lead to the accumulation of platelets and the formation of a thrombus. This initial process is dynamic. Evidence indicates that in patients undergoing myocardial infarction, opening and closing of the artery is common and is related partly to vasoconstriction and partly to thrombus formation and dissolution [6]. Rupture of an unstable plaque may not always lead to a coronary event and may be unnoticed by the patient. But plaque rupture is common in persons dying suddenly [7]. Some cases of sudden death may not be related to ischemia from the thrombus but to the electrophysiological consequences of a platelet embolus passing further down the coronary tree or to disease unrelated to atheroma [8]. Furthermore, rupture of a plaque does not necessarily occur at severely stenosed lesions. Coronary angiography after infarction shows that the lesion at the site of the thrombosis may be small. Rupture of an unstable plaque may depend more on the nature of the plaque (calcified, fibrotic, lipid laden) that on the severity of occlusion of the coronary artery.

These concepts regarding the initiation of coronary events in arteries diseased with atheroma in man have major consequences for the interpretation of results from experimental work in animals.

During the last 25 years, much work has been undertaken in attempts either to reduce infarct size in the myocardium following occlusion of a coronary artery or to delay the development of tissue necrosis. Much has been learned. In retrospect, it is difficult to understand how the concept of reduction of infarct size without any change of coronary flow was so easily accepted in a tissue, such as the heart, which is critically dependent on blood flow for its proper function. What has become evident is that maintained or restored blood flow is a necessary prerequisite for the long-term survival of cardiac cells. This increase of blood flow must arise from removal of the occlusion, flow through pre-existing collaterals, or opening or growth of new collaterals.

The meaning of words

Cardiologists are fond of inventing new terms and phrases. Examples include reversible and irreversible damage, jeopardised myocardium, threatened myocardium, lethal ischemia, borderzone, salvaged myocardium, infarct size and area at risk. More recent examples are stunned myocardium [9], stuttering ischemia [10], hibernating myocardium [11], ischemic preconditioning and total ischemic burden [12]. Some of the concepts contained in these phrases are similar to the earlier concept of chronic ischemia. Such phrases are useful shorthand but have almost no other value. Many of the terms are poorly defined. The best example is the distinction implied by the use of the phrases reversible and irreversible damage during ischemia. The presence of irreversible damage can only be established by reperfusion of the myocardium and later quantitation of the amount of necrotic tissue. There is no means of characterizing myocytes as irreversibly damaged during ischemia, since key events may occur at the moment of reperfusion and an intervention may be discovered which can reduce the amount of subsequent necrotic tissue. The only exception is the presence of a total loss of cell organisation or disruption of the sarcolemma during ischemia. That is a late event and not useful to the clinician or experimentalist.

Clinical results

The GISSI trial of streptokinase [13] in patients with myocardial infarction has established that thrombosis is an important process in the pathology of myocardial infarction, that reperfusion of the myocardium is advantageous, and that the duration of the ischemic period is a critical determinant of the sequelae of infarction. The results have since been confirmed in four additional trials using a variety of thrombolytic agents [14–17]. The endpoint of the GISSI trial was death, an unquestionable endpoint with immediate impact on clinician, patient and the public. Other studies have demonstrated reduction of infarct size and improved myocardial function after thrombolytic therapy.

These clinical trials have confirmed what has been established over the last two decades by experimental scientists, namely that infarct size was determined by (1) the duration of the ischemic period, (2) the amount of muscle dependent for blood flow on the occluded artery, (3) the presence of residual blood flow through the native vessels, (4) the blood flow through collateral vessels, and (5) the oxygen consumption at the moment of occlusion (Table 1). The problems now facing the clinician are (Table 2) whether other drug interventions at the moment of reperfusion can limit the ultimate extent of myocardial necrosis, whether blood flow after thrombolysis is maximal (reflow is not synonomous with patency – the no-reflow phenomenon is a real entity), whether immediate recurrence of the thrombosis can be prevented, and whether manipulation of the repair processes and inflammation following infarction is beneficial or harmful. What is unquestionable is that reperfusion soon after occlusion of a coronary artery is advantageous. Permanent total

Table 1. Determinants of myocardial infarct size.

1. Duration of ischemic episode
2. Anatomical distribution of the occluded artery
3. Presence and extent of existing collaterals
4. Residual flow through native vessels – 'stuttering ischemia'
5. Oxygen consumption at the moment of occlusion

Table 2. Recanalization – the clinical problems.

---

1. Therapy at time of thrombolysis to delay cell death
2. Establish reflow after recanalization
3. Prevention of early restenosis
4. Modification of inflammatory and repair processes
5. Timing of investigation and possible angioplasty
6. Long term prevention of atheroma
7. Long term prevention of recurrent cardiac events

---

occlusion will always lead to more cell death than partial occlusion or late reperfusion.

Experimental models and disease in man

In broad terms, experimental results in animals have provided information relevant to the pathology of myocardial infarction in man but most experimental animal models are grossly over-simplistic. Perhaps the three major considerations are, first, that in man myocardial infarction usually occurs in the presence of previous disease or, at least, of atheroma in more than one coronary artery. Chronic obstruction to flow will have allowed collaterals to develop and flow may be limiting in other areas of heart muscle when a given part of the myocardium ceases to function because of coronary occlusion. Second, the occlusion and re-opening of an artery is related to plaque rupture and thrombosis [6] and is almost never as acute as in experimental models [4–6]. Experimentally, reperfusion of coronary arteries is usually achieved by release of some form of constrictor. Rapid reperfusion in this way is more harmful to the myocardium than slow restoration of flow [18]. In man, in the context of myocardial infarction, the process is more complex and can be intermittent [6] i.e. stuttering ischemia. Ischemia may be terminated either by natural thrombolysis or thrombolytic therapy, both of which are slow processes in comparison to the release of an occluder. Third, most infarctions in man appear to be associated with episodes of ischemia and reflow at the onset of infarction (stuttering ischemia) so that the 'preconditioning effect' [19, 20] needs more consideration.

No-reflow phenomenon

The patency of a coronary artery is not synonomous with reperfusion. Following a transient period of ischemia, flow is increased (the hyperemic response). After more prolonged ischemia, flow on release of the occlusion is greatly reduced and this is referred to as the no-reflow phenomenon [21–24]. If myocardium is maximally vasodilated before a period of ischemia, then both ischemia and hypoxia progressively increase coronary resistance. The increase of flow after short periods of ischemia only occurs because initial tone in the coronary arteries is present. Many mechanisms contribute to the increase of resistance. These include smooth muscle contraction [22], extra-vascular forces such as myocardial oedema [25] and contracture of myocytes [22], plugging of arterioles [26], oedema of endothelial cells and damage to the endothelium. Hemorrhage can occur in dogs following sudden restoration of flow, but seems to be a rare event in man.

Reperfusion damage

Reperfusion of heart muscle after more than a few minutes of ischemia is accompanied by a transient rise of resting tension, release of intracellular enzymes, persisting functional abnormalities, influx of calcium, disruption of cell membranes and eventual necrosis of at least a proportion of the tissue. This entity has been called 'reperfusion damage'. The damage is believed to be the consequence of events occurring at the moment of reperfusion and not the result of biochemical changes during the period of ischemia. The litera-ture has been reviewed [27]. The existence of reperfusion damage has been challenged, the entity being regarded as the expression of events occurring during ischemia which become evident when flow is re-established; yet that is an unlikely explanation, since an identical phenomenon occurs on reoxygena-tion [28]. Reperfusion damage has also been considered as damage which would otherwise inevitably occur over time but which was evident in a short period of time.

The proof of the existence of reperfusion damage depends on the descrip-tion of the mechanism or the demonstration that the phenomenon can be prevented by an intervention at the moment of reperfusion. The latter condition is pivotal. Numerous pharmacological interventions have been shown to increase recovery of the myocardium after a period of ischemia, but most need to be introduced before the onset of ischemia and thus have limited clinical application. Such interventions exert a benefit by a cardioplegic effect (reduction of myocardial contraction resulting in a lower rate of consumption of adenosine triphosphate), alteration of coronary flow at the moment of reperfusion, change of systemic hemodynamics to alter oxygen consumption or alteration of residual flow through the native coronary vessel or collaterals.

In the dog, the infusion of superoxide dismutase and catalase at the moment of reperfusion results in a reduction of infarct size [29]. The effect appears to be independent of the other variables previously mentioned although these are notoriously difficult to measure and hold constant in the canine model. In other models superoxide dismutase does increase coronary flow on reperfusion [30, 31].

The most convincing evidence comes from experiments where the calcium concentration in the perfusate is manipulated at the time of reperfusion.

Table 3. Major factors in reperfusion or reoxygenation injury.

Factor	Consequence
1. Reactive radicals	Damage to lipid membranes
	Modulation of membrane proteins
2. Sodium-calcium exchange Sodium-hydrogen exchange	Calcium overload
3. Activation of phospholipases Lipid accumulation	Increased membrane permeability
4. Osmotic forces and cell swelling Intercellular mechanical forces	Cell membrane disruption

Increased recovery of mechanical function has been reported in the working rat heart preparation [32] and improvement of both function and biochemical parameters in the arterially perfused septum of the rabbit [33, 34]. These experiments seem to establish that reperfusion damage is a real phenomenon due to events affecting the myocyte at the moment of reperfusion.

Hypotheses to explain reperfusion damage

Many hypotheses have been put forward to account for reperfusion damage. Some are shown in Table 3.

The oldest and best known hypothesis is the calcium hypothesis. This supposes that the sudden influx of calcium on reperfusion is the primary cause of subsequent cell death. Certainly, calcium does accumulate immediately in the reperfused myocardium [35–38]. The net gain is due to an increase of influx not reduction of efflux and the degree of cell damage relates to the total tissue calcium. The essential question is what brings about the increased influx of calcium and whether the influx is a consequence of damage to the cell membrane and movement of calcium down its concentration gradient (extracellular calcium 10^{-3}M, intracellular calcium 10^{-6}M) or a result of the normal function of physiological ion control mechanisms in the presence of pathological ionic gradients. Calcium accumulation in the myocyte does not always lead to necrosis. A small net gain of calcium can be ejected by the cell's normal mechanisms for the control of intracellular calcium [39].

The calcium influx occurs in the absence of gross disruption of the cell membrane (see below) and is not inhibited by calcium antagonists, high extracellular potassium, quiescence or alpha-blockade [37, 38, 40]. It can be inhibited by nickel ions [38] and is mimicked by hydrogen or cumene peroxide but not lysophosphatidylcholine [40]. These observations support the idea that calcium influx is at least in part due to modification of the cell membrane at the moment of reoxygenation or reperfusion resulting in a massive influx of calcium.

Damage to the cell membrane may result from mechanical stresses from adjacent cells on the cell membrane which develop contracture as a result of a small inward movement of calcium [41]. Osmotic pressure changes on reperfusion may cause the cell to be disrupted and calcium to flow into the cell down its concentration gradient [42]. These mechanisms are probably not of central importance since influx of calcium can occur without markers gaining access to the intracellular space [38]. Total destruction of the cell membrane is a late event in myocardial ischemia and not a determining factor in the development of necrosis.

Alterations in the lipid structure have been described and lead to the formation of blebs and enzyme loss [43]. Recently it has been shown that sarcolemmal vesicles are sensitized to the effects of oxygen radicals by these lipids [44].

Lazdunski and colleagues [45] have put forward the hypothesis that sodium-hydrogen exchange is inhibited during ischemia by the low extracellular pH. On reperfusion hydrogen ions move out of the cell in exchange for sodium. The increase in the intracellular sodium concentration activates sodium-calcium exchange. The overall consequence is an increased calcium influx due to a net exchange of hydrogen and calcium ions. This hypothesis in its simplest form is unlikely to be correct since calcium influx occurs on reoxygenation and reperfusion and during hypoxia the extracellular pH is not greatly altered. Nevertheless, it is conceivable that sodium-calcium exchange is a relevant mechanism and other factors initiate this series of ionic events.

The most fashionable idea for the cause of reperfusion damage is that the function of the cell membrane by oxygen or other radicals generated at the moment of reperfusion. Calcium influx can be mimicked by peroxides [40]. During ischemia, the enzyme systems used by the cell to protect itself from radicals are reduced in activity. Some evidence does exist for the increased production of radicals [47]. Much of the evidence for this hypothesis has rested on experiments using inhibitors of questionable specificity and affecting only one mechanism of radical production. Radicals could be generated from white cells, the endothelium, in the cell membrane or in mitochondria. White cells are absent from many preparations in which reperfusion damage has been demonstrated. Several studies have shown a beneficial effect of adding superoxide dismutase to the perfusate or blood before reperfusion [29, 31]. This substance can alter coronary blood flow [30, 31] so that not all its effects are necessarily due to the destruction of radicals. The enzyme may not cross the cell membrane and it could be that in some models where no effect of superoxide dismutase has been observed [48] radicals are formed in mitochondria or the inner surface of the cell membrane and are inaccessible to the enzyme.

Few experiments exist in which the effects of reperfusion have unquestionably been prevented. For this to be shown, the intervention must be introduced at the moment of reperfusion or just before. The manipulation of the extracellular calcium concentration [32–34] and the addition of superoxide dismutase [29] are two interventions which appear to be beneficial at least in some models.

Conclusion

Reperfusion damage is a real entity and can be modified. There is evidence for reperfusion damage in man [49]. Reperfusion is always beneficial since increase of the duration of ischemia is harmful, but the benefits of reperfusion are small after 60 minutes total occlusion. The effects of ischemia are dependent on residual or collateral flow so that the time before the onset of cell necrosis can be greatly extended by a small residual coronary flow. The mechanism of reperfusion damage is complex and probably multifactorial. Calcium accumulation usually accompanies reperfusion damage and is probably not just a marker of such damage but also a cause of the damage. At present no effective therapeutic intervention has been identified but the principle has been established that intervention at the time of reperfusion can influence the occurrence of damage.

References

1. Heberden W (1772) Some account of a disorder of the breast. Med Trans Coll Phys (London) 2: 59–67
2. Obrastzow WP, Straschenko ND (1910) Zur Kenntis der Thrombose der Koronararterien des Herzens. Z Klin Med 71: 116–125
3. Herrick JB (1912) Clinical features of sudden obstruction of the coronary arteries. JAMA 59: 2015–2020
4. DeWood MA, Spores J, Notske R, Mouser LT, Burroughs R, Golden MS, Lang HT (1980) Prevalence of total coronary occlusion during the early hours of transmural myocardial infarction. N Engl J Med 303: 897–902
5. DeWood MA, Stifter WF, Simpson CS, Spores J, Eugster GS, Judge TP, Hinnen ML (1980) Coronary arteriographic findings soon after non-Q-wave myocardial infarction. N Engl J Med 315: 417–423
6. Davies GJ, Cherchia S, Maseri A (1986) Prevention of myocardial infarction by very early treatment with intra-coronary streptokinase. N Engl J Med 311: 1488–1492
7. Davies MJ, Thomas A (1986) Thrombosis and acute coronary-artery lesions in sudden cardiac death. New Engl J Med 310: 1137–1140
8. Thomas AC, Knapman PA, Krikler DM, Davies MJ (1988) Community study of the causes of 'natural' sudden death. Br Med J 297: 1453–1456
9. Braunwald E, Kloner RA (1982) The stunned myocardium: prolonged, postischemic ventricular dysfunction. Circulation 66: 1146–1149
10. Poole-Wilson PA (1986) What causes cell death? In: DJ Hearse, DM Yellon (eds) Therapeutic approaches to myocardial infarct size limitation. Raven Press: New York pp 43–60
11. Rahimtoola SH (1985) A perspective on the three large multicenter randomised clinical trials of coronary bypass surgery for chronic stable angina. Circulation 72 (suppl 5): 123–135

23

12. Cohn PF (1986) Total ischemic burden: definition, mechanisms, and therapeutic implications. Am J Med 81: 2–6
13. GISSI Study (1986) Effectiveness of intravenous thrombolytic treatment in acute myocardial infarction. Lancet 1: 397–401
14. The ISAM Study Group (1986) A prospective trial of intravenous streptokinase in acute myocardial infarction (ISAM). Mortality, morbidity, and infarct size at 21 days. N Engl J Med 314: 1465–1471
15. ISIS-2 Collaborative Group (1988) Randomised trial of intravenous streptokinase, oral aspirin, both, or neither among 17187 cases of suspected acute myocardial infarction: ISIS-2. Lancet 2: 349–360
16. AIMS Trial Study Group (1988) Effect of intravenous APSAC on mortality after acute myocardial infarction: preliminary report of a placebo-controlled trial. Lancet 1: 545–549
17. Wilcox RG, Olsson CG, Skene AM, Von der Lippe G, Jensen G, Hampton JR (1988) Trial of tissue plasminogen activator for mortality reduction in acute myocardial infarction. Lancet 2: 526–530
18. Yamazaki S, Fujibayashi Y, Rajogopalan RE, Meerbaum S, Corday E (1986) Effects of staged versus sudden reperfusion after acute coronary occlusion in the dog. J Am Coll Cardiol 7: 564–572
19. Neely JR, Grotyohann LW (1986) Role of glycolytic products in damage to ischemic myocardium. Dissociation of adenosine triphosphate levels and recovery of function of reperfused ischemic hearts. Circ Res 55: 816–824
20. Murry CE, Jennings RB, Reimer KA (1986) Preconditioning with ischemia: a delay of lethal cell injury in ischemic myocardium. Circulation 74: 1124–1136
21. Kloner Ra, Reimer KA, Willerson JT, Jennings RB (1976) The 'no-reflow' phenomenon after temporary coronary occlusion in the dog. J Clin Invest 54: 1496–1508
22. Fleetwood G, Poole-Wilson PA (1986) Diastolic coronary resistance in the isolated rabbit heart during and after ischaemia: contribution of extracellular forces. Cardiov Res 20: 883–890
23. Humphrey SM, Gavin JB, Herdson PB (1980) The relationship of ischemic contracture to vascular reperfusion in the isolated rat heart. J Mol Cell Cardiol 12: 1397–1406
24. Johnson WB, Malone SA, Pantely GA, Anselone CG, Bristow JD (1988) No reflow and extent of infarction during maximal vasodilatation in the porcine heart. Circulation 78: 462–472
25. Vogel WM, Cerel AW, Apstein CS (1986) Post-ischaemic cardiac chamber stiffness and coronary vasomotion: the role of edema and effects of dextran. J Mol Cell Cardiol 18: 1207–1218
26. Engler RL, Schmid-Schonbein GW, Pavalel RS (1983) Leukocyte capillary plugging in myocardial ischaemia and reperfusion in the dog. Am J Pathol 111: 98–111
27. Hearse DJ (1977) Reperfusion of the ischemic myocardium. J Mol Cell Cardiol 9: 605–616
28. Hearse DJ, Humphrey SM, Bullock GR (1978) The oxygen paradox and the calcium paradox: the two facets of the same problem? Cardiology 10: 641–668
29. Jolly SR, Kane WJ, Bailie MB, Abrams GD, Lucchesi BR (1986) Canine myocardial reperfusion injury: its reduction by the combined administration of superoxide dismutase and catalase. Circ Res 54: 227–285
30. Gaudel Y, Duvelleroy MA (1986) Role of oxygen radicals in cardiac injury due to reoxygenation. J Mol Cell Cardiol 16: 459–470
31. Ambrosio G, Weisfeldt ML, Jacobus WE, Flaherty JT (1987) Evidence for a reversible radical-mediated component of reperfusion injury: reduction by recombitant human superoxide dismutase administered at the time of reflow. Circulation 75: 282–291
32. Kuroda H, Ishiguro S, Mori T (1986) Optimal calcium concentration in the initial reperfusate for post-ischaemic myocardial performance (calcium concentration during reperfusion). J Mol Cell Cardiol 18: 625–633
33. Shine KI, Douglas AM, Ricchiuti NV (1978) Calcium, strontium, and barium movements during ischemia and reperfusion in rabbit ventricle. Implications for myocardial preservation. Circ Res 43: 712–720

34. Shine KI, Douglas AM (1983) Low calcium reperfusion of ischemic myocardium. J Mol Cell Cardiol 15: 252–260
35. Shen AC, Jennings RB (1972) Myocardial calcium and magnesium in acute ischemic myocardial injury. Am J Pathol 67: 417–440
36. Bourdillon PD, Poole-Wilson PA (1982) The effects of verapamil guiescence and cardioplegia on calcium exchange and mechanical function in ischemic rabbit myocardium. Circ Res 50: 360–368
37. Bourdillon PDV, Poole-Wilson PA (1981) Effects of ischaemia and reperfusion on calcium exchange and mechanical function in isolated rabbit myocardium. Cardiov Res 15: 121–130
38. Poole-Wilson PA, Harding DP, Bourdillon PDV, Tones MA (1986) Calcium out of control. J Mol Cell Cardiol 16: 175–187
39. Murphy E, Aiton JF, Horres CR, Lieberman M (1983) Calcium elevation in cultured heart cells: its role in cell injury. Am J Phy 245: C316–C321
40. Tones MA, Poole-Wilson PA (1985) Alpha-adrenoceptor stimulation, lysophosphoglycerides, and lipid peroxidation in reoxygenation induced calcium uptake in rabbit myocardium. Cardiov Res 19: 228–236
41. Ganote CE, Kaltenbach JP (1979) Oxygen-induced enzyme release: early events and a proposed mechanism. J Mol Cell Cardiol 11: 389–406
42. Jennings RB, Reimer KA, Steenbergen C (1986) Myocardial ischaemia revisited. The osmolar load, membrane damage, and reperfusion. J Mol Cell Cardiol 18: 769–780
43. Post JA, Lamers JMJ, Verdouw PD, ten Cate FJ, van der Giessan WJ, Verkleij AJ (1987) Sarcolemmal destabilisation and destruction after ischaemia and reperfusion and its relation with long-term recovery of regional left ventricular function in pigs. Eur Heart J 8: 423–430
44. Mak IT, Kramer JH, Weglicki WB (1986) Potentiation of free radical-induced lipid peroxidation injury to sarcolemmal membranes by lipid amphihiles. J Biol Chem 261: 1153–1157
45. Lazdunski M, Frelin C, Vigne P (1985) The sodium/hydrogen exchange system in cardiac cells: its biochemical and pharmacological properties and its role in regulating internal concentrations of sodium and internal pH. J Mol Cell Cardiol 17: 1029–1042
46. Cobbold PH, Bourne PK (1986) Aequorin measurements of free calcium in single cells. Nature 312: 444–446
47. Rao PS, Cohen MV, Mueller HS (1983) Production of free radicals and peroxides in early experimental myocardial ischaemia. J Mol Cell Cardiol 15: 713–716
48. Richard VJ, Murry CE, Jennings RB, Reimer KA (1988) Therapy to reduce free radicals during early reperfusion does not limit the size of myocardial infarcts caused by 90 minutes of ischaemia in dogs. Circulation 78: 473–480
49. Ferrari R, Ceconi C, Curello S, Cargnoni A, Condorelli E, Belloli S, Albertini A, Visioli O (1988) Metabolic changes during post-ischaemic reperfusion. J Mol Cell Cardiol 20 (suppl 2): 119–133

PART II

The role of energy deficiency

The critical ATP threshold hypothesis

P.G. SPIECKERMANN
Institute of Medical Physiology, University of Vienna, A-1090, Schwarzspanierstraße 17, Austria

Introduction

Despite the discussions in other sections of this book on the final causes of cell death, this chapter will analyse whether any correlation exists during ischemia between the cellular energetic situation and disturbances of functions, metabolism and structure of myocardial cells. In this context, the question arises as to whether a critical cellular ATP level marks the transgression from a living to a dead cell, marking a 'point of no return'.

This necrotic cell is the end-result of a multifactorial process which follows from an imbalance between energy demand and energy supply. In the myocardium, the balance of energy can be equalized only under aerobic conditions. During ischemia, anaerobic glycolysis can satisfy only part of the myocardial energy demand. This automatically causes a deficiency in energy, which manifests itself in the disturbance of all energy consuming processes and finally leads to irreversible damage of the tissue. Because function, metabolism and structure of tissue are closely inter-related, impairments are to be expected in all three areas.

The energy deficiency leads to a breakdown of high energy phosphates, to changes in intermediary metabolism, to disturbances in the contractile function of the heart, to electrolyte shifts with alterations of the electrophysiological processes and to cell swelling. Additionally, structural lesions occur in contractile structures as well as in the different membrane systems of the cell. An excellent review is given by Reimer and Jennings [1]. Today, knowledge of these processes and their time course is of great clinical importance. The widespread use of cardioplegic solutions in cardiac surgery results from these concepts. Interest arose also with the introduction of PTCA and thrombolytic therapy in the management of coronary heart disease. The central question is always the tolerance of the tissue to ischemia under the different prevailing conditions. The concept of reanimation physiology will therefore now be discussed.

This concept is based mainly on findings in experiments with global total ischemia in order to standardize the experimental conditions and to minimize

H.M. Piper (ed.) Pathophysiology of severe ischemic myocardial injury, 27–39.
© *1990 Kluwer Academic Publishers, Dordrecht –*

inhomogeneity problems. Sometimes – to follow the changes in 'slow motion' – the energy requirements of the myocardium were reduced by hypothermia, cardioplegia or both.

Functional changes during ischemia

The functional disturbances which appear after cessation of oxygen and fuel supply to the heart occur in a distinct characteristic sequence [2–4]. Certain metabolic and structural changes can be correlated with the individual functional phases. Three distinct phases can be differentiated: undisturbed, disturbed and suspended function.

Phase of undisturbed function

This phase, sometimes called 'period of latency', lasts only a few seconds, during which the contractions are undisturbed [5–9]. This is because the oxygen reserve available ($\sim$1 ml O_2/100g) allows the heart to work aerobically until a critical pO_2 in the tissue is reached [10]. Because 1 contraction needs approximately 0.1 ml O_2/100 g tissue weight, this reserve lasts for approximately 10 contractions. After reaching the critical pO_2 of $\sim$1–5 mmHg [11, 12] the 'phase of disturbed function' begins. Related to energy demand, the duration of this latency may be between 3 and 30 seconds.

Phase of disturbed function

This phase, together with phase 1, can be defined as 'survival time' [13]. The first changes in myocardial contractions appear after 6 to 10 heart cycles following the beginning of ischemia [5–9]. This number corresponds very well with data from PTCA [14]. The beating of the heart becomes irregular and the function insufficient. Often after a phase of fibrillation the heart finally stops beating. At this point, the phase of suspended function begins. As phase 1, the survival time is also dependent on myocardial energy demand and may last several minutes [5, 6, 9, 15].

Phase of suspended function

The sum of phases 1, 2 and 3 is known as 'reanimation' or 'resuscitation time'. In phase 3 function is only suspended but the tissue is not destroyed. This period has definitely ended when reanimation of the organ is no longer possible, even if oxygen supply is restored. The myocardium is then irreversibly damaged and rigor mortis of the heart has developed (so called 'stone heart' [16]). If during the survival time (phase 2) the myocardium is once again supplied with oxygen, it can recover its function to full efficiency. The heart muscle in phase 3, however, is not immediately able to resume the work of circulation. It now requires a *recovery time* for processes of reparation and resynthesis, during which the circulation must be assisted by heart massage or by by-pass methods. The duration of the recovery period is in approximate exponential correlation with the duration of preceding ischemia. The theoretical limit of reanimation time is by definition accompanied by an infinite or endless recovery time.

This point makes the experimental determination of the reanimation time or the evaluation of the tolerance of the heart to ischemia very problematic. It is only possible in retrospect from the success or failure of reanimation by reperfusion, during which additional damage may be induced (reperfusion damage). Further, by definition of reanimation time the time for recovery should be infinite.

These difficulties explain the considerably differing values for the duration of maximally tolerated ischemia times between 5 and 60 minutes [17–20]. The matter is further complicated by the differing experimental models and the important fact that the reanimation time depends critically on myocardial energy demand before and during energy deficiency. Pathologic-anatomic findings speak especially for a critical time between 20 and 30 minutes [1, 19].

Creatinphosphate, ATP and lactate during ischemia

The continuously increasing energy deficiency manifests itself in the breakdown of high-energy compounds, especially CP and ATP. These high-energy phosphates (HEP) are not physiological energy reserves in the strictest sense – as is, for example, glycogen – but these compounds are necessary for the maintenance of function and structure of the tissue. The lack of energy is the principal cause of functional and structural changes during oxygen deficiency. The levels of high energy phosphates may therefore be used as an index of the extent of ischemic burden of the myocardium.

Figure 1 shows the behaviour of CP, ATP and lactate in the myocardium of the left ventricle in dogs during normothermic ischemia under deep halothane narcosis [21]. Ischemia is initiated by transection of the ascending aorta. After that, a sharp decrease in CP and a slower breakdown of ATP occurs. The fast increase of lactate – only 0.1 of the total content could be drawn in – is significant and the result of an intensive anaerobic glycolysis.

The individual phases of the metabolic changes can be more easily distinguished if the metabolic activity of tissue is reduced by hypothermia and cardioplegia. Figure 2 presents mean values for CP, ATP and lactate from 20 ischemia experiments in which the heart was arrested by a hypothermic (15 °C) selective coronary perfusion with a cardioplegic solution for 10 minutes [21]. As a result, the cardiac energy demand was reduced 50 times compared with

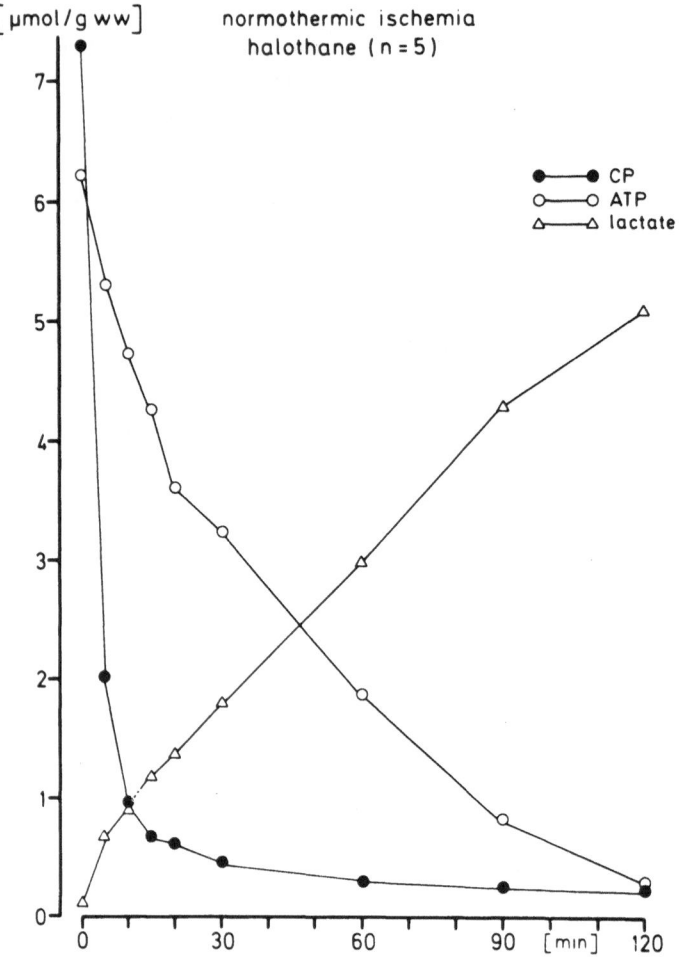

Fig. 1. The decrease in CP and ATP and the production of lactate in the normothermic myocardium of the left ventricle during ischemia under halothane (n=5).

normal heart function under resting conditions (therefore a logarithmic time scale was necessary). The metabolites are shown in relation to the calculated intramyocardial PO_2 derived from myocardial oxygen consumption and oxygen reserve [22].

In the first phase of ischemia, the tissue content of metabolites remains constant. Only after the intramyocardial oxygen pressure falls to a very low critical value does breakdown of high energy phosphates occur. To begin with, it is more a breakdown of CP and only a small fraction of ATP which seems to be in equilibrium with CP in the LOHMANN reaction. At the same time, anaerobic glycolysis is activated and lactate content increases sharply. If CP is reduced to a value under 3 µmol/g ww, a faster breakdown of ATP occurs. This corresponds with the findings of Eggleton and Eggleton in 1929 (!) [23].

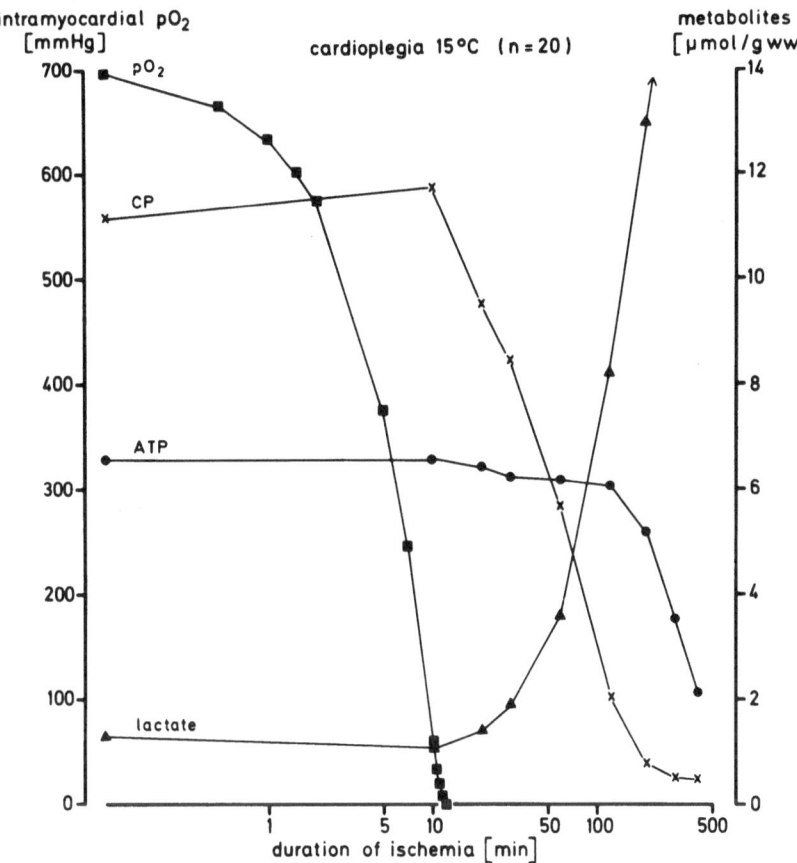

Fig. 2. Time course of CP, ATP, and lactate with respect to the calculated oxygen tension in the myocardium of the left ventricle during hypothermic ischemia. The hearts were arrested by a selective coronary perfusion with a 15°C cardioplegic solution.

The slight reduction of ATP during the fall of CP – 8% within 120 minutes – is interpreted by us as relating to the breakdown of that small ATP pool, which has a high turnover rate, is coupled to Creatinephosphate/Creatine and is responsible for the contraction of the muscle. The value of 8% corresponds with the findings of Hohorst *et al.* (1962) for skeletal muscle [24]. When these pools of CP and the small ATP fraction are decomposed during oxygen deficiency, no chemical energy remains for the contraction and the heart stops beating (end of survival time).

A synopsis of metabolic, functional and additionally structural alteration (albeit simplified) during myocardial ischemia is given in Fig. 3 [21]. The high-energy phosphate content of the tissue remains unaltered during the period of latency (phase 1) because the heart, due to the amount of oxygen in reserve, continues to function aerobically. During the second phase, of increasingly disturbed function (early pump failure), a small amount of ATP, and a large amount of CP begin to break down. If CP is reduced to a value of

32

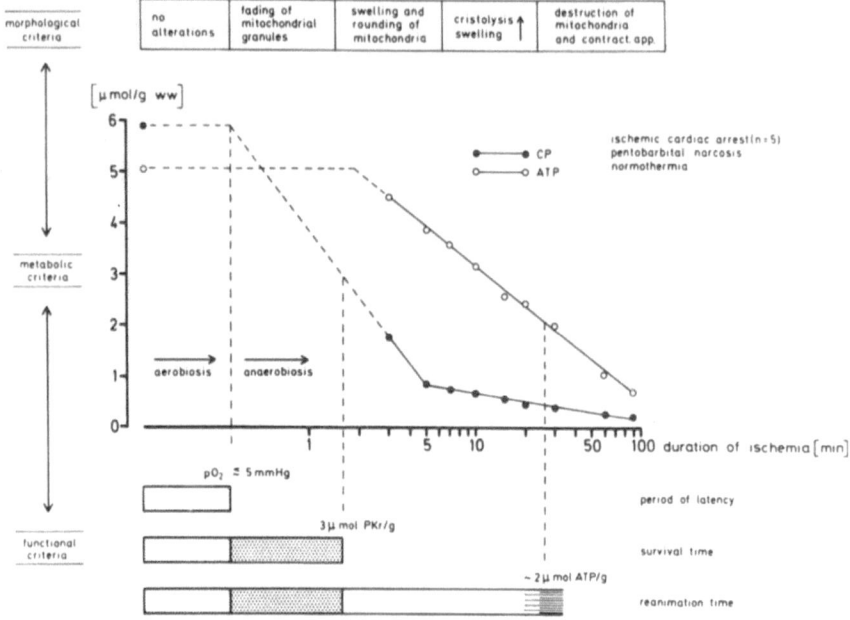

Fig. 3. A synopsis of the morphological (above), metabolic (middle), and functional (below) disturbances and changes during normothermic myocardial ischemia under pentobarbital. A logarithmic chart of the time axis was chosen for didactic reasons.

about 3 µmol/g ww, the major part of ATP begins to split. The third phase is ended when ATP decreases to very low values, smaller than 1–2 µmol/g ww. The heart can at this point no longer be revived, for the limit of the reanimation period, the point of no return has been reached. This limit is not thought of as a defined border, but rather as a continuous transition from a catabiotic to an irreversibly damaged cell. From this state of irreversibility, return is not possible.

Morphological changes which principally affect the mitochondria appear simultaneously with the functional and metabolic disturbances. During CP breakdown, only the mitochondrial granules fade, marked structural changes begin with the decay of ATP and the mitochondria and the contractile apparatus and the sarcolemma are destroyed. Damage appears to be irreversible if the ATP level is less than 1–2 µmol/g ww of tissue [1, 21, 25].

Index of reanimation potential

Because the function of an organ and its potential for reanimation are coupled with the tissue content of HEPs, the respective metabolic state can be appraised as an index of the degree of tissue damage. The time needed to reach a given metabolic state of HEPs can therefore be used as an index for

the tissue's tolerance to ischemia. This designated metabolic state can be chosen relatively arbitrarily. Using linear interpolation of the breakdown curves during ischemia, we determine the time it takes for CP to break down to a value of 3 μmol/g ww and ATP to 4 μmol/g ww. We designate these times as t-CP and t-ATP, respectively. The t-CP corresponds to the end of the survival time (phase 2) and t-ATP to a point of time during the phase of suspended function (phase 3), when recovery time has in fact been prolonged, but has a tolerable value (20–30 minutes) even under clinical conditions, for example after cardiac arrest during heart surgery with extracorporal circulation. Transgressing this time leads to a steep exponential prolongation of recovery, to more or less severe functional complications relative to the length of the preceding ischemia and to marked structural changes of the cell. The time to reach a precise metabolic state is dependent on two factors:
1. the starting levels of HEPs before ischemia and
2. the reduction rate of these compounds during ischemia.
Both factors vary with the myocardial energy demand before and during ischemia.

Dependence of HEP content on myocardial energy demand

As a result of splitting and resynthesis processes, a variation in the equilbrium is dependent on myocardial energy demand. In Fig. 4 the levels of CP, ATP, ADP and AMP from more than 50 experiments are plotted against the corresponding myocardial oxygen consumption, showing that the higher the myocardial energy demand, the smaller the equilibrium content in the tissue. The variation in oxygen consumption is achieved by changes in mechanical stress, different types of ischemia and various methods of induced cardiac arrest [26].

Dependence of HEP splitting rate on myocardial energy demand before and during oxygen deficiency

The higher the energetic stress on the myocardium before and during oxygen deficiency, the faster the HEPs, breakdown. Figure 5 compares the time course of ATP-breakdown and lactate production in different experimental groups. CP is not included for reasons of clarity; however, the curves progress correspondingly.

Exsanguination by severing of the aorta relieves the work-load of the heart. During barbiturate anesthesia, transection of the aorta produces a metabolic state of 4 μmol/g myocardium (t-ATP) after about 5 minutes. During coronary litigation, however, a condition in which the affected myocardial area maintains its function as long as possible, the ATP in the infarcted zone is reduced to this value after only 2 minutes [27].

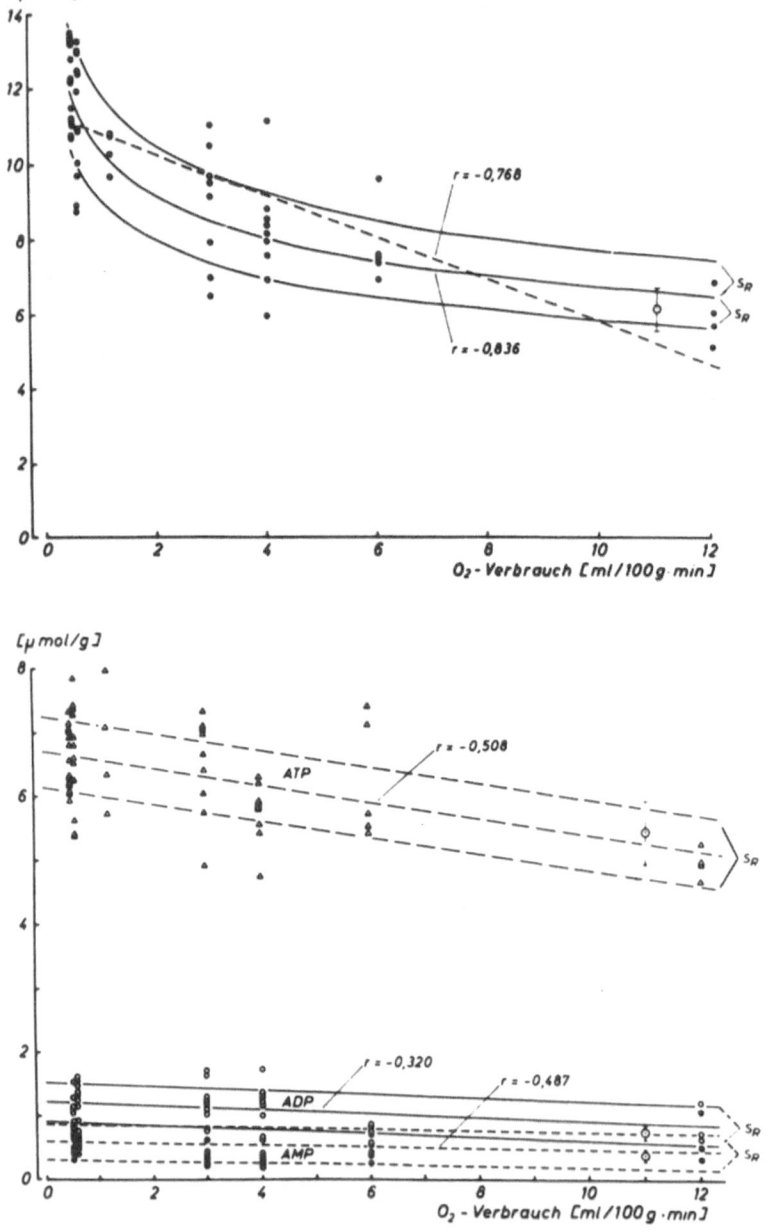

Fig. 4. Dependence of myocardial tissue content of CP (above), ATP, ADP, and AMP (below) on oxygen consumption of the heart. The variation in myocardial oxygen demand is produced by changes in mechanical stress, variation of anesthetics, and different forms of cardioplegia.

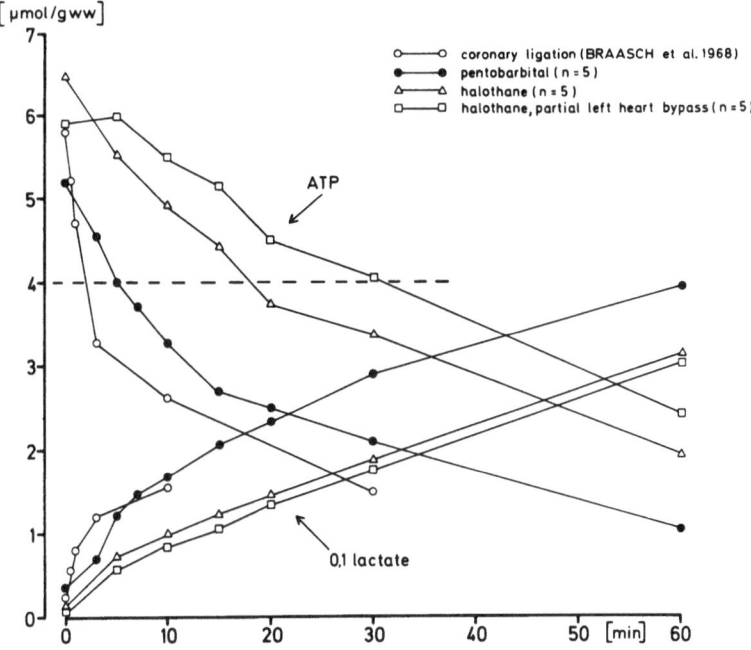

Fig. 5. ATP breakdown and production of lactate in the myocardium of the left ventricle during normothermic ischemia under the following experimental conditions: (1) coronary ligation, (2) barbiturate anesthesia, (3) halothane anesthesia, and (4) pre-ischemic relief of the heart by a partial left ventricular bypass under halothane.

The remaining curves of Fig. 5 punctuate the influence of pre-ischemic stress on the metabolism of HEPs during ischemia. Due to the quasi beta-receptor-blocking effect of halothane, the myocardial energy demand under this agent is reduced: t-ATP amounts to about 16 minutes. However, t-ATP extends to over 30 minutes if, before ischemia (but otherwise under the same experimental conditions), the mechanical stress of the left heart is reduced by an additional partial left ventricular bypass.

The relations between myocardial tolerance to ischemia and the energy metabolism of the heart can be briefly summarized as follows:

A sufficient HEP content of the heart muscle is important for myocardial reanimation. The higher the myocardial energy demand, the lower the starting level of the phosphates and the faster their breakdown. Thus, limited tolerance to ischemia results at high levels of activity, and a prolonged tolerance results at low levels. All conditions with an increased myocardial oxygen consumption shorten the length of time during which the tissue can tolerate an oxygen deficiency. However, decreasing myocardial oxygen demand is one possible means of myocardial protection.

Discussion

It is now considered trivial to state that HEPs, especially ATP, are necessary for normal function and maintenance of structure of a cell. ATP is, therefore, also necessary for reanimation of an organ after an ischemic insult. It is not surprising that the transgression to irreversibility after ischemic damage is coupled with a critical ATP content of the tissue [22, 28–30]. This level is always estimated at smaller than 1–2 µmol/g ww [21, 22, 31–34]. It may depend on the experimental model chosen and vary from species to species. The assumption of a critical ATP content does not mean that a sharp, precisely defined border exists but that it must be interpreted as a range for the transgression process from reversibly injured to irreversibly damaged cells. In this region, the probability of revivability drops markedly and tends towards zero, the recovery time to infinite or endless. ATP availability is without doubt a necessity for reanimation but it is not the only requirement. This explains why the critical ATP hypothesis is sometimes questioned [35, 36]. In principle, the essential role of ATP in cell function and reanimation is accepted, but in addition several important contributory factors to the damage process need to be emphasized. Neely and Grotjohann [35] wrote: 'It seems clear that decreased oxidative production of ATP and the associated loss of adenine nucleotides, if allowed to progress until adenine nucleotides are critically low, can in itself result in irreversibility. Even when ATP levels are not totally depleted, a good negative correlation between residual ATP and cellular function has been reported for several models of ischemia'. As contributory factors, structural damage to membranes or contractile structures, ionic imbalances, especially overloading the cells with calcium, cell swelling, activation or inhibition of key enzymes – also discussed in other chapters of this book – are of key importance.

The following arguments and findings support the concept proposed.

1. A correlation can be shown between ATP content and myocardial structure and function. However, under certain experimental conditions, a dissociation between morphology and energetic situation may exist [37].
2. With increasing ATP depletion, ATP resynthesis will be delayed [21, 30, 38–43]. ATP can only be restored to the order of the sum of adenine nucleotides before reoxygenation. This is due to rapid loss of degradation products of adenine nucleotides and the low rate of adenosine de novo synthesis [43]. The same can be shown in isolated cardiocytes [44] and may be the metabolic correlation to the prolonging of recovery time with ischemic burden.
3. A variety of mitochondrial functional defects have been observed during ischemic injury. They all progress in correlation with decreasing ATP [1, 45].
4. Electrophysiological disturbances and ionic shifts [46] can be related to the individual phases of reanimation time.
5. In the time course of ischemia, lactate production slows down and ceases

under 2 μmol ATP/g ww. This may be due to a lack of phosphate for the phosphorylation of fructose-6-phosphate. Anaerobic glycosis is no longer a source of ATP production [22].

6. ATP is essential for the maintenance of myofibrillar relaxation. With loss of ATP the myocardial tone increases and ultimately the so-called 'stone heart' develops [47–49].

References

1. Reimer KA, Jennings RB (1986) Myocardial Ischemia, Hypoxia and Infarction. In: HA Fozzard *et al.* (ed) The Heart and Cardiovascular System. New York, p 1133
2. Opitz E, Schneider M (1950) Über die Sauerstoffversorgung des Gehirns und den Mechanismus von Mangelwirkungen. Ergebn Physiol 46: 126
3. Schneider M (1958) Über die Wiederbelebung nach Kreislaufunterbrechung. Thoraxchirurgie 6: 95
4. Schneider M (1964) Die Wiederbelebungszeit verschiedener Organe nach Ischämie. Langenbecks Arch Klin Chir 308: 252
5. Kreuzer H, Schoeppe W (1963) Der Myokarddruck bei veränderter Koronardurchblutung und bei Ischämie. Pflügers Arch ges Physiol 278: 209
6. Prinzmetal M, Schwarzt LL, Corday E, Spritzler R, Bergmann HC, Krüger HE (1949) Studies on the coronary circulation. VI. Loss of cardiac contractility after coronary artery occlusion. Ann intern Med 31: 429
7. Sayen JJ, Sheldon WF, Peirce G, Kuo PT (1958) Polarographic oxygen in experimental acute regional ischemia of the left ventricle. Circulat Res 6: 779
8. Sayen JJ, Sheldon WF, Peirce G, Kou PT (1954) Motion picture studies of ventricular muscle dynamics in experimental localized ischemia, correlated with myocardial oxygen tension and electrocardiograms. J Clin Invest 33: 962
9. Tennant R, Wiggers CJ (1935) The effect of coronary occlusion on myocardial contraction. Amer J Physiol 112: 351
10. Bretschneider HJ (1964) Überlebenszeit und Wiederbelungszeit des Herzens bei Normo- und Hypothermie. Verh Dtsch Ges Kreislaufforsch 30: 11
11. Fabel H, Lübbers DW, Rybak R (1964) Die Bestimmung des Myoglobingehaltes und des kritischen Sauerstoffdruckes am schlagenden Kaninchenherzen 'in situ'. Pflügers Arch ges Physiol 279: R32
12. Lübbers DW (1968) Intercapillärer O$_2$-Transport und intracelluläre Sauerstoffkonzentration. In: Biochemie des Sauerstoffs. 19. Colloquium der Gesellschaft für Biologischie Chemie (Berlin – Heidelberg – New York) S 67
13. Sugar O, Gerard RW (1938) Anoxia and brain potentials. J Neurophysiol 1: 558
14. Serruys PW, Meester GT (eds) (1986) Coronary Angioplasty: A controlled model for ischemia. Dordrecht – Boston – Lancaster
15. Porter WT (1894) On the ligation of the coronary arteries. J Physiol 15: 121
16. Cooley DA, Reul GJ and Wukasch DC (1972) Ischemic contracture of the heart: 'Stone heart.' Am J Cardiol 29: 575
17. Rusch H (1898) Experimentelle Studien über Ernährung des isolierten Säugerherzens. Pflügers Arch ges Physiol 7: 533
18. Blumgart AL, Gittigan DR, Schlesinger MJ (1941) Experimental studies on the effect of temporary occlusion of coronary arteries. II. The production of myocardial infarction. Am Heart J 22: 374
19. Jennings RB, Baum JH, Herdson PB (1965) Fine structural changes in myocardial ischemic injury. Arch Path 79: 135
20. Milnes RF, Woude RV, Sloan H (1958) Extended asystole. Arch Surg 77: 13

21. Spieckermann PG, Überlebens- und Wiederbelebungszeit des Herzens. Anaesthesiology and Resuscitation Vol 66. Berlin: Springer
22. Kübler W and Spieckermann PG (1970) Regulation of glycolysis in the ischemic and anoxic myocardium. J Mol Cell Cardiol 1: 351
23. Eggleton CP and Eggleton P (1929) A method of estimating phosphagen and some other phosphorous compounds in muscle tissue. J Physiol 68: 193
24. Hohorst HJ, Reim M and Bartels H (1962) Studies on the creatine kinase equilibrium in muscle and the significance of ATP and ADP levels. Biochem Biophys Res Commun 7: 142
25. Hübner G (1971) Electron microscopic investigation of cardioplegia: Electron microscopy of various forms of cardiac arrest in correlation with myocardial function. Methods Archiev Exp Pathol 5: 518
26. Kübler W, Grebe D, Orellano LE, Spieckermann PG and Bretschneider HJ (1968) Zur Bewertung des Gewebsgehaltes der energiereichen Phosphate für die Pathogenese der Herzinsuffizienz.In: Reindell H, Keul J, and Doll E (eds Herzinsuffizienz: Pathophysiologie und Klinik. Stuttgart: Thieme p 226
27. Braasch W, Gudbjarnason S, Puri PS, Ravens KG and Bing RJ (1968) Early changes in energy metabolism in the myocardium following coronary artery occlusion in anesthetized dogs. Circ Res 23: 429
28. Gudbjernason S, Mathes P, Ravens KG (1970) Functional compartmentation of ATP and creatine phosphate in heart muscle. J Mol Cell Cardiol 1: 325
29. Jennings RB, Hawkins HK, Lowe JE, Hill ML, Klotman S, Reimer KA (1977) Relation between high energy phosphate and lethal injury in myocardial ischemia in the dog. Am J Pathol 92: 187
30. Reibel DK, Rovetto MJ (1979) Myocardial adenosine salvage rates and restoration of ATP content following ischemia. Am J Physiol 237: H247
31. Isselhard W (1968) Einfluß von Prenylamin auf Herz- und Gehirnstoffwechsel und auf die Myokardfunktion. In: Moser K, Lujf A (eds) Beta-Rezeptorenblockade in Klinik und Experiment. Wien p 87
32. Kammermeier H (1964) Verhalten von Adenin-Nucleotiden und Kreatinphosphat im Herzmuskel bei funktioneller Erholung nach länger dauernder Asphyxie. Verh dtsch Ges Kreisl-Forsch 30: 206
33. Jennings RB, Reimer KA (1981) Lethal myocardial injury. Am J Pathol 102: 241
34. Grinwald PM, Hearse DJ, Segal MB (1980) A possible mechanism of glycolytic impairment after adenosine triphosphate depletion in the perfused rat heart. J Physiol 301: 337
35. Neely JR, Grotjohann LW (1984) Role of glycolytic products in damage to ischemic myocardium. Circ Res 55: 816
36. Poole-Wilson PA (1984) What causes cell death. In: Hearse DJ, Yellon DM (eds) Therapeutic approaches to myocardial infarct size limitation. New York p 43
37. Bretschneider HJ, Gebhard MM, Preusse CJ (1984) Cardioplegia, Principles and Problems. In: Sperelakis N (ed) Physiology and Pathophysiology of the heart. Boston
38. Isselhard W, Mäurer W, Stemmel W, Krebs J, Schmitz H, Neuhof H, Esser A (1970) Stoffwechsel des Kaninchenherzens in situ während Asphyxie und in der postasphyktischen Erholung. Pflügers Arch ges Physiol 316: 164
39. Kammermeier H (1964) Verhalten von Adeninnucleotiden und Kreatinphosphat im Herzmuskel bei funktioneller Erholung nach länger dauernder Asphyxie. Verh dtsch Ges Kreisl-Forsch 30: 206
40. De Boer LWV, Ingwall JS, Kloner RA, Braunwald E (1989) Prolonged derangements of canine myocardial purine metabolism after a brief coronary artery occlusion not associated with anatomic evidence of necrosis. Proc Natl Acad Sci (USA) 77: 5471
41. Zimmer HG, Ibel H (1984) Ribose accelerates the repletion of the ATP pool during recovery from reversible ischemia of the rat myocardium. J Mol Cell Cardiol 16: 863
42. Humphrey SM, Holiss DG, Seelye RN (1985) Myocardial adenine pool depletion and recovery of mechanical function following ischemia. Am J Physiol 248: H644

43. Zimmer HG, Trendelenburg C, Kammermeier H, Gerlach E (1973) De novo synthesis of myocardial adenine nucleotides in the rat. Circ Res 32: 635

44. Piper HM, Schwartz P, Hütter JF, Spieckermann PG (1984) Energy metabolism and enzyme release of cultured adult rat heart muscle cells during anoxia. J Mol Cell Cardiol 16: 995

45. Piper HM, Sezer O, Schleyer M, Schwartz P, Hütter JF, Spieckermann PG (1985) Development of ischemia induced damage in defined mitochondrial subpopulations. J Molec Cell Cardiol 17: 125

46. Gettes LS (1986) Effect of ischemia on cardiac electrophysiology. In: Fozzard HA et al. (ed) The heart and cardiovascular system. New York p 1317

47. Holubarsch C, Alpert NR, Goulette R, Mulieri LA (1982) Heat production during hypoxic contracture of rat myocardium. Circ Res 51: 777

48. Lewis MJ, Housmans PR, Claes VA, Brutsaert DL, Henderson AH (1980) Myocardial stiffness during hypoxic and reoxygenation contracture. Cardiovasc Res 14: 339

49. Ventura-Clapier R, Vassort G (1981) Rigor tension during metabolic and ionic rises in resting tension in rat heart. J Mol Cell Cardiol 13: 551

Importance of glycolytically produced ATP for the integrity of the threatened myocardial cell

Lionel H. Opie

Medical Research Council, Heart Research Unit, University of Cape Town, Medical School, CAPE TOWN 7925, South Africa

Summary

The hypothesis that glycolytically produced ATP has a special role in the preservation of myocardial cells is critically examined. Considerable indirect evidence supports this proposal, although the electrophysiological data remain controversial and capable of different interpretations. Thus far the most convincing evidence favoring the concept of compartmentation comes from data relating rates of glycolytic flux to enzyme release from the isolated heart or from isolated myocytes and from the regulation of the onset of ischemic contracture. More direct evidence has now been obtained in isolated cardiac myocytes. The hypothesis formed the basis of a metabolically orientated approach towards decreasing severity of myocardial ischemic injury. Nonetheless, until analytical methods become available for the specific measurement of a membrane-related pool of ATP, the hypothesis will be supported by indirect rather than direct evidence.

Introduction

Interest in the possible benefits of glycolytic flux for the ischemic myocardium dates back to the pioneering work of Sodi-Pallares *et al.* [1] which Owen, Thomas and I took as the basis for our studies on the effects of ischemia on the regional extraction of glucose by the myocardium [2]. The metabolism of glucose could be beneficial to the ischemic myocardium [3] by several possible mechanisms: increasing the rate of anaerobic glycolysis, reversing ion loss, by a direct membrane effect, by altering the extracellular volume, and by decreasing circulating FFA concentrations. Later the concept was expanded to suggest that glycolytically produced ATP could play a special role in the protection of the sarcolemma, especially during ischemia [4], as well as in the promotion of myocardial relaxation [5]. Even more recently [6], the hypothesis has been evolved further to suggest that the rate of glycolysis ultimately helps to determine cell viability in ischemia.

H.M. Piper (ed.) Pathophysiology of severe ischemic myocardial injury, 41–65.

Before reviewing evidence for and against these proposals, it is first necessary to delineate the effects of ischemia on glycolytic flux.

Pathways of glycolysis

Glycolysis may be defined as that metabolic pathway (Emden-Meyerhorf) converting glucose 6-phosphate to pyruvate. From the point of view of utilization and production of ATP, the pathways of glycolysis can be divided into two parts. Firstly, glycolysis converts glucose 6-phosphate derived from glucose or glycogen into fructose 1,6-diphosphate, using 1 molecule of ATP; another 1 molecule of ATP is used in the phosphorylation of glucose but not in glycogen breakdown. In the second phase of the process, glycolysis converts each 6-carbon hexose into two trioses, thereby making 4 molecules of ATP (without any O_2 requirement) for each glucose 6-phosphate ultimately converted to pyruvate. Thus, when glucose is the source of glycolysis, the whole glycolytic path uses 2 ATP and produces 4 ATP, i.e. the net production is 2. But when glycogen is the source, ATP production is 3 per molecule passing through glycolysis.

During normal oxygenation, glucose uptake and glycolysis are inhibited by the metabolism of non-glucose substrates such as free fatty acids, lactate or ketone bodies. Lack of oxygen, on the other hand, activates glucose uptake and glycolysis both directly and indirectly, the latter effect because of the inhibition of the oxidation of the alternate non-glucose substrates.

Glucose uptake

A major control point in glycolysis is the rate of transport of glucose across the sarcolemma, which is directly accelerated by anaerobiosis. For glucose to enter the heart cell requires: (1) an adequate rate of delivery of glucose to the heart cell by the coronary blood flow; (2) the transport of glucose from the blood across the capillary membrane into the interstitial space; and (3) the transport of glucose across the sarcolemma into the cytosol of the heart cell. During experimental hypoxia and mild ischemia, it is the third process which is accelerated. However, during severe ischemia, the delivery of glucose (the first process) can be much reduced because of the severe limitation of the coronary blood flow [7].

Phosphorylation of glucose

After transport across the sarcolemma, the next step in the metabolism of glucose is its irreversible phosphorylation to glucose 6-phosphate, controlled by the enzyme hexokinase which has properties such that intracellular glucose is phosphorylated as rapidly as it is transported in through the sarcolemma. Even when the rate of transport of glucose into the cell is increased by hypoxia, free glucose does not accumulate within the cell.

Further metabolism of glucose 6-phosphate can in turn be either directed to the formation of its isomer fructose 6-phosphate and thence into the glycolytic pathway, or to another isomer glucose 1-phosphate eventually to form glycogen. These three isomers (glucose 6-phosphate, fructose 6-phosphate, and glucose 1-phosphate) are freely interchangeable and function as the hexosemonophosphate pool.

Regulation of glycolysis

The flow through glycolysis in the myocardium can be increased several fold by severe hypoxia [8]. An important rate-limiting enzyme is *phosphofructo-kinase*; when its activity increases as in anoxia, hexosemonophosphates are converted to fructose 1,6-phosphate; thus the cellular content of glucose 6-phosphate falls, the inhibition of hexokinase is relieved, more glucose is phosphorylated and more glucose taken up. During anoxia, glucose uptake, glucose phosphorylation and the activity of phosphofructokinase may all change harmoniously to accelerate glucose uptake and glycolysis during anoxia because of the co-ordinated control of the initial part of glycolysis [9].

Two factors accelerate the activity of phosphofructokinase during anoxia [10]. First, the energy status of the cell is of major importance. During conditions of adequate oxygenation and substrate supply, the cellular content of ATP is high and the enzyme is ATP-inhibited. During anoxia, ATP levels fall, those of ADP and AMP rise, as does that of Pi (the latter also being derived from breakdown of creatine phosphate). Hence the inhibition of ATP is relieved both by the fall in ATP and by de-inhibition by the breakdown products of ATP. Also during hypoxia, lack of oxidative metabolism decrease citrate levels and relieves the inhibition of citrate on phosphofructokinase.

Another important factor regulating phosphofructokinase activity is pH; a rise stimulates activity and a fall inhibits. The inhibitory effect of acidosis is one factor explaining the difference between the effects of severe ischemia which inhibits glycolysis, and mild ischemia which accelerates glycolysis. A crucial difference is whether or not the coronary flow is adequate (as in mild ischemia) to wash out most of the accumulated protons, or inadequate, as in severe ischemia, with accumulation of protons and inhibition of phosphofruc-tokinase.

Triose metabolism

The next steps of glycolysis lie in triose metabolism, whereby the 6-carbon structure resulting from the activity of phosphofructokinase is converted to two trioses, each of which then ultimately forms pyruvate (from which the exits to glycolysis are either to lactate or to the citrate cycle). The rate-controlling step is catalysed by the enzyme glyceraldehyde-3-phosphate dehydrogenase, an enzyme subject to feedback inhibition by the products of glycolysis including $NADH_2$ and lactate. Therefore, during severe ischemia, both phosphofructokinase and glyceraldehyde-3-phosphate dehydrogenase are inhibited by the end-products (lactate, protons, $NADH_2$).

Glycolysis: Effects of degree of ischemia

During mild ischemia, the cellular contents of ATP and citrate are low, inorganic phosphate is high, and the result is that phosphofructokinase is accelerated, glycolytic flux enhanced, and there are high rates of production of glycolytic ATP. During severe ischemia, the cellular effects of hypoxia are combined with those of severely restricted flow. Now an accumulation of protons, $NADH_2$ and lactate inhibits phosphofructokinase, despite the acceleration caused by the decreased levels of ATP and citrate. Furthermore, glyceraldehyde-3-phosphate dehydrogenase is inhibited as already outlined. Two opposing factors at work: reduction of coronary flow indirectly reduces delivery of oxygen which will stimulate glycolysis, while the severe reduction of flow allows accumulation of products of glycolysis to the ischemic cells by the very low of coronary flow also decreases glucose uptake in severe ischemia.

Glucose uptake and severity of ischemia

The above metabolic facts explain why, as coronary flow decreases, there is a bimodal effect on glucose uptake. A modest fall in coronary flow (mild ischemia) increases glucose uptake and a more major fall (severe ischemia) decreases uptake. Therefore, as the coronary flow rate progressively falls, there will be a critical flow level at which increased glucose uptake switches to decreased uptake. Thus an increased glucose uptake reflects modest ischemia and a decreased uptake reflects severe ischemia. A recent hypothesis [6] proposes that an increase of glucose uptake reflects continued cell viability and a decreased uptake reflects loss of viability of the ischemic cells. On this basis cells threatened by ischemia could be divided by their patterns of glucose uptake into those with increased values (viable) or decreased values (non-viable). Thus (1) any benefits of enhanced glycolysis are likely to be limited to zones of moderate or mild flow restriction and (2) in zones of severe ischemia, coronary flow would first have to be improved by thrombolytic reperfusion or revascularization, or similar procedures, to achieve the desired benefit.

Proposed benefits of glycolytic ATP in ischemia

In experimental mild ischemia, there are situations in which production of glycolytic ATP can be related to membrane function, as defined by electrogenesis and rates of enzyme release, and also to the development of calcium-dependent ischemic contracture. Some evidence for these points of view will now be provided.

Glycolytic ATP and electrogenesis

The general hypothesis is that ATP produced by glycolysis could be related to electrogenesis. ATP in or near the plasma membrane may play a role in the promotion of the slow inward current associated with the plateau of the action potential. In ischemia, such ATP is thought to exist in a compartment not exchanging readily with ATP produced by residual mitochondrial metabolism, but rather to be generated by glycolysis. The rates of glycolytically generated ATP in the normally oxygenated heart are negligible from the point of view of the overall energy requirements of the heart, but this hypothesis would nevertheless accord a special role to such glycolytic ATP especially in ischemia. The hypothesis has been referred to in earlier reviews [11, 12].

Prasad and MacLeod [13] used anoxic papillary muscle to show that the rate of lactate production correlated with the duration of the action potential. Eisenberg *et al.* [14] showed that the action potential duration was shortened by dinitrophenol, then lengthened as glucose in a high concentration was added, and then shortened again when glucose was omitted. However, these data in oxygen-limited hearts, or in hearts with mitochondrial inhibition, cannot be extrapolated to normally oxygenated hearts. Some data of Prasad and MacLeod [13] and the recent experiments by Hayashi *et al.* [15] suggest that, in the adult heart, mitochondrially produced ATP enters the same compartment as glycolytically produced ATP to maintain the action potential duration.

To examine whether mitochondrially produced ATP could maintain the action potential in normally oxygenated perfused rat hearts, Girardier and I compared the action potential obtained by a floating microelectrode when the rat heart was perfused with pyruvate, compared with glucose perfusions [16]. In the presence of pyruvate, glycolytic flux from glycogen was totally inhibited. Several electrical changes were found including shortening of the action potential duration (Fig. 1). At first sight, the data support the concept of ATP compartmentation with the possibility that glucose was providing ATP in a compartment accessible to the cell membrane for electrical activity. Yet all the changes found could be explained by an increase of citrate during pyruvate perfusions, with a consequent decrease of intracellular calcium and

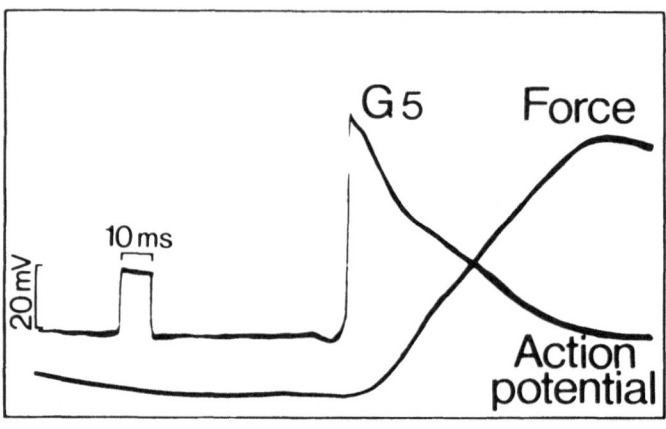

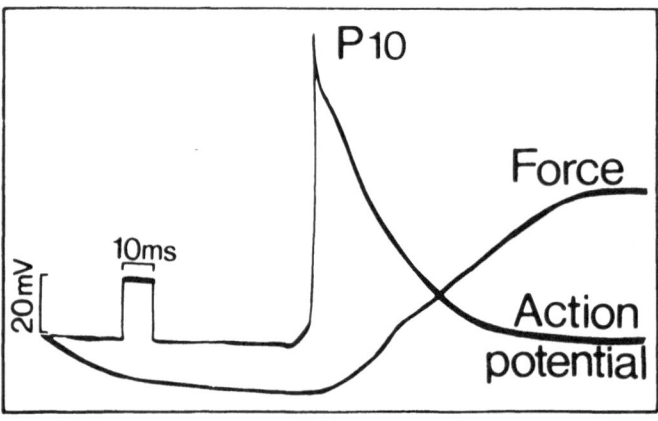

Fig. 1. An apparently simple observation, that glucose prolongs the action potential duration of the isolated perfused rat heart, has a complex explanation. The upper panel shows data obtained with glucose 5 mM as external substrate and the lower panel with pyruvate 10 mM as external substrate. Note with glucose the wider action potential duration and the increased force of contraction as well as the delayed conduction time (interval between stimulation artefact and upstroke of action potential). Note with pyruvate the greater amplitude of action potential upstroke. The most likely explanation of these changes does not lie in compartmentation of ATP in relation to glycolysis, but in a decreased intracellular cytosolic calcium concentration with pyruvate perfusions, resulting from an increased intracellular citrate level, because all the pyruvate-induced changes were reversed by the addition of ouabain.
From collaborative work with L. Giradier. For details see [16].

a decreased force of contraction [16]. In normoxic papillary muscles in which glycolysis was inhibited by metabolic block (and therefore no increase in citrate could be expected), there was no change in the action potential duration [15]. When whole heart underperfusion caused ischemia, glucose inhibited and pyruvate promoted the incidence of reperfusion arrhythmias and enzyme release, and the differences could be related to the varying rates of anaerobic ATP production during the ischemic period [4]. In cultured fetal cells, the results support the concept of a role for glycolytic ATP in electrogenesis [17] yet may not be extrapolated directly to the different metabolic patterns in the adult heart because fetal cells are generally more dependent on glycolytic metabolism than those of the adult heart. Thus, in summary, the overall electrophysiological evidence, based on the relation between glucose and the action potential duration, does not provide unequivocal evidence for the concept of ATP compartmentation, as there can be alternative explanations for at least some of the findings.

Glycolytic ATP and the ATP-sensitive potassium channel

More convincing evidence links glycolytically produced ATP to the activity of the ATP-sensitive potassium channel. There are many potassium channels in the myocardium, of which one is ATP-sensitive and normally 'closed' by the ambient cellular levels of ATP. Severe depletion of ATP 'opens' this channel [18]. The level of ATP required to 'close' the channel is very low, much lower than that found at levels and durations of ischemia associated with potassium leakage, so that it has been doubted that 'opening' of this channel could play an important role in the potassium loss found in the myocardium during early ischemia. Nevertheless, the potassium loss of ischemia responds to agents 'closing' potassium channels such as glibenclamide [19] showing that the potassium channel can 'open' at ATP levels so high that (1) compartmentation must be evoked so that there could be a very low local level of ATP or (2) effects of any given level of ATP must be modified by other factors such as the level of ADP and GTP [20, 21]. A third and convincing possibility is that glycolytic ATP is more able than mitochondrial ATP to provide the energy required for channel closure [22]. The latter studies give strong support to the concept of compartmentation of cytosolic ATP.

Glycolytic ATP and enzyme release

De Leiris *et al.* [23] and Opie and Bricknell [24] showed that coronary ligated rat hearts released the enzymes lactate dehydrogenase (LDH) and creatine kinase (CK) and that such release of enzymes was decreased when glucose was added to non-glucose perfusates (Fig. 2). The calculated rate of glycolytic flux in the heart could be inversely related to the rate of enzyme release. Changes in the levels of high-energy phosphate compounds were not relevant. Higgins *et al.* [25, 26] showed that (1) release of enzymes from cultured

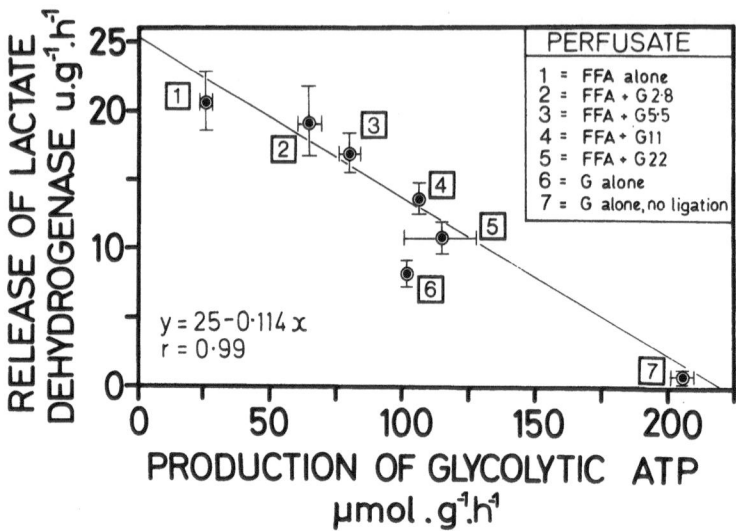

Fig. 2. Relationship between rate of production of glycolytic ATP and release of lactate dehydrogenase from coronary ligated rat heart perfused with various substrates. Free fatty acids (FFA) alone = palmitate 0.5 mM, albumin 0.1 mM, (G) = glucose 2.8 mM–22 mM, G G alone = glucose 11 mM. Ins = addition of insulin, 2 mU/ml. All groups had coronary ligation. Note inverse relationship between production of glycolytic ATP and release of enzyme.
Reproduced from [24] with permission of Cardiovascular Research.

neonatal myocytes was inversely related to the glycolytic flux rate and that (2) the resistance of cardiac sarcolemma to attack by phospholipases was dependent on the energy status. Earlier, Gudbjarnason *et al.* [27] had postulated an inhibition of intracellular energy transfer in ischemic muscle which might be explained by a breakdown of the unidirectional phosphocreatine energy shuttle to result in ATP compartmentalization. These data are consonant with the hypothesis that glycolytic ATP helps to protect the myocardial cell membrane without, however, providing direct proof for the hypothesis.

Glycolytic ATP and ischemic contracture

Impressive links exist between the onset of ischemic contracture in underperfused isolated hearts and glycolytic flux. Bricknell *et al.* [28] investigated the relationship between tissue ATP, ischemic contracture, and glycolysis. The source of ATP production was varied in potassium-arrested globally underperfused rat hearts, so that ATP was derived from either glycolysis or from mitochondrial sources (Fig. 3). Iodoacetate or deoxyglucose was used to block glycolysis and atractyloside to block transfer of ATP outward from the mitochondria (for method, see [4, 28]). ATP produced by glycolysis was

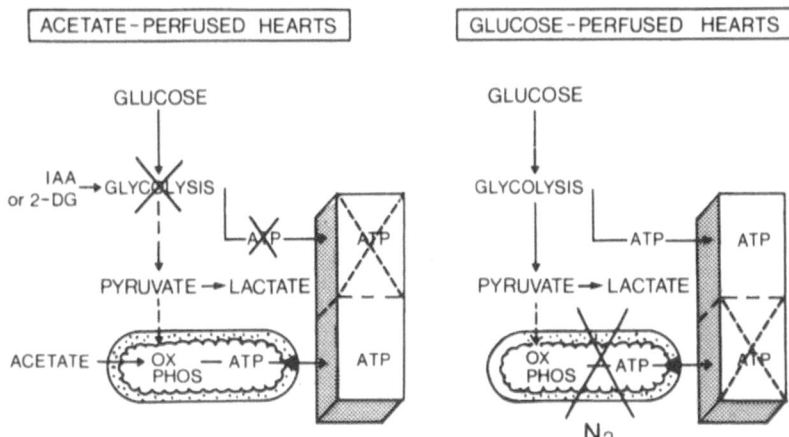

Fig. 3. A simplified scheme of the energy-producing metabolic pathways and the points where the inhibitors are thought to act. IAA, iodoacetic acid, sodium salt; 2-DG, 2-deoxyglucose; ATP, adenosine triphosphate; OX PHOS, oxidative phosphorylation (intramitochondrial). The 'box' represents the cytosolic ATP while the division represents the hypothetical compartmentalization. Total tissue ATP is the sum of the cytosolic ATP and the mitochondrial ATP. (a) Acetate-perfused hearts; (b) glucose-perfused hearts. Acetate-perfused hearts with blocked glycolysis developed ischemic contracture more readily than glucose-perfused hearts with blocked mitochondrial production of ATP. Thus it is the source of the ATP and not the total ATP level that is of importance in this model. Reproduced from [28] with permission of the Journal of Molecular and Cellular Cardiology.

better able to delay or prevent contracture than ATP produced by oxidative phosphorylation. From the theoretical point of view, ischemic contracture is caused by either inadequate ATP to dissociate the actin-myosin cross-bridges or by an increase of resting cytosolic calcium levels [29]. Several workers, notably Hearse *et al.* [30], have proposed a critical tissue level of ATP at which ischemic contracture develops. In contrast, others have dissociated tissue ATP levels from the development of contracture and have argued that glycolytic ATP production is of particular importance in the prevention of ischemic contracture [31–33].

Our unpublished rat heart data show that ischemic contracture in low-flow ischemia consistently developed when non-glycolytic substrates were provided or when glucose flux was inhibited by (1) addition of 2-deoxyglucose or iodoacetate (Fig. 4) or (2) by low external concentrations of glucose. We were able to dissociate changes in levels of tissue ATP from the development of ischemic contracture. We also showed that provision of glucose during low-flow ischemia delayed the onset of ischemic contracture, although the total tissue level of ATP fell to lower values than those found at onset of acetate-induced contracture. The total tissue content of ATP at the onset of ischemic contracture was too high for the development of rigor so that substantial subcellular compartmentation of ATP had to be postulated.

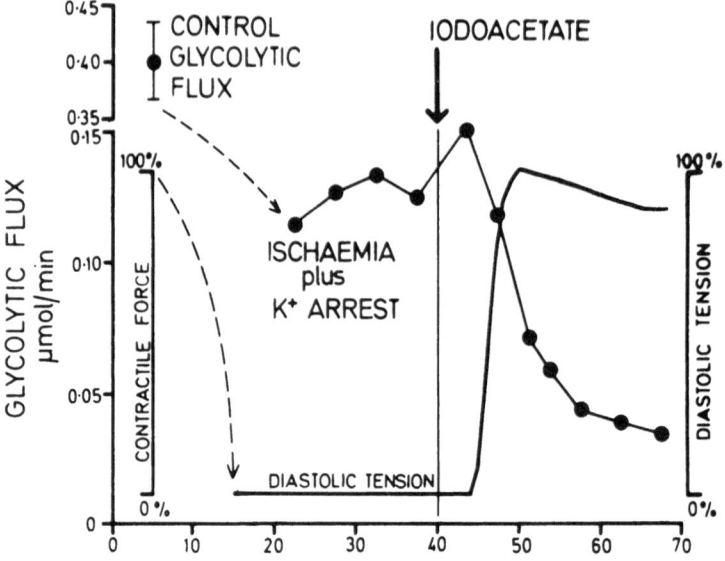

Fig. 4. Role of glycolysis in prevention of ischemic contracture in isolated rat heart. Upon potassium arrest, the contractile force fell to zero diastolic tension, and glycolytic flux decreased. Upon further addition of iodoacetate, an inhibitor of glycolysis, two changes occurred: (a) glycolytic flux fell rapidly towards zero and (b) diastolic tension rose rapidly. These unpublished data support a role for glycolytic flux in the prevention of ischemic contracture. For methods, see [28].

Several reports indicate that the source and turnover of ATP are more important than the concentration of ATP in the prevention of ischemic contracture [31, 33] and in the maintenance of normal contractile activity [5, 16]. We therefore calculated rates of ATP production from glycolysis (glucose and glycogen) and from residual mitochondrial metabolism. The consistent distinguishing feature of those hearts in which ischemic contracture did not develop was the production of ATP from glucose at rates of about 2.0 μmol ATP/g/min or higher.

My co-workers and I proposed [34] that glycolysis provides a small but crucial supply of cytosolic ATP that is accessible to the contractile process but does not influence the total tissue ATP content. Alternatively, glycolytically produced ATP may meet the energy requirements for calcium uptake by the sarcoplasmic reticulum (Fig. 5) or calcium extrusion by the sarcolemma, thus maintaining a state of relaxation during ischemia. Bing and Fishbein [35] studied hypoxic contracture in isolated rat papillary muscles. When glycolytic inhibition was produced by iodoacetate, more severe electronmicroscopic damage appeared than with hypoxia alone, a result in general agreement with our findings. However, there was no direct proof that glycolytic and not mitochondrial ATP was protective.

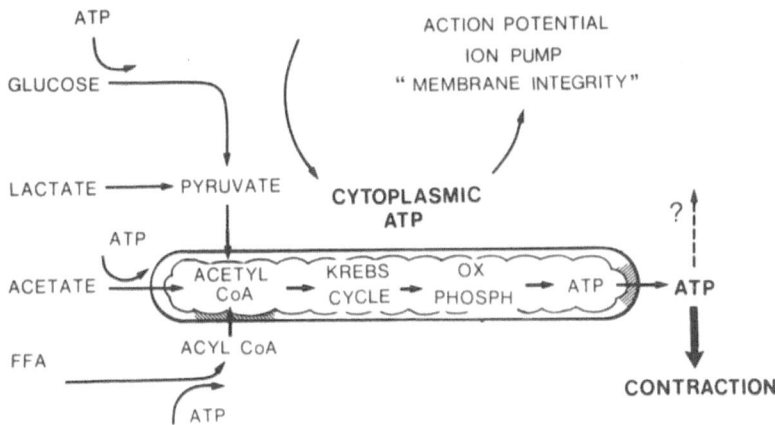

Fig. 5. Hypothetical role of glycolysis in providing cytoplasmic ATP for maintenance of ion gradients, including those of the sarcoplasmic reticulum.
Fig. © LH Opie.

Glycolytic ATP and reperfusion damage

The rate of production of glycolytic ATP during the ischemic period also appears to be a factor in the prevention of reperfusion damage as evidenced by the decreased release of enzymes and fewer arrhythmias during the early reperfusion period [4]. At the end of the ischemic period, perfusion with glucose or pyruvate as external substrates gave similar values for the tissue contents of ATP and creatine phosphate, whereas reperfusion damage was much less in glucose-perfused hearts [4].

Evidence against ATP compartments

If there were a 'critical' level of ATP (total tissue content) below which irreversible damage occurs, then there could not be significant compartmentation of ATP. Thus Kubler and Spieckermann [36] found that as myocardial ATP fell below 3.5 µmol/g wet weight in hearts arrested by ischemia at 15°C, lactate production ceased because of ATP lack for the conversion of fructose 6-phosphate to fructose 1,6-bisphosphate (phosphofructokinase reaction). That ATP level also defined the theoretical limit of myocardial ischemia that could be tolerated with recovery of adequate cardiac function after rewarming and reperfusing the heart. Hearse *et al.* [30] has claimed a similar limit for recovery from whole heart ischemia induced by aortic clamping. In non-cardiac cells, Trump [37, 38] has shown that the decline in the level of ATP during cell injury could be correlated with the development of mitochondrial swelling. Jennings *et al.* [39] have linked irreversible ultrastructural changes to ATP levels of about 0.4–0.6 µmol/g fresh wt. Similarly, endocardial ATP levels of 0.6 µmol/g fresh wt are linked to irreversible pathological changes [40]. Such severe degrees of ATP depletion are probably associated with such severe decreases in coronary flow that many other complex metabolic changes must be happening at that time and it is difficult to ascribe a dominant role to ATP depletion. Opposing the concept of a critical level of ATP, Gudbjarnason *et al.* [27] found that in the non-infarcted zone after coronary ligation in the dog, ATP could drop as low as 1.5 to 2.0 µmol/g and the heart could contract and survive. In reperfusion after cardiac arrest, Schaper *et al.* [41] found cardiac survival even after ATP levels had fallen to below 1 µmol/g wet wt. When heart cells were deprived of glycolysis by substrate starvation [42], there is an entirely different situation, so that their conclusion that total ATP production rather than glycolytic ATP production is of prime importance, may hold for that particular experimental situation.

There must be some overall correlation between life and death of the cell and the presence or absence of ATP (taking extremes) and hence some correlation of the fall of ATP decrease with irreversibility. Thus the overall evidence from the studies cited above does not disprove the concept of compartmentalization.

Apparent failure of glycolytic ATP to benefit in ischemia

An important negative study, oft-quoted, is that of Neely and Grotyohann [43]. They studied cardiac recovery after total ischemic arrest, and found that mechanical recovery was inversely related to the extent of lactate accumulation in the ischemic period. They also studied glycogen depleted hearts, perfused with various lactate concentrations before arrest, and found decreased recovery as the perfusate lactate rose. Hence they reasoned that decreased glycolysis had a protective effect during ischemia, and vice versa. However, it should be noted that they specifically studied a situation of zero flow (total global ischemia) when all glycolytic ATP production must have ceased; they did not specifically measure rate of glycolysis during the ischemic period, so that their data neither disprove nor prove any hypothesis relating glycolytic flux to protection of the membrane during ischemia.

Glycogen depletion: a rebuttal

Furthermore, Lagerstrom *et al.* [44] specifically studied the effects of prior glycogen depletion on post-ischemic recovery, in an attempt to confirm or deny the Neely-Grotyohann hypothesis. In the system of Lagerstrom *et al.* [44] preservation of cardiac glycogen improved recovery, whereas high tissue lactate levels were not associated with mechanical deterioration during the recovery period. There were a number of experimental differences in that Lagerstrom *et al.* [44] used rabbits and not rats, and their perfusate had a relatively high calcium concentration of 2.5 mM versus the normal 1.25 mM of Neely and Grotyohann [43]. The study of Lagerstrom *et al.* [44] is important in that the beneficial and protective role of cardiac glycogen stores is clearly shown; presumably glycolytic ATP was produced for longer in hearts with high cardiac glycogen, but, once again, rates of glycolytic ATP production were not measured, so that this paper cannot be used as direct evidence favoring the glycolytic ATP hypothesis.

Therefore, it seems that no data have yet been accumulated to show that an *increased glycolytic flux* during the ischemic period fails to achieve some benefit.

A further proposal, recently presented, is that glycolytic flux may actually help to maintain tissue viability during ischemia.

Hypothesis: Glycolysis and cell viability

The hypothesis now being proposed [6] is that the *rate of glycolysis has an intimate relationship to the severity of myocardial ischemia and helps to determine ultimate cell viability*. As the coronary flow rate progressively falls, there will be a critical flow level at which increased glucose uptake switches to decreased uptake (Fig. 6). It is proposed that an increase of glucose uptake reflects continued cell viability and a decreased uptake reflects loss of viability of the ischemic cells. Ischemia cells could be divided by the differences in glucose uptake into those with increased values (viable) or decreased values (non-viable) (see Fig. 7).

Glucose uptake as a determinant of or contributor to cell viability

(This and the following four sections are reproduced from Opie [6] with permission of the publishers of J Appl Cardiol).

In myocardial ischemia of mild to moderate severity, the ongoing metabolism of glucose appears to have a direct effect in determining myocardial cell viability. Thus factors increasing glycolytic flux decrease ischemic injury, whereas factors decreasing flux tend to augment ischemic injury (Tables 2 and 3; [6]). In particular, the following associations should be noted: (a) in the ischemic myocardium, the rate of glycolytic flux can be critical in preventing ischemic contracture [4] and glycolysis is a more effective source of energy than is oxidative phosphorylation [28]; (b) glycolysis may govern the electrophysiological properties of the ischemic cell and, in particular, glycolysis is more effective than oxidative phosphorylation in preventing ATP-sensitive K^+-channels from opening [22]; (c) increasing rates of glycolysis decrease enzyme release from the ischemic coronary-ligated isolated heart [24]; (d)

54

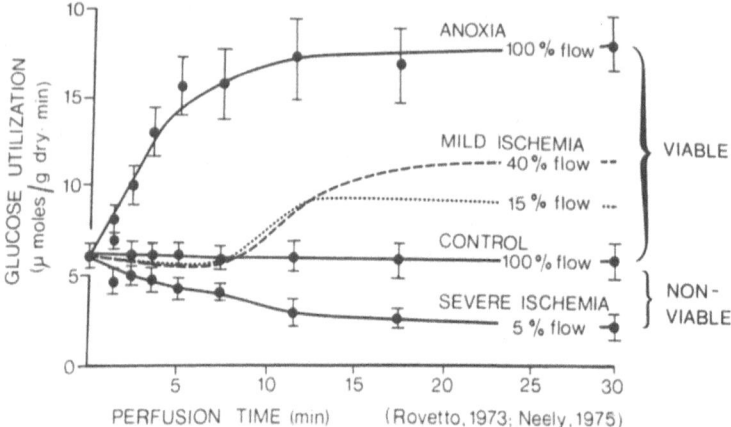

Fig. 6. Effect of coronary flow rate on glucose uptake of isolated perfused rat heart. Note the increased glucose uptake during anoxia with maintained coronary flow and washout of inhibitory metabolites. As coronary flow decreases and ischemia progresses, the inhibitory products of anaerobic glycolysis accumulate so that the glucose uptake falls progressively. For data sources see [64, 65]. These approximate values for coronary flow, based on isolated rat heart data, cannot directly be extrapolated to man.

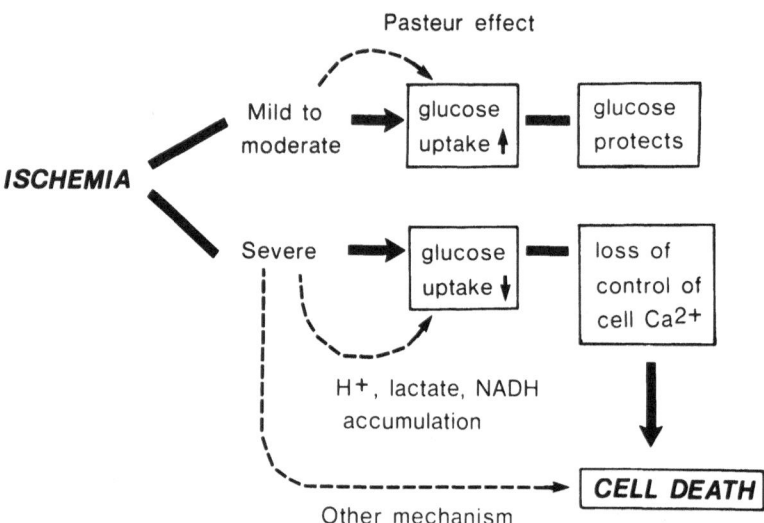

Fig. 7. The hypothesis relating rate of glycolysis to cell death. During mild to moderate ischemia (see Fig. 5) glucose uptake is increased providing the benefit of increased glycolytic ATP. During severe ischemia the accumulation of protons, lactate and NADH inhibits glycolysis and glucose uptake. Consequently there is a loss of control of intracellular calcium with the formation of ischemic contracture [4, 49].
Fig. © LH Opie.

Table 1. Effects of substrate on enzyme release and comparison of content of tissue metabolites in infarcting zone with non-infarcting zone in hearts perfused with glucose, palmitate-albumin, or palmitate-albumin plus glucose and insulin. Biopsies taken by drill method 60 min after coronary artery ligation. Biopsies taken at the end of 15 min initial Langendorff perfusion gave ATP values of 3.66 ± 0.51 (8); after 15 min work (immediately preligation), ATP values were 3.50 ± 0.24 (4); values ± SEM in micromoles per gram. Concentrations of substrates: glucose 11 mmol l^{-1}; palmitate 0.5 mmol l^{-1} (bound to albumin 0.1 mmol l^{-1}; insulin added as 2 mU cm^{-3}). Units: grams fresh weight (= dry weight × 5). From [6] with permission of J Appl Physiol.

Enzyme release and tissue metabolite	Tissue zone	Glucose	P	Palmitate	P	Pyruvate + glucose + insulin
LDH release ($g^{-1}h^{-1}$)	Whole heart	6.6	<<0.001	23.5	<0.001	12.8
ATP (μmol g^{-1})	Ischemic	0.72	NS	0.69	NS	0.88
	Non-ischemic	2.89	NS	2.35	NS	2.23
Creatine phosphate (μmol g^{-1})	Ischemic	0.88	NS	1.15	NS	0.91
	Non-ischemic	4.16	NS	3.48	NS	2.76
Lactate (μmol g^{-1})	Ischemic	7.32	NS	5.03	<0.001	16.03
	Non-ischemic	3.88	NS	2.81	<0.001	5.72
Glycogen (μmol C6 g^{-1})	Ischemic	2.97	NS	2.84	<0.005	8.4
	Non-ischemic	8.68	NS	8.93	<0.001	23.9

Reproduced from [24] with permission of Cardiovascular Research.

Table 2. Relationship between factors decreasing glycolytic flux and the extent of ischemic injury.

Factor decreasing flux	Effect on ischemic injury	Reference
Fasting	No data	
Diabetes (alloxan)	Increase	[66]
Alternative fuels:		
FFA	Increase	[67]
Lactate	Increase	[50]
		[68]
		[49]
Ketones	Increase	[66]
Acidosis, severe	Increase	[69]
Decreased heart work	Decrease[1]	[70]

1. Decreased heart work decreases ischemic injury, showing that mechanical reduction of O_2 demand is more important than the metabolic effect on glycolysis.
From [6] with permission of J Appl Physiol.

Table 3. Relationship between factors increasing glycolytic flux and the extent of ischemic injury.

Factor increasing flux	Effect on ischemic injury	Reference
Fed state	No data	
Insulin	Decrease	[67]
Glucose	Decrease	[71]
		[59]
		[23]
Antilipolytic agents	Decrease	[72]
Acidosis, mild	Decrease	[73]
Alkalosis	Decrease	[69]
Activation of pyruvate dehydrogenase	Decrease	[74]
Increased heart work	Decrease[1]	[70]

1. See footnote to Table 1.
From [6] with permission of J Appl Physiol.

glycolysis can help to maintain normal resting tension in hypoxic ventricular strips [5]; (e) infusions of glucose, insulin and potassium help to protect the infarcting dog heart against necrosis [45]; and (f) enhanced glycolytic flux helps to maintain mitochondrial function during ischemia and reperfusion, possibly by scavenging free radicals [46]. However, an increased severity of myocardial ischemia removes the protective effect of glycolysis during ische-mia [47], presumably by feedback inhibition of glycolysis by glycolytic end-products [43].

Mechanisms relating decreased glycolytic flux to myocardial cell necrosis

Two basic mechanisms could explain why a decreased glucose uptake would lead to myocardial cell necrosis: First, ischemic contracture, an irreversible end-point, is delayed or totally inhibited by adequate rates of glycolytic flux [48]. Because the development of ischemic contracture is not dependent on the myocardial levels of ATP and phosphocreatine [28], the probable mechanism is by a rise of intracellular calcium [4, 49]. It is postulated that glycolytic ATP may have a special function in the control of intracellular calcium levels during ischemia [48] and also in the maintenance of normal gradients of other ions such as potassium [22]. Excess loss of potassium, by removing the transmembrane resting potential, will lead to electrical death of the cell. Secondly, during severe ischemia, a decreased glucose uptake is caused by an intracellular accumulation of $NADH_2$, protons and lactate [43], each of which may have disadvantageous metabolic consequences. For example, $NADH_2$ in excess inhibits oxidative enzymes so that even the residual O_2 uptake in the ischemic zone can no longer be fully used for adequate rates of ATP production. Proton accumulation can lead to an intracellular acidosis, which in turn, if severe enough, can activate lysosomes, with consequent breakdown of cellular proteins. Accumulation of lactate, even if neutral, can damage mitochondria [50] through mechanisms which still need to be clarified.

Provisional experimental evidence favoring hypothesis

The above propositions could be tested by (1) relating the severity of cell necrosis to glucose uptake in a model of developing myocardial infarction; (2) relating myocardial viability to increased extraction of labelled deoxyglucose in patients with ischemic heart disease, using the technique of positron emission tomography; or by (3) at a relatively fixed flow, the rate of provision of glucose to the ischemic myocardium could be altered and thereby the extent of necrosis should change. The first of these three experimental proposals has not yet been attempted, to the knowledge of the present author. The second and third proposals are already supported by three different sets of experimental evidence.

In two studies, the uptake of F-18-labelled deoxyglucose was used to determine cell viability 4–20 hours after reperfusion, which was instituted after 3 hours of left anterior descending coronary occlusion in dogs [51–53]. First, glucose uptake has been related to necrosis in a dog model with left anterior descending coronary artery occlusion by balloon inflation [51].

In the second study, the uptake of glucose was close to 100% in the area which was ischemic after reperfusion. The myocardial blood flow was 41% of the control value in that area. However, in the necrotic area, glucose uptake was only about one-third of the control and myocardial blood flow about 5% of the control. In the zones of patchy necrosis, glucose uptake in the epicardium (167%) was greater than in the endocardium (85%). Hence, as the myocardial blood flow fell by over half in the ischemic zones, glucose uptake was retained at normal levels, showing a relative increase of glucose uptake to the myocardial blood flow in the reperfused myocardium. Even in the necrotic myocardium, glucose uptake was high in relation to the coronary blood flow, presumably the result of admixture of severely and less severely ischemic myocardial cells.

In both studies, glucose uptake was determined by F-18-labelled deoxyglucose. Sochor et al. [52] found that a modest degree of necrosis was associated with a glucose uptake which had increased relative to the control value. As the glucose uptake decreased, more necrosis was evident. In zones with predominant necrosis (more than 80%) glucose uptake, as indirectly measured by FDG, is very low, in conformity with the proposed hypothesis. Such severe necrosis was associated with a reduction of below 15% in the myocardial blood flow [52].

Of particular interest was the finding in the study by Sochor et al. (1985) [51] that viable tissue could be delineated by a combination of increased glucose uptake and modest or no increase in pyrophosphate extraction, whereas necrotic tissue is delineated by a decrease in FDG uptake and a considerable increase in pyrophosphate extraction (pyrophosphate is thought to combine with intracellular calcium, which would support the proposals in Fig. 7).

Patient data

There are also data in patients linking the uptake of FDG to the viability of ischemic segments. Tillisch et al. [54] showed that the combination of PET estimations of FDG and N-13 ammonia (the latter used as a mark of coronary flow) could distinguish between (1) normal myocardium with uniform distribution of both tracers; (2) infarcted myocardium with concordant reduction of both tracers; and (3) ischemic myocardium with an increase of FDG in relation to the uptake of N-13 ammonia [55]. The results of revascularization were predicted with a greater than 80% accuracy using the radiolabelled techniques. Using similar techniques, there is evidence for viable tissue in some infarct regions obtained by PET [56]. In contrast, measurements made by ECG (presence or absence of Q-waves) and echocardiogram (wall motion studies) were relatively unreliable as a means of determining the degree of viable myocardium.

Critical flow rate and glycolysis

Taken together, the above data suggest a strong association between increased glucose uptake and reversible ischemia. It follows that the uptake of glucose by ischemic cells may not only be a marker of viability but actively contribute to their viability. This conclusion has important consequences. First, there is a requirement for ongoing glycolysis in the ischemic myocardium to prevent cell necrosis. However, as the coronary flow falls to a certain critical level, enhanced glucose uptake will lead to an accumulation of adverse metabolic products and there will be no benefit or possibly even harm from glycolysis [43]. Data from rat and dog heart studies suggest that the 'critical' flow rate lies between 5 (Fig. 5) and 20% [51]. Once this 'critical' level is reached, then the only way to obtain improved benefit from glycolysis would be by revascularization. In zones of more modest ischemia, promotion of glucose metabolism either directly (glucose and insulin) or indirectly (by β-blockade, see [57]) should help to achieve the same aim.

Glucose-insulin-potassium in isolated heart studies

Although GIK has consistently been shown to be beneficial in large animal studies with the hearts *in situ* (see Dalby *et al.*, 1981 [58]), the mechanism could be by inhibition of rates of free fatty acid uptake [59]. Therefore, studies in isolated hearts at fixed circulating levels of FFA are more germane to the hypothesis that production of glycolytic ATP may protect membrane integrity.

Apparent failure of GIK in isolated pig heart

Liedtke *et al.* [60] used isolated pig hearts to test the effect of increasing glucose from 8.6 mM to 'excess' levels of 27 mM, together with insulin, on the performance of the globally ischemic pig heart perfused with FFA levels of about 1.25 mM. The excess glucose and insulin did not enhance mechanical activity, despite a considerable increase of glucose uptake and, hence, by implication of glycolytic flux. Thus there was a dissociation between glycolytic flux and mechanical effects of ischemia.

Rebuttal experiments

To further examine the Liedtke data, we perfused isolated rat hearts with a high FFA concentration (1.25 mM bound to albumin 0.25 mM) and added insulin or various concentrations of glucose (Fig. 8) after the induction of regional ischemia by coronary artery ligation. We found a decrease of enzyme release induced by the simple addition of glucose (or of insulin), with the glucose effect increasing as the concentration rose from 5.5 to 11 mM. However, upon further increasing the glucose concentration to 27.5 mM, no further decrease of enzyme release could be obtained. We therefore propose

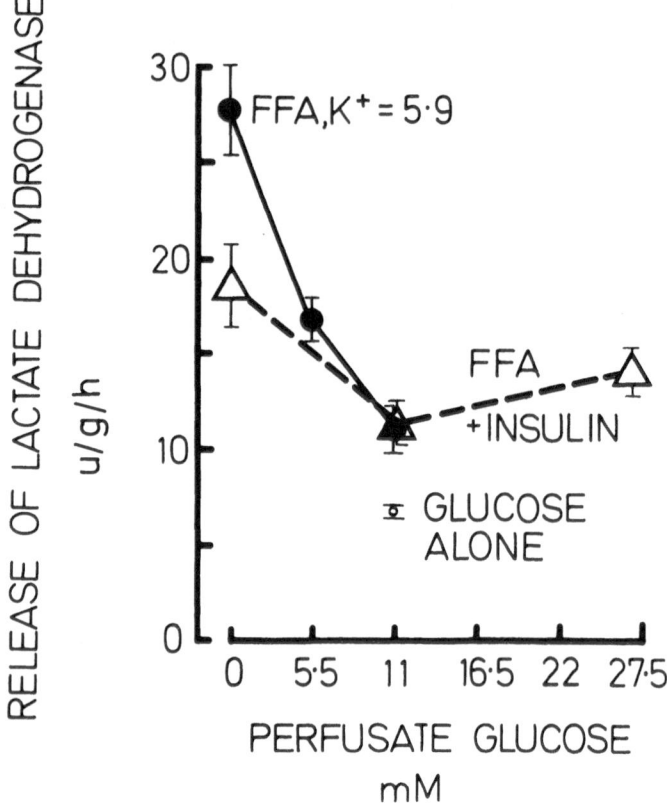

Fig. 8. Effect of glucose and/or insulin on coronary-ligated working hearts perfused with FFA (for conditions,see [61]).FFA = palmitate 1.5 mM bound to albumin 0.25 mM. Note: (1) addition of insulin even in the absence of glucose decreases release of lactate dehydrogenase (LDH); (2) peak effects of glucose reached at 11 mM; an increased concentration of 27.5 mM even in the presence of added insulin caused no further decrease in enzyme release. Unpublished data.

that the apparently negative data of Liedtke *et al.* [60] could be explained by postulating that the rate of glycolysis achieved in their low-glucose hearts was already sufficiently high to yield maximal benefit from glycolysis. In addition, it should be noted that the end-point of their study was mechanical function, whereas in our study the major end-point was enzyme release. We also went on to show that the benefits of addition of glucose to hearts perfused with FFA included an improved mechanical function as well as enzyme release [61] and that the benefit was lost at a low perfusate concentration of potassium, 3.0 mM, which depressed the cardiac output substantially in FFA-perfused hearts. Thus it appears that a *high-normal plasma potassium is required*, at least in isolated perfused hearts, to allow the benefit of glycolysis to be translated into improved cardiac output and lessened enzyme release. We also showed that at a relatively high potassium perfusate concentration of 5.9

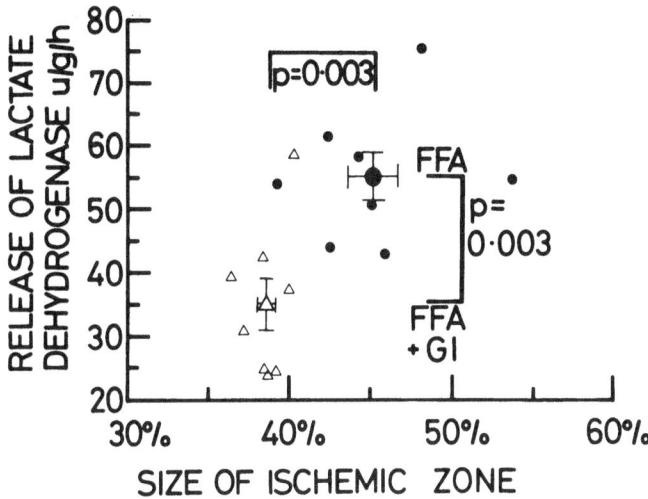

Fig. 9. Relation between rate of release of lactate dehydrogenase and size of ischemic zone (measured roughly by disulphan blue) in coronary-ligated isolated working rat hearts. FFA = free fatty acids as palmitate 1.5 mM bound to albumin 0.25 mM. GI = glucose 11 mM and insulin 2 mU/ml. Note greater rate of release of LDH and bigger size of ischemic zone in hearts perfused with FFA than those perfused with addition of glucose and insulin. Unpublished data.

mM, the increased rate of glycolytic flux was inversely related to the extent of enzyme release (Fig. 9). Finally, we assessed the effects of added glucose-insulin on the size of the ischemic zone in the isolated coronary ligated rat heart model (Fig. 9); both ischemic size and enzyme release were reduced.

Nuclear magnetic resonance data

More recently, Hoekenga *et al.* [62] showed that GIK decreased the rate of glycogen mobilization during ischemia without the overall rate of glycolysis being altered in an isolated guinea-pig heart system. They proposed that the glycogen-sparing effect could be of relevance in a clinical setting by prolonging the availability of glycolytic substrate supply. However, no attempts were made to relate variations in glycolytic flux rate to any protection during ischemia or thereafter.

Glycolytic flux and GIK in isolated hearts

Thus the data reviewed in the preceding section show that relatively small amounts of glucose are required to protect the myocardium from ischemia in isolated hearts. Circulating concentrations of approximately 9 mM to 11mM may give adequate protection. For protection to be achieved requires the

62

presence of a relatively high potassium concentration (approximately 6 mM). The site of action of GIK in hearts with regional ligation cannot be defined and might vary from the ischemic zone to the adjacent aerobic heart muscle [63].

References

1. Sodi-Pallares D, Testelli MR, Fishleder BR, *et al.* (1962) Effects of an intravenous infusion of a potassium-glucose-insulin solution on the electrocardiographic signs of myocardial infarction. A preliminary clinical report. Am J Cardiol 9: 166–181
2. Owen P, Thomas M, Opie LH (1969) Relative changes in free fatty acid and glucose utilisation by ischemic myocardium after coronary artery occlusion. Lancet i: 1187–1190
3. Opie LH (1970) The glucose hypothesis: Relation to acute myocardial ischemia. J Mol Cell Cardiol 1: 107–115
4. Bricknell OL, Opie LH (1978) Effects of substrates on tissue metabolic changes in the isolated rat heart during underperfusion and on release of lactate dehydrogenase and arrhythmias during reperfusion. Circ Res 43: 102–115
5. Anderson GL, Morris RG (1978) Role of glycolysis in the relaxation process in mammalian cardiac muscle: Comparison of the influence of glucose and 2-deoxyglucose on maintenance of resting tension. Life Sci 23: 23–32
6. Opie LH (1989) Hypothesis: Glycolytic rates control cell viability in ischemia. J Appl Cardiol, in press
7. Achs MJ, Garfinkel D (1977) Computer stimulation of energy metabolism in anoxic perfused rat heart. Am J Physiol 232: R164–R174
8. Opie LH (1971/72) Substrate utilization and glycolysis in the heart. Cardiology 56: 2–21
9. Newsholme EA (1971) The regulation of phosphofructokinase in muscle. Cardiology 56: 22–34
10. Opie LH (1968) Metabolism of the heart. I. Metabolism of glucose, glycogen, free fatty acids and ketone bodies. Am Heart J 76: 685–698
11. Opie LH (1975) Metabolism of free fatty acids, glucose and catecholamines in acute myocardial infarction. Relation to myocardial ischemia and infarct size. Am J Cardiol 36: 938–953
12. Opie LH (1983) High energy phosphate compounds. In: Drake-Holland AJ, Noble MIM (eds) Cardiac Metabolism. John Wiley and Sons Ltd, 279–307
13. Prasad K, MacLeod DP (1969) Influence of glucose on the transmembrane action potential of guinea-pig papillary muscle. Circulation 24: 939–950
14. Eisenberg G, Vereecke J, van der Heyden G, Carmeleit E (1983) The shortening of the action potential by DNP in guinea-pig ventricular myocytes is mediated by an increase of a time-independent K conductance. Pflugers Arch 397: 251–259
15. Hayashi H, Watanabe T, McDonald TF (1987) Action potential duration in ventricular muscle during selective metabolic block. Am J Physiol 253: H373–H379
16. Opie LH, Tuschmidt R, Bricknell OL, *et al.* (1980) Role of glycolysis in maintenance of the action potential duration and contractile activity in isolated perfused rat heart. J Physiol (Paris) 76: 821–829
17. Cheneval JP, Hyde A, Blondel B, *et al.* (1972) Heart cells in culture. Metabolism, action potential and transmembrane ionic movements. J Physiol (Paris) 64: 413–430
18. Noma A, Shibasaki T (1985) Membrane current through adenosine-triphosphate-regulated potassium channels in guinea-pig ventricular cells. J Physiol (Lond) 363: 463–480
19. Kantor P, Coetzee WA, Carmeleit E, *et al.* (1989) Reduction in ischemic K^+ loss and arrhythmias: The effect of the sulfonylurea, glibenclamide. Circ Res, in press

20. Dunne MJ, Petersen OH (1986a) Intracellular ADP activates K^+ channels that are inhibited by ATP in an insulin secreting cell line. FEBS Let 208: 59–62
21. Dunne MJ, Petersen OH (1986b) GTP and GDP activation of K^+ channels that can be inhibited by ATP. Pflugers Arch 407: 564–565
22. Weiss JN, Lamp ST (1987) Glycolysis preferentially inhibits ATP-sensitive K^+ channels in isolated guinea pig cardiac myocytes. Science 238: 67–69
23. De Leiris J, Lubbe WF, Opie LH (1975) Effects of free fatty acid and glucose on enzyme release in experimental myocardial infarction. Nature 153: 746–747
24. Opie LH, Bricknell OL (1979) Role of glycolytic flux in effect of glucose in decreasing fatty-acid induced release of lactate dehydrogenase from isolated coronary ligated rat heart. Cardiovasc Res 13: 693–702
25. Higgins TJC, Bailey PJ, Allsopp D (1981) The influence of ATP depletion on the action of phospholipase C on cardiac myocyte membrane phospholids. J Mol Cell Cardiol 13: 1027–1030
26. Higgins TJC, Allsopp D, Bailey PJ, D'Souza EDA (1981) The relationship between glycolysis, fatty acid metabolism and membrane integrity in neonatal myocytes. J Mol Cell Cardiol 13: 599–615
27. Gudbjarnason S, Mathes R, Ravens KG (1970) Functional compartmentation of ATP and creatine phosphate in heart muscle. J Mol Cell Cardiol 1: 325–339
28. Bricknell OL, Daries PS, Opie LH (1981) A relationship between adenosine triphosphate, glycolysis and ischemic contracture in the isolated rat heart. J Mol Cell Cardiol 13: 941–945
29. Katz AM, Tada M (1977) The 'stone heart' and other challenges to the biochemist. Am J Cardiol 39: 1073–1077
30. Hearse DJ, Garlick PB, Humphrey SM (1977) Ischemic contracture of the myocardium: mechanism and prevention. Am J Cardiol 39: 986–993
31. Lipasti JA, Nevalainen TJ, Alanen KA, Tolvanen MA (1984) Anaerobic glycolysis and the development of ischemic contracture in isolated rat heart. Cardiovasc Res 18: 145–148
32. Allen DG, Morris PG, Orchard CH, Pirolo JS (1985) A nuclear magnetic resonance study of metabolism in the ferret heart during hypoxia and inhibition of glycolysis. J Physiol 361: 185–204
33. Bittl JA, Balschi J, Ingwall JS (1987) Contractile failure and high-energy phosphate turnover during hypoxia: ^{31}P-NMR surface coil studies in living rat. Circ Res 60: 871–878
34. Owen P, Dennis SC, Opie LH (1989) Glucose flux rate regulates onset of ischemic contracture in globally underperfused rat hearts. Circ Res, in press
35. Bing OHL, Fishbein MC (1979) Mechanical and structural correlates of contracture induced by metabolic blockade in cardiac muscle from the rat. Circ Res 45: 298–308
36. Kubler W, Spieckermann PG (1970) Regulation of glycolysis in the ischemic and the anoxic myocardium. J Mol Cell Cardiol 1: 351–357
37. Laiho KU, Trump BF (1975) Studies on the pathogenesis of cell injury – effects of inhibitors of metabolism and membrane function on the mitochondria of Ehrlich ascites tumor cells. Lab Invest 32: 163–182
38. Trump BF, Mergner WJ, Kahng MW, et al. (1976) Studies on the subcellular pathophysiology of ischemia. Circulation 53 (Suppl 1): 17–26
39. Jennings RB, Hawkins HK, Lowe JE, et al. (1978) Relation between high energy phosphate and lethal injury in myocardial ischemia in the dog. Am J Pathol 92: 187–207
40. Lowe JE, Jennings RB, Reimar KA (1979) Cardiac rigor mortis in dogs. J Mol Cell Cardiol 11: 1017–1031
41. Schaper J, Mulch J, Winkler B, Schaper W (1979) Ultrastructural, functional, and biochemical criteria for estimation of reversibility of ischemic injury: a study on the effects of global ischemia on the isolated dog heart. J Mol Cell Cardiol 11: 521–541
42. Haworth RA, Hunter DR, Berkoff HA (1981) Contracture in isolated adult rat heart cells. Role of Ca^{2+}, ATP and compartmentation. Circ Res 49: 1119–1128
43. Neely JR, Grotyohann LW (1984) Role of glycolytic products in damage to ischemic

myocardium. Dissociation of adenosine triphosphate levels and recovery of function of reperfused ischemic hearts. Circ Res 55: 816–824

44. Lagerstrom CF, Walker WE, Taegtmeyer H (1988) Failure of glycogen depletion to improve left ventricular function of the rabbit heart after hypothermic ischemic arrest. Circ Res 63: 81–86

45. Rose A, Opie LH, Bricknell O (1976) Evaluation of histologic criteria of early experimental myocardial infarction. Comparison with biochemical and electrocardiographic parameters. Arch Pathol 100: 516–571

46. Ferrari R, Curello S, Ceconi C (1986) Glucose and FFA as myocardial substrate during ischemia: Effects on glutathione status (Abstract). J Mol Cell Cardiol 18 (Suppl 1): 108

47. Apstein CS, Gravino FN, Haudenschild CC (1983) Determinants of a protective effect of glucose and insulin on the ischemic myocardium. Circ Res 52: 515–526

48. Opie LH, Owen EP, Dennis SC (1985) Glycolysis prevents ischemic contracture (Abstract). Circulation 72 (Suppl III): 349

49. Allen DG, Lee JA, Smith GL (1988) The effects of simulated ischaemia on intracellular calcium and tension in isolated ferret ventricular muscle. J Physiol 400: 91P–92P

50. Armiger LC, Gavin JB, Herdson PB (1974) Mitochondrial changes in dog myocardium induced by neutral lactate in vivo. Lab Invest 31: 29–33

51. Sochor H, Schwaiger M, Schelbert HR, et al. (1985) Assessment of tissue viability in reperfused canine myocardium by a multiple radiotracer technique (Abstract). J Am Coll Cardiol 5: 451

52. Sochor H, Schwaiger M, Schelbert HR, et al. (1987) Relationship between Tl–201, Tc–99m (Sn) pyrophosphate and F-18 2-deoxyglucose uptake in ischemically injured dog myocardium. Am Heart J 114: 1066–1077

53. Melin JA, Wijns W, Keyeux A, et al. (1988) Assessment of thallium-201 redistribution versus glucose uptake as predictors of viability after coronary occlusion and reperfusion. Circulation 77: 927–934

54. Tillisch J, Brunken R, Marshall R, et al. (1986) Reversibility of cardiac wall-motion abnormalities predicted by positron tomography. New Engl J Med 314: 884–888

55. Marshall RC, Tillisch JH, Phelps ME, et al. (1983) Identification and differentiation of resting myocardial ischemia and infarction in man with positron computed tomography, ^{18}F-labeled fluorodeoxyglucose and N-13 ammonia. Circulation 67: 766–778

56. Brunken R, Tillisch J, Schwaiger M, et al. (1986) Regional perfusion, glucose metabolism and wall motion in patients with chronic electrocardiographic Q-wave infarctions: evidence for peristence of viable tissue in some infarct regions by positron emission tomography. Circulation 73: 951–963

57. Opie LH, Thomas M (1976) Propranolol and experimental myocardial infarction: substrate effects. Postgrad Med J 52 (Suppl 4): 124–132

58. Dalby AJ, Bricknell OL, Opie LH (1981) Effect of glucose-insulin-potassium infusions on epicardial ECG changes and on myocardial metabolic changes after coronary artery ligation in dogs. Cardiovasc Res 15: 588–598

59. Opie LH, Owen P (1976) Effect of glucose-insulin-potassium infusions on arteriovenous differences of glucose and of free fatty acids and on tissue metabolic changes in dogs with developing myocardial infarction. Am J Cardiol 38: 310–321

60. Liedtke AJ, Hughes HC, Neely JR (1976) Effects of excess glucose and insulin on glycolytic metabolism during experimental myocardial ischemia. Am J Cardiol 38: 17–27

61. Opie LH (1988) Sympathetic stimulation of ischemic myocardium: Role of plasma free fatty acids and potassium. J Cardiovasc Pharmacol 12 (Suppl 1): S31–S38

62. Hoekenga DE, Brainard JR, Hutson JY (1988) Rates of glycolysis and glycogenolysis during ischemia in glucose-insulin-potassium-treated perfused hearts: A ^{13}C, ^{31}P nuclear magnetic resonance study. Circ Res 62: 1065–1074

63. Liedtke AJ, Nellis SH, Whitesell LF (1982) Effects of regional ischemia on metabolic function in adjacent aerobic myocardium. J Mol Cell Cardiol 14: 195–205

64. Rovetto MJ, Whitmer JT, Neely JR (1973)   Comparison of effects of anoxia and whole heart ischemia on carbohydrate utilization in isolated working rat hearts. Circ Res 22: 699–711

65. Neely JR, Liedtke AJ, Whitmer JT, *et al.* (1975)   Relationship between coronary flow and adenosine triphosphate production from glycolysis and oxidative metabolism. In: Roy PR, Harris P (eds) Recent Advances in Studies on Cardiac Structure and Metabolism. Baltimore: University Park Press, 301–321

66. Sinclair-Smith B, Opie LH (1978)   Effect of diabetic ketosis on enzyme release from isolated perfused rat hearts with experimental myocardial infarction. J Mol Med 10: 221–234

67. De Leiris J, Feuvray D (1977)   Ischaemia-induced damage in the working rat heart preparation. The effect of perfusate substrate composition upon subendocardial ultrastructure of the ischaemic left ventricular wall. J Mol Cell Cardiol 9: 365–373

68. Wissner SB (1974)   The effect of excess lactate upon the excitability of the sheep Purkinje fiber. J Electrocardiol 7: 17–26

69. Regan, TJ, Effros RM, Haider B, *et al.* (1976)   Myocardial ischaemia and cell acidosis: Modification by alkali and the effects on ventricular function and cation composition. Am J Cardiol 37: 501–507

70. Maroko PR, Kjekshus JK, Sobel BE, *et al.* (1971)   Factors influencing infarct size following experimental coronary artery occlusions. Circulation 43: 67–82

71. Maroko PR, Libby P, Sobel BE, *et al.* (1972)   Effect of glucose-insulin-potassium infusion on myocardial infarction following experimental coronary artery occlusion. Circulation 45: 1160–1175

72. Oliver MF, Rowe MJ, Luxton MR, *et al.* (1976)   Effect of reducing circulating free fatty acids on ventricular arrhythmias during myocardial infarction and on ST-segment depression during exercise-induced ischaemia. Circulation 53: 1–210

73. Bing OHL, Brooks WW, Messer JV (1973)   Heart muscle viability following hypoxia: protective effect of acidosis. Science 180: 1297–1298

74. Mjos OD, Miller NE, Riemersma RA, *et al.* (1976)   Effects of dichloroacetate on myocardial substrate extraction, epicardial ST-segment elevation, and ventricular blood flow following coronary occlusion in dogs. Cardiovasc Res 10: 427–436

PART III

The search for critical cellular structures

Loss of sarcolemmal integrity in ischemic myocardium

MARCEL BORGERS

Department of Life Sciences, Janssen Research Foundation, B–2340 Beerse, Belgium

Introduction

When reporting the ultrastructural changes in the heart during ischemia and post-ischemic reperfusion, the sarcolemma (SL) usually receives little attention in comparison with other subcellular organelles of cardiac myocytes. The reason for this is obviously related to the slow onset of appearance: SL-changes are subtle, if noticeable at all, during the early periods of ischemia and when they become fully expressed they only appear in the picture long after other 'spectacular' changes have been witnessed in other organelles. Hence, understandably, the SL is seldom given the front page coverage which, in my opinion, it rightfully deserves. This is illustrated by the fact that of a list of 47 metabolic, functional and structural alterations which occur within seconds and minutes after the onset of severe ischemia [1] none have been related to the sarcolemma. Cell membrane deterioration occurs only once among 17 events taking place within hours of ischemia and is considered to be a terminal event preceding cell death. The question of which events precisely determine the point of 'no return' during ischemic injury is difficult to answer in view of the complexity of the interrelation between the functions of the different subcellular entities: an impaired mitochondrial function may have direct consequences for the functional behavior of the SL and vice versa. There are, however a number of observations that point directly to the SL as one of the major subcellular entities in controlling cell survival: (a) the coincidence of the structural breakdown of the SL during prolonged ischemia and the lack of functional recovery of the heart after post-ischemic reperfusion [2–4]; (b) the loss of volume regulation, due to increased SL permeability, coincides with irreversible ischemic injury [2, 5]; and (c) when structural SL-changes are induced by other means than ischemia the cell loses its ability to regulate ion-fluxes and becomes irreversibly damaged [6–8]. SL characterization during preterminal stages of ischemic injury by means other than classic electronmicroscopy is necessary in order to clarify some of the many unanswered questions. In order to relate early intracellular deteriorative events with sarcolemmal impairment, methodologies like freeze-fracture [9, 10] and

H.M. Piper (ed.) Pathophysiology of severe ischemic myocardial injury, 69–89.
© *1990 Kluwer Academic Publishers, Dordrecht –*

distribution of calcium at the ultrastructural level, have been used [11, 12] and will be summarized in this paper.

Although cells can be injured by a variety of pathways and no single cause of cell death suffices to explain all lethal events, the loss of SL integrity resulting in the dissipation of transmembrane electrolyte gradients, most probably constitutes the final pathway of cell injury. Ischemia induces a complex series of noxious alterations such as energy depletion [13], cellular acidosis [14], oxygen free radical generation [15–17], formation of amphiphiles such as free fatty acids, fatty acid esters and lysophospholipids [18, 19] which may all contribute to the loss of cellular ion homeostasis. Much attention has been focused on the central role of Ca^{2+} in mediating and propagating ischemic cell injury, finally causing myocardial cell death [7, 14 20–22]. The hypothesis that disturbances in intracellular Ca^{2+} overload may be detrimental to cells has many theoretical backgrounds.

Transients of Ca^{2+} into the cell during ischemia/reperfusion cause significant increases in cytosolic free Ca^{2+}, resulting in an activation of CA^{2+}-dependent intracellular metabolic processes. Phospholipases will be activated by free cytosolic Ca^{2+}, resulting in a breakdown of cell. ATPases are regulated by Ca^{2+} and their activation will lead to denaturation of proteins and excessive depletion of ATP [14]. The scavenging of Ca^{2+} by mitochondria will lead to overload, uncoupling of the oxidative phosphorylation and potentiation of the damaging effects of oxygen radicals on mitochondrial energy transport. It is therefore not too difficult to envisage how an unrestrained increase in $(Ca^{2+})_i$ can upset the homeostasis of cellular messengers, electrolytes and energy. Because ischemic tissue contains large amounts of Ca^{2+} and because protective effects are observed for different classes of Ca^{2+} antagonists in experimental and clinical conditions, the hypothesis that ischemia causes an uncontrolled increase in total cell Ca^{2+} and that augmented cytosolic free Ca^{2+} initiates the cascade of deleterious events leading to cell death is clearly feasible.

Structure and composition of the sarcolemma

The myocytes from the heart form a syncytium through the interconnection of branched cells by specialized cell surface membrane parts, the gap junctions of the intercalated disks. The cell surface of the cardiomyocytes consists of a 60 nm thick sarcolemma-glycocalyx complex. Its structure comprises the sarcolemma (a unit membrane or lipid bilayer) and the glycocalyx, which is mainly composed of mucopolysaccharides. This 50 nm thick layer is usually subdivided into an electron lucent surface coat and a moderately dense external lamina. The surface coat is an integral part of the sarcolemma and many of its glycoproteins penetrate into or through the lipid bilayer. Both components of the glycocalyx contain fixed negatively charged sites, mainly due to an abundance of sialic acid [24].

The sarcolemma (SL) is a 9–10 nm thick layer which is composed of lipids and proteins, the lipids being arranged in a bilamellar leaflet [25]. Membrane lipids are mainly phosphatidylcholine, phosphatidylethanolamine, sphingomyelin and the acidic lipids phosphatidylserine and phosphatidylinositol. Phospholipids of the SL are thought to play an important role in the physiology as well as the pathology of the heart [9, 19, 23].

In addition, the importance of sarcolemmal phospholipids in Ca^{2+} binding and their possible contribution in the control of contraction is indicated or suggested by a series of studies [26–28]. These studies have shown the existence of a strong correlation between SL bound Ca^{2+} and the contractile force. At least 80% of the SL bound Ca^{2+} can be attributed to phospholipid binding [28]. In order to further characterize SL Ca^{2+}, it is necessary to know the phospholipid composition and its distribution within the SL. Recent investigations have focused on the distribution of the phospholipid classes between the two monolayers of the SL [29, 30]. The SL, isolated by 'gas-dissection' technique, contains 38% of the total cellular phospholipid, which in turn is composed of phosphatidylethanolamine (PE) 24.9%, phosphatidylcholine (PC) 52%, phosphatidylserine/phosphatidylinositol (PS/PI) 7.2%, sphingomyelin (Sph) 3.5%. The cholesterol/phospholipid ratio of the SL is 0.5.

The distribution of the phospholipids between the inner and the outer monolayer was defined with the use of two phospholipases A_2, sphingomyelinase C and trinitrobenzene sulfonic acid as lipid membrane probes. The phospholipid classes were found to be asymmetrically distributed: the negatively charged phospholipids, PS/PI, were located exclusively in the inner or cytoplasmic leaflet; 75% of PE in the inner leaflet; 93% of Sph in the outer leaflet; and 43% of PC is located in the outer leaflet. The same authors also determined the plasmalogen content and the distribution within the SL. They showed that the inner SL leaflet is highly enriched with PC and PE plasmalogens. The predominance of PS/PI, PE and most of the PC and PE plasmalogens at the cytoplasmic SL side was discussed in relation to the phospholipid-ionic binding, the control of cellular Ca^{2+} homeostasis and the response of the cardiac cell to ischemia-reperfusion (*vide infra*).

The proteinateous parts embedded in the lipid bilayer which are of interest in the study of ischemic and post-ischemic reperfusion damage mainly concern enzymes, carriers and channels, especially those involved with Ca^{2+} handling. Under normal physiological conditions the myocardial cell has a complex system to control the transsarcolemmal Ca^{2+} fluxes. Among these are the Ca^{2+} ATPase, Na^+/K^+ ATPase, Na^+/Ca^{2+} exchanger, Na^+/H^+ exchanger and the slow Ca^{2+} channel. It has been suggested that the negatively charged phospholipid molecules form a lipid annulus around ion pumps (i.e. Na^+/K^+ ATPase) and Ca^{2+}/Mg^{2+} ATPase at the inner surface of the SL [30]. If these observations and the proposed hypothesis are true, then this class of phospholipids may play a determinant role in the regulation of Ca^{2+} release and Ca^{2+} rebinding during the course of an action potential, in the regulation of enzyme activity and in the maintenance of membrane impermeability. A number of SL cation channels have been well established, although their relative contribution in the overall ion homeostasis is not entirely clear. As far as their contribution to pathological ion shifts are concerned this is merely a black box [31]. Using cytochemical methodology [32], Ca^{2+} has been localized at the inner leaflet of the SL in normoxic cardiomyocytes of man, dog, rabbit, guinea-pig, hamster and rat [11, 12, 33, 34]. This cytochemically demonstrated Ca^{2+} is thought to represent the Ca^{2+} pool which is bound to acidic phospholipids which exclusively inhabit the cytoplasmic face of the bilayer. 20-nanometer deposits line the SL (Figs. 1 and 2), SL derived vesicles, T-tubules (Fig. 3) and the entire intercalated disk area. A special type of deposition is present at gap junctions where the Ca^{2+} is seen in a paired position (Fig. 4). Direct topographical confirmation of the existence of this pool has been given in the work of Wheeler-Clark and Tormey [35] showing that the SL contained as much Ca^{2+} as the sarcoplasmic reticulum and that both organelles did participate in Ca^{2+}-loading during inotropic interventions, a theory proposed earlier by both Lüllmann and Peters [26] and Langer [28].

Sarcolemmal changes during ischemia and postischemic reperfusion

Points currently under debate and addressed here are the structural equivalent of reversible versus irreversible damage and the question of whether or not oxygen is a necessary component in the production of irreversible injury. Few criteria have been considered as valid morphological signs of irreversibility [2, 13]. Although severe swelling of the matrix with concurrent disruption of cristae in mitochondria have been described as indicators of severe damage, only the presence of flocculent densities in the mitochondrial matrix has been considered as a sign of irreversibility [36]. The formation of contraction bands and interruptions of the SL have been reported as terminal morphologic events of injury [37, 38]. At present, it is not clear how far these ultimate changes are past the point of no return. The structural changes at the SL during and after ischemia usually differ from those seen after other insults which compromise cardiac cell survival such as Ca^{2+}-free/Ca^{2+}-rich perfusion. The formation of liquid filled blebs which separate the two layers of the glycocalyx has been demonstrated after global normothermic ischemia and reperfusion [39], in chronically ischemic human myocardium [40], after regional myocardial ischemia and prolonged reperfusion, and upon reoxygenation after prolonged anoxic perfusion [3, 7, 41]. In all these conditions, and contrary to the Ca^{2+}-paradox situation, the separation of the outer glycocalyx layer is seen either focally or concerns only a limited number of cells. If present, EL-SC spaces are, in contrast to the Ca^{2+}-paradox situation, often filled with membranous blebs derived from the SL. This indicates that prolonged oxygen shortage not only perturbs the glycocalyx but also the lipid

Figs. 1–4. Dog. Ultrastructural distribution of SL-bound Ca^{2+}.

    1. Black deposits of ± 20 nm thickness line the inner leaflet of the bilayer (arrow) (× 33705).

    2. High magnification of a portion of the SL (× 61965).

    3. T-tubular profiles (T) show deposits, exclusively facing the cytoplasm (× 52245).

    4. Gap junction. The deposits are distributed in a paired fashion (arrow) facing each the cytoplasmic side of the membrane (× 104985).

bilayer. Interruptions of this lipid bilayer are frequent after prolonged ischemia and become very pronounced during post-ischemic reperfusion [2, 4, 39]. The fact that the two layers of the glycocalyx are not separated in the majority of damaged cells does not mean that they have retained their ion barrier function or even that the anchoring system is left intact. The absence of liquid filled blebs under these conditions may be due to intracellular accumulation of fluid. This is in strong contrast with the Ca^{2+}-paradox situation where cell shrinking is generally observed.

More commonly observed after prolonged ischemia are the changes to the SL itself, either confined to the lipid bilayer structure, the intramembranous (proteinateous) particles (IMP) or the anchoring systems of the SL with the cytoskeleton. Ischemia and subsequent reperfusion damages the lipid bilayer, morphologically characterized by density changes of the SL, interruptions of the bilayer and the presence of phospholipid-like blebs in between the SL and the glycocalyx [4, 39, 42, 43]. These alterations have been attributed to the action of Ca^{2+}-activated phospholipases, oxygen derived free radicals, insertion of endogenous amphiphiles or to acidosis (*vide infra*).

Freeze-fracture techniques which reveal the internal composition of the SL have shown that redistribution of IMP in the SL can take place as soon as 5 minutes after normothermic ischemia, although in a reversible manner [10]. This alteration is paralleled by an acute loss of cellular K^+ and by marked but reversible electrophysiological changes. Such changes are not matched with detrimental alterations in classical thin section electron microscopy. In the search for additional criteria to determine morphological changes at the point of irreversibility some cytochemical methods to localize different intracellular sites of Ca^{2+} have been applied [12].

A correlation between the failure to recover function during post-ischemic reperfusion and the inability of the SL to bind Ca^{2+} has been established. It has been proposed that Ca^{2+} which is bound to the inner aspect of the lipid bilayer plays an important role in the integrity of the SL. This hypothesis has been verified in the dog made ischemic for 60 minutes [44], in rabbit isolated working heart after periods of normothermic ischemia ranging from 15 to 75 minutes [12] and in rat isolated cardiomyocytes exposed to anoxia for 30 to 120 minutes [22]. The effects of reperfusion or reoxygenation have been studied in all these situations and ultrastructural changes, combined with changes in Ca^{2+} distribution, have been used as criteria for assessment of the degree of ischemic damage to the SL.

In a study with isolated cardiomyocytes [11] the time-related redistribution of Ca^{2+} during anoxia concerned the initial increase of SL associated Ca^{2+} and mitochondrial matrix Ca^{2+}. These alterations were most pronounced after 60 minutes of anoxia. Simultaneously with the global shape change of the cells (contracture), the SL bound Ca^{2+} disappeared, and clustered Ca^{2+} deposits accumulated in the mitochondria. These changes occurred in about 35% of the cells after 120 minutes of anoxia and were interpreted as changes at the point of irreversibility corresponding to an inability of the cells to recover metabolically.

The initial increase in Ca^{2+} binding to the SL, in addition to the scavenging of Ca^{2+} by the mitochondria, has been interpreted as a cellular rescue reaction in order to keep the cytosol Ca^{2+} as low as possible. The loss of SL's ability to bind Ca^{2+} after prolonged anoxia, similar to that seen in ischemic hearts of the dog (Fig. 5) [44] and rabbit (Fig. 6) [12], is considered as the first sign of irreversible loss of the cells' Ca^{2+} homeostasis. This observation is interpreted as a prelude to cytosolic Ca^{2+}-overload because it occurs during the ischemic phase, prior to reperfusion and precedes any other structural sign of membrane degeneration. An exception to the general observation of the loss of SL Ca^{2+} binding is formed by the gap junction area. This site, in contrast to other parts of the SL, retains its Ca^{2+} binding at the end of a 60 minute normothermic ischemia. It is possible that the gap junctional Ca^{2+} represents a different pool from that at the other parts of the SL, being more tightly bound and functioning as a shut-down mechanism between the interconnected cells in order to rescue neighbouring cells. Indeed, under pathological conditions of Ca^{2+} overload, an excessive increase in Ca^{2+} will effectively disconnect metabolically compromised and defective cells from their normally functioning neighbours by a rapid shut-down of gap junctional conductance and intercellular communication [45].

However, after reperfusion, when the injury to the cells becomes fully expressed, a total loss of membrane-bound Ca^{2+} is seen. This is always associated with a marked increase in the amount of Ca^{2+} precipitates inside the damaged mitochondria (Figs. 7 and 8).

Thus, there appears to be a close correlation between the structural changes of the SL, including the loss of bound Ca^{2+}, and the increased transmembrane Ca^{2+}-influx that leads to mitochondrial Ca^{2+}-overload.

The time sequence of reversible and irreversible ultrastructural changes and the shifts in Ca^{2+} distribution which parallel these events as seen in the isolated rabbit working heart [12] are given in Table 1.

The whole scale of changes was already present after 15 minutes of ischemia, despite involving only a limited number of cells. All shifts from the normal distribution pattern of Ca^{2+} were found to be linearly related with time. Transmural involvement was complete from 60 minutes ischemia onward, meaning that no cells regained the normal distribution pattern after reperfusion. However, it must be noted that after ischemic periods which lasted longer than 45 minutes the post-ischemic reperfusion is far from uniform. The non-reperfusability of some areas, especially in the mid zone, was very obvious in the 60 and 75 minute ischemic hearts.

Reperfusion after 30 and 45 minutes of ischemia resulted in a marked exacerbation of the structural injury to most subcellular entities: sarcomeres were often hypercontracted; nuclei showed margination of heterochromatin and the SL demonstrated a general lack of recovery of Ca^{2+} binding.

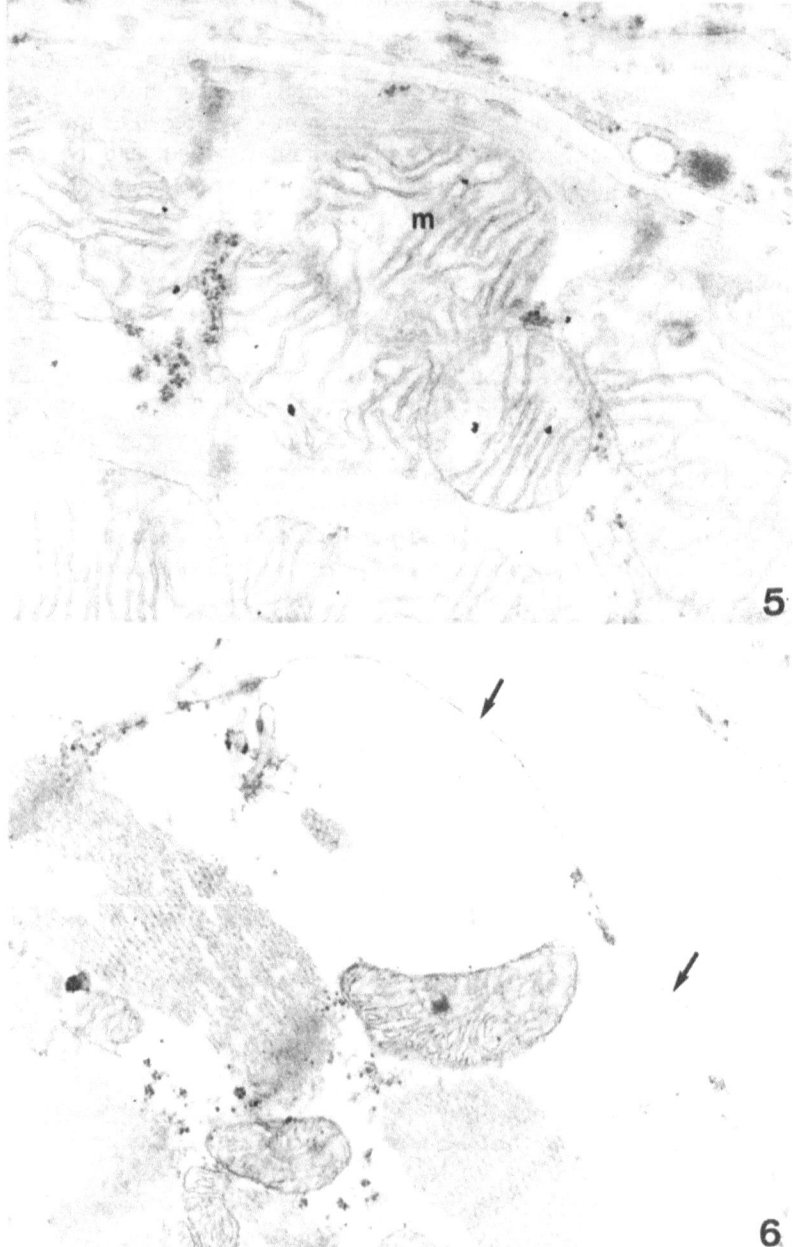

Fig. 5. Dog. Shifts of Ca²⁺ are seen after 60 min of normothermic ischemia, prior to reperfusion. Note absence of SL Ca²⁺ deposits, also the swollen mitochondria (m) are virtually devoid of Ca²⁺ (× 36936).

Fig. 6. Rabbit. Severely edematous cell shows clear interruption of the SL (arrows) after 90 min of ischemia. The fuzzy glycocalyx coat although less dense than normal remains in close apposition to the SL (× 26730).

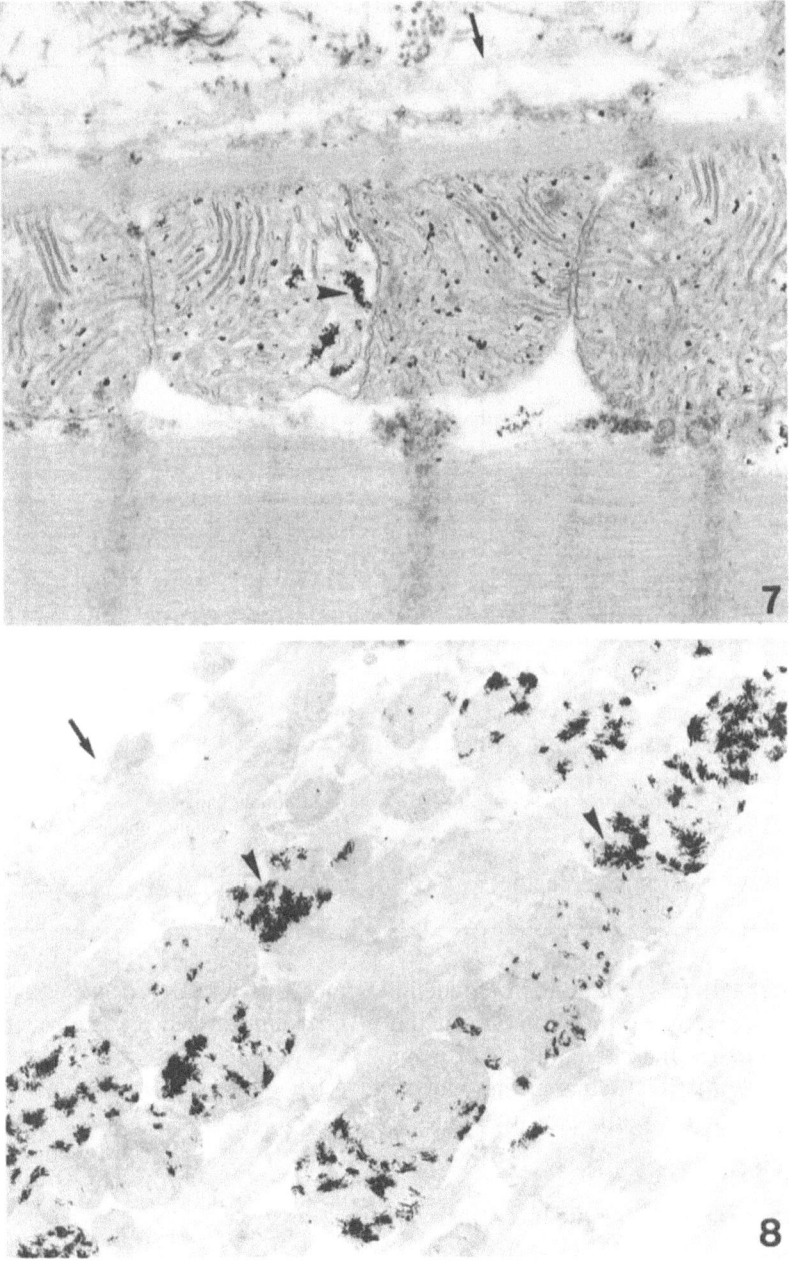

Fig. 7. Dog. Degeneration of the SL with separation of the glycocalyx (arrow) after 5 min of reperfusion following 60 min of normothermic ischemia. Swollen mitochondria have accumulated clusters of Ca^{2+} (arrowhead) ($\times$ 30375).

Fig. 8. Rat. Necrotic cell after 30 min of ischemia and 30 min postischemic reperfusion. The SL is completely degenerated (arrow), the fluid filled cytoplasm contains highly swollen mitochondria with clustered Ca^{2+} deposits (arrowheads) ($\times$ 10080).

Table 1. Time-related ultrastructural changes and Ca^{2+} shifts during ischemic and postschemic reperfusion.

Ischemia	Reperfusion
15–30 min	
• Loss of mitochondrial matrix granules • Decrease in number of SL bound Ca^{2+} deposits	• Recovery of structure and normal to increased Ca^{2+} binding at the SL
• Swelling of mitochondrial matrix • Intracellular fluid accumulation	• Increase in single Ca^{2+} in mitochondria • Reappearance of mitochondrial matrix granules
(Reversible changes)	(Reversible changes)
30–45 min	
• Swelling of mitochondrial matrix with interruptions of cristae • Loss of SL bound Ca^{2+} without intracellular Ca^{2+} accumulation • Loss of definition of SL-glycocalyx structure • Focal degeneration of cells with interruptions of SL • Presence of mitochondria with flocculent densities	• No recovery of SL Ca^{2+} deposits • Accumulation of Ca^{2+}-deposits in mitochondria • Contraction of band necrosis • Nuclear pyknosis • SL disintegration (Irreversible changes)
(Partly reversible changes)	
60–75 min	
• Absence of SL bound Ca^{2+} deposits • Disruption of SL • Occurrence of flocculent densities in all mitochondria • Degeneration of cells with contraction band necrosis and/or cytolysis (Irreversible changes)	• No additional changes (Irreversible changes)

After 60 and 75 minutes of ischemia, there was no longer any essential difference between the structure of the myocardium at the end of ischemia and that after post-ischemic reperfusion.

As for the SL, breaks in the bilayer have been frequently observed after these prolonged periods of ischemia.

Biochemical basis for the loss of sarcolemmal integrity

Although structural changes at the SL during ischemia are not easily detectable with transmission electron microscopy, changes in the permeability of the SL to ions take place prior to reperfusion. It is generally thought that cytosolic Ca^{2+} overload, caused by the failure of SL to maintain ion homeostasis and the lack of intracellular sequestration of Ca^{2+}, both highly energy dependent processes, form the basis of cellular dysfunction and cell death during prolonged exposure to oxygen shortage [14]. An increase in free cytosolic Ca^{2+} will activate Ca^{2+} dependent phospholipases resulting in a breakdown of cell membranes and loss of ionic gradients [23]. Furthermore, it has been suggested that an intracellular accumulation of hydrogen ions, due to anaerobic metabolism, plays an important role in the reversible/irreversible transition [46].

Biochemical analysis shows that after prolonged ischemia the activity of proteinateous components of the ionic homeostasis system such as Na^+/K^+ ATPase and Ca^{2+} ATPase is depressed [47–51], which might cause an increase in intracellular Ca^{2+} concentration. Moreover, the reversal of the Na^+/Ca^{2+} exchanger may contribute to an overload in cytosolic Ca^{2+} [52–53].

Parts of the SL other than the pumps, carriers and channels, may also play a role in the ion regulation. The lipid bilayer, which serves as an impermeable barrier for ions, together with the glycocalyx, exert a powerful role in the ion homeostasis. Consequently, whenever these layers become impaired, a major influx of Ca^{2+} along this route is likely.

The sequence of causal events leading to the ultimate damage is not yet fully understood. Impairment of SL Ca^{2+} binding may be a critical event on the edge of irreversibility, although it could be an epiphenomenon of another critical change. The SL itself may represent an important 'buffer' in sequestering cytosolic Ca^{2+} [26]. Loss of this buffer capacity may influence cellular Ca^{2+} homeostasis directly, but also indirectly since recent evidence suggests that Ca^{2+} ATPase loses function when the SL becomes seriously depleted of Ca^{2+} [54].

Cytochemical evidence for a change in Ca^{2+} binding by acidic phospholipids during ischemia and post-ischemic reperfusion has been presented above. The biochemical counterpart of these changes has been presented by Philipson and Ward [19], Verkley and Post [25] and Post et al. [29]. The hypothesis proposed concerned the destabilization of the lipid bilayer during an ischemic insult and a further exacerbation of the lesion during post-ischemic reperfusion. Again, a central role in these events has been allotted to Ca^{2+}. Bersohn et al. [48] have shown that periods of ischemia lasting between 10 and 60 minutes, which cause inhibition of Na^+/K^+ ATPase and adenylcyclase and failure of Na^+/Ca^{2+} exchange, were not paralleled by changes in total phospholipid and cholesterol content of the SL, although changes in relative amounts of specific phospholipids were not excluded. Degradation of SL phospholipids could only be observed after long periods of ischemia [23, 55], when the point of no return was exceeded. The peculiar asymmetric distribution of acidic phospholipids and the 'non-bilayer' preferring phosphatidylethanolamine in the inner part of bilayer (vide supra), led Post et al. [29] to formulate the hypothesis that the decrease of pH during ischemia causes lateral phase segregation of the phospholipids in the inner monolayer. An increase in intracellular Ca^{2+} during early reperfusion aggravates the phase segregation of phospholipids in the inner monolayer of the SL. This induces a destabilization of the inner monolayer of the SL, causing uncontrolled fusion processes, a destruction of the membrane and an additional Ca^{2+} gain and loss of cellular integrity.

Distributional alterations of phospholipids are necessary to involve rearrangement of the integral SL proteins expressed as clustering of IMP. It has been demonstrated that a redistribution of IMP in biomembranes can be induced by lowering of the temperature [56] or the pH [57] or by increasing the Ca^{2+} concentration [56, 58]. Since intracellular pH may drop to 5.65 during ischemia [59], lowering of pH may be the most important factor responsible for particle aggregation during ischemia. Ca^{2+} may be involved in the continuing aggregation during reperfusion.

Acidosis and Ca^{2+} may induce particle aggregation by reducing the repulsing forces between the proteins by charge neutralization [57]. Alternatively, Ca^{2+} and protons could solidify the negatively charged lipids phosphatidylserine and phosphoinositides in the bilayer [60], which are both present in the inner monolayer of the SL [29, 61]. Crystallization of these lipids will lead to lateral phase separation of solid and fluid lipid domains, whereby the intramembranous particles will be squeezed into the fluid domains [56]. The disruption of the SL and the formation of unilamellar or multilayered myelin-like blebs [25] has been interpreted as the consequence of a destabilized bilayer configuration. The Zwitter-ionic phosphatidylethanolamine will adopt the hexagonal II phase thus inducing uncontrolled fusion events leading to irreversible disruption of the SL [25, 62].

An alternative explanation of the loss of SL integrity during ischemia is provided by the endogenous amphiphile theory. Amphiphiles, such as free fatty acids, fatty acid esters and lysophospholipids which are generated during ischemia are considered as mediators in the genesis of SL injury [18, 63, 64]. These endogenously produced amphiphiles can be inserted into the bilayer either as monomers or aggregates (micelles). Apart from increasing the volume of the membrane and altering the conformation of membrane proteins, the insertion of amphiphiles into the SL may displace Ca^{2+} from negatively charged sites of the phospholipids because of a change in the orientation of the polar head group [18, 63]. The cytochemically demonstrated loss of SL Ca^{2+}-binding may well be the result of such a displacement.

The observations that the insertion of cationic amphiphiles such as polymyxin B compromise cardiac cell survival and displace SL bound Ca^{2+} [22, 65] strongly favor the amphiphile theory. Similar changes are observed after exposure of cardiomyocytes to reactive oxygen species [22, 66]. The damaging effects of peroxidative events on membranes by oxygen free radicals during ischemia [67] and especially during post-ischemic reperfusion [15–18] have been well documented and have been proposed as likely causes of the detrimental changes to the SL.

Insults to the sarcolemma resembling ischemic damage

Among those conditions which lead to irreversible myocardial degeneration and in which the SL is centrally involved, the Ca^{2+} paradox phenomenon is the best documented [68–72].

When Ca^{2+} is removed from the buffer, perfusing isolated hearts, the permeability of the cell membrane to Ca^{2+} is increased. When Ca^{2+} is again added to the extracellular milieu, there is an explosive Ca^{2+} entry into the cell, resulting in cellular Ca^{2+} overload and irreversible hypercontracture. During exposure to the Ca^{2+} free environment the SL becomes totally depleted of cytochemically demonstrable Ca^{2+} [72] with the exception of the gap junctions. The external lamina of the glycocalyx is separated from the rest of the SL leaving large liquid filled blebs in between. In this situation, the cells are in a completely relaxed state, possess high energy levels and show no other morphological signs of degeneration of the SL lipid bilayer. A factor common to the oxygen paradox (ischemia/reperfusion) and the Ca^{2+}-paradox, is that the SL, irrespective of its ultrastructural appearance, loses its ability to bind Ca^{2+}. More importantly, this loss apparently precedes the massive degeneration of other subcellular organelles.

Other stimuli which induce irreversible dysfunction of myocardial cells that show similar shifts in SL bound Ca^{2+} are:

a) oxygen free radicals (*vide supra*) generated during xanthine oxidase/ hypoxanthine-xanthine exposure or during illumination of the photosensitive dye rose bengal [66],

b) high external K^+ (Fig. 9) which causes persistent depolarization [73],

c) veratridine which by prolonging the open state of the Na^+ channel activates the reversed Na^+/Ca^{2+} exchanger [22],

d) ouabain which inhibits the Na^+/K^+ pump [22, 73],

e) prolonged exposure to high concentrations of epinephrine [73],

f) amphiphiles such as palmitoylcarnitine and polymyxin B [22, 65].

Again the common change in the SL which accompanies irreversible cell damage is the inability of the SL to retain its Ca^{2+} binding. In the cardiomyopathic Bio-hamster, Olbrich et al. [34] recently showed that Ca^{2+} overload can be detected cytochemically in early stages of the hamster cardiomyopathy, i.e. in myocardium appearing morphologically normal. This suggests that intracellular Ca^{2+} overload precedes myocardial necrosis in the cardiomyopathic hamster. There appeared to be a striking parallel in morphological changes and Ca^{2+} redistribution between the cardiomyopathic hamster heart and a myocardium subjected to transient ischemia and exhaustive catecholamine stimulation. The authors concluded that the lack of Ca^{2+} precipitate on the SL in myocytes undergoing necrosis supported the hypothesis that the loss of SL Ca^{2+} binding seems to be a crucial event in the development of irreversible cell injury.

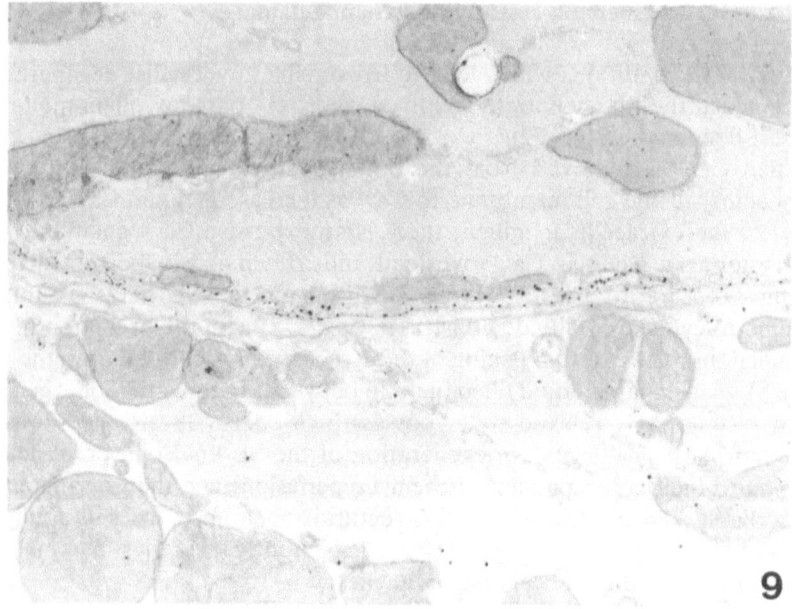

9

Fig. 9. Rat. Persistent depolarization with high K$^+$ for 5 min. Area showing a severely injured cell (lower) with loss of SL Ca^{2+} binding whereas the other (upper) looks structurally intact with normal Ca^{2+} deposits at the SL ($\times$ 20475).

Pharmacological protection against ischemia through intervention at the sarcolemma

There are a number of interventions which either directly or indirectly preserve the surface integrity of ischemic and anoxic myocardium [74]. Interventions such as hypothermia, ß-adrenergic blockade and possibly Ca^{2+}-entry blockers may exert membrane protection indirectly through their energy sparing effect, so that sufficient energy remains available to maintain ionic homeostasis and hence alleviate cellular injury.

Direct interactions with the cell surface components, resulting in the stabilization of the SL during ischemia, have been proposed for glucocorticosteroids, nucleoside transport inhibitors, local anesthetics and some subclasses of Ca^{2+}-antagonists such as the diarylalkylpiperazines [33]. Ultrastructural studies on myocardial ischemia in man, dog and rabbit clearly point to a protective role of diarylalkylpiperazines at the level of the SL [39, 40, 75]. Whereas mitochondrial alterations such as matrix swelling and cristae disruption could not be prevented at the end of the ischemic period, there was retention of SL bound Ca^{2+} in the treated hearts, but none at all in the untreated ones. Thus, during ischemia, the structural preservation of the SL coincided with stabilization of cytochemically demonstrable Ca^{2+} at the

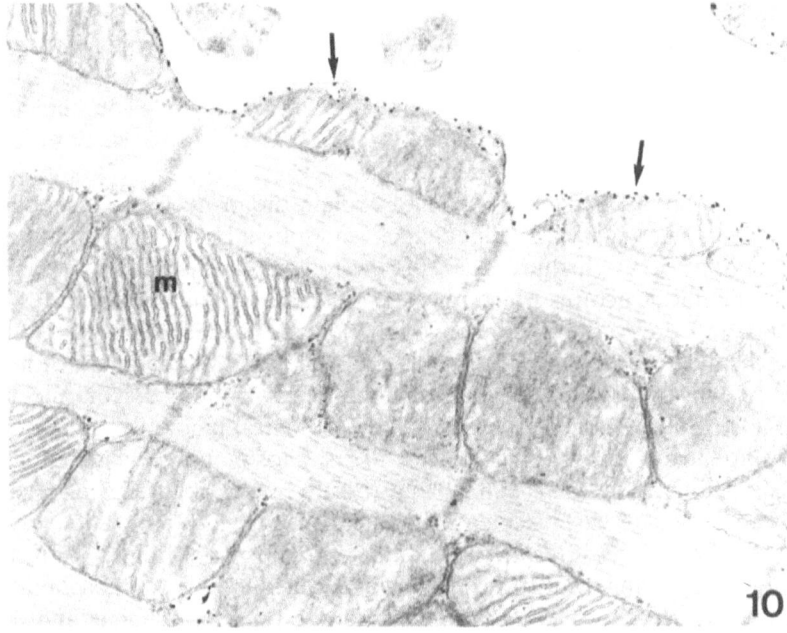

Fig. 10. Rat. Langendorff heart perfused with the diarylalkylpiperazine lidoflazine (1 mg.l⁻¹)
for 30 min followed by ischemia for 60 min, no reperfusion. Note that despite the cytoplasmic
alterations such as mitochondrial swelling (m) the SL looks intact with Ca^{2+} present in
normal amounts (arrows) ($\times$ 27945).

SL-level (Fig. 10). During post-ischemic reperfusion, the SL structure stayed
intact. This was clearly demonstrated by the maintenance of the close apposition of the different surface layers, the absence of intracellular fluid accumulation, and the presence of SL Ca^{2+}. Several studies have confirmed these
initial observations and have also indicated that the diarylalkylpiperazines
flunarizine, cinnarizine, lidoflazine and mioflazine provide significant protection against cell damage imposed by other pathological stimuli which induce
cytosolic Ca^{2+}-overload [22, 44, 75]. In contrast to this, only a weak degree
of protection could be obtained with those Ca^{2+}-antagonists possessing a
high degree of affinity for the slow channels [22]. These observations suggest
that in many of the pathological conditions, including ischemia/reperfusion,
the bulk of Ca^{2+} that crosses the SL is not mediated through the physiological
slow channels. However, the more lipophilic dihydropyridine nicardipine and
verapamil, at high concentrations, do afford protection against myocardial
cell damage. These effects have been attributed to membrane stabilization
[22]. The exact mode by which protective drugs stabilize the SL during
ischemia, thereby counteracting the increased permeability to ions such as
Ca^{2+} and possibly K^+ and Na^+ (enabling volume regulation), is not clearly
understood at present. A possible clue to their mechanism of action might be
the observation that these drugs stabilize the binding of Ca^{2+} to acidic

phospholipids at the inner membrane surface. Janero *et al.* [76] recently showed that various Ca^{2+}-antagonists, although differing in potency, protect cardiac membrane phospholipids against oxidative injury. In another study, nisoldipine or chlorpromazine pretreatment has been shown to counteract the decrease of phosphatidylethanolamine existing at the cytosolic side of the SL during prolonged periods of ischemia [77].

The hypothesis I personally favor to explain the protective effects of the above -mentioned diarylalkylpiperazines and possibly of highly lipophilic compounds of other chemical classes is the following: diarylalkylpiperazines are amphiphilic structures which can be inserted into the inner portion of the lipid bilayer thereby altering the physical properties of the membrane. When such a chemical amphiphile is incorporated in the SL it will compete with and hinder the insertion of endogenous amphiphiles (monomers or micelles) which are produced during ischemia. This topological hindrance of free fatty acids, fatty acid esters, acylcarnitines and lysophospholipids which alter the bilayer configuration (*vide supra*) may result in the following effects: 1) prevention of Ca^{2+} displacement from the bilayer; 2) stabilization of the phospholipid annulus surrounding channel and enzyme proteins; 3) preserving the bilayer configuration of the asymmetrically distributed phospholipids, a situation which becomes severely compromised during ischemia and post-ischemic reperfusion. Striking in this respect is the observation that the same diarylalkylpiperazines which provide protection against ischemic damage also prevent structural and functional impairment of myocardial cells during oxygen free radical attack during which amphiphiles may be acting in some way identical to the ischemic reperfusion insult. Also supporting the hypothesis of drug partition in the lipid bilayer is the fact that these protective drugs are slow to take effect, but remain effective over a long period. On the other hand, direct protection of the proteinateous components of the SL which may suffer from free radical damage during ischemia/reperfusion [78, 79] cannot be excluded.

Conclusions

The various time related involutional events at the SL during ischemia and post-ischemic reperfusion are complex and not yet clearly understood. The relative contribution of the different components of the SL mucopolysaccharide coat, phospholipid bilayer, cholesterol, integral proteins (channels, carriers, enzymes) in subserving the ionic gradients is merely a black hole. There is, however, general agreement concerning the direct relationship between irreversible myocardial damage and the loss of cellular Ca^{2+}-homeostasis. The latter principally involves the SL. Structural and functional degeneration of the myocardium as seen after ischemia can be mimicked by a number of pathological stimuli that compromise SL integrity. They have as a common denominator cytosolic Ca^{2+}-overload which is preceded by the inability of the SL to bind Ca^{2+}.

A number of drugs have been identified which, most probably, exert their beneficial action by stabilizing phospholipid asymmetry and bilayer configuration during the ischemic/reperfusion insult. A mechanism by which protective amphiphilic chemicals compete with endogenously formed amphiphiles is proposed as a possible mode of protection.

A large number of essential questions still remain unanswered and many controversial issues still have to be dealt with. Among these are those relating to:

1) the role of specialized areas of the SL such as the gap junction in propagating or stopping myocardial cell degeneration;
2) the anchoring system between cytoskeletal elements and the SL in relation to IMP redistribution and ultimate SL damage;
3) the relative contribution of oxygen free radical production during ischemia whereby the SL may be weakened prior to reperfusion;
4) the ways of free radical production that damage the SL, other than the one mediated by the xanthine oxidase;
5) the further documentation of the molecular mode by which cardioprotective drugs interact with SL components;
6) the relative contribution of subtypes of slow channels (T and L) and the Na^+/Ca^{2+} exchanger as underlying causes of Ca^{2+} overload;
7) the role of the glycocalyx as buffer for ions, storage compartment or ion exchanger;
8) the further elucidation of the underlying causes for the species differences in vulnerability against ischemia;
9) the role of plasmalogen content of the lipid bilayer in relation to differences in distribution between inner and outer lipid layer and differences between species with different vulnerability to ischemic damage; and
10) the study of repair mechanisms of the SL after the ischemic insult.

References

1. Hearse DJ (1988) Ischemia at the Crossroads? Cardiovasc Drugs and Ther 2: 9–15
2. Jennings RB, Ganote CE (1974) Structural changes in myocardium during acute ischemia. Circ Res 34/35: 156–172
3. Ganote CE, Sebra-Gomes R, Nayler WG, Jennings RB (1975) Irreversible myocardial injury in anoxic perfused rat hearts. Am J Pathol 80: 419–438
4. Schaper J (1979) Ultrastructure of the myocardium in acute ischemia. In: W Schaper (ed) The Pathophysiology of Myocardial Perfusion. Elsevier, Amsterdam
5. Di Bona DR, Powell WJ (1980) Quantitative correlation between cell swelling and necrosis in myocardial ischemia in dogs. Circ Res 47: 653–665
6. Crevey BJ, Langer GA, Frank JS (1978) Role of Ca^{2+} in maintenance of rabbit myocardial cell membrane structural and functional integrity. J Mol Cell Cardiol 10: 1081–1100
7. Hearse DJ, Humphrey SM, Bullock GR (1979) Reoxygenation, reperfusion and the calcium

paradox: Studies of cellular damage and enzyme release. In: DJ Hearse and J de Leiris (eds) Enzymes in Cardiology. Diagnosis and Research. John Wiley

8. Ruigrok TJC, Zimmerman ANE (1979) Effect of calcium on myocardial tissue damage and enzyme release. In: DJ Hearse and J de Leiris (eds) Enzymes in Cardiology. Diagnosis and Research. John Wiley

9. Post JA, Lamers JMJ, Verdouw PD, Ten Cate FJ, Van der Giessen WJ, Verkleij AJ (1987) Sarcolemmal destabilization and destruction after ischaemia and reperfusion and its relation with long-term recovery of regional left ventricular function in pigs. Eur Heart J 8: 423–430

10. Frank JS, Beydler S, Wheeler N, Shine KI (1988) Myocardial sarcolemma in ischemia: a quantitative freeze-fracture study. Am J Physiol 225 (Heart Circ Physiol 24): H467–H475

11. Borgers M, Piper HM (1986) Calcium-shifts in anoxic cardiac myocytes. A cytochemical study. J Mol Cell Cardiol 18: 439–448

12. Borgers M, Liu GS, Xhonneux R, Thoné F, Van Overloop P (1987) Changes in Ultrastructure and Ca^{2+} distribution in the isolated working rabbit heart after ischemia. Am J Pathol 126: 92–102

13. Jennings RB, Reimer KA, Steenbergen C (1986) Myocardial ischemia revisited. The osmolar load, membrane damage, and reperfusion. J Mol Cell Cardiol 18: 769–780

14. Nayler WG, Panagiotopoulos S, Elz JS, Daly MJ (1988) Calcium-mediated damage during post-ischaemic reperfusion. J Mol Cell Cardiol 20 (suppl II): 41–54

15. Guarnieri C, Flamigni F, Calderera CM (1980) Role of oxygen in the cellular damage induced by reoxygenation of hypoxic heart. J Mol Cell Cardiol 12: 797–808

16. Gauduel Y, Duvelleroy MA (1984) Role of oxygen radicals in cardiac injury due to reoxygenation. J Mol Cell Cardiol 16: 459–470

17. McCord JM (1985) Oxygen-derived free radicals in postischemic tissue injury. N Engl J Med 312: 159–164

18. Corr PB, Gross RW, Sobel BE (1984) Amphipathic metabolites and membrane dysfunction in ischemic myocardium. Circ Res 55: 135–154

19. Philipson KD, Ward R (1984) Effects of fatty acids on Na^+–Ca^{2+} exchange and Ca^{2+} permeability of cardiac sarcolemmal vesicles. J Biol Chem 260: 9666–9671

20. Katz AM, Reuter H (1979) Cellular calcium and cardiac cell death. Am J Cardiol 44: 168–170

21. Poole-Wilson PA, Harding DP, Bourdillon PDV, Tones MA (1984) Calcium out of control. J Mol Cell Cardiol 16: 175–188

22. Borgers M, Ver Donck L, Vandeplassche G (1988) Pathophysiology of cardiomyocytes. Ann New York Academy Sciences 5: 433–453

23. Chien KR, Reeves JP, Buja LM, Bonte F, Parkey RW, Willerson JT (1981) Phospholipid alterations in canine ischemic myocardium. Temporal and topographical correlations with Tc-99m-PPi accumulation and an in vitro sarcolemmal Ca^{2+} permeability defect. Circ Res 48: 711–719

24. Langer, GA (1978) The structure and function of myocardial cell surface. Am J Physiol H461–H468

25. Verkleij AJ, Post JA (1986) Physico-chemical properties and organization of lipids in membranes: their possible role in myocardial injury. In: H Stam, GJ van der Vusse (eds) Lipid Metabolism in the normoxic and ischaemic heart. Steinkopff Verlag, Darmstadt

26. Lüllman H, Peters T (1977) Plasmalemmal calcium in cardiac excitation-contraction coupling. Clin Exp Pharmac Physiol 4: 49–57

27. Philipson KD, Langer GA (1979) Sarcolemmal bound calcium and contractility in the mammalian myocardium. J Mol Cell Cardiol 11: 857–875

28. Langer GA (1986) Role of sarcolemmal-bound calcium in regulation of myocardial contractile force. J Am Coll Cardiol 8: 65A–68A

29. Post JA, Langer GA, Op den Kamp JAF, Verkleij AJ (1988) Phospholipid asymmetry in cardiac sarcolemma. Analysis of intact cells and 'gas-dissected' membranes. Biochem Biophys Acta 943: 256–266

30. Post JA (1989) Lipid organization in myocardial sarcolemma and ischemia/reperfusion damage. PhD Thesis, Utrecht

31. Catterall WA (1988) Structure and function of voltage-sensitive ion channels. Science 242: 50–61

32. Borgers M, Thoné F, Verheyen A, Ter Keurs HEDJ (1984) Localization of calcium in skeletal and cardiac muscle. Histochem J 16: 295–309

33. Borgers M (1983) The role of the sarcolemma-glycocalyx complex in myocardial cell function. In: DeBakey and Gotto (eds) Factors influencing the course of myocardial ischemia. Elsevier Science Publishers.

34. Olbrich HG, Borgers M, Thoné F, Frotscher M, Mutschler E, Schneider M, Kober G, Kaltenbach M (1988) Ultrastructural localization of calcium in the myocardium of cardiomyopathic syrian hamsters. J Mol Cell Cardiol 20: 753–762

35. Wheeler-Clark ES, Tormey JMcD (1987) Electron probe X-ray microanalysis of sarcolemma and junctional sarcoplasmic reticulum in rabbit papillary muscles: low sodium-induced calcium alterations. Circ Res 60: 246–250

36. Shen AC, Jennings RB (1972) Myocardial calcium and magnesium in acute ischemic injury. Am J Pathol 67: 417–440

37. Ganote CE (1983) Contraction band necrosis and irreversible myocardial injury. J Mol Cell Cardiol 15: 67–73

38. Jennings RB, Schaper J, Hill ML, Steenbergen C, Reimer KA (1985) Effect or reperfusion late in the phase of reversible ischemic injury. Circ Res 56: 262–278

39. Flameng W, Daenen W, Borgers M, Thoné F, Xhonneux R, Van de Water A, Van Belle H (1981) Cardioprotective effects of lidoflazine during 1 hour normothermic global ischemia. Circulation 64: 796–807

40. Flameng W, Borgers M, Van der Vusse GJ, Demeyere R, Vandermeersch E, Thoné F, Suy R (1983) Cardioprotective effects of lidoflazine in extensive aorta-coronary bypass grafting. J Thorac Cardiovasc Surg 85: 758–768

41. De Leiris J, Feuvray D (1979) Morphological correlates of myocardial enzyme leakage. In: DJ Hearse and J de Leiris (eds) Enzymes in Cardiology. Diagnosis and Research. John Wiley, London

42. Nayler WG, Grinwald P (1981) Calcium entry blockers and myocardial function. Fed Proc 40: 2855–2861

43. Jennings RB, Reimer KA (1979) Biology of experimental, acute myocardial ischaemia and infarction. In: DJ Hearse and J de Leiris (eds) Enzymes in Cardiology. Diagnosis and Research. John Wiley, London

44. Flameng W, Xhonneux R, Van Belle H, Borgers M, Van de Water A, Wouters L, Wijnants J, Thoné F, Van Daele P, Janssen PAJ (1984) Cardioprotective effects of mioflazine during 1 h normothermic global ischemia in the canine heart. Cardiovasc Res 18: 528–537

45. Matthews EK (1986) Calcium and membrane permeability. Brit Med Bull 42: 391–397

46. Neely JR, Grotyohann LW (1984) Role of glycolytic products in damage to ischemic myocardium. Circ Res 55: 816–824

47. Beller GA, Conroy J, Smith TW (1976) Ischemia-induced alterations in myocardial (Na^+ + K^+)-ATPase and cardiac glycoside binding. J Clin Invest 57: 341–350

48. Bersohn MM, Philipson KD, Fukushima JY (1982) Sodium-calcium exchange and sarcolemmal enzymes in ischemic rabbit hearts. Am J Physiol 242 (Cell Physiol. 11): C288–C295

49. Krause S, Hess ML (1984) Characterization of cardiac sarcoplasmic reticulum dysfunction during short-time, normothermic, global ischemia. Circ Res 55: 176–184

50. Sordahl LA, Stewart ML (1980) Mechanism of altered mitochondrial calcium transport in acutely ischemic canine hearts. Circ Res 47: 814–820

51. Vasdev SC, Biro GP, Narbaitz R, Kako KJ (1980) Membrane changes induced by early myocardial ischemia in the dog. Can J Biochem 58: 1112–1119

52. Poole-Wilson PA, Tones MA (1988) Sodium exchange during hypoxia and reoxygenation in the isolated rabbit heart. J Mol Cell Cardiol 20 (suppl II): 15–22

53. Grinwald PM, Brosnahan C (1987) : Sodium imbalance as a cause of calcium overload in posthypoxia reoxygenation injury. J Mol Cell Cardiol 19: 487–495

54. Preuner F (1985) Functional alterations of the sarcolemma in Ca^{2+}-free perfused hearts. Basic Res Cardiol 80 (suppl 2): 19–23

55. Steenbergen C, Jennings RB (1984) Relationship between lysophospholipid accumulation and plasma membrane injury during total in vitro ischemia in dog heart. J Mol Cell Cardiol 16: 605–621

56. Verkleij AJ, Ververgaert PHJT (1978) Freeze fracture morphology of biological membranes. Biochim Biophys Acta 515: 303–327

57. Elgsaeter A, Shutton D, Branton D (1976) Intramembrane particle aggregation in erythrocyte ghosts. II. The influence of spectrin aggregation. Biochim Biophys Acta 426: 101–122

58. Gerritsen WJ, Verkleij AJ, Van Deenen LLM (1979) The lateral distribution of intramembrane particles in the erythrocyte membrane and recombinant vesicles. Biochim Biophys Acta 555: 26–41

59. Bailey IA, Radda GK, Seymour AL, Williams SR (1982) The effects of insulin on myocardial metabolism and acidosis in normoxia and ischaemia. A ^{31}P-NMR study. Biochim Biophys Acta 720: 17–27

60. Papahadjopoulos D, Vail WJ, Newton C, Nir S, Jacobsen K, Poste G, Lazo R (1977) Studies on membrane fusion. III. The role of calcium-induced phase changes. Biochim Biophys Acta 465: 579–598

61. Philipson KD, Bers DM, Nishimoto AY (1980) The role of phospholipids in the Ca^{2+} binding of isolated sarcolemma. J Mol Cell Cardiol 12: 1159–1173

62. Verkleij AJ (1984) Lipidic intramembraneous particles. Biochim Biophys Acta 779: 43–63

63. Katz AR, Messineo FC (1981) Lipid-membrane interactions and the pathogenesis of ischemic damage in the myocardium. Circ Res 48: 1–16

64. Fink KL, Gross RW (1984) Modulation of canine myocardial sarcolemmal membrane fluidity by amphiphilic compounds. Circ Res 55: 585–594

65. Burt JM, Langer GA (1983) Ca^{2+} displacement by polymyxin B from sarcolemma isolated by 'gas dissection' from cultured neonatal rat myocardial cells. Biochem Biophys Acta 729: 44–52

66. Ver Donck L, Van Reempts J, Vandeplassche G, Borgers M (1988) A new method to study activated oxygen species induced damage in cardiomyocytes and protection by Ca^{2+}-antagonists. J Mol Cell Cardiol 20: 811–823

67. Rao PS, Cohen M, Mueller HS (1983) Production of free radicals and lipid peroxides in early experimental myocardial ischaemia. J Mol Cell Cardiol 15: 713–716

68. Zimmerman ANE, Daems W, Hulsman WC, Snyder J, Wisse E, Durrer D (1967) Morphological changes of heart muscle caused by successive perfusion with calcium-free and calcium-containing solutions (calcium paradox). Cardiovasc Res 1: 201–209

69. Hearse DJ, Humphrey SM, Boink ABTJ, Ruigrok TJ (1978) The calcium paradox: metabolic electrophysiological, contractile and ultrastructural characteristics in four species. Eur J Cardiol 7: 241–249

70. Grinwald PM, Nayler WG (1981) Review: Calcium entry in the calcium paradox. J Mol Cell Cardiol 13: 867–880

71. Ganote CE, Sims MA (1984) Parallel temperature dependence of contracture-associated enzyme release due to anoxia, 2,4-dinitrophenol (DNP) or caffeine and the calcium paradox. Am J Pathol 116: 94–106

72. Borgers M, Van Belle H (1985) Intracellular Ca^{2+} shifts during the Ca^{2+} paradox. Bas Res Cardiol 80 (suppl 2): 25–30

73. Borgers M, Thoné F, Ver Donck L (1985) Sarcolemma-bound calcium. Its importance for cell viability. Bas Res Cardiol 80 (suppl 1): 31–36

74. Kloner RA, Braunwald E (1980) Observations on experimental myocardial ischaemia. Cardiovasc Res 14: 371–395

75. Liu GS, Borgers M, Xhonneux R, Van Overloop P, Thoné F, Wouters L, Leijssen L (1986)

Evaluation of protective effects of lidoflazine and mioflazine in cardiac ischemia. Drug Dev Res 8: 407–416

76. Janero DR, Burghardt B, Lopez R (1988) Protection of cardiac membrane phospholipid against oxidative injury by calcium antagonists. Biochem Pharmacol 37: 4197–4203

77. Takahashi, K, Kako, K.J. (1986) The effects of myocardial ischemia and nisoldipine pretreatment on the asymmetric distribution of phosphatidylethanolamine in a canine heart sarcolemmal preparation. Biochem Med Metabol Biol 35: 308–321

78. Kako KJ (1987) Free radical effects on membrane protein in myocardial ischemia/ reperfusion injury. J Mol Cell Cardiol 19: 209–211

79. Dean RT (1987) Free radicals, membrane damage and cell-mediated cytolysis. Br J Cancer 55 (suppl VIII): 39–45

Mitochondrial injury in the oxygen-depleted and reoxygenated myocardial cell

HANS MICHAEL PIPER

Physiologisches Institut I, Universität Düsseldorf, Moorenstr. 5, D-4000 Düsseldorf 1, FRG

Introduction

The myocardium cannot maintain its normal energetic state without oxidative energy production by the mitochondria. Therefore, during insufficient oxygen supply, the myocardial cell becomes progressively depleted of its energy reserves and ultimately deteriorates. Recovery of the myocardium from a period of oxygen depletion requires sufficient preservation of mitochondrial function. Apart from their central role in energy metabolism, mitochondria also perform a vital function in cellular Ca^{2+} homeostasis, since the mitochondria represent the largest intracellular compartment for the sequestration of excess Ca^{2+} from the cytosol. Control of cytosolic Ca^{2+} concentration becomes disturbed in energy deficiency and can be re-normalized when mitochondrial energy production is restored. For these reasons, damage of the mitochondria may be of crucial importance for recovery from states of cellular oxygen deprivation (anoxia, ischemia).

Since mitochondrial functions cannot be investigated in detail in experiments with intact cells or tissue, many of the current concepts about mitochondrial injury are derived from studies on mitochondria isolated from injured hearts. In most of these studies, mitochondrial functions were found to be progressively impaired in the course of ischemic or anoxic tissue injury. But some caution is required when the function of mitochondria in the isolated state is extrapolated to their function in tissue. It must be asked whether the isolation procedure adds or detracts anything from the functional defects the mitochondria had in the intact cell. Even if this can be, it is important to know to what extent mitochondrial malfunction could jeopardize the survival of the cell. The two major problems in relying on studies on isolated mitochondria are, first, that they might not demonstrate the real extent of injury, and, second, that they might be irrelevant because the full capacity of mitochondrial function is not required for the survival of the intact cell. To a certain extent, data from *in vitro* studies can be scrutinized by the study of cell functions that depend on a sufficient metabolic function of the mitochondria.

H.M. Piper (ed.) Pathophysiology of severe ischemic myocardial injury, 91–113.
© *1990 Kluwer Academic Publishers, Dordrecht* –

The central question of this review is whether mitochondria could be the limiting cell structure for the reversibility of ischemic or anoxic cell injury.

Role of mitochondria in anaerobic metabolism

O_2-sensitivity of myocardial energy metabolism

In mitochondria, the energy stored in oxidizable substrates can be transformed into energy stored in ATP. When substrates and oxygen are present in sufficient concentrations, these substrates become oxidized by transferring electrons to O_2 (for an extensive review see [1]). Thus, by the catalysis of the cytochrome c oxidase, oxygen is reduced to water. The transfer of electrons is mediated by the elements of the respiratory chain in the inner mitochondrial membrane. It results in outward transport of protons from the matrix space, thus creating an electrochemical gradient across the inner membrane. The energy contained in this gradient is used to synthesize ATP from ADP and inorganic phosphate; but it can also be used for other reactions requiring energy such as sequestration of Ca^{2+} into the matrix space. Synthesis of ATP takes place at the F_1 subunit of the multisubunit enzyme H^+-ATPase. ATP is extruded to the cytosol in a 1:1 exchange for ADP via the adenine nucleotide translocator.

It has been demonstrated that, in the individual heart muscle cell, mitochondrial respiration does not stop and glycolytic flux does not increase unless exogenous pO_2 has dropped below 1 torr [2]. This means that the oxygen consumption of the cell as a whole is almost as sensitive to low oxygen tension as the oxygen uptake of the isolated mitochondrion. The presence of myoglobin as an oxygen binding capacity in the cytosol prevents the formation of a distinct cytosolic gradient for oxygen [2]. In comparison to normal arterial oxygen tension, failure of oxidative metabolism in the individual myocardial cell occurs at extremely low oxygen tension and comes close to the K_m of the cytochrome c oxidase (0.2 torr; [3, 4]). Unlike single isolated cardiomyocytes. the perfused heart responds metabolically in a gradual fashion to lowering of the oxygen tension. This can be explained as a statistical phenomenon: the lower the total amount of oxygen supplied to the heart per unit of time, the fewer cells along the perfusion path can satisfy their oxygen demand.

When the myocardial cell becomes deprived of oxygen, by cessation of perfusion (ischemia) or lack of oxygen in the perfusate (anoxia), electron flux ceases and the mitochondrial transmembrane gradient dissipates. Dissipation of the mitochondrial membrane potential in the ischemic myocardium has been demonstrated in the ischemic heart using a potential-sensitive fluorescent dye (DASPMI) partitioning over the mitochondrial inner membrane [5].

Anaerobic energy production

If mitochondrial respiration ceases, the myocardial cell has lost its most efficient way of producing energy, i.e. by oxidation of substrate. All FAD-dependent substrates, such as fatty acids, cannot be utilized further. Glucose, however, can still be converted into lactate, but instead of 38 only 2 mol ATP per mol exogenous glucose (or 3 mol ATP per mol glucose-6-phosphate if derived from glycogen) are obtained. A lowering of the phosphorylation potential, i.e. of the ratio (ATP/ADP × P_i), is the signal for increasing glycolytic flux. The supply of glucose-6-phosphate is improved since glucose uptake is accelerated and netglycogenolysis begins. The rate limiting enzyme of the Embden-Meyerhof pathway under normoxic conditions, phosphofructokinase, is activated and the rate control for glycolytic flux is shifted downstream to the point of glyceraldehyde-3-phosphate dehydrogenase (GAPDH) [6, 7]. Since cytosolic reduction equivalents can no longer be reoxidized by transferring them to the respiratory chain, the cytosolic NADH/NAD ratio increases. The near-equilibrium reaction catalysed by the lactate dehydrogenase is forced into the direction of lactate production. Production of lactate is the most important escape mechanism for an early cessation of glycolysis since NADH can thus be reoxidized. Thereby NAD, needed as co-substrate for the GAPDH reaction, is regenerated.

Lactate, however, is not the only end-product of anaerobic energy metabolism. To a lesser degree, mitochondria can also contribute to anaerobic energy production in that they synthesize succinate as an anaerobic end-product. Under ischemic conditions, succinate is synthesized from glutamate and this may account for 20% of the ATP produced by substrate level phosphorylation [8].

ATPase activity of de-energized mitochondria

When the oxygen tension falls below 0.5 torr and electron transfer ceases, the electrochemical gradient across the inner mitochondrial membrane dissipates and the mitochondrial ATP synthetase is turned into an ATP hydrolase by a conformational change [9, 10]. Under some conditions, the energy released by the hydrolysis of ATP can be utilized to generate some electrochemical gradient, but whether this applies to mitochondria in ischemic and anoxic tissue is not known. The contribution of the mitochondrial ATPase to the loss of energy in the oxygen depleted myocardial cell is well documented. It was demonstrated by the use of the specific inhibitor oligomycin [11, 12] that this mechanism may account for 80% of ATP breakdown during 20 minutes of ischemia. Thus, one major effect by which mitochondria contribute to the aggravation of hypoxic cellular injury consists of the inversion of a normal physiological function.

Interestingly, the activity of the mitochondrial ATPase is reduced when the cytosolic pH drops [13]. Thus, acidosis of ischemic tissue, which has the negative effect of decreasing anaerobic glycolytic energy production, also opposes a too rapid energy loss; and this, to a certain extent, can compensate for the aforementioned effect. It has been suggested [13] that the effect of pH on the ATPase in de-energized mitochondria is due to improved binding conditions for its natural inhibitor protein [9].

Ultrastructural alterations

Disappearance of native matrix granules

The most prominent early ultrastructural indication of energy depletion in cardiomyocytes is the gradual disappearance of the small native matrix granules [14, 15]. These consist of phospholipids with proteins, among them cytochrome c oxidase [16]. They disappear not only in hypoxia, but also during stages of increased energy demand. It has been hypothesized [16] that the granules contain components of the inner mitochondrial membrane which become incorporated into the inner membrane when disappearing. Physiologically, the granules may serve as a structural reserve for energy production. The common feature of high energy demand with hypoxia is a decreased ATP/ADP ratio in the cytosol. It can be speculated that this ratio determines the mobilization of the granules.

Swelling and membrane fractionation

When conventional fixation techniques (glutaraldehyde and osmium tetroxide) for electron microscopy are applied, mitochondria of well-energized tissue contain a regular pattern of parallel cristae structures, which are folds of the inner mitochondrial membrane. In energy depleted heart cells [15, 17] mitochondria appear less dense due to the opening of translucent spaces between the cristae; the mitochondria appear swollen. Mitochondria start swelling when a third of the normoxic ATP content is lost [15]. Interestingly, the onset of mitochondrial swelling is not synchronous throughout the cell, suggesting the existence of two intermixed mitochondrial populations which differ in sensitivity to hypoxic metabolic changes [15]. The pathophysiological significance of mitochondrial swelling is not clear. Swelling of the mitochondria is not one of the first signs of structural injury of the myocardial cell. In isolated cardiomyocytes protrusion of small 'microblebs' from the cell's surface starts earlier [15] indicating a weakening of the cytoskeletal anchoring of the sarcolemma.

In the further course of cellular injury, mitochondrial membrane structures become more and more irregular. Mitochondria swell enormously and the cristae often appear fractured and distorted [17]. In tissue prepared for electron microscopy by a technique which reduces protein denaturation [18] structural alteration of membrane structures takes on a different appearance; the cristae become dissolved to diffuse material rather than fracturing into small membrane sheets. The difference in the results obtained by different techniques of specimen preparation raises some doubt about the reality of the ultrastructural alterations found by current electron microscopic techniques. The results of different approaches are consistent in that they demonstrate an extensive change in the physical condition of mitochondria in ischemia and hypoxia. But the structural alterations observed may be partly artifactitious.

Crystalline deposits

When myocardium is reoxygenated after an extended period of oxygen depletion, ultrastructural injury worsens. In mitochondria, crystalline deposits rapidly appear and these have been identified as deposits of calcium and phosphate [19, 20]. They are suspected to be the consequence of the cell flooding with calcium after disruption of the sarcolemma, i.e. to indicate a state of already irreversible cell injury. In isolated cardiomyocytes, hypercontracted after anoxia-reoxygenation, these deposits are atypical [15]. But in contrast to myocardial cells in tissue, isolated cells maintain an intact sarcolemma and can re-establish a normal Ca^{2+} homeostasis even when hypercontracted [21, 22].

Malfunction of mitochondria isolated from injured myocardium

Changes in chemical composition

The lipid composition of mitochondria isolated from ischemic tissue before the onset of irreversible injury was found to be altered. In the phospholipid fraction, the fatty acid composition of lysophosphatidyl choline, lysophosphatidyl ethanolamine and sphingomyeline was different [23], possibly indicating the activation of phospholipases. The cholesterol content of the mitochondria which normally has low levels, increased. This may be due to a redistribution of cholesterol within the cell, since the cholesterol content of the sarcolemma decreased in ischemic hearts [24]. An altered composition of the mitochondrial inner membranes may contribute to their increased permeability, as for Ca^{2+} (see below).

In mitochondria isolated from ischemic tissue, components of the respiratory chain (Fig. 1) are progressively lost or denatured. Among cytochromes [25], the loss is most pronounced in cytochrome c, known to be only loosely bound at the outer surface of the inner mitochondrial membrane (Fig. 2). But integral components of the membrane structure, such as cytochromes aa_3, are

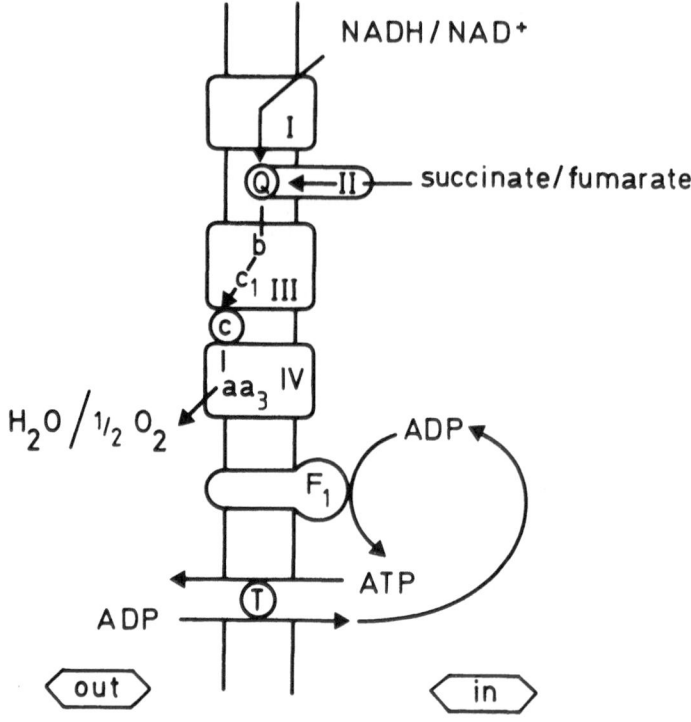

Fig. 1. Schematic representation of the respiratory chain. Abbreviations: in/out, inside/outside the inner mitochondrial membrane; I–IV, complexes I–IV; b, c_1, c, aa_3, cytochromes; Q, coenzyme Q; F_1, F_1–ATPase; T, adenine nucleotide translocase.

also extensively lost. In low-flow ischemic hearts perfused with fatty acids, a characteristic loss of cytochrome b was observed [26].

The loss of structural elements from mitochondrial membranes may be the cause of limited recovery of mitochondrial function after restoration of normoxic conditions. In mitochondria from ischemic hearts, the number of adenine nucleotide translocator units decreases, either by loss or denaturation. Indeed, with respect to the adenine nucleotide translocator, a close correspondence between the recovery of activity and the remaining amount of non-denatured protein was found [25]. This, however, was only in the case of recovery from mild ischemia. After prolonged ischemia, the specific activity of the translocator units could no longer be recovered within 30 minutes reperfusion.

Adenine nucleotide contents

Parallel to the loss of adenine nucleotides from the whole cells, adenine nucleotide contents of mitochondria isolated from ischemic tissue also de-

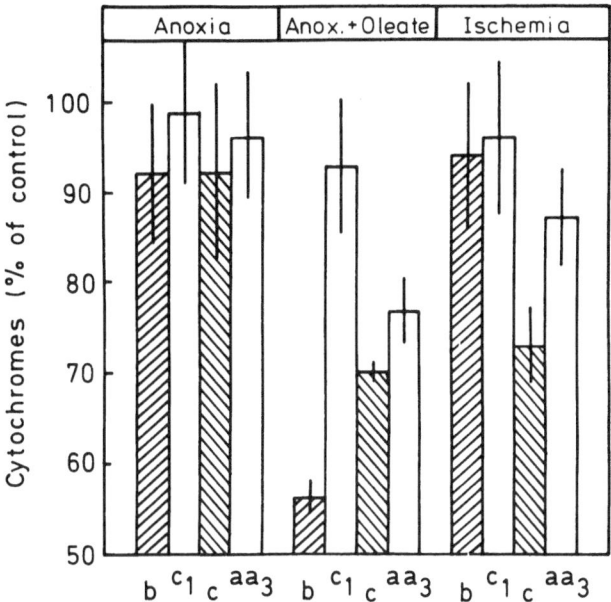

Fig. 2. Mitochondria from isolated guinea pig hearts after 60 min low-flow anoxia ± 0.4 mM oleate and 45 min complete ischemia: Loss of cytochromes b, c_1, c, aa_3, expressed as percentages of aerobic control values. The methods are described in ref. [26]. ($\bar{x}$ ± S.D., n = 5.)

crease [25, 27] (Fig. 3). Experiments by Asimakis *et al.* show [28, 29] that adenine nucleotides, but not adenosine, are lost from mitochondria under respiratory inhibition. The release can be blocked by inhibition of the adenine nucleotide translocator, and stimulated by an increase in the extramitochondrial phosphate concentration [29]. These results suggest that mitochondria become depleted of adenine nucleotides because inorganic phosphate accumulates when high-energy phophates become broken down in the cytosol.

Respiratory chain functions

NADH reductase (complex I of the respiratory chain) is impaired early in hypoxic myocardium [25, 30–32] (Fig. 4). Since it is particularly sensitive to acidosis [31], the oxidation of NAD-dependent substrates is reduced most noticeably in mitochondria from ischemic tissue. This early impairment, however, is still a reversible phenomenon. At this early stage, uncoupled respiration is still unchanged, indicating a defect in the coupling of complex I to ADP phosphorylation [25]. Subsequently, the functions of the coenzyme Q-reductase (complex III) and of succinate dehydrogenase (complex II) also become affected so that both the oxidation of NAD- and FAD-dependent substrates are reduced. The activity of the mitochondrial ATP synthetase

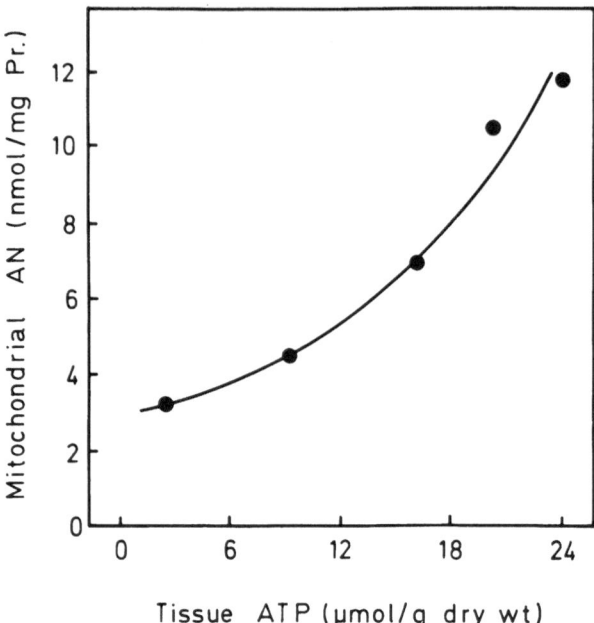

Fig. 3. Mitochondria from isolated guinea pig hearts in complete ischemia: Relation between myocardial ATP content and mitochondrial contents of adenine nucleotides. The methods are described in ref. [25]. ($\bar{x}$, n = 5.)

(complex V) has been shown to be reduced considerably by acidosis [13]. Other parts of the respiratory apparatus are only slightly affected. Thus, the activity of cytochrome c oxidase (complex IV) remains almost unchanged during the reversible phase of complete and low-flow ischemia [25, 32].

In most studies, the capability of mitochondria for oxidative phosphorylation in vitro was analyzed in the absence of extramitochondrial Na^+, Ca^{2+}, and Mg^{2+}. Myocardial cells injured by oxygen depletion and reoxygenation take up Na^+ and Ca^{2+}. In isolated myocardial cells, a pronounced cation uptake is already observed during anoxic incubation [33]. The ischemic myocardial cell is protected from a large uptake of cations due to the limitation of the interstitial space. Here, large cation movements are observed with reperfusion [34]. To what extent free Mg^{2+} concentrations change in hypoxic or ischemic and reoxygenated myocardial cells is not yet clear [35].

At high cytosolic Ca^{2+} concentrations, mitochondria use respiratory energy for uptake of Ca^{2+} which can be inhibited by Mg^{2+} [36]. Na^+ stimulates Ca^{2+} efflux from heart mitochondria which in turn enhances the cycling of Ca^{2+} across the inner mitochondrial membrane [37, 38]. Futile Ca^{2+} cycling may contribute to slow recovery or complete failure of the reoxygenated cell because it dissipates respiratory energy. Since the exact compostion of the

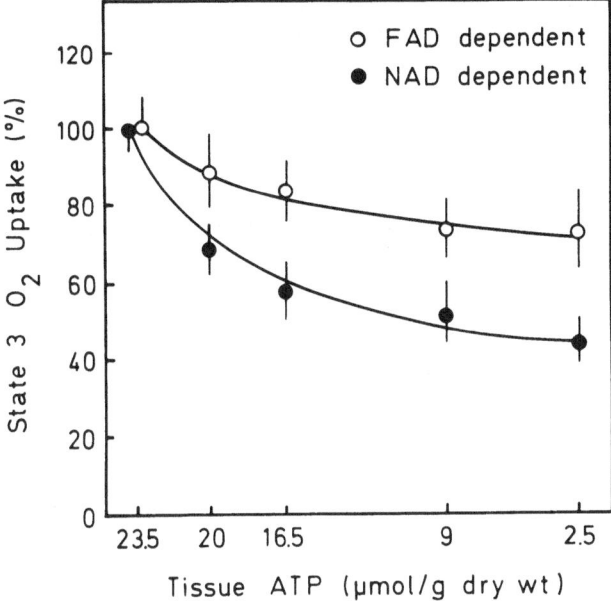

Fig. 4. Mitochondria from isolated guinea pig hearts in complete ischemia: State 3 respiration with glutamate (NAD-dependent) and succinate plus rotenone (FAD-dependent) in relation to the myocardial ATP content. Values are expressed as percentages of aerobic control values. The methods are described in ref [25]. ($\bar{x} \pm$ S.D., n = 5).

extramitrochondrial milieu is not known, estimates of the energy costs of mitochondrial Ca^{2+} movements in the reoxygeneated heart cell remain speculative.

Adenine nucleotide translator

The impairment of the adenine nucleotide translocator in mitochondria from ischemic myocardium has received much attention [39]. It has been hypothe-sized that increased levels of long-chain acyl coenzyme A (CoA) esters in the ischemic tissue are responsible for the reduction of this carrier's activity [40–42]. This hypothesis is based on the finding that, when ß-oxidation stops, long-chain acyl CoA accumulate in the mitochondrial matrix [43]. It has been demonstrated with inner mitochondrial membranes turned inside-out (submitochondrial particles), that long-chain acyl CoA do indeed inhibit the translocase from within the matrix space [44]. It is, however, unclear whether free concentrations of these compounds ever reach the inhibitory levels in mitochondria of ischemic cells. This is because the intracellular distribution of these amphiphilic compounds cannot be exactly determined. In the cell, long-chain acyl compounds bind not only to mitochondrial membranes, but also to other cell structures and soluble proteins, as e.g. the fatty acid binding protein [45], and there is no established way to preserve this distribution in cell fractionation.

It has also been demonstrated that the activity of the adenine translocator is related to mitochondrial contents of adenine nucleotides, in mitochondria depleted of adenine nucleotides *in vitro* as well as by the impact of ischemia *in vivo* [25, 28, 46]. Since free matrix concentrations of adenine nucleotides and acyl CoA are not known, the causal mechanism remains uncertain. Increased long-chain acyl CoA levels and reduced adenine nucleotide contents may both contribute to the observed reduction in adenine nucleotide translocase activity. This is because, in the matrix space, the concentration of substrate for the transporter is reduced and that of the inhibitor is increased.

Ca^{2+} sequestration

During the early phase of ischemia, mitochondria become progressively permeable to sequestered Ca^{2+} [25]. The basic Ca^{2+} permeability of mitochondria is increased by a mechanism different from the physiological Na^+ dependent release mechanism. Supply of ischemic hearts with fatty acids further enhances mitochondrial Ca^{2+} leakage [26]. These results suggest that the ability of mitochondria in the reoxygenated cell to remove Ca^{2+} from the cytosol is impaired by their increased permeability. This defect will also influence their capability for oxidative phosphorylation, since Ca^{2+} release and re-uptake constitute a vicious cycle, wasting respiratory energy.

A number of conditions are known to induce efflux of Ca^{2+} from energized mitochondria *in vitro* by other ways than through the Na^+ dependent efflux mechanism; namely, depletion of mitochondrial adenine nucleotides [47–49]; fixation of the adenine nucleotide translocase in the c-state conformation, (with the nucleotide binding side in outward orientation [50, 51]; high extramitochondrial concentrations of Ca^{2+} plus inorganic phosphate [51], pyrophosphate [52], long-chain acyl-coA [53], lysophospholipids [48, 54], pro-oxidants [51, 55], and oxidation and hydrolysis of the mitochondrial pyridine nucleotides [55, 56]. There are also ways of neutralizing these effects; for example incubation of mitochondria with high concentrations of ATP and ADP [49]; fixation of the adenine nucleotide translocase in the m-state conformation (with the nucleotide binding side in inward orientation [50]); oligomycin [51]; inhibition of mitochondrial phospholipase A_2 [48] and free-radical scavengers [51, 55]. At present the mechanisms involved in these states of increased Ca^{2+} permeability are under investigation. As key factors the activation of phospholipase A_2, fixation of the adenine nucleotide conformation in the c-state. and oxygen radical effects have been hypothesized [50, 51, 55].

Mitochondria from ischemic myocardium exhibit a striking correlation

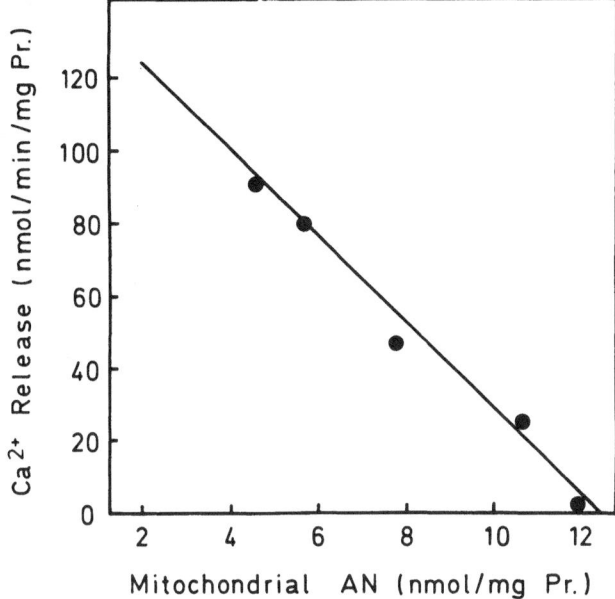

Fig. 5. Mitochondria from isolated guinea pig hearts in complete ischemia: Relation between passive Ca^{2+} release and mitochondrial content of adenine nucleotides. Mitochondrial release of Ca^{2+} was determined after prior accumulation of 100 nmol Ca^{2+}/mg protein and blockage of further uptake by ruthenium red. The methods are desribed in ref. [25]. ($\bar{x}$, n = 5.)

between adenine nucleotide contents and passive Ca^{2+} efflux (Fig. 5). Furthermore, the contents of long-chain acyl CoA and lysolipids are also increased in preparations of mitochondria with greater Ca^{2+} efflux [23, 26, 43]. These and other factors inducing Ca^{2+} leakage *in vitro*, may be responsible for the weakness of mitochondria isolated from injured cells, but this has not yet been established conclusively.

The finding of increased leakage of Ca^{2+} in mitochondria from ischemic myocardium is in apparent contrast [57] to the fact that mitochondria can accumulate large amounts of Ca^{2+} in the reoxygenated cell [21, 58]. But most of this accumulated Ca^{2+} is deposited as a complex of Ca^{2+} with phosphate, so that an increase in total mitochondrial Ca^{2+} is not indicative of high intramitochondrial concentrations of ionized Ca^{2+} [38]. *In vitro*, mitochondria can accumulate considerable amounts of Ca^{2+} in the form of insoluble precipitates with phosphate and yet still retain their metabolic functions [38]. It is not yet completely understood why, in mitochondria isolated from injured myocardium, the capacity for respiratory energy production is the more reduced the higher their total calcium load [59, 60].

The cause of the mitochondrial deposition of Ca^{2+} in reperfused myocardium is not known in any detail. It is possible that the increased concentrations of cytosolic inorganic phosphate represent the major driving force. The putative morphological correlates of accumulated Ca^{2+}, i.e. electron-dense crystalline intramitochondrial deposits, have been regarded as signs of irreversible cell injury [21, 22]. But the occurrence of calcium precipitates is not a sign of irreversible injury of the mitochondria. Instead, it demonstrates their preserved metabolic competence because the accumulation of Ca^{2+} by mitochondria requires respiratory energy and the precipitation of Ca^{2+} and phosphate depends on the net uptake of adenine nucleotides by mitochondria [38]. Therefore, the condition of mitochondria which start to develop crystalline deposits in reperfused myocardium is unlikely to be the cause of irreversibility. This view is supported by the finding that inhibition of mitochondrial Ca^{2+} accumulation by ruthenium red upon reoxygenation can retain control rates of mitochondrial ATP re-synthesis [61]. Further, the respiratory inhibition of mitochondria from ischemic-reperfused myocardium can be partly reversed by incubation with Ca^{2+} chelators [59].

The calcium content of mitochondria isolated from ischemic tissue varies only slightly, whereas mitochondria from tissue reperfused after prolonged ischemia have a 2- to 3-fold increase in calcium content [57, 59, 60]. This relative difference was found in mitochondria isolated with and without a Ca^{2+} chelator, even though in the absence of the latter, mitochondrial Ca^{2+} contents were generally higher [57, 59]. It is doubtful whether any of the techniques applied to isolate mitochondria can preserve the true Ca^{2+} content that the mitochondria contain within the cell [38, 62]. Nevertheless, the increased Ca^{2+} contents of mitochondria isolated from reperfused myocardium correspond to the frequency of crystalline mitochondrial deposits in electron microscopic pictures of reperfused myocardium.

The effect of long-chain fatty acids

When fatty acids are present in low-flow ischemia, myocardial damage is more pronounced than when they are not present [25, 26]. This is not due to any single cause, since the presence of fatty acids already reduces the rate of glycolytic energy production during anoxia [63] and enhances mitochondrial injury which becomes relevant reoxygenation [25]. The presence of fatty acids not only aggravates but also alters the type of ischemic mitochondrial damage, in that sites in the respiratory chain become affected which would otherwise remain stable [26]. Cytochrome b which is embedded in the lipophilic phase of complex III is normally stable in mitochondria from anoxic and ischemic myocardium. But when ischemic hearts are supplied with fatty acids it is extensively reduced, exceeding even the loss of cytochrome c (Fig. 2). Under ischemic conditions without exogenous fatty acids the cytochrome c oxidase activity of complex IV is the most stable part of the respiratory chain. But as a result of the action of the fatty acids, cytochrome c oxidase activity becomes reduced. It has been shown [64] that fatty acids do not directly impair the function of the cytochrome c oxidase, but interfere with the interaction of this complex with the surrounding membrane lipids. Under the influence of fatty acids in ischemic tissue, the capability of mitochondria to actively take up Ca^{2+} is also reduced. In addition, the passive leakage of Ca^{2+} from mitochondria is greatly enhanced [26]. One may speculate that a greater expenditure of energy for enhanced futile Ca^{2+} cycling contributes to the poor recovery of myocardium from ischemia with fatty acid supply.

In ischemic hearts perfused with fatty acids, the mitochondrial content of long-chain acyl CoA is clearly increased and the content of long-chain acyl carnitine remains low [26, 30, 31]. This suggests that the additional damage to mitochondria, caused by the presence of fatty acids in ischemia, is due to the physicochemical interaction of long-chain acyl CoA with the inner mito-chondrial membrane. Physiological long-chain fatty acyl species differ in their effect on mitochondria. The unsaturated oleic acid was found to be more harmful than palmitic acid for mitochondrial function [26], corresponding to a greater affinity of this fatty acid moiety to mitochondrial membranes [65]. The described effects of fatty acids are not due to a true "detergent effect" [39]. If they permeabilized mitochondrial membranes, the ATP/O rations should decrease. But in mitochondria isolated from fatty acid perfused hearts, the ATP/O ratio remained constant [26]. In many biochemical experiments, mitochondria have been exposed to high fatty acid concentrations *in vitro*, but these are very unlikely to occur during the reversible phase of ischemia or anoxia in the cytosol of the heart muscle cell.

Structure dependent injury of long-chain acyl moieties has also been reported in studies in which mitochondria were exposed *in vitro* to non-esterified fatty acids [66] or acyl carnitines [67]. In these experiments the oleyl moiety always caused more damage than the palmitoyl moiety. The similarity of results for fatty acids and their acylcarnitine esters suggested that mito-chondria were affected by a physicochemical interaction of the acyl residues with mitochondrial membranes. But from a quantitative estimate of free fatty acids and acyl carnitines in the cytosol of myocardial tissue, it was concluded that extramitochondrial concentrations which cause damage *in vitro*, are too high to occur in the cytosol during the reversible phase of ischemia [66, 67].

Mitochondria as a source for oxygen radicals

The role of free radicals in severe myocardial injury has been extensively discussed during recent years. The term 'free radicals' refers to molecules with an unpaired electron, most of which are chemically highly reactive. Chemical radicals are intermediates of a number of biochemical reactions, and usually the cell is protected from their potentially deleterious effects [68, 69]. A crucial role of free radicals in myocardial injury could relate to an increase in free radical formation, greater toxicity of the species formed, and defects in the defense system. According to the most favoured theory, oxygen radicals represent a crucial factor in reperfusion/reoxygenation injury due to both their enhanced formation and to a weakening of the normal cellular defence mechanisms during ischemic or hypoxic stress. Indeed, in ischemic and reperfused myocardium the concentration of glutathione and the activities of superoxide dismutase, catalase, and glutathione peroxidase were found to be reduced [70–72].

In ischemic-reperfused and hypoxic-reoxygenated myocardium free radicals may be generated by a 'leaking' electron chain [73–75]. In heart mitochondria, oxygen radicals can also be formed by the enzyme NADH oxidoreductase, which is not an integral part of the respiratory chain [76]. Increased electron leakage at oxygen tensions too low for the cytochrome c oxidase, similar to electron leakage in isolated mitochondria under antimycin blockade [73, 84], might be the cause of increased formation of carbon- and oxygen-centered radicals [77] in ischemic tissue. Mitochondria have also been suggested to be the source of the burst of oxygen radicals formed immediately when ischemic or hypoxic tissue is reoxygenated. Persistent impairment in cytochrome oxidase activity and the initially reduced state of respiratory chain elements have been suggested as causal factors [72, 78]. It has also been hypothesized that perturbation of the respiratory chain in ischemic cells favours mitochondrial electron leakage [78]. In contrast to this hypothesis, hydrogen peroxide formation indicating such leakage was found to be reduced in mitochondria isolated from 1 h globally ischemic rabbit hearts ± 1 hour reperfusion [79]. In another study, the production of hydroxyl radicals by mitochondria isolated from 45 and 90 minutes globally ischemic rabbit hearts was examined [80]. At 90 minutes ischemia, a depression was also found, but in mitochondria isolated at 45 minutes ischemia, hydroxyl radical formation was increased by 30% in comparison with mitochondria from aerobic control hearts. This may indicate that mitochondrial radical formation plays a role in ischemia-reperfusion injury only within a defined 'time window'. If so, it seems unlikely that increased oxygen radical formation by the mitochondria in reperfused/reoxygenated myocardium is the primary cause of reperfusion injury, since this is even more pronounced after 90 minutes than 45 minutes ischemia in the rabbit heart (unpublished observation).

Mitochondria as targets for free radical attack

Mitochondria can be attacked by free radicals originating in the cytosol as well as in the mitochondrium itself. Mitochondria possess their own defense system against free radical attack. Superoxide radicals can dismutate via the mitochondrial matrix superoxide dismutase to hydrogen peroxide which in turn is reduced to water by glutathione peroxidase. This way oxygen radicals are detoxified. In mitochondria isolated from ischemic-reperfused hearts, the ability to degrade oxygen radical enzymatically activity is apperently compromised, since the activities of these defensive enzymes are diminished [79]. This may also explain why mitochondria from ischemic myocardium in which hydroxyl radical formation was found to be increased could be stimulated to a normal rate of ATP production by the addition of superoxide dismutase and catalase [80].

At high rates of oxygen radical formation, even the use of the detoxification system has its price. Oxidized glutathione, produced by the glutathione peroxidase, becomes further reduced by the glutathione reductase which in turn increases the fraction of oxidized pyridine nucleotides. Once oxidized, pyridine nucleodtides can be hydrolysed by a transhydrogenase reaction to ADP-ribose and nicotinamide which in turn is lost from the mitochondria [55]. This loss of pyridine nucleotides from mitochondria is accompanied by an increase in passive Ca^{2+} efflux (see above). This can cause excessive Ca^{2+} cycling across the inner mitochondrial membrane, by which mitochondria deteriorate. It seems, therefore, that mitochondria will deteriorate in any case when forced to cope with increased oxygen radical formation.

In vitro, oxygen radicals have been shown to enhance mitochondrial permeability, inhibit electron transport, and reduce the activities of the F_1-ATPase and the adenine nucleotide translocase [51, 55]. These effects are not limited to the presence of Ca^{2+}, but Ca^{2+} does intesify the damage [81]. Such results of experiments with isolated mitochondria are compatible with a causal role of oxygen radicals in mitochondrial injury in ischemia-reoxygenation, but they do not prove it beyond doubt.

Respiratory competence of the reoxygenated myocardial cell

Capability for oxidative phosphorylation after brief periods of oxygen depletion

Relatively brief periods of ischemia insufficient to cause irreversible cell injury may nevertheless cause prolonged depression of myocardial contractility ('stunned myocardium' [82]). It has been demonstrated that the inability to perform mechanical work is not due to impaired mitochondrial function [83–85]. Oxygen consumption in such hearts is increased [84] or only slightly reduced [85] in spite of a pronounced depression of the contractile performance. This increased oxygen consumption may partly be due to increased utilization of fatty acids, but not to mitochondrial uncoupling since the ATP/O ratio remains unaltered [84]. These results suggest that myocardial stunning is due to inefficiency of ATP utilitization but not ATP production.

Capability for oxidative phosphorylation after extended periods of oxygen depletion

After extended periods of ischemia or hypoxia, resupply of the myocardium with oxygen and substrates does not promote cell recovery but exacerbates the already existing injury, a phenomenon termed 'oxygen paradox' [86]. The

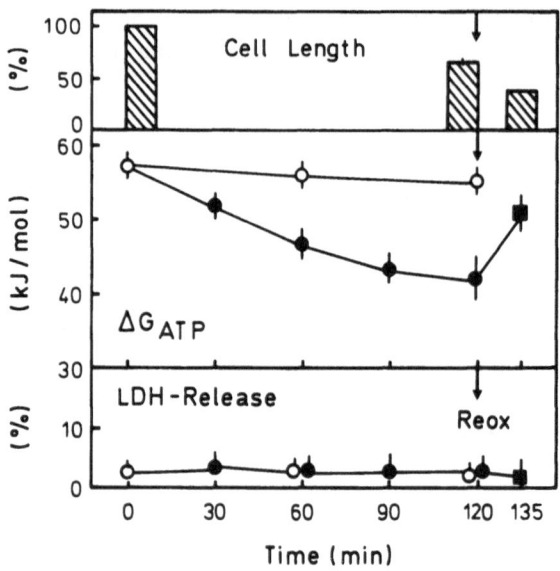

Fig. 6. Isolated adult cardiomyocytes from rat in substrate free anoxia-reoxygenation: Top: Average cell length of cardiomyocytes, in percent of normoxic control length. Middle: Free energy change of ATP hydrolysis, ΔG_{ATP}. Bottom: extracellular activity of lactate dehydrogenase in cardiomyocyte cultures, in percent of total activity of dish content. Average cell length was determined from 40 cells in each experiment. Closed symbols: 0–120 min anoxia with subsequent 15 min reoxygenation in glucose-free medium. Open symbols: Normoxic control incubation with 5 mM glucose. The methods are described in ref. [19]. ($\bar{x} \pm$ S.D., n = 5.)

oxygen paradox is characterized by a sudden onset of contracture and massive enzyme release. It does not occur when oxidative energy production is completely diminished [87], for it requires a relative preservation of mito-chondrial metabolic function. In the natural course of the oxygen paradox, disruption of the sarcolemma and massive influx of Ca^{2+} into the cell soon terminate mitochondrial ATP production. By blocking the compulsory Ca^{2+} uptake of mitochondria with ruthenium red, added to the reperfusion me-dium, it has been demonstrated that, under conditions of the oxygen paradox, the mitochondria are still capable of producing ATP [61].

Isolated cardiomyocytes exhibit only a partial oxygen paradox. In response to late reoxygenation, they hypercontract [11] but retain an intact sar-colemma as demonstrated by the absence of enzyme release [19] (Fig. 6). They therefore represent a suitable model to investigate whether restoration of mitochondrial function after extended anoxia is sufficient to re-establish the cell's normal energetic state.

The cytosolic energetic state of the cell can be characterized by ΔG_{ATP}, the free energy change of ATP hydrolysis [88, 89]: $\Delta G_{ATP} = \Delta G°_{ATP} + R \cdot T \cdot \ln$ ([ATP] / [ADP] · [P$_i$]), where $\Delta G°_{ATP}$ denotes the absolute value of the standard free energy change, R the universal gas constant, T the absolute

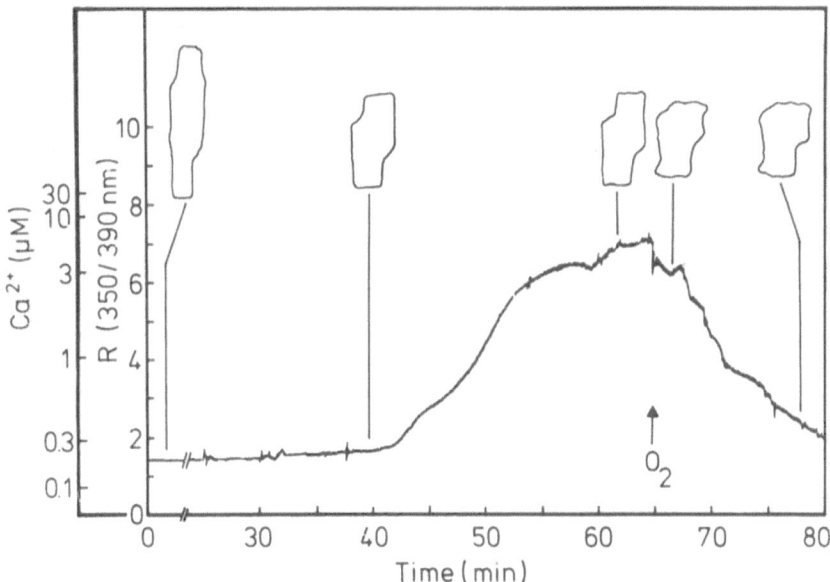

Fig. 7. Single isolated adult cardiomyocyte from rat in substrate free anoxia-reoxygenation: Cell shape and free cytosolic Ca^{2+}. The ordinate shows the ratio of fura-2 fluorescence at 350 and 390 nm excitation and the calibrated estimate of the Ca^{2+} concentration. Data were presented in ref. [20].

temperature, and symbols in brackets free cytosolic metabolite concentrations. The equation shows that the 'energetic value' of ATP depends on the advancement of ATP hydrolysis. When isolated cardiomyocytes were re-oxygenated after 120 minutes in substrate-free anoxia, they hypercontracted to a round cell remnant. In spite of the drastic morphological changes, the cytosolic concentrations of ADP and P_i were rapidly reduced, and within 15 minutes the free energy change of ATP hydrolysis recovered to 90% of the normoxic control value which was 57 kJ/mol ATP [19] (Fig. 6). Since the free energy change defines the possibility of high-energy reactions, its recovery enables the cells to regain control of such basic functions as cation homeostasis. Indeed, reoxygenated and hypercontracted isolated cardiomyocytes can reactivate the pump mechanisms which clear the cytosol from accumulated Ca^{2+} and re-establish normal resting levels of cytosolic Ca^{2+} [20] (Fig. 7). These results are in accordance with previous studies indicating that in cardiomyocytes, after an extended period of oxygen depletion, mitochondrial metabolism is less disturbed than other aspects of energy metabolism [90, 91].

Oxidative phosphorylation and reoxygenation-induced hypercontracture

It has been found in anoxic-reoxygenated cardiomyocytes, that a cytosolic Ca^{2+} concentration of 2–3 μM marks an important threshold level for the recovery of a normal Ca^{2+} homeostasis [92]. Beyond this level, a rapid re-establishment of normal Ca^{2+} homeostasis cannot be achieved, and hyper-contracture is inevitable when the cardiomyocyte is reoxygenated. In studies on isolated mitochondria, however, it has been shown that this concentration is the mitochondrial starting point for active Ca^{2+} accumulation. Beyond this threshold, Ca^{2+} uptake into the mitochondria competes with ATP produc-tion for respiratory energy [38]. Consequently, the supply of ATP to the Ca^{2+} pumps of the sarcolemma and the sarcoplasmic reticulum diminishes. The mitochondrial capacity for Ca^{2+} accumulation alone is not sufficient to regain control of cytosolic Ca^{2+} homeostasis. In single cardiomyocytes, hypercon-tracture as an immediate response to reoxygenation at high cytosolic Ca^{2+} concentrations occurs only when oxidative phosphorylation is active. Thus, both high cytosolic Ca^{2+} levels and some metabolic energy are required for eliciting this reoxygenation phenomenon. These are the requirements for a Ca^{2+}-induced contracture which is the result of a rapid, energy-consuming crossbridge cycling [33].

Conclusions

The impairment of mitochondrial respiratory functions may become apparent on reperfusion of hypoxic or ischemic tissue. Since, under anaerobic condi-tions, the mitochondria do not respire, damage to the respiratory chain acquired during ischemia does not contribute to the progression of cell damage. But the extrapolation of the results obtained on mitochondria isolated from ischemic/hypoxic-reoxygenated tissue to the role of mitochon-dria in the reoxygenated cell has a great degree of uncertainty, for a number of reasons:

1. Studies on isolated mitochondria can have a technical bias in that the subfraction of mitochondria isolated from normoxic tissue may differ from that isolated from injured tissue. Attempts have been made to overcome this problem by investigating the ischemia-induced changes in defined mitochondrial subpopulations [25].
2. The metabolic behavior of isolated mitochondria may be influenced by the loss of internal contents during the isolation procedure (e.g. ions, lipids).
3. *In vitro*, mitochondrial functions are investigated in certain fixed func-tional states which may differ considerably from their functional state in the intact cell.

The results of different laboratories are largely consistent with respect to the sites of mitochondrial injury. They are, however, not consistent in the way they relate these changes to certain stages of tissue injury. In one of these studies [25], in which the mitochondrial injury was followed in defined subpopulations, extensive impairment of mitochondrial function was already documented during the initial phase of reversible ischemia. In other studies, the properties of mitochondria seemed unaltered during the early phase of ischemia. It is conceivable that injury affecting only part of the mitochondria initially may remain undetected if the isolation procedure applied always select the most intact mitochondria. The results from different laboratories are also consistent in that a point in time at which mitochondrial respiratory functions would suddenly and markedly deteriorate was not identified. Therefore, studies on isolated mitochondria lend no support to the idea that a certain degree of reduced mitochondrial function determines the point of no-return in cellular injury.

For these and other reasons, results from studies on isolated mitochondria have to be interpreted with some caution. They certainly give the most detailed biochemical results, but their relevance in understanding mitochondrial function in the injured cell remains, in most cases, unclear. Thus the mitochondrial capability for oxidative phosphorylation may be found to be reduced by 40% at a time when tissue ATP has dropped from 24 to 17 $\mu mol/g$ dry weight in the ischemic guinea pig heart [25]. But this defect may not be responsible for the inability of the heart to function after reperfusion. This is because even in a heart functioning at normal work load, only part of the total respiratory capacity of normal mitochondria is used; but after an ischemic or hypoxic period functional insufficiency already becomes apparent at low levels of energy demand.

The ultrastructural analysis of mitochondrial injury by electron microscopic techniques has not provided a more direct criterion for detecting critical functional failure. It has not been proven unambiguously that the ultrastructural changes detected by standard techniques are not, at least partly, artefacts of the procedures of fixation and embedding. It therefore remains unclear how a certain state of structural injury, as visualized by these techniques, relates to functional impairment. In particular, electron microscopy seems unable to determine when mitochondrial injury definitely becomes irreversible.

The results on myocardial metabolism of ischemic-reperfused hearts and anoxic-reoxygenated cardiomyocytes are not compatible with the role of the mitochondria as the primary failing cell structure. Instead, mitochondria retain sufficient functional competence at times when other crucial cell functions have already failed. Even the elicitation of the oxygen paradox depends on a sufficient preservation of the metabolic competence of mitochondria. In isolated cardiomyocytes, mitochondrial function survives deterioration of large parts of the cytoskeletal ultrastructure.

Acknowledgement

This study was supported by the Deutsche Forschungsgemeinschaft, grant Pi 162/2–1.

110

References

1. Hatefi Y (1985) The mitochondrial electron transport chain and oxidative phosphorylation. Annu Rev Biochem 54: 1015–1069
2. Wittenberg BA, Wittenberg JB (1985) Oxygen pressure gradient in isolated cardiac myocytes. J Biol Chem 260: 6548-6554
3. Chance B (1965) Reaction of oxygen with the respiratory chain in cells and tissue. J Gen Physiol 49: 163–188
4. DeGroot H, Noll T, Sies H (1985) Oxygen dependence and subcellular partitioning of hepatic menadione-mediated oxygen uptake. Arch Biochem Biophys 243: 556–562
5. Fuchs J, Zimmer G, Bereiter-Hahn J (1987) A multiparameter analysis of the perfused rat heart: responses to ischemia, uncouplers and drugs. Cell Biochem Funct 5: 245–253 Drug Res 37: 1030–1034
6. Kübler W, Spieckermann PG (1970) Regulation of glycolysis in the ischemic and the anoxic myocardium. J Mol Cell Cardiol 1: 351–377
7. Rovetto MJ, Lamberton WF, Neely JR (1973) Mechanism of glycolytic inhibition in ischemic rat hearts. Circ Res 37: 742–751
8. Wiesner RJ, Deussen A, Borst M, Schrader J, Grieshaber K (1989) Glutamate degradation in the ischemic dog heart: contribution to anaerobic energy production. J Mol Cell Cardiol 21: 49–59
9. Schwerzmann K, Pedersen P (1986) Regulation of the mitochondrial ATP Synthase/ATPase complex. Arch Biochem Biophys 250: 1–18
10. Gomez-Puyou MT, Martins OB, Gomez-Puyou A (1987) Synthesis and hydrolysis of ATP by the mitochondrial ATP synthase. Biochem Cell Biol 66: 677–682
11. Haworth RA, Hunter DR, Berkoff HA (1981) Contracture in isolated adult rat heart cells: role of CA^{2+}, ATP and compartmentation. Circ Res 49: 1119–1128
12. Rouslin W, Erickson JL, Solaro RJ (1986) Effects of oligomycin and acidosis on rates of ATP depletion in ischemic heart muscle. Am J Physiol 250: H503–H508
13. Rouslin W (1983) Protonic inhibition of the mitochondrial oligomycin-sensitive adenosine 5'-triphosphatase in ischemic and autolyzing cardiac muscle. J Biol Chem 258: 9657–9661
14. Hatt PY, Moravec J (1971) Acute hypoxia of the myocardium. Ultrastructural changes. Cardiology 56: 73–84
15. Schwartz P, Piper HM, Spahr R, Spieckermann PG (1984) Ultrastructure of adult myocardial cells during anoxia and reoxygenation. Am J Pathol 115: 349–361
16. Hertsens RC, Bernaert I, Joniau M, Jacob WA (1986) Immunohistochemical investigation of native matrix granules of the rat heart mitochondrion. J Ultrastruct Mol Struct Res 94: 1–15
17. Reimer KA, Jennings RB (1986) Myocardial ischemia, hypoxia and infarction. In: Fozzard HA, Haber E, Jennings RB, Katz AM, Morgan HE (eds) The Heart and Cardiovascular System. New York, Raven Press, pp 1133–1201
18. Sjostrand F, Allen BS, Buckwald GD, Okamoto F, Young H, Bugyi H, Beyersdorf F, Barnard J, Leaf J (1986) Studies of controlled reperfusion after ischemia. IV. Electron microscopic studies: Importance of embedding techniques in quantitative evaluation of cardiac mitochondrial structure during regional ischemia and reperfusion. J Thorac Cardiovasc Surg 92: 513–524
19. Siegmund B, Koop A, Klietz T, Schwartz P, Piper HM (1989) Sarcolemmal integrity and metabolic competence of cardiomyocytes under anoxia-reoxygenation. Am J Physiol 258: in press
20. Piper HM, Jacobson SL, Schwartz JL, Mealing GAR, Whitfield JF (1988) Disturbance of Ca^{2+} homeostasis in restrained cardiomyocytes under anoxia and reoxygenation. J Mol Cell Cardiol 20, suppl V: 35
21. Trump BF, Mergner WJ, Kahng MW, Saladino AJ (1976) Studies on the subcellular pathophysiology of ischemia. Circulation 53, suppl I: 18–26
22. Jennings RB, Ganote CE (1976) Mitochondrial structure and function in acute myocardial ischemic injury. Circ Res 38, suppl I: I80–I90

23. Lochner A, Sanan D, Victor T, Bester R, Kotze JCN, van der Merwe N, Schabort I (1985) Mitochondrial and sarcolemmal function in the ischemic myocardium. In: Berman MC, Gevers W, Opie LH (eds) Membranes and Muscle. Oxford, IRL Press, pp 309–325

24. Bester R, Lochner A (1988) Sarcolemmal phospholipid fatty acid composition and permeability. Biochim Biophys Acta 941: 176–186

25. Piper HM, Sezer O, Schleyer M, Schwartz P, Hütter JF, Spieckermann PG (1985) Development of ischemia-induced damage in defined mitochondrial subpopulations. J Mol Cell Cardiol 17: 186–198

26. Piper HM, Das A (1987) Detrimental actions of endogenous fatty acids and their derivatives. A study of ischaemic mitochondrial injury. Basic Res Cardiol 82, suppl 1: 187–196

27. Asimakis GK, Conti VR (1984) Myocardial ischemia: correlation of mitochondrial adenine nucleotide and respiratory function. J Mol Cell Cardiol 16: 439–448

28. Asimakis GK, Sordahl LA (1981) Intramitochondrial adenine nucleotides and energy-linked functions of heart mitochondria. Am J Physiol 241: H672–H681

29. Asimakis GK, Wilson DE, Conti VR (1985) Release of AMP and adenosine from rat heart mitochondria. Life Sci 37: 2373–2380

30. Lochner A, van Niederkerk I, Whitesell LF (1981) Mitochondrial acyl-CoA, adenine nucleotide translocase activity and oxidative phosphorylation in myocardial ischemia. J Mol Cell Cardiol 13: 991–997

31. Kotaka K, Miyazaki Y, Ogawa K, Satake T, Sugiyama S, Ozawa T (1982) Reversal of ischemia-induced mitochondrial dysfunction after coronary reperfusion. J Mol Cell Cardiol 14: 223–231

32. Rouslin W (1983) Mitochondrial complexes I, II, III, IV, and V in myocardial ischemia and autolysis. Am J Physiol 244: H743–H748

33. Piper HM (1989) Energy deficiency, calcium overload or oxidative stress: Possible causes of irreversible ischemic myocardial injury. Klin Wschr 67: 465–476

34. Walsh LG, Tormey J McD (1988) Subcellular electrolyte shifts during in vitro myocardial ischemia and reperfusion. Am J Physiol 255: H197–H928

35. Garfinkel L, Altschuld RA, Garfinkel D (1986) Magnesium in cardiac energy metabolism. J Mol Cell Cardiol 18: 1003–1013

36. Jacobus WE, Tiozzo R, Lugli G, Lehninger AL, Carafoli E (1975) Aspects of energy-linked calcium accumulation by rat heart mitochondria. J Biol Chem 250: 7863–7870

37. Nicholls DG, Crompton M (1980) Mitochondrial calcium transport. FEBS Lett. 111: 261–268

38. Carafoli E (1985) The homeostasis of calcium in heart cells. J Mol Cell Cardiol 17: 203–212

39. Katz AM, Messineo FC (1981) Lipid-membrane interactions and the pathogenesis of ischemic damage in the myocardium. Circ Res 48: 1–16

40. Pande SV, Blanchaer MC (1971) Reversible inhibition of mitochondrial adenosine diphosphate phosphorylation by long chain acyl coenzyme A esters. J Biol Chem 246: 402–411

41. Shug AL, Lerner C, Elson O, Shrago E (1971) The inhibition of adenine nucleotide translocase by oleoyl CoA and its reversal in rat liver mitochondria. Biochem Biophys Res Commun 43: 557–563

42. Shug AL, Shrago E, Bittar N, Folts JD, Roke JR (1975) Acyl CoA inhibition of adenine nucleotide translocation in ischemic myocardium. Am J Physiol 228: 689–692

43. Idell-Wenger JA, Grotyohann LW, Neely JR (1978) Coenzyme A and carnitine distribution in normal and ischemic hearts. J Biol Chem 253: 4310–4318

44. Woldegiorgis G, Shrago E (1979) The recognition of two specific binding sites of the adenine nucleotide translocase by palmityl CoA in bovine heart mitochondria and submitochondrial particles. Biochem Biophys Res Commun 89: 837–844

45. Glatz JFC, Veerkamp JH (1985) Intracellular fatty acid binding proteins. Int J Biochem 17: 13–22

46. LaNoue KF, Watts JA, Koch CD (1981) Adenine nucleotide transport during cardiac ischemia. Am J Physiol 241: H663–H671

47. Harris EJ (1979) Modulation of Ca^{2+} efflux from heart mitochondria. Biochem J 178: 673–680

112

48. Harris EJ, Cooper MB (1981) Calcium and magnesium losses in response to stimulants of efflux applied to heart, liver and kidney mitochondria. Biochem Biophys Res Commun 788–796

49. Sordahl LA, Stewart ML (1980) Mechanism(s) of altered mitochondrial calcium transport in acutely ischemic canine hearts. Circ Res 47: 814–820

50. Le Quoc K, Le Quoc D (1988) Involvement of the ATP/ADP carrier in calcium-induced perturbations of the mitochondrial inner membrane permeability: Importance of the orientation of the nucleotide binding site. Arch Biochem Biophys 265: 249–257

51. Carbonera D, Azzone GF (1988) Permeability of inner mitochondrial membrane and oxidative stress. Biochim Biophys Acta 943: 245–255

52. D'Souza MP, Wilson DF (1982) Adenine nucleotide efflux in mitochondria induced by inorganic pyrophosphate. Biochim Biophys Acta 680: 28–32

53. Palmer JW, Pfeiffer DR (1981) The control of Ca^{2+} release from heart mitochondria. J Biol Chem 256: 6742–6750

54. Beatrice MC, Stiers O, Pfeiffer DR (1982) Increased permeability of mitochondria during Ca^{2+} release induced by t-butyl hydroperoxide or oxalacetate. J Biol Chem 257: 7161–7171

55. Richter C, Frei B (1988) Ca^{2+} release from mitochondria induced by prooxidants. Free Rad Biol Med 4: 365–375

56. Lehninger AL, Vercesi A, Bababunmi EA (1978) Regulation of Ca^{2+} release from mitochondria by the oxidation-reduction state of pyridine nucleotides. Proc Natl Acad Sci USA 75: 1690–1694

57. Lochner A, van der Merwe N, de Villiers M, Steinmann C, Kotze JCN (1987) Mitochondrial Ca^{2+} fluxes and levels during ischaemia and reperfusion: possible mechanisms. Biochim Biophys Acta 927: 8–17

58. Ashraf M, Bloor CM (1976) X-ray microanalysis of mitochondrial deposits in ischemic myocardium. Virchows Arch B Cell Pathol 22: 287–297

59. Peng CF, Kane JJ, Murphy ML, Straub KD (1977) Abnormal mitochondrial oxidative phosphorylation of ischemic myocardium reversed by Ca^{2+}-chelating agents. J Mol Cell Cardiol 9: 897–908

60. Ferrari R, Williams A, Di Lissa F (1988) The role of mitochondrial function in the ischemic and reperfused myocardium. In: Caldarera CM, Harris P (eds) Advances in Studies on Heart Metabolism. Bologna, CLUEB, pp 245–255

61. Ferrari R, Di Lissa F, Raddino R, Visioli O (1982) The effects of ruthenium red on mitochondrial function during post-ischemic reperfusion. J Mol Cell Cardiol 14: 737–740

62. Coll KE, Joseph SK, Corkey BE, Williamson JR (1982) Determination of free Ca^{2+} concentration and kinetics of Ca^{2+} efflux in liver and heart mitochondria. J Biol Chem 257: 8696–8704

63. Piper HM, Das D (1986) The role of fatty acids in ischemic tissue injury: difference between oleic and palmitic acid. Basic Res Cardiol 81: 373–383

64. Nagami M, Yoshida S, Saitoh T, Takeshita M, Ogawa T (1988) Effect of oleic acid on mitochondrial cytochrome c oxidase activity. Biochem Int 17: 763–771

65. Spector AA, Brennan DE (1972) Effect of free fatty acid structure on binding to rat liver mitochondria. Biochim Biophys Acta 260: 433–438

66. Piper HM, Sezer O, Schwartz P, Hütter JF, Spieckermann PG (1983) Fatty acid-membrane interactions in isolated cardiac mitochondria and erythrocytes. Biochim Biophys Acta 732: 193–203

67. Piper HM, Sezer O, Schwartz P, Hütter JF, Schweickhardt C, Spieckermann PG (1984) Acyl-carnitine effects on isolated cardiac mitochondria and erythrocytes. Basic Res Cardiol 79: 186–198

68. Slater TF (1984) Free radical mechanisms in tissue injury. Biochem J 222: 1–15

69. Sies H, Cadenas E (1985) Oxidative stress: damage to intact cells and organs. Phil Trans R Soc Lond B 311: 617–631

70. Guarnieri C, Flamigni F, Caldarera CM (1980) Role of oxygen in the cellular damage induced by re-oxygenation of hypoxic heart. J Mol Cell Cardiol 12: 797–808

71. Meerson FZ, Kagan VE, Kozlov YP, Belkina LM, Arkhipenko YV (1982) The role of lipid peroxidation in pathogenesis of ischemic damage and the antioxidant protection of the heart. Basic Res Cardiol 77: 465–485

72. Ferrari R, Ceconi C, Curello S, Guarnieri C, Caldarera CM, Albertini A, Visioli O (1985) Oxygen-mediated myocardial damage during ischemia and reperfusion: role of cellular defences against oxygen toxicity. J Mol Cell Cardiol 17: 973–945

73. Turrens JF, Boveris A (1980) Generation of superoxide anion by the NADH dehydrogenase of bovine heart mitochondria. Biochem J 191: 421–427

74. Nohl H, Jordan W, Hegner D (1982) Mitochondrial formation of OH radicals by an ubisemiquinone-dependent reaction. An alternative pathway to the iron-catalysed Haber-Weiss cycle. Hoppe-Seyler's Z. Physiol Chem 363: 599–607

75. Nohl H, Jordan W (1986) The mitochondrial site of superoxide formation. Biochem Biophys Res Commun 138: 533–539

76. Nohl H (1987) A novel superoxide radical generator in heart mitochondria. FEBS Lett 214: 269–273.

77. Arroyo CM, Kramer JH, Leiboff RH, Mergner GW, Dickens BF, Weglicki WB (1987) Spin trapping of oxygen and carbon-centered free radicals in ischemic canine myocardium. Free Rad Biol Med 3: 313–316

78. McCord JM (1988) Free radicals and myocardial ischemia: Overview and outlook. Free Rad Biol Med 4: 9–14

79. Shlafer M, Myers CL, Adkins S (1987) Mitochondrial hydrogen peroxide generation and activities of glutathione peroxidase and superoxide dismutase following global ischemia. J Mol Cell Cardiol 19, 1195–1206

80. Otani H, Tanaka H, Inoue T, Umemoto M, Omoto K, Tanaka K, Sato T, Osako T, Masuda A, Nonoyama A, Kagawa T (1984) In vitro study on contribution of oxidative metabolism of isolated rabbit heart mitochondria to myocardial reperfusion injury. Circ Res 55: 168–175

81. Malis CD, Bonventre JV (1986) Mechanisms of calcium potentiation of oxygen free radical injury to renal mitochondria. J Biol Chem 261: 14201–14208

82. Braunwal E, Kloner RA (1982) The stunned myocardium: prolonged postischemic ventricular dysfunction. Circulation 66: 1146–1149

83. Ambrosio G, Jacobus WE, Bergman CA, Weisman HF, Becker LC (1987) Preserved high-energy phosphate metabolic reserve in globally 'stunned' hearts despite reduction of basal ATP content and contractility. J Moll Cell Cardiol 19: 953–964

84. Sako EY, Kingsley-Hickman PB, From AHL, Foker JE, Ugurbil K (1988) ATP synthesis kinetics and mitochondrial function in the postischemic myocardium as studies by ^{31}P NMR. J Biol Chem 263: 10600–10607

85. Liedtke AJ, DeMaison L, Eggleston AM, Cohen LM, Nellis SH (1988) Changes in substrate metabolism and effects of excess fatty acids in reperfused myocardium. Circ Res 62: 535–542

86. Hearse DJ, Humphrey SM, Chain EB (1973) Abrupt reoxygenation of the anoxic potassium-arrested perfused rat heart: A study of mitochondrial enzyme release. J Mol Cell Cardiol 5: 395–407

87. Ganote CE (1983) Contraction band necrosis and irreversible myocardial injury. J Mol Cell Cardiol 15: 67–73

88. Veech RL, Lawson JWR, Cornell NW, Krebs HA (1979) Cytosolic phosphorylation potential. J Biol Chem 254: 551–561

89. Siegmund B, Koop A, Piper HM (1989) The use of the creatine kinase reaction to determine free energy change of ATP hydrolysis in anoxic cardiomyocytes. Pflügers Arch 413: 435–437

90. McDonough KH, Spitzer JJ (1983) Effects of hypoxia and reoxygenation on adult rat heart cell metabolism. Proc Soc Exp Biol Med 173: 519–526

91. Cheung JY, Leaf A, Bonventre JV (1986) Mitochondrial function and intracellular calcium in anoxic cardiac myocytes. Am J Physiol 250: C18–25

92. Allshire A, Piper HM, Cuthbertson KSR, Cobbold PH (1987) Cytosolic free Ca^{2+} in single rat heart cells during anoxia and reoxygenation. Biochem J 244: 381–385

Lysosomal integrity in ischemic, hypoxic and recovering heart

ROBERT S. DECKER[1,2] and MARLENE L. DECKER[1]

Department of [1]Medicine (Cardiology) and [2]Cell, Molecular and Structural Biology, Northwestern University Medical School, Chicago, Illinois 60611, USA

Lysosomal hypothesis of ischemic injury

The early experiments of de Duve and his colleagues first implicated the lysosome as a potential mediator of ischemic cell injury [1, 2]. Ligating a branch of the hepatic artery was accompanied by a marked subcellular redistribution of lysosomal enzyme activity in the ischemic liver. Since de Duve [1] had recently documented that the lysosome represented a latent storehouse of catabolic acid hydrolases, such alterations in lysosomal properties prompted considerable speculation that these organelles might represent a population of subcellular 'suicide bags' which, in theory, could provoke intracellular damage if 'activated' by appropriate changes in the intracellular environment [3]. Such provocative observations encouraged numerous investigations aimed at identifying whether alterations in 'lysosomal integrity' were, in any way, temporally correlated with evolving ischemic damage in the heart and other tissues [3–7].

Coronary artery occlusion is accompanied by a broad spectrum of metabolic lesions which develop rapidly in the ischemic myocardium (this book). Deprivation of oxygen quickly depletes the myocardium of its high energy phosphates, promotes the accumulation of lactate and protons, elevates lysophospholipids and arachidonic acid, liberates free radicals and disturbs the regulation of cell volume and ion content among others (this book). All these metabolic abnormalities develop during the reversible phase of cell injury. If, however, the interruption of blood flow or oxygen deprivation is prolonged, then irreversible ischemic damage and cell death ensue [8–10]. At or near the point of irreversible injury, ATP and creatine phosphate stores are nearly exhausted [11, 12], mitochondrial failure is apparent [9], cell volume and ion regulation are lost [13–15] and lysosomal disruption [7] can be documented in the failing myocardium. Which, if any, of the phenomena enumerated above transforms the reversibly injured myocyte into a necrotic one remains an elusive target.

Alterations in cardiac lysosomal properties continue to foster considerable debate about the potential role that the intracellular release of lysosomal acid

H.M. Piper (ed.) Pathophysiology of severe ischemic myocardial injury, 115–145.
© 1990 Kluwer Academic Publishers, Dordrecht –

Table 1. The 'lysosomal hypothesis' of ischemic cell injury.

1. Ischemia produces lowered ATP, lowered pH, accumulation of membrane-active fatty acids, etc.
2. These events, in turn, produce a reduction in membrane integrity (including lysosomal membranes).
3. Enzymes that are normally latent (e.g., lysosomal hydrolases) leak out from their normal membrane delimited sites.
4. This results in abnormal degradation of certain cellular constituents because of (a) abnormal contact between hydrolytic enzymes and potential substrates, and (b) the presence during ischemia of a decreased pH (nearer the pH optima of most lysosomal hydrolases).
5. If severe enough, this abnormal hydrolysis of cellular constituents could contribute to the development of further cell injury including additional membrane damage and further release and activation of latent hydrolases.
6. This positive feedback cycle could continue until irreversible damage develops.

hydrolases might play in provoking cell injury [4, 5, 7]. Time and again investigators have speculated as to whether the release of lysosomal acid proteinases and phospholipases, for example, might initiate myofibrillar and sarcolemmal damage of the variety encountered during an ischemic or hypoxic insult. From such discussions, the 'lysosomal hypothesis of ischemic injury' evolved into an experimentally testable paradigm (Table 1). This hypothesis focused attention on verifying (1) whether lysosomal enzyme release preceded irreversible injury or merely represented a post-necrotic event [4, 5] and (2) whether the redistribution of such degradative enzymes attends evolving intracellular damage. This chapter will summarize some of the unique properties of the cardiac lysosomal vacuolar apparatus [16], review those experiments that validly test the lysosomal hypothesis and provide evidence supporting a role for the lysosomal vacuolar apparatus in repair processes that accompany restitution of coronary blood flow or re-oxygenation.

Properties of the cardiac lysosomal vacuolar apparatus

For years, classical subcellular fractionation protocols employed to prepare enriched lysosomal fractions failed to reveal that a similar population of organelles could be isolated from heart or skeletal muscle [4, 17]. Even though lipofucsin granules were recognized as normal constituents of the cardiac myocyte and displayed lysosomal acid hydrolase activity [4], the conflicting biochemical behavior of myocardial acid hydrolases and the observation that the majority of the lysosomal enzyme activity resided in the cardiac interstitial cell complement questioned the biochemical existence of a lysosomal vacuolar apparatus in the cardiac myocyte [4, 7]. However, modification of lysosomal isolation schemes and the development of improved cytochemical and immunocytochemical approaches have clarified many of the cardiac lysosomal intricacies [7].

Smith and Bird [8] first demonstrated that a bimodal distribution of acid hydrolase enriched particles could be isolated from ventricular homogenates and confirmed the presence of distinct lysosomal populations in the heart. Nevertheless, the yield of intact lysosomes was poor and a significant amount of lysosomal enzymatic activity remained membrane-bound but sedimented not in the light mitochondrial fraction, but, rather in a less dense membranous compartment that was clearly not lysosomal in the true sense of the word. From such preparations, it was also not possible to confirm an intracellular redistribution of lysosomal enzyme activity during the first hour of ischemia [4, 7]. Subsequently, it was discovered that much of this confusion arose because the isotonic sucrose employed to prepare cardiac lysosomes failed to solubilize the contractile apparatus, thus trapping lysosomes and minimizing their yield. Furthermore, in many homogenates much of the lysosomal enzyme activity could be found in the non-sedimentable state, suggesting that a significant proportion of the intact lysosomes were disrupted during isolation. Therefore, such preparations precluded any thorough assessment of lysosomal latency during the early phases of ischemic or hypoxic injury. However, the introduction of an isotonic or hypertonic KCl extraction medium effectively solubilized the myofibrils, markedly enhanced the recovery of intact lysosomes and improved conditions for the optimal study of lysosomal latency [19, 20]. Moreover, fractionation of post-nuclear KCl extracts convincingly revealed the presence of detergent releaseble lysosomal enzyme activity in a subcellular fraction enriched with sarcoplasmic reticulum [20, 21], demonstrating the existence of another compartment exhibiting lysosomal properties. Thus, this simple modification made it possible to disclose subtle, but significant, changes in lysosomal stability that were impossible to discern previously [21–24].

In as much as biochemical attempts to trace lysosomal enzyme redistribution are fraught with complications even under the best of circumstances, a parallel cytochemical and/or immunocytochemical visualization of representative lysosomal enzyme becomes an essential element in unraveling the organization of the lysosomal vacuolar apparatus in the cardiac myocyte [7]. Cytochemical and immunocytochemical techniques complement each other. The former reveals the existence of active enzyme by depicting the distribution of an enzymatic reaction product, while the latter relies on immune recognition to localize the enzyme, itself. Theoretically, such a combined approach would provide precise information on the specific location of a lysosomal enzyme and whether it retains its enzymatic activity. When combined with an accurate biochemical assessment of lysosomal properties, a considerably clearer picture of the cardiac lysosomal vacuolar apparatus emerges [7].

The presence of a heterogeneous population of organelles that stained positively for acid phosphatase, aryl sulfatase and several other lysosomal enzymes has been recognized for many years in the heart; however, it was not until, perhaps, ten years ago that a more thorough characterization of the lysosomal vacuolar apparatus was completed using refined cytochemical and immunocytochemical techniques [7]. In addition to the now classical perinuclear distribution of lysosomal dense and residual bodies and autophagic vacuoles, two other subcellular compartments stained positively for acid phosphatase and aryl sulfatase – one anticipated, the other not [25–30]! Since lysosomal enzymes are glycoproteins whose N-linked oligosaccharides undergo post-translational modification in the Golgi apparatus [31–33], it was not surprising to discover acid phosphatase and aryl sulfatase at this site. However, Topping and Travis [25] only reported the presence of these enzymes in the trans-Golgi network (TGN) of the endoplasmic reticulum [34, 35], previously termed GERL by Novikoff [36]. Primary lysosomes and autophagic vacuole membrane were believed to emanate from this region. Our observations also implicated the trans-elements of the Golgi apparatus as well as the TGN in lysosomal biogenesis in fetal [37, 38], neonatal [39] and adult cardiac myocytes [40, 41] with acid phosphatase and/or aryl sulfatase positive coated vesicles (primary lysosomes) developing from the Golgi cisternae and the TGN, whereas acid hydrolases destined for autophagic vacuoles and dense bodies appear to be derived from the TGN [7, 37, 38]. The sarcoplasmic reticulum represents a third major repository of acid phosphatase and aryl sulfatase activity [25, 26, 28, 40, 41]. Both junctional and non-junctional elements display acid hydrolase reaction products [26, 41] and Topping and Travis [25] provided tentative evidence supporting their involvement in lysosomal formation. The presence of lysosomal enzyme activity at this locale correlates positively with biochemical determinations indicating the presence of these enzymes in subcellular fractions enriched with sarcoplasmic reticulum [20, 21].

Although much of our knowledge concerning the organization of the cardiac lysosomal vacuolar apparatus has evolved from studies on acid phosphatase and aryl sulfatase, enzymes whose role in catabolic activities and whose *in vivo* substrates are poorly understood, the introduction of newly developed cytochemical [42–45] and immunocytochemical [46–49] approaches to investigate the distribution of the lysosomal proteinases, cathepsins B and D, made it possible, for the first time, to examine enzymes with the potential to damage proteins and disrupt vital cell functions. Both techniques place these acid proteinases in the cardiac lysosomal vacuolar apparatus [40, 41, 50], but the conjugation of anti-cathepsin D antibodies to either fluorescein or horseradish peroxidase [46] provided, perhaps, the best probes to study this protein. Figures 2 and 3 illustrate the distribution of cathepsin D by fluorescence and immunoelectron microscopy. Much of the acid proteinase is present in a perinuclear population of autophagic vacuoles and dense bodies in both ventricular myocytes and interstitial cells [30, 40, 41]. In addition, such probes have placed cathepsin D in the sarcoplasmic reticulum and the TGN of myocytes obtained from fasted [41] and thyrotoxic [50] rabbit hearts.

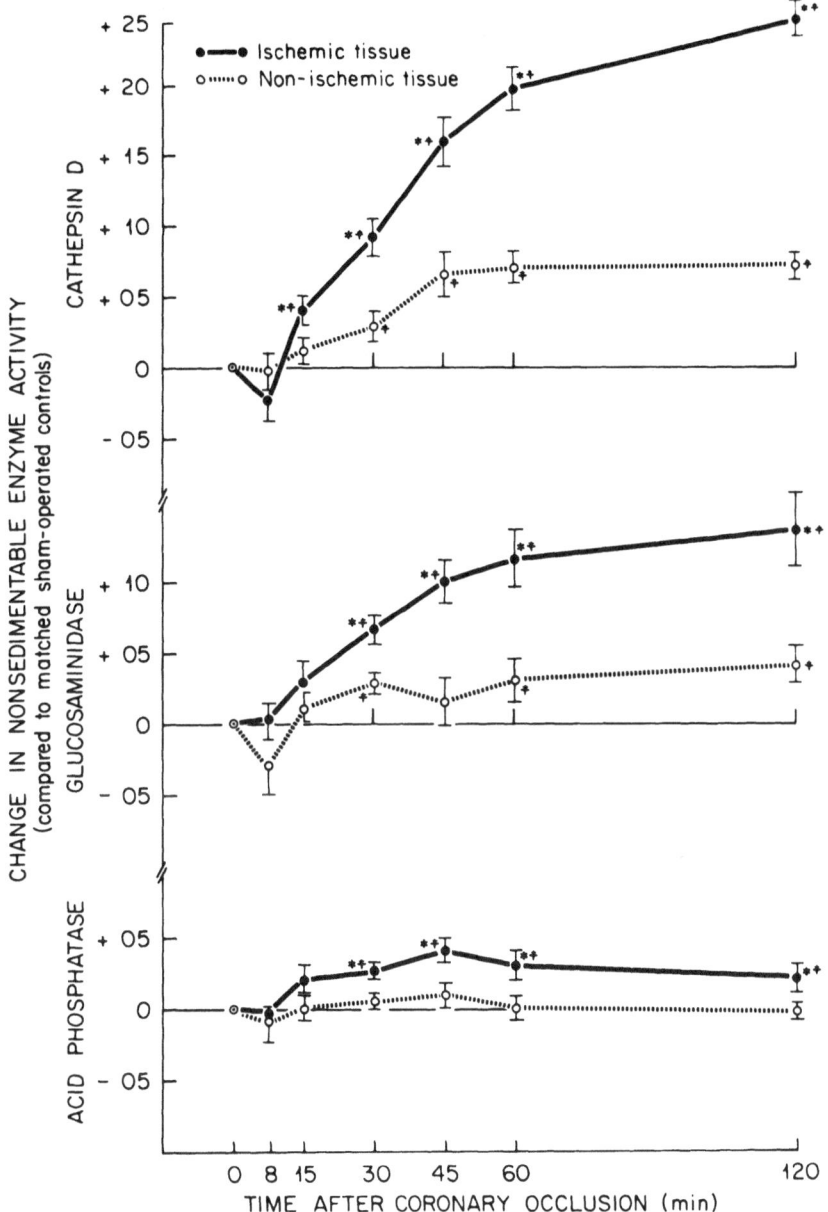

Fig. 1 Effect of coronary ligation for 8 to 120 minutes on on-sedimentable activities of cathepsin D, N-acetyl-, β, D-glucosaminidase, and acid phosphatase in ischemic and non-ischemic tissue. Results are plotted as the mean ± 1 standard error of the mean of values for non-sedimentable activity divided by total (non-sedimentable plus sedimentable) activity, expressed as the difference from age-match, sham-operated controls. Mean vaules at all times for sham-operated animals were: cathepsin D = 0.29; glucosaminidase = 0.57; acid phosphatase = 0.78; ‡ = p<0.05 compared to sham-operated controls; * = p<0.05 compared to matched non-ischemic tissue.

The future development of monoclonal antibodies and implementing the use of active-site directed inhibitors [44, 45] to trace the presence of active enzyme will further enhance our ability to unravel the remaining structural and functional complexities of the lysosomal vacuolar apparatus in the cardiac myocyte.

Lysosomal alterations in ischemic and hypoxic heart

Almost immediately after coronary artery ligation, the myocardium supplied by that occluded vessel becomes cyanotic, contractile activity subsides, ion fluxes are disrupted and the ischemic myocytes commence respiring anaerobically [51]. As the myocytes accumulate lactate and become acidotic, morphological evidence of cell injury develops [9, 10, 28, 29], and if coronary flow is not re-established in the acutely ischemic myocardium within 20–40 minutes, then the cells become irreversibly injured and die. Reversibly damaged myocytes, however, develop a unique set of structural changes that include: (1) depletion of intracellular glycogen; (2) mitochondrial dilation with a concomitant loss of matrix; and (3) condensation of nuclear chromatin. Each of these morphological features of cell injury is reversible upon reperfusion [7, 8, 52]. Conversely, the appearance of mitochondrial osmiophilic densities [8, 9], lysosomal rupture [22] and sarcolemmal discontinuities [8, 10, 52] signals the impending development of irreversible cell injury. The temporal appearance of these functional and structural deficits also characterizes other models of ischemic-like injury, including global ischemia, autolysis and hypoxic perfusion with or without substrate depletion and acidosis [53–56]. If the lysosomal hypothesis in its present form (Table 1) plays a pivotal role in the evolution of irreversible cell injury, then the release of acid hydrolases from the lysosomal vacuolar apparatus must transpire prior to the appearance of structural and functional evidence indicative of irreversible damage.

Early studies documented a marked subcellular redistribution of lysosomal enzyme activity in homogenates of ischemic heart and lent support to the lysosomal hypothesis [4]. However, these early investigations were controversial for the enhanced levels of non-sedimentable acid hydrolase activity developed after prolonged periods of ischemia [57, 58]. As protocols for the measurement of lysosomal latency improved (see preceding section), significant changes in non-sedimentable lysosomal enzyme activity could be demonstrated within 1–2 hours after acutely ligating a coronary artery or perfusing hearts in hypoxic media [59–70]. Prolonged ischemic or hypoxic episodes also induced the appearance of lysosomal activity in the interstitum, cardiac lymph and blood in animals [71–73] and patients [74, 75]. The presence of this extracellular acid hydrolase activity, in all probability, reflected a diffusion of enzyme in post-necrotic, infarcted tissue.

In most instances, little attempt was made to critically correlate lysosomal changes with the progression of ischemic injury. Weglicki's laboratory coupled the use of radioactive microspheres with KCl extraction of lysosomes to demonstrate that the redistribution of lysosomal activity was directly proportional to reduced coronary flow and the severity of the cardiac ischemia [21]. Others also illustrated that in the same canine model, low coronary flow and the depletion of acid phosphatase and aryl sulfatase reaction products from the sarcoplasmic reticulum appeared to parallel one another [26, 62, 76]. Similar results have also been obtained from Katagiri's laboratory [65, 66] and in this instance were compared with the ultrastructural progression of ischemic injury [77].

Even though such reports provide circumstantial evidence supporting the lysosomal hypothesis of ischemic injury, the interpretation of such observations is complicated by several factors. First, even with improved lysosomal extraction [19, 20], the rise in non-sedimentable enzyme activity might merely reflect an enhanced susceptibility of a dilated lysosomal complement [3, 7, 55] to mechanical shear force rather than a true diffusion of the acid hydrolases into ischemic myoplasm. A further important caveat to such biochemical measurements is that, by themselves, this experimental approach cannot distinguish changes in myocytic lysosomes from those that might develop within the interstitial population, which has a well developed lysosomal vacuolar apparatus [22, 28]. Secondly, while acid phosphatase and aryl sulfatase are considered classic histochemical markers for the lysosome and are, therefore, useful in the study of cardiac lysosomal behavior, they are unlikely to be meaningfully involved in the degradation of cardiac membranous and myofibrillar proteins, for example [78, 79]. Although our laboratory [28, 29] as well as others [3, 26, 27, 37, 38, 65, 66, 77] have successfully employed acid hydrolase cytochemistry to monitor lysosomal alterations in ischemic and hypoxic heart and liver, careful interpretation of such observations is crucial in verifying the lysosomal hypothesis. For example, the depletion and redistribution of acid phosphatase and sulfatase reaction products in ischemically damaged myocytes [26, 28, 29, 66, 77] and hepatocytes [80] may, in fact not reflect true enzyme release, rather the differential inactivation of lysosomal enzyme activity during tissue preparation. Since cytochemically generated reaction products are also known to diffuse from enzymatic reaction sites [81], the presence of lead or barium precipitates does not *a priori* reveal the location of the enzyme itself. Third and perhaps most germane to the present discussion, much of the lysosomal enzyme redistribution reported in the literature appears to develop after 1–5 hours of ischemia and, therefore, probably represents post-necrotic damage. Although significant lysosomal changes accompany ischemic injury, previous experimental approaches have lacked the appropriate sensitivity to affirm or refute the lysosomal hypothesis of ischemic injury.

Our laboratory has established several criteria that we believe to be crucial in testing the lysosomal hypothesis. (1) A biochemical redistribution of lysosomal enzyme activity must precede the development of irreversible cell injury. (2) The lysosomal change must be of myocytic origin and the enzyme protein in question must be localized at an intracellular site displaying structural evidence of damage. (3) If possible, an approach should be employed to demonstrate that the enzyme itself is in a catalytically active state [44, 45]. (4) The enzyme(s) should proteolyze and/or hydrolyze 'significant' cardiac macromolecules both *in vitro* and *in vivo*. (5) Lastly, and perhaps most difficult, some attempt should be made to correlate the hydrolysis of specific macromolecules with the loss of vital cell function. Employing these standards, our laboratory has expended a considerable effort in documenting the redistribution of a major lysosomal proteinase, cathepsin D, in ischemic heart. We have advanced the notion that a proteolytic attack on crucial myocyte proteins might conceivably interfere with vitally important subcellular activities. Cathepsin D was chosen not because it was 'the proteinase' responsible for mediating irreversible damage, but because it is a well characterized acidic endopeptidase [79] located principally in cardiac myocytes [41, 47] and has been documented to degrade myofibrillar proteins *in vitro* [43, 82–84]. This acid proteinase fulfills several of our criteria and, thus, represents a degradative enzyme amenable to experimental evaluation.

After occluding the circumflex branch of the left coronary artery, serial measurements of non-sedimentable cathepsin D activity (Fig. 1) and paired immunofluorescence experiments (Fig. 4) revealed that redistribution of cathepsin D [22, 24] could be demonstrated prior to structural evidence of irreversible ischemic injury [22, 28]. Within 30 minutes of the onset of coronary artery ligation, cathepsin D could be visualized within dilated lysosomes and in the neighboring myoplasm [40]. Anti-cathepsin D immunoperoxidase reaction products appear preferentially associated with adjacent myocyte membranes and elements of the contractile apparatus (Fig. 5). Although the morphology of these ischemic myocytes is distorted and suboptimal because of the stringent requirements for localizing cathepsin D, the enzyme could be routinely observed outside the confines of the lysosome prior to that time when mitochondria acquired osmiophilic densities and sarcolemmal lesions appeared [28], which are structural abnormalities indicative of irreversible damage [8, 10]. If the ischemic insult is prolonged beyond 30 minutes then evidence of diffusely distributed cathepsin D (Fig. 6) can be routinely observed on myofibrillar elements and associated with disruptions of the sarcolemma (Fig. 7). Furthermore, using fluorescein-conjugated active site directed inhibitors of the dinitrophenyl-pepstatin category [45], we suggest that the cathepsin D localized to non-lysosomal intracellular sites represents native enzyme capable of proteolytic activity (Fig. 8). This novel approach provides the first documented evidence that this acid proteinase can remain functional within an ischemic environment. Extending the period of ischemia beyond one hour results in further diffusion of cathepsin D with a concomitant decline in recognizable, intact lysosomes; however, under such circumstances, the lysosomal complement of the interstitial cell population displays no apparent loss in lysosomal integrity [22]. Our observations clearly

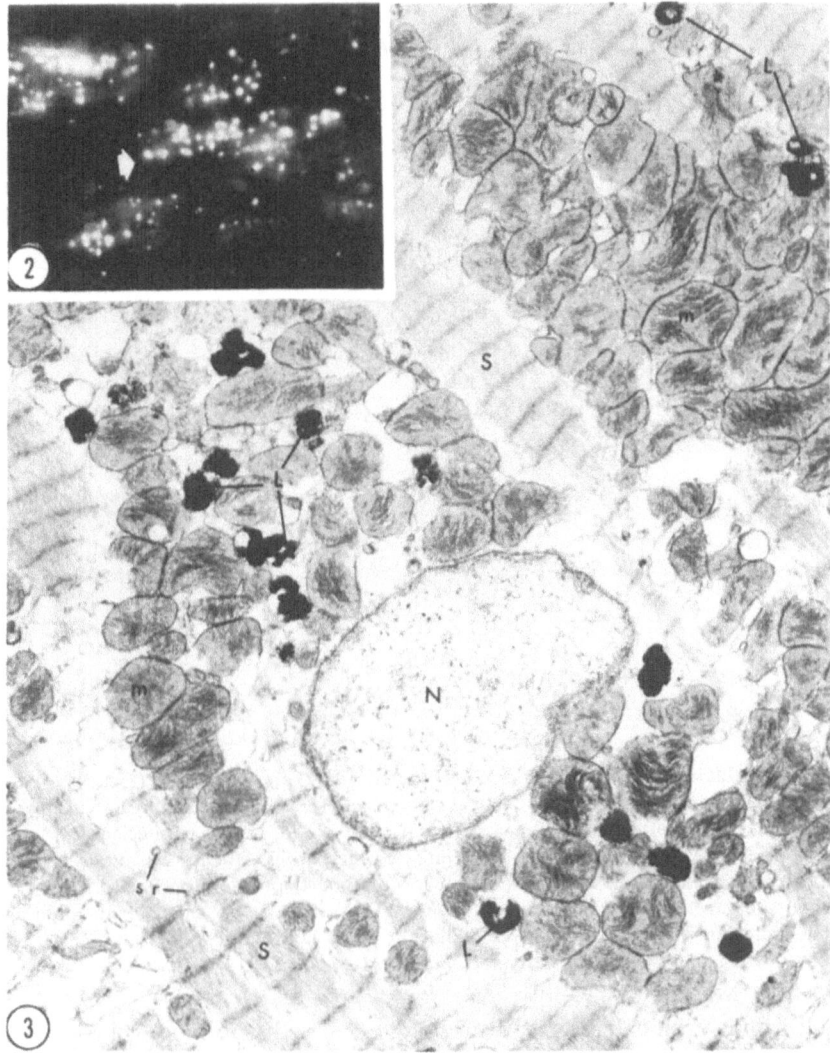

Figs. 2 and 3. Figures illustrate the normal distribution of cathepsin D in the fluorescence (Fig. 2) and electron (Fig. 3) microscopes. Immunofluorescence reveals numerous aggregates (arrows) of brightly staining granules, most of which exhibit a perinuclear location. In the electron microscope, vivid deposits of peroxidase reaction product are observed on many secondary lysosomes (L), partially surrounding myocytic nuclei (N). Other positively stained lysosomes are interspersed among mitochondria (m) and myofibrils (S). Elements of the sarcoplasmic reticulum (sr) do not contain significant amounts of reaction product in normal myocytes. Figure 2 = x720; Figure 3 = x12,150.

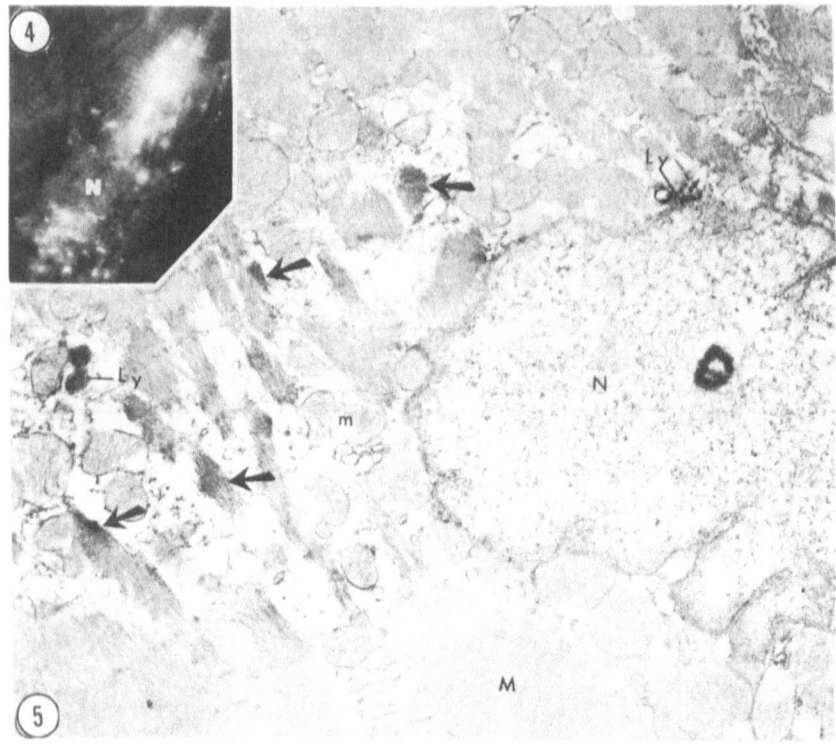

Figs. 4 and 5. Illustrate the distribution of fluorescein (Fig. 4) and peroxidase (Fig. 5) labelled antibodies directed against lysosomal cathepsin D in subendocardial myocytes 30 minutes after ligation of the circumflex coronary artery. Note the diffuse perinuclear (N) location of the enzyme (arrows) within the injured myocytes (Fig. 4). Ultrastructurally, many lysosomes (L) appear dilated and peroxidase reaction product appears distributed on neighboring organelles and myofibrils (arrowheads). This most likely accounts for the diffuse immunofluorescent staining pattern. Note the lack of amorphous matrix as densities in the mitochondria. Figure 4 = x900; Figure 5= x22,500.

establish that a biochemical and morphological redistribution of lysosomal cathepsin D develops before structural evidence of irreversible injury is apparent in acutely ischemic rabbit subendocardium. Diffusion of this enzymatically active acid proteinase is a specific myocytic response to ischemic injury and provides evidence which supports the lysosomal hypothesis of ischemic injury (Table 1). Such observations should, nevertheless, be tempered with some degree of caution for, while the release of cathepsin D is compatible with the lysosomal hypothesis, it does not demonstrate causality. These results may merely reflect an early feature of a more generalized cell damage which accompanies ischemia [10, 15].

The inherent biological variation that accompanies the occlusion of a coronary artery in animal models has prompted the study of isolated perfused

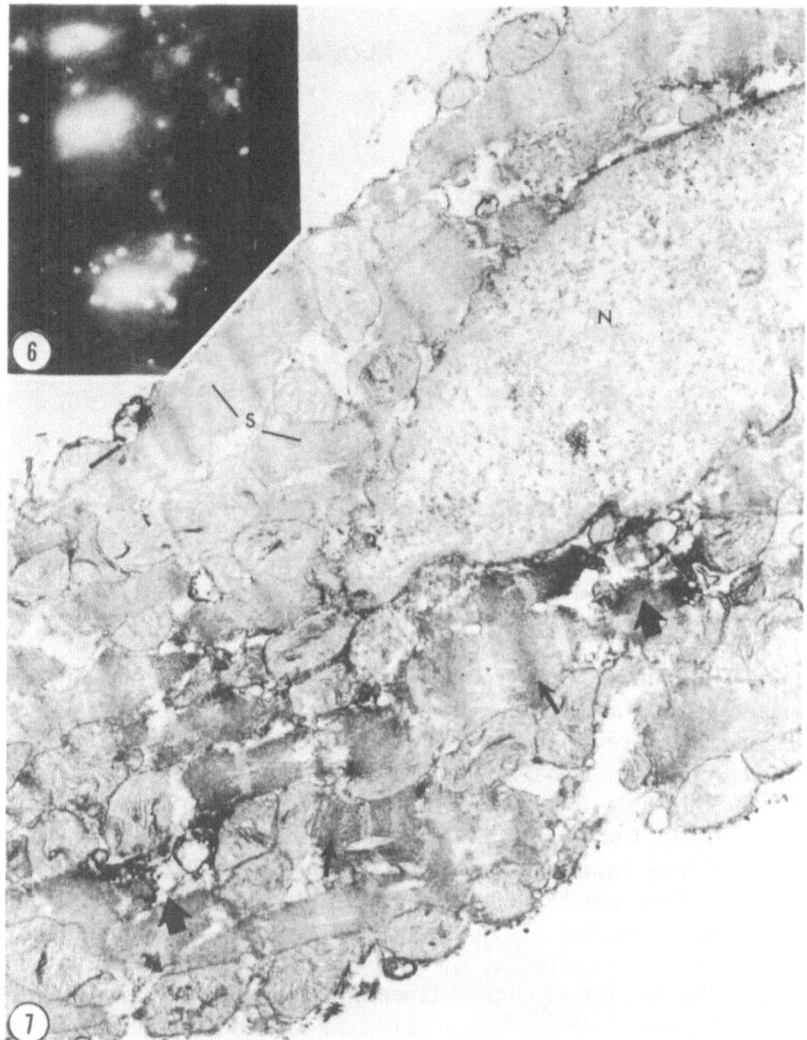

Figs. 6 and 7. Demonstrate the diffuse distribution of cathepsin D that attends irreversible cell injury. Imunofluorescence microscopy illustrates cathepsin D positive halos and dilated lysosomes (Fig. 6) while peroxidase reaction product is apparent throughout the myoplasm at one hour of ischemia. Figure 6 = 850x; Figure 7 = 25,500x.

hearts under precisely controlled conditions. While such preparations circumvent, for the most part, heterogeneous cell injury that characterizes *in vivo* ischemia, they can only approximate *in vivo* ischemia by either globally reducing coronary flow or by perfusing under hypoxic and/or substrate deprived conditions. Welman and Peters [63] as well as Chua and associates [64] documented a significant increase in non-sedimentable acid hydrolase

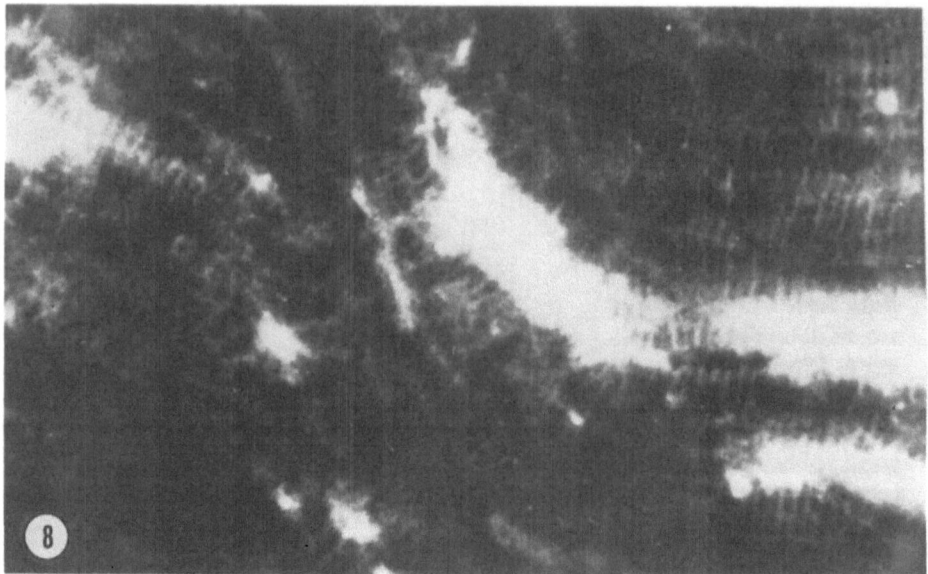

Fig. 8. This figure reveals that fluorescein labeled pepstatin binds to lysosomal and myofibrillar cathepsin D, demonstrating the presence of active enzyme. Figure 8 = 1500x.

during the first hour of either hypoxic perfusion or global ischemia. However, no structural studies accompanied these biochemical experiments, making the conclusions drawn regarding changes in lysosomal latency difficult, at best, to interpret. McCallister *et al.* [55], though, illustrated that low flow, global ischemia promotes the formation of autophagic vacuoles in rat hearts during the first 30 minutes of perfusion. Therefore, the redistribution of lysosomal enzyme activity in this model may either reflect a true subcellular release of enzyme or the appearance of a more fragile class of lysosomes that are readily disrupted during isolation [3, 7]. When a biochemical and immunofluorescence analysis was conducted on hypoxic, substrate-depleted perfused rabbit hearts, marked elevations in non-sedimentable cathepsin D were recognized within 20–40 minutes (Table 2) but such changes in lysosomal latency were *not* accompanied by enzyme release [7, 56]. Like globally ischemic rat hearts, autophagic vacuoles develop within the first 30 minutes of hypoxia [56] – a phenomena *not* mimicked in ischemic rabbit myocardium [28]. If hypoxia was extended beyond one hour, a biochemical and immunofluorescence redistribution of cathepsin D can be readily appreciated in these injured myocytes [7]. However, at this juncture the damage incurred appears irreversible for contractile function cannot be restored upon reoxyganation. Thus, in this hypoxic model early changes in lysosomal latency appear correlated with the formation of a fragile complement of lysosomes and *not* enzyme release *per se*. Only after irreversible injury is lysosomal rupture apparent, implying that in hypoxic heart, irreversible damage may proceed without significant redistribution of lysosomal enzymes. Although *in vitro* preparations offer the advantage of a reproducible and homogeneous response to controlled changes in

Table 2. Influence of hypoxia and reoxygenation on the biochemical distribution of cathepsin D activity in rabbit hearts.

Normoxia	Hypoxia × 20min	Hypoxia × 20min + Reoxygenation × 30min	Hypoxia × 40min	Hypoxia × 40min + Reoxygenation × 30min	Hypoxia × 60min	Hypoxia × 60min + Reoxygenation × 30min
38±2%	43±3%	41±6%	46±3%*	41±6%	56±4%*	58±7%*

Each value represents the mean ± 1 SEM of 10 hearts, expressed as the percentage of total (sedimentable + non-sedimentable) cathepsin D activity that was present in the non-sedimentable fraction.
* 0.01 by Students' t-test for unpaired samples, compared to normoxia.

the extracellular environment, clearly release of cathepsin D develops earlier in ischemic myocardium than in hypoxic heart.

Modification of lysosomal responses in ischemic and hypoxic heart

A variety of therapeutic interventions have been employed to minimize the spread of intracellular damage that develops in ischemic or hypoxic heart [85–87]. Most are administered to improve coronary flow, thereby enhancing oxygen supply and eliminating harmful metabolites or decreasing myocardial demand for oxygen while simultaneously stimulating anaerobic pathways. Since major alterations in membrane structure and permeability are a prominent characteristic of ischemically injured myocytes, others have employed a variety of agents which are believed to act directly on phospholipid membranes in an effort to 'stabilize' them and, presumably, afford such 'stabilized membranes' some degree of protection from 'ischemic attack'. A variety of pharmacologic approaches have been employed to prevent lysosomal enzyme release and to inhibit lysosomal and non-lysosomal proteinases and phospholipases in ischemic myocardium.

Glucocorticoids were among the first group of reported membrane stabilizing agents employed to ameliorate ischemic myocyte damage. The efficacy of their use was based upon Weissmann's [88, 89] experiments which demonstrated that certain steroids prevented the rupture of lysosomes when they were exposed to thermal activation or osmotic stress *in vitro*. Since many of these natural and synthetic glucocorticoids inhibited the release of lysosomal enzymes from activated neutrophils, Weissmann [89] concluded that steroids also interfered with membrane traffic in these phagocytes. These two observations represent the premise upon which glucocorticoids were subsequently used to 'stabilize' cell membranes, i.e., they limited the movement of proteins in and out of membrane-bound compartments and inhibited intracellular membrane flow.

Corticosteriod therapy has been implemented extensively to stabilize cardiac lysosomes in ischemic and hypoxic myocardium with rather mixed results [7]. Several groups purported to demonstrate lysosomal stabilization and a reduction of ischemic necrosis [27, 90–92] while other carefully conducted studies revealed no correlations between steroid treatment and non-sedimentable lysosomal activity [73, 93]. Experiments in our laboratory appear to have resolved some of these discrepancies, which we believe reflect the use of different ischemic models and modes of steroid administration [23, 29]. Parallel use of biochemical, immunofluorescence and fine structural techniques to investigate the redistribution of cathepsin D revealed that therapeutic doses of the synthetic glucocorticoid, methylprednisolone, stabilized lysosomes and inhibited the rise in non-sedimentable acid hydrolase activity, prevented the immunohistochemical leakage of cathepsin D from such stabilized organelles (Figs. 9–12) and slowed structural signs of irreversible cell injury [29]. However, at one hour enzyme redistribution was apparent in ischemic homogenates, cathepsin D appeared intracellularly and myocytes displayed overt signs of irreversible damage. Our observations convey the impression that steroids can only influence lysosomal integrity and delay ischemic injury transiently in a model where coronary flow is reduced more than 85% as measured by the distribution of radioactive microspheres. Although corticosteroids may be more effective in protecting less severely ischemic myocardium, it seems probable that in regions of acutely ischemic heart, methylprednisolone only postpones the onset of lysosomal enzyme release and irreversible cell injury. Even though the delay in cathepsin D redistribution and the development of cell injury are compatible with the lysosomal hypothesis, our observations might reflect other mechanisms that secondarily stabilize the lysosome and other membranous elements of the myocyte. Therefore, our 'positive' results do not directly resolve this cause and effect issue [5].

Lysosomotropic weak bases like chloroquine also markedly alter lysosomal properties [94] including those in the heart [95]. Such compounds elevate intralysosomal pH [39, 96, 97], inhibit protein degradation [35, 98, 99] and inactivate lysosomal cathepsin B activity [35, 97, 98] in cardiac myocytes and other cell types. In response to these combined actions, the cardiac lysosomal vacuolar apparatus dilates significantly [38, 95] and rates of proteolysis are markedly depressed [38, 99]. At the doses employed to provoke these lysosomal alterations, lysosomal stabilization is an early consequence of chloroquine treatment in cultured hearts [95]. Welman and Peters [92] further reported that chloroquine prevented increases in non-sedimentable lysosomal enzyme activity that are normally encountered in anoxic guinea pig hearts. The degree of stabilization was similar to that obtained when anoxic perfusion medium was supplemented with corticosteroids rather than the weak base. Although such results suggest that chloroquine is a useful lysosomal membrane stabilizer, our laboratory demonstrated that prolonged exposure to this lysosomotropic agent, in fact, promotes a loss in lysosomal latency that

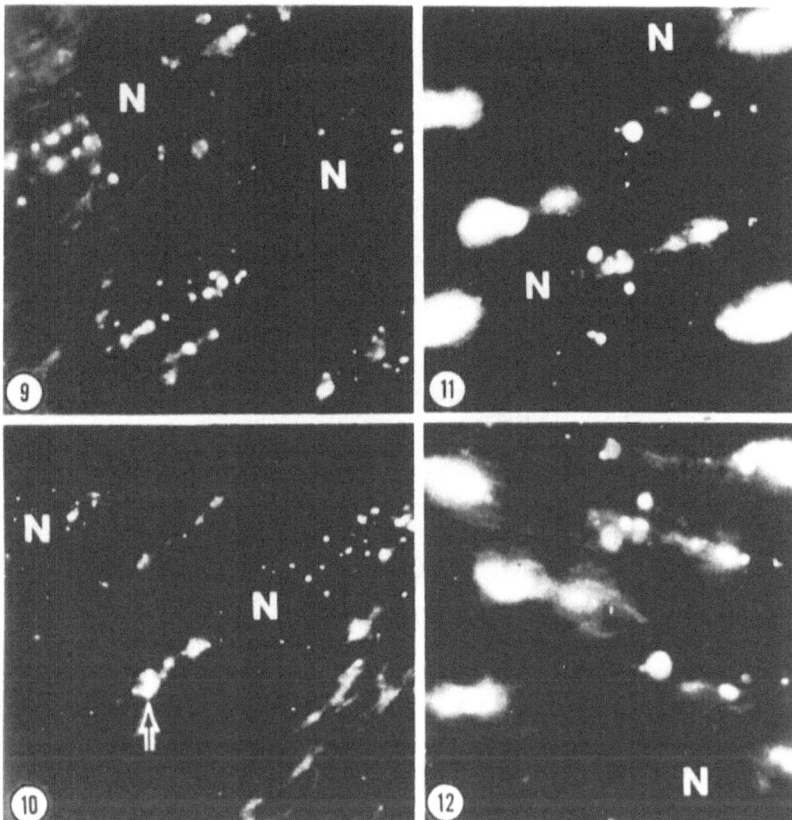

Figs. 9–12. Disclose changes in the distribution in lysosomal cathepsin D during ischemia and the effects of methylprednisolone on cathepsin D localization. Fig. 9 (30 minute ischemia), Fig. 10 (45 minute ischemia), and Fig. 11 (60 minute ischemia) demonstrate that the steroid protects cardiac lysosomes for 45 minutes (compare Fig. 4); at 1 hour prominent fluorescent halos are apparent in steroid-treated myocytes (Fig. 11), and these cells are indistinguishable from untreated cells after 1 hour of ischemia (Fig. 12). Myocyte Nuclei (N). Figures 9–12 = x578.

appears positively correlated with continued vacuolar swelling [95]. Thus, while weak bases may stabilize lysosomes in perfused hearts, their long term use at doses required to influence lysosomal structure and function, limits their usefulness in a therapeutic role.

Critical alterations in phospholipid metabolism are also closely correlated with the development of irreversible ischemic injury in liver [3, 100, 101] and heart [102]. *In vivo* pretreatment with chlorpromazine, a potent inhibitor of several phospholipases, including some of lysosomal origin [103–105], decreased cell injury, reduced phospholipid degradation and prevented calcium influx [106] in ischemic liver and partially suppressed phospholipid breakdown and changes in membrane permeability in ischemic myocardium [102,

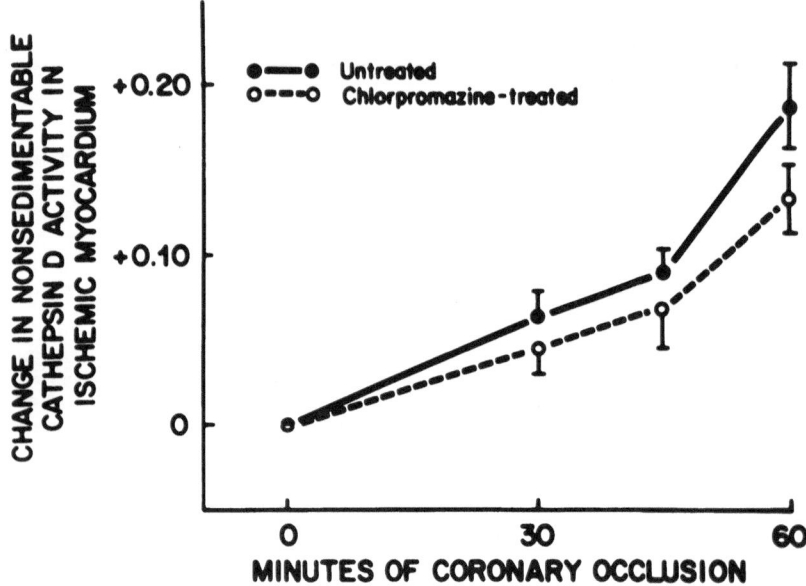

Fig. 13 Redistribution of cathepsin D activity in ischemic myocardium of untreated (•) and chlorpromazine-treated (o) rabbits. Differences between the fraction of non-sedimentable cathespin D activity in ischemic and non-ischemic sections of each heart are displayed. Each point represents the mean ± 1 SEM of 11–15 hearts.

107, 108]. Chien and Farber proposed that phospholipid breakdown was mediated by membrane delimited phospholipases that were activated as intracellular calcium levels rose during ischemia. Perhaps the release of latent phospholipases with acidic pH optima might be especially detrimental in this regard [105, 109].

Since chlorpromazine has been documented to stabilize lysosomes prepared from ischemic liver [3, 80], our laboratory investigated the redistribution of cardiac lysosomal cathepsin D in rabbits pretreated with chlorpromazine prior to coronary artery ligation. Employing doses of chlorpromazine comparable to those used in the ischemic liver models, only minimal stabilization of lysosomal cathepsin D could be documented in ischemic rabbit heart (Fig. 13). Although this 'protective effect' was statistically significant, the temporal development of diffuse cathepsin D staining and the evolution of structural damage that attended irreversible ischemic injury were not altered by drug treatment [110]. Furthermore, it is clear that chlorpromazine is significantly less effective than methylprednisolone, for example, in stabilizing lysosomes in the same rabbit model [7, 23]. The question remains, however, which of chlorpromazine's well-known pharmacologic actions are operative in the ischemic myocardium. If the release of membrane-delimited hydrolases is of functional importance in contributing to the development of ischemic injury, drugs in the chlorpromazine group may not offer a rational approach to reducing ischemic injury in the heart.

A variety of other therapeutic agents which are reported to stabilize cardiac lysosomes also reduce ischemic or hypoxic damage. The β adrenergic blocker, propranolol, reportedly stabilizes lysosomes in anoxically perfused guinea pig hearts to about the same degree as corticosteroids and lysosomotropic compounds [111]. Moreover, this β blocker reputedly blocks the degradation of myofibrillar proteins and appears to inhibit the release of lysosomal cathepsins B, D, L that develop in ischemic canine myocardium [68]. Propranolol is also reported to inhibit a variety of cardiac phospholipases, thereby reducing phospholipid degradation during ischemic injury [112, 113]. Mepindolol, a newly introduced β blocker, also appears to preferentially reduce phospholipid breakdown in ischemic heart [114]. The calcium channel blockers, nifedipine [115] and diltiazem [116], also limit lysosomal cathepsin D redistribution in hypoxic cat and rat heart as well as preserving high energy phosphates in the damaged hearts. Such observations imply that calcium loading labilizes lysosomal membranes. Monoamine oxidase inhibitors [71], prostaglandins E_1 and E_2 [117] and prostacyclin [118] among others, are all linked with lysosomal stabilization during ischemic and hypoxic injury. Lastly, when the thiol proteinase inhibitor, Ep459 [79], is administered prior to coronary occlusion, the degradation of myosin heavy chain, α actinin and troponin I normally observed in ischemic dog heart is significantly reduced by this active site-directed inhibitor [119]. Since the electrophoretic pattern of 'infarcted myofibrils' is similar to the pattern obtained when myofibrillar proteins are degraded by partially purified lysosomal cathepsins B and L, it implicates these proteinases in contractile protein damage of the variety visualized in ischemic heart [40, 119]. It must be emphasized, however, that Ep459 is likely to inhibit the calcium-dependent cysteine proteinases present in the heart, which also appear to be activated during ischemia [120].

From this brief summary it is clear that a variety of therapeutic agents with unique pharmacologic properties appear to stabilize lysosomal structure and preserve myocardial integrity during an ischemic or hypoxic insult. The implication from these diverse observations is that the release of lysosomal enzymes mediates the evolving intracellular damage. Such assumptions are unlikely, for any intervention that limits ischemic injury will prevent lysosomal disruption. For example, ligating a coronary artery of a heart from a rabbit deprived of food, results in little structural evidence of irreversible ischemic injury or lysosomal enzyme release for up to 90 minutes (Fig. 14) after occlusion [40]. Whatever pathophysiologic changes of fasting that confer this degree of protection and allow the starved rabbit heart to resist ischemia, increases in non-sedimentable cathepsin D still transpire in association with irreversible injury. Therefore, correlations between lysosomal stabilization and the alleviation of ischemic damage should not be assumed to imply a lysosomal or membrane action of the agent being examined in the absence of

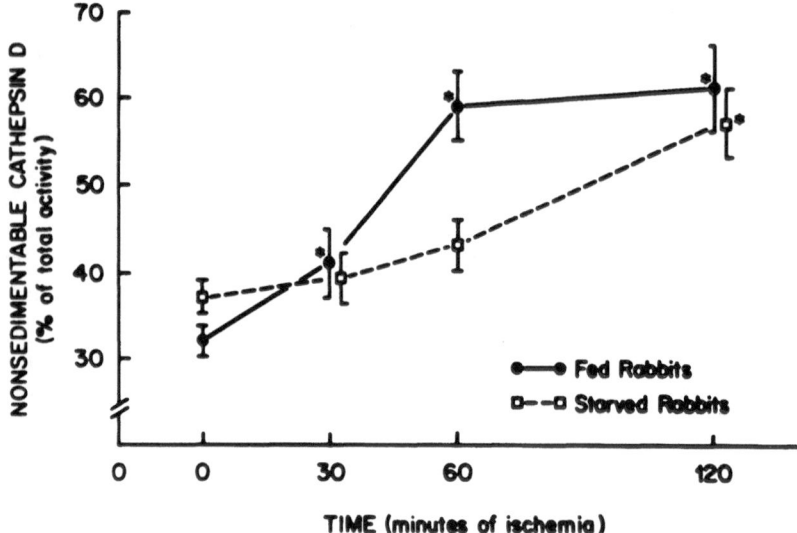

Fig. 14. Changes in the biochemical distribution of cathepsin D activity in ischemic myocardium of fed and starved rabbits. Each point represents the mean − 1 standard error of the mean of at least six animals with values expressed as the proportion of total enzyme activity (non-sedimentable + sedimentable) that was present in the non-sedimentable fraction. Asterisk, p<0.05 compared to non-ischemic tissue in the same group.

some other compelling reason to suggest a primary influence of the intervention on lysosomal latency. Even when an agent seems to directly act upon the lysosome, it remains plausible that the stabilization encountered may represent a totally unrelated action.

Lysosomal responses in reperfused and reoxygenated hearts

When the duration of the ischemic or hypoxic episode is relatively brief, restitution of coronary flow or reoxygenation results in little or no cell death and complete recovery of contractile function (121, 122). If, however, the insult is prolonged, reversibly injured myocytes pass the 'point of no return' and upon reperfusion or reoxygenation, die [10, 15]. Only by re-establishing coronary flow or reoxygenating the perfusate can reversible injury be truly distinguished from irreversible injury by monitoring myocardial structure and function [8, 54]. Even though occluding a coronary artery for as little as 20 minutes significantly depletes high energy phosphate stores [11] and elicits major structural changes in the myocardium [10], upon reperfusion, oxidative phosphorylation resumes and normal contractile function rapidly redevelops [8]. Similarly, hypoxic hearts display essentially the same properties after reoxygenation [53]. Such hearts display little evidence of cell death; moreover, within 15 minutes of reperfusion or reoxygenation, the structural changes that develop in the ischemic or hypoxic myocardium are completely reversed and/or repaired. If, however, either insult is prolonged to 40–60 minutes and beyond, irreversible damage is apparent in an increasing number of myocytes. Under such conditions, irreversibly damaged myocytes swell explosively, develop pycnotic nuclei, contraction bands, mitochondrial amorphous matrix densities, major sarcolemmal discontinuities and lysosomal rupture [7, 10, 53, 121, 122]. These structural lesions are accompanied by hypercontraction, loss of ion regulation, edema, extracellular release of cytoplasmic enzymes like creatine kinase and lactate dehydrogenase and lysosomal enzymes.

During the first day following a myocardial infarction induced by ligating a coronary artery, lysosome-laden neutrophils and macrophages invade the necrotic tissue and phagocytose tissue debris. The removal of these dead myocytes is accompanied by an increase in lysosomal enzyme activity [58, 123], but such changes clearly reflect post-necrotic events not directly involved with the development or repair of ischemic damage in injured myocytes. Nevertheless, several recent investigations suggest that lysosomal alterations which occur during the early phases of hypoxic and ischemic injury and during the recovery from such insults may be primarily concerned with subcellular repair rather than in provoking intracellular damage [3, 7]. Since considerable variability attends coronary occlusion and reflow, our investigations concerning the potential role of lysosomes in the repair of myocytic damage have focused on the perfused hypoxic heart and the cultured fetal mouse heart where more uniform injury and recovery can be controlled and where interventions designed to specifically study lysosomal activity can be monitored carefully [7].

When rabbit hearts are subjected to hypoxic perfusion for one hour, myocytes display morphological signs of irreversible cell injury [56] including the diffusion of cathepsin D from dilated lysosomes [122]. Reoxygenation fails to restore contractility but does initiate an oxygen paradox similar to that noted in reperfused ischemic [8] and reoxygenated hypoxic [53] heart. Lysosomal cathepsin D remains diffusely distributed and non-sedimentable acid proteinase activity continues to increase in reoxygenated hearts (Table 2). Clearly under these conditions, prolonged hypoxia followed by reoxygenation only amplifies the damage to lysosomes as it does to other cell organelles [53, 124].

Conversely, hypoxic perfusions of a briefer duration (20–40 minutes) followed by reoxygenation produces structural and functional damage that is reversible [56]. Like the results obtained by McCallister et al. [55] in globally ischemic rat heart and those in the ischemic liver [3, 80], lysosomal autophagic vacuoles develop early in the course of hypoxia (at 20 minutes). However, reversibly injured rabbit myocytes display a marked autophagic response that develops within 15 to 30 minutes of reoxygenation and is associated with a decline in non-sedimentable cathepsin D activity [122]. Prolonging hypoxia to 40 minutes exacerbates intracellular damage, but reoxygenated hearts resume beating and reacquire normal ultrastructural features that include the development of large autophagic vacuoles which have sequestered damaged mitochondria (Fig. 15). At 30 minutes of reoxygenation, such lysosomes display evidence of lysosomal enzyme reaction products (Fig. 16) confirming that they truly represent autophagic vacuoles [7]. Recovering hearts also reveal diminished levels of non-sedimentable acid proteinase activity (Table 2), indicating that the autophagic vacuoles that appear in recovery are more stable than their hypoxic counterparts. Our results suggest that reversibly injured myocytes appear to employ their lysosomal vacuolar apparatus to eliminate damaged organelles during recovery from hypoxia. The appearance of autophagic vacuoles during the early phases of hypoxia and global ischemia may reflect an early attempt at repair that fails to proceed when ATP and creatine phosphate levels decline, because the sequestration of cell organelles is an energy requiring event. Conversely, irreversibly injured myocytes that exhibit ruptured lysosomes are incapable of initiating an autophagic response during the oxygen paradox [56].

Perfused hearts lack the long-term stability to thoroughly follow the fate of the autophagic vacuoles that develop during reoxygenation. Of major concern is whether the organelles that are sequestered during the early phases of recovery are ultimately degraded and the observations gleaned from perfused hearts, in actuality, represent the repair of subcellular hypoxic injury. To answer this question we turned to another ischemic model, the well characterized fetal mouse heart [125]. When subjected to hypoxia and glucose deprivation for 1–3 hours, ATP levels decline, morphological evidence of hypoxic damage develops (Fig. 17) but no major shifts in lysosomal latency have been documented [125, 126]. The resupply of oxygen and substrate facilitates recovery which can be studied for at least 24 hours. As in the adult hypoxic heart, reversibly injured fetal hearts commence beating and exhibit a dramatic lysosomal response during recovery [37]. At as early as five minutes of reoxygenation lysosomal dense bodies appear and the Golgi apparatus hypertrophies (Fig. 18). Autophagic vacuoles sequester these damaged organelles over the next 15 minutes (Fig. 19) and appear to become activated when they fuse with enzyme-laden dense bodies. Once this event transpires these large autophagic vacuoles gradually disappear as their contents are, presumably, degraded to constituent amino acids and fatty acids by resident lysosomal proteinases and phospholipases [37]. The entire process appears to be completed within six hours when the lysosomal size profile returns to a value that is indistinguishable from normoxic hearts (Fig. 20). These observations strongly support the contention that the lysosomal vacuolar apparatus is intimately involved with the resolution of subcellular damage incurred in reversibly injured hearts [37]. The disruption of this complex membranous compartment that transpires at or near the point of irreversible cell injury would, in all likelihood, preclude mounting any effective lysosomally mediated repair processes upon reperfusion or reoxygenation. Thus, lyso-

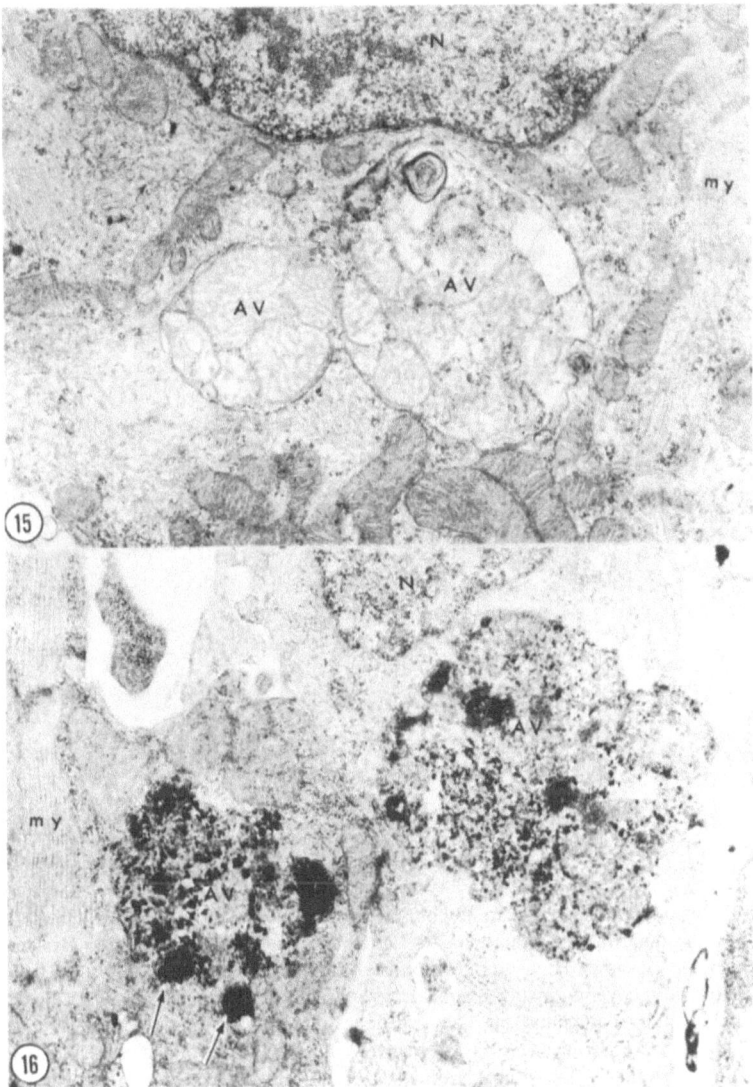

Figs. 15 and 16. Depict the autophagic vacuoles that developed within 30 min of reoxygenation following 40 minutes of hypoxic perfusion. Figure 15 reveals the presence of damaged mitochondria and membranous elements within these vacuoles (AV) in the perinuclear region of the myocyte. Figure 16 demonstrates the presence of acid phosphatase reaction product within such lysosomal vacuoles (AV). Figures 15, 16 = x 20,000.

somal rupture just prior to the onset of irreversible injury might be expected to hasten intracellular damage, while simultaneously eliminating a major repairative pathway [7, 37].

Since a variety of lysosomally active agents are known to stabilize or alter lysosomal activity in ischemic or hypoxic hearts [7], a similar pharmacologic

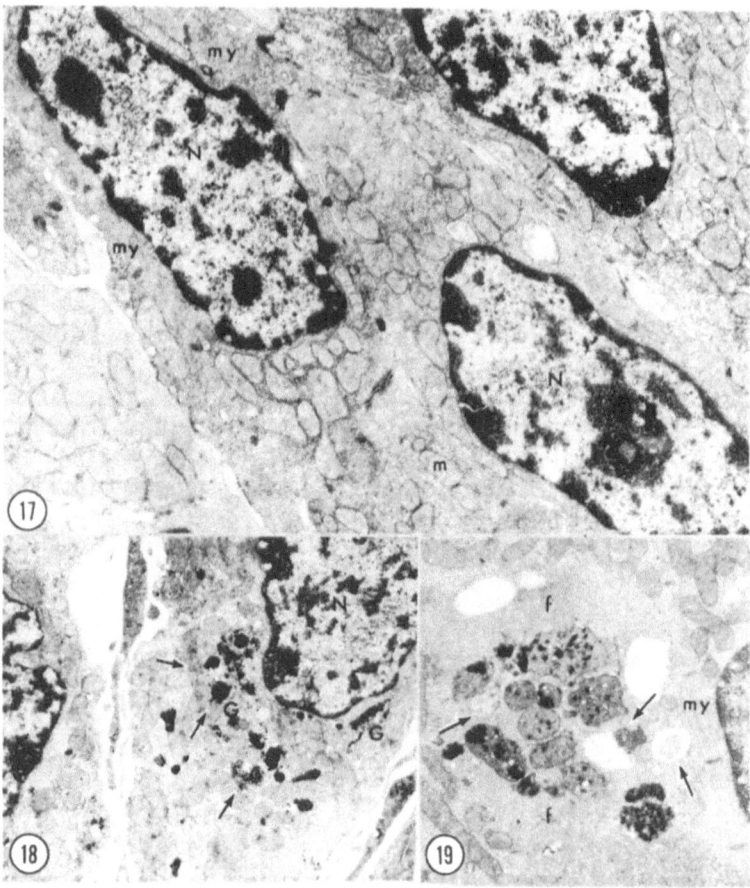

Figs. 17–19. Reveals the effect of a one hour anoxic insult on fetal myocyte structure (Fig. 17) and the lysosomal response that appears within 15 minutes of reoxygenation (arrows) (Fig. 18). Figure 19 shows damaged mitochondria just prior to their removal by autophagic mechanisms. The recovering myocyte appears to upregulate lysosomal packaging (Fig. 18) while simultaneously segregating damaged organelles (arrows) for ultimate removal and degradation (Fig. 19). Nucleus (N), myofibrils (my), mitochondria (m), microfilaments (f). Figures 17–19 = x8,000.

approach was employed to determine whether 'lysosomal stabilization' prior to and during recovery might jeopardize the development of this putative repair pathway. The reoxygenated, hypoxic fetal hearts were exposed to therapeutic doses of chloroquine, colchicine, leupeptin and corticosteroid and recovery was monitored cytochemically and morphologically [38]. In the presence of the lysosomotropic weak base, which stabilizes fetal heart lysosomes [95], inhibits proteolysis [127] and elevates intralysosomal pH [39], the lysosomal response normally encountered does not develop during recovery and damaged organelles remain randomly scattered throughout the myo-

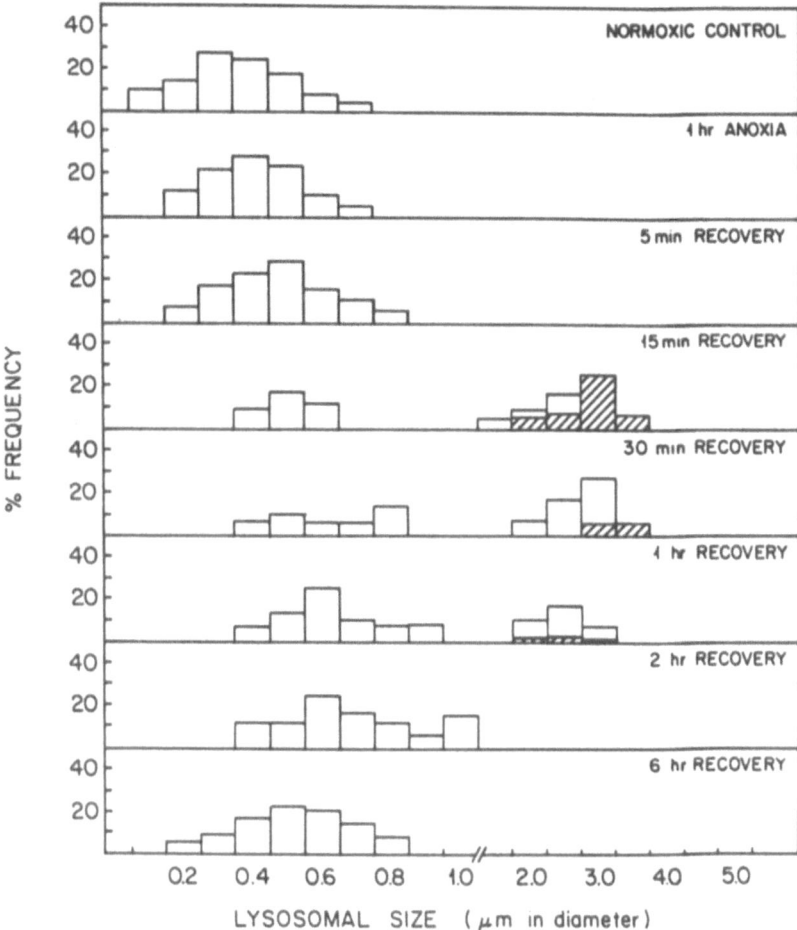

Fig. 20. Illustrates the change in diameter of fetal myocyte lysosomes in normoxic, anoxic and reoxygenated fetal hearts. Large autophagic vacuoles develop within 15 minutes of recovery and persist for 30–90 minutes. After six hours the lysosomal size distribution reveals that the lysosomal population of normoxic and recovered hearts are indistinguishable. The diameter of all lysosomes was measured from 50 randomly selected electron micrographs obtained from normoxic, anoxic and recovering hearts. The % frequency of the lysosomal population is plotted against lysosomal size. Cross-hatched bars represent lysosomes that fail to exhibit acid hydrolase activity.

plasm of recovering fetal myocytes. Similarly, colchicine also inhibits the formation of autophagic vacuoles [128]. Although this alkaloid is not known to directly stabilize lysosomal membranes, its ability to prevent microtubule assembly may interfere with the formation of autophagic vacuoles and the delivery of lysosomal enzymes to them in a manner similar to that reported for neutrophils where phagocytic vacuoles fail to develop in the presence of colchicine [129, 130]. Colchicine also depresses cardiac protein degradation in fetal hearts [127], further implicating microtubules as, perhaps, a central structural element regulating autophagy.

Conversely, recovering fetal hearts treated with either leupeptin or hydrocortisone appear to generate autophagic vacuoles, but both drugs delay or prevent their resorption and disappearance [38]. Since leupeptin is known to inhibit the lysosomal cysteine proteinases cathepsins B, H and L (78, 79) and suppress protein degradation in fetal hearts [127], it is likely that the autophagic vacuoles that develop probably function inefficiently because several of the enzymes responsible for proteolysis are inhibited. Hydrocortisone also prevents the regression of these lysosomes; however, in this instance the mechanism of corticosteroid action is not clear. Recovering fetal hearts retain an enlarged population of autophagic vacuoles when these hearts are allowed to recover in the presence of the corticosteroid [38]. These vacuoles lack demonstrable acid hydrolase activity even though positively stained dense bodies are frequently encountered in the neighborhood [38]. Such results suggest that the fusion of dense bodies, which probably provide the acid hydrolases required for degradation, is inhibited in the presence of the steroid [88, 89]. This phenomena may well be related to the generally poor healing that accompanies steroid therapy following myocardial infarctions [131]. Although the use of these therapeutic interventions do not directly implicate the lysosome in the repair of hypoxic damage, the present observations strongly support their role in this activity [3, 7].

The lysosomal hypothesis – future directions

Observations collected over the last decade clearly demonstrate that a major subcellular redistribution of lysosomal acid hydrolases accompanies the progression of ischemic and hypoxic myocardial injury. Further, these enzymes which are normally sequestered away from cytoplasmic constituents, diffuse into the surrounding acidotic environment at or just prior to the development of irreversible cell injury. The presence of one lysosomal proteinase, cathepsin D, which has been located in its native-active state at sites of overt subcellular damage, is compatible with the lysosomal hypothesis of ischemic injury. If the lysosomal hypothesis is expanded to include other hydrolytic enzymes that are known to reside in the sarcoplasmic reticulum (for example, the neutral phospholipases) or those cytoplasmic phospholipases [105, 109] and the calcium-dependent neutral proteinases which have been implicated in mediating cytoskeletal damage in ischemic and hypoxic hearts [132, 133], then it is not difficult to imagine that the activation of latent and non-latent proteinases and phospholipases might mediate the degradation of key macromolecules transforming a reversibly damaged myocyte into a necrotic one.

Nevertheless, it should be re-emphasized that the release of acid or neutral hydrolases into the acidotic milieu of an ischemic myocyte does not prove that the damage observed is the direct result of their release and action; it is equally likely that these changes may result from some other injurious event and that the temporal association between enzyme redistribution and evolving damage is purely coincidental. For example, free radical generating systems promote lysosomal membrane lipid peroxidation and the release of lysosomal acid hydrolases [134]; moreover, antioxidants appear to inhibit lysosomal enzyme redistribution [135]. Observations such as these tend to support this contention. Similarly the stabilization of lysosomes mediated by other pharmacologic agents (pp. 127–132) also conforms to the lysosomal hypothesis; but such beneficial influences might be mediated through an independent mechanism which improves cell viability and preserves lysosomal integrity. Thus, current approaches have documented clearly that major lysosomal changes attend ischemic and hypoxic injury, but these studies cannot presently distinguish cause from effect. If, however, the lysosomal hypothesis is false even in its broadest sense, then it may be possible to dissociate changes in lysosomal latency from evolving damage. Further modifications of the hypothesis will require an intensified effort to determine whether such a dissociation can be identified under differing experimental conditions.

Whether it is ultimately established that the release of latent lysosomal enzymes mediates cell death, recent evidence clearly suggests that an intact, functional lysosomal vacuolar apparatus plays an important role in subcellular repair during recovery from sublethal hypoxia and ischemic-like stresses. Activation of an autophagic response represents an early feature of recovery and appears responsible for the sequestration and ultimate degradation of damaged organelles. Further, if future efforts to specifically stabilize lysosomes or inhibit their resident enzymes do indeed reduce or delay the development of ischemic necrosis, it is conceivable that such an improvement may ultimately interfere with the myocardium's repairative processes; therefore, future efforts must continue to be directed towards elucidating the basic cellular mechanism(s) which underlie ischemic and hypoxic injury and repair.

Acknowledgements

The authors are indebted to the effort and support of Drs. Kern Wildenthal, Robin Poole and John Dingle whose role in these investigations was crucial from their inception to their completion. The studies reported here were funded by grants from the National Heart, Lung and Blood Institute, the Moss Heart Fund and the American Heart Association.

References

1. de Duve C (1959) Lysosomes. In: T Hayashi (ed) Subcellular Particles pp 128–159 Ronald Press, New York.

140

2. de Duve C and Beaufay H (1955) Tissue fractionation studies. Influence of ischemia on the state of some bound enzymes in rat liver. Biochem J 73: 610–616

3. Wattiaux R and Wattiaux-DeConinck S (1984) Effects of ischemia on lysosomes. Int Rev Exp Path 26: 85–106

4. Wildenthal K (1975) Lysosomes and lysosomal enzymes in the heart. In: JT Dingle and RT Dean (eds) Lysosomes in Biology and Pathology. Vol 4. North Holland Publ. Co., Amsterdam pp 167–190

5. Wildenthal K (1978) Lysosomal alterations in ischemic myocardium: Result or cause of myocellular damage? J Mol Cell Cardiol 10: 595–603

6. Weismann G. Hoffstein S, Gennaro D and Fox AC (1977) Lysosomes in ischemic myocardium, with observations on the effects of methylprednisolone. In: AM Lefer, GJ Kelliker and MJ Rovetto (eds) Pathophysiology and Therapeutics of Myocardial Ischemia Spectrum Publ. Inc., New York pp 367–379

7. Decker RS and Wildenthal K (1980) Role of lysosomes and latent hydrolytic enzymes in ischemic damage and repair of the heart. In: K Wildenthal (ed) Degradative Processes in Heart and Skeletal Muscle. Elsevier-North Holland Biomed. Press, Amsterdam pp 389–418

8. Kloner RA, Ganote CE, Whalen DA Jr and Jennings RB (1974) Effects of a transient period of ischemia on myocardial cells. II. Fine structure during the first few minutes of reflow. Am J Pathol 399–422

9. Trump BF, Mergner WJ, Kahng MW and Saladino AJ (1976) Studies on the subcellular pathophysiology of ischemia. Circ 53 (Suppl 1): 17–26

10. Jennings RB and Hawkins HK (1980) Ultrastructural changes in acute myocardial ischemia. In: K Wildenthal (ed) Degradative Processes in Heart and Skeletal Muscle. Elsevier-North Holland Biomed. Press, Amsterdam pp 295–346

11. Jennings RB, Hawkins HK, Lowe JE, Hill ML, Klotman S and Reimer KA (1978) Relation between high energy phosphate and lethal injury in myocardial ischemia in the dog. Am J Pathol 92: 187–214

12. Reimer KA, Jennings RB, and Hill ML (1981) Total ischemia in dog hearts in vitro. 2. High energy phosphate depletion and associated defects in energy metabolism, cell volume regulation and sarcolemmal integrity. Circ Res 49: 901–911

13. Nayler WG (1981) The role of calcium in the ischemic myocardium. Am J Pathol 102: 262–273

14. Buja LM, Burton KP, Hagler HK and Willerson JT (1983) Quantitative x-ray microanalysis of the elemental composition of individual myocytes in hypoxic rabbit myocardium. Circ 68: 872–874.

15. Jennings RB, Reimer KA and Steenbergen C Jr (1986) Myocardial ischemia revisited. The osmolar load, membrane damage and reperfusion. J Mol Cell Cardiol 18: 769–780

16. de Duve C and Wattiaux R (1966) Functions of Lysosomes. Ann Rev Physiol 28: 435–492

17. Bird JWC (1975) Skeletal muscle lysosomes. In: JT Dingle and RT Dean (eds) Lysosomes in Biology and Pathology, Vol 4. North Holland Publ Co., Amsterdam pp 75–109

18. Smith AL and Bird JWC (1975) Distribution and particle properties of the vacuolar apparatus of cardiac muscle lysosomes and the isolation and characterization of acid, neutral and alkaline proteases. J Mol Cell Cardiol 7: 39–61

19. Kao R, Rannels DE, and Morgan HE (1975) Preparation of homogenates of heart muscle for assay of lysosomal enzyme activity. In: JT Dingle and RT Dean (eds) Lysosomes in Biology and Pathology, Vol 4. North Holland Publ. Co., Amsterdam pp 184–197

20. Ruth RC, Kennett FF and Weglicki WB (1978) A new technique for isolation of particulate lysosomal activity from canine and rat myocardium. J Mol Cell Cardiol 10: 739–751

21. Kennett FF and Weglicki WB (1978) Effects of well-defined ischemia on myocardial lysosomal and microsomal enzymes in a canine model. Circ Res 43: 750–758

22. Decker RS, Poole AR, Griffin EE, Dingle JT and Wildenthal K (1977) Altered distribution of lysosomal cathepsin D in ischemic myocardium. J Clin Invest 59: 911–921

23. Decker RS, Poole AR, Single JT and Wildenthal K (1978) Influences of methylprednisolone

on the sequential redistribution of cathepsin D and other lysosomal enzymes during myocardial ischemia in rabbits. J Clin Invest 62: 797–804

24. Wildenthal K, Decker RS, Poole AR, Griffin EE and Dingle JT (1978) Sequential lysosomal alterations during cardiac ischemia. I. Biochemical and immunohistochemical changes. Lab Invest 38: 656–661

25. Topping TM and Travis DF (1974) An electron cytochemical study of mechanisms of lysosomal activity in the rat left ventricular mural myocardium. J Ultrastruct Res 46: 1–22

26. Hoffstein S, Gennaro DE, Weissmann G, Hirsch J, Streuli F and Fox AC (1975) Cytochemical localization of lysosomal enzyme activity in normal and ischemic dog myocardium. Am J Pathol 79: 193–206

27. Hoffstein S, Weissmann G and Fox AC (1976) Lysosomes in myocardial infarction: Studies by means of cytochemistry and subcellular fractionation, with observations on the effects of methylprednisolone. Circ 53 (Suppl 1): 34–44

28. Decker RS and Wildenthal K (1978) Sequential lysosomal alterations during cardiac ischemia. II. Ultrastructural and cytochemical changes. Lab Invest 38: 662–673

29. Decker RS and Wildenthal K (1978) Influences of methylprednisolone on ultrastructural and cytochemical changes during myocardial ischemia: Selective effects of various cell inclusions and organelles including lysosomes. Am J Pathol 92: 1–22

30. Decker RS and Wildenthal K (1981) Lysosomal alterations in the heart, skeletal muscle and liver of hyperthyroid rabbits. Lab Invest 44: 455–465

31. Rosenfeld MG, Kreibich G, Popov D, Kato K and Sabatini DD (1982) Biosynthesis of lysosomal hydrolases: Their synthesis in bound polysomes and the role of co- and post-translational processing in determining their subcellular distribution. J Cell Biol 93: 135–143

32. Goldberg D, Gabel C and Kornfeld S (1984) Processing of lysosomal enzyme oligosaccharide units. In: JT Dingle and RT Dean and W Sly (eds) Lysosomes in Biology and Pathology, Vol 7. Elsevier, Amsterdam pp 45–62

33. Samarel AM, Ferguson AG, Worobec SW and Lesch M (1984) Transport and proteolytic processing of rabbit cardiac cathepsin D. Ann J Physiol 248: C135–C144

34. Geuze HJ, Slot JW, Strous JAM, Hasilik A and Von Figura K (1985) Possible pathways for lysosomal enzyme delivery. J Cell Biol 101: 2253–2262

35. Farquhar MG (1985) Progress in unraveling pathways of Golgi traffic. Ann Rev Cell Biol 1: 447–488

36. Novikoff, PM, Novikoff AB, Quintana N and Hauw J-J (1971) Golgi apparatus, GERL, lysosomes of neurons in rat dorsal root ganglion studied by thick and thin section cytochemistry. J Cell Biol 50: 859–886

37. Ridout RM, Wildenthal K and Decker RS (1986) Lysosomal responses of fetal mouse hearts recovering from anoxia and substrate depletion. J Mol Cell Cardiol 18: 853–865

38. Ridout RM, Wildenthal K and Decker RS (1986) Influence of agents that alter lysosomal function on fetal mouse hearts recovering from anoxia and substrate depletion. J Mol Cell Cardiol 18: 867–876

39. Decker RS, Decker ML, Thomas V and Fuseler JW (1985) Responses of cultured cardiac myocytes to lysosomotropic compounds and methylated amino acids. J Cell Sci 74: 119–135

40. Decker RS, Poole AR and Wildenthal K (1980) Distribution of lysosomal cathepsin D in normal, ischemic and starved rabbit cardiac myocytes. Circ Res 46: 485–494

41. Decker RS, Decker ML, Herring GH, Morton PC and Wildenthal K (1980) Lysosomal vacuolar apparatus of cardiac myocytes in heart of starved and refed rabbits. J Mol Cell Cardiol 12: 1125–1139

42. Smith RE and Van Frank RM (1975) The use of amino acid derivatives of 4-methoxy-B-napthalamine for assay and subcellular localization of tissue proteinases. In: JT Dingle, RT Dean (eds) Lysosomes in Biology and Pathology, Vol 4. North Holland Publ. Co., Amsterdam pp 193–250

43. Bird JWC, Spanier AM and Schwartz WN (1978) Cathepsins B and D: Proteolytic activity and ultrastructural localization in skeletal muscle. In: H Segal (ed) Protein Turnover and

Lysosome Function. Academic Press, New York pp 589–604

44. Matthews ITW, Decker RS and Knight GK (1981) Bimane-labelled pepstatin, a fluorescent probe for the localization of cathepsin D. Biochem J 199: 611–617

45. Matthews ITW, Decker RS, Hornebeck W and Knight GK (1983) Dinitrophenyl-pepstatins as active-site-directed localization reagents for cathepsin D. Biochem J 211: 139–147

46. Poole AR (1977) Antibodies to enzymes and their uses with particular reference to lysosomal enzymes. In: JT Dingle (ed) Lysosomes: a laboratory handbook, 2nd ed. North-Holland Publ. Co., Amsterdam pp 246–311

47. Wildenthal K, Poole AR and Dingle JT (1975) Influence of starvation on the activities and localization of cathepsin D and other lysosomal enzymes in hearts of rabbits and mice. J Mol Cell Cardiol 9: 859–866

48. Decker RS, Decker ML and Poole AR (1980) The distribution of lysosomal cathepsin D in rabbit heart. J Histochem Cytochem 28: 231–237

49. Mort JS, Poole AR and Decker RS (1981) Immunofluorescent localization of cathepsins B and D in human fibroblasts. J Histochem Cytochem 29: 649–658

50. Parmacek MS, Decker ML, Lesch M, Samarel AM and Decker RS (1986) Lysosomal changes during thyroxine-induced left ventricular hypertrophy in rabbits. Am J Physiol 251: C737–C747

51. Neely JR, Rovetto MJ, Whitner JT and Morgan HE (1973) Effects of ischemia on function and metabolism of the isolated working rat heart. Am J Physiol 225: 651–658

52. Jennings RB and Ganote CE (1974) Structural changes in myocardium during acute ischemia. Circ Res 35 (Suppl 3): 156–168

53. Ganote CE, Seabra-Gomes R, Nayler WG and Jennings RB (1975) Irreversible myocardial injury in anoxic perfused rat hearts. Am J Pathol 80: 419–450

54. Herdson PB, Sommers HM and Jennings RB (1965) A comparative study of the fine structure of normal and ischemic dog myocardium with special reference to early changes following temporary occlusion of a coronary artery. Am J Pathol 46: 367–386

55. McCallister LP, Munger BL, Neely JR (1977) Electron microscopic observations and acid phosphatase activity in the ischemic rat heart. J Mol Cell Cardiol 9: 353–364

56. Decker RS and Wildenthal K (1980) Lysosomal alterations in hypoxic and reoxygenated hearts. I. Ultrastructural and cytochemical changes. Am J Pathol 98: 425–444

57. Brachfeld N (1969) Maintenance of cell viability. Circ 40 (Suppl IV): 202–215

58. Ravens KG and Gudbjarnason S (1969) Changes in the activities of lysosomal enzymes in infarcted canine muscle. Circ Res 24: 851–856

59. Ricciutti MA (1972) Myocardial lysosome stability in the early acute stages of ischemic injury. Am J Cardiol 30: 492–497

60. Ricciutti MA (1972) Lysosomes and myocardial cellular injury. Am J Cardiol 30: 498–502

61. Spath JA, Lane DL and Lefer AM (1974) Protective action of methylprednisolone on the myocardium during experimental myocardial ischemia in the cat. Circ Res 35: 44–51

62. Gottwik MG, Kirk ES, Hoffstein S and Weglicki WB (1975) Effect of collateral flow on epicardial and endocardial lysosomal hydrolases in acute myocardial ischemia. J Clin Invest 56: 914–923

63. Welman E and Peters TJ (1977) Enhanced lysosomal fragility in anoxic perfused guinea pig heart. Effects of glucose and mannitol. J Mol Cell Cardiol 9: 101–120

64. Chua B, Kao RL, Rannels DE and Morgan HE (1979) Inhibition of protein degradation by anoxia and ischemia in perfused rat hearts. J Biol Chem 254: 6617–6623

65. Sasai Y, Nakamura N, Kobayaski Y and Katagiri T (1982) Studies on intracardiac acid hydrolases in the ischemic myocardial necrosis. Jap Circ J 46: 1137–1344

66. Katagiri T, Sasai Y, Nakamura N, Minatoguchi H, Yokayama M, Katayashi T, Takeyama Y, Ozawa K and Niitani H (1983) Acid hydrolases in the initiation of ischemic myocardial necrosis. Adv Myocardiol 4: 363–369

67. Okamatsu S and Lefer AM (1983) The protective effects of nifedipine in the isolated cat heart. J Surg Res 35: 35–40

68. Tsuchida K, Yamazaki R, Kanecko K and Aihara H (1986)   Effects of propranolol on tissue necrosis in experimental myocardial infarction in dogs. J Pharmocobiodym 9: 836–841

69. Kono N, Yamagishita T, Geshi E and Katagiri T (1987)   Degradation of cardiac sarcoplasmic reticulum in acute myocardial ischemia. Jap Circ J 51: 411–420

70. Ichikara K, Haneda T, Onodena S and Abiko Y (1987)   Inhibition of ischemia-induced subcellular redistribution of lysosomal enzymes in the perfused rat heart by the calcium entry blocker, diltiazem. J Pharmacol Exp Ther 242: 1109–1113

71. Laborit H and London A (1969)   Role des lysosomes dans les lisions de l'infarctus experimental du myocarde et dans l'action protective des inhibitenurs da la monoamine oxydase. Agressologie 10: 303–308

72. Araki H and Takenaka F (1975)   An increase of cathepsin D activity in cardiac lymph and pericardial fluid induced by experimental myocardial ischemia in the dog. Life Sci 17: 613–618

73. Ali M, Ellis A and Glick G (1977) Effects of methylprednisolone on cardiac lymph in acute ischemia in dogs. Am J Physiol 232: H602–H607

74. Welman E, Selwyn AP, Peters TJ, Colbeck JF and Fox KM (1978)   Plasma lysosomal enzyme activity in acute myocardial infarction. Cardiovasc Res 12: 99–105

75. Welman E, Peters TJ and Fox KM (1979)   Lysosomal and cytosolic enzyme release in acute myocardial infarction: effects of methylprednisolone. Circ 59: 730–733

76. Gottwick MG, Kirk ES, Kennett FF and Weglicki WB (1978)   Release of lysosomal enzymes during ischemic injury of canine myocardium. In: Kobayashi T, Ito Y and Rona G (eds) Recent Advances in Studies on Cardiac Structure and Metabolism, Vol 12. University Park Press, Baltimore pp 431–438

77. Nakamura N, Sasai Y, Takeyama Y and Katagiri T (1983)   Electron microscopic cytochemical studies on acid phosphatase activity in acute myocardial ischemia. Jap Heart J 24: 595–606

78. Barrett AJ (1980)   The many forms and functions of cellular proteinases. Fed Proc 39: 9–14

79. Kirschke H and Barrett AJ (1987)   The chemistry of lysosomal proteases. In: H Glaumann and FJ Ballard (eds) Lysosomes: Their Role in Protein Breakdown. Academic Press, New York pp 193–238

80. Wattiaux R, Wattiaux-DeConinck S and Dubois F (1982)   Prevention by chlorpromazine of lysosomal enzyme release caused by a transitory ischemia, effect of hypothermia. Biochem Pharmacol 31: 1167–1171

81. Brunk VT and Ericsson JLE (1972)   Cytochemical evidence for the leakage of acid phosphatase through ultrastructurally intact lysosomal membranes. Histochem J 4: 479–485

82. Schwartz WN and Bird JWC (1977)   Degradation of myofibrillar proteins by cathepsins B and D. Biochem J 167: 811–817

83. Ogunro EA, Lanman RB, Spencer JR, Ferguson AG and Lesch M (1979)   Degradation of canine cardiac myosin and actin by cathepsin D isolated from homologus tissue. Cardiovasc Res 13: 621–629

84. Jones TL, Ogunro EA, Samarel AM, Ferguson AG and Lesch M (1983)   Susceptibilities of cardiac myofibrillar proteins to cathespin D-catalyzed degradation. Am J Physiol 245: H294–299

85. Hillis LD and Braunwald E (1977)   Myocardial ischemia. N Eng J Med 296: 1034–1041

86. Rude R, Miller E and Braunwald E (1981)   Efforts to limit the size of myocardial infarcts. Ann Int Med 95: 736–761

87. Opie L (1985)   The Heart: Physiology, Metabolism, Pharmacology and Therapy. Grune and Stratton, London pp 351–372

88. Weissmann G (1973)   Effects of corticosteroids on the stability and fusion of biomembranes. In: KF Austin and L Fichtenstein (eds) Asthma. Academic Press, New York pp 221–233

89. Weissmann G (1976)   Corticosteroids and membrane stabilization. Circ 53: 171–172

90. Busuttil RW, George WJ and Hewitt RL (1975)   Protective effect of methylprednisolone on the heart during ischemic arrest. J Thorac Cardiovasc Surg 70: 955–965

91. Spath JA and Lefer AM (1975)   Effects of dexamethysone on myocardial cells in the early phase of acute myocardial infarction. Am Heart J 90: 50 55

92. Welman E and Peters TJ (1977) Prevention of lysosome disruption in anoxic myocardium by chloroquine and methylprednisolone. Pharmacol Res Comm 9: 29–38

93. Kennett FF and Weglicki WB (1978) Lack of effect of methylprednisolone on lysosomal and microsomal enzymes after two hours of well defined canine myocardial ischemia. Circ Res 43: 759–768

94. de Duve D, De Borsy T, Poole B, Trouet A, Tulkens P and Van Hoof F (1974) Lysosomotropic agents. Biochem Pharmacol 23: 357–376

95. Ridout RM, Decker RS and Wildenthal K (1978) Chloroquine induced lysosomal abnormalities in cultured fetal mouse hearts. J Mol Cell Cardiol 10: 175–183

96. Ohkuma S and Poole B (1978) Fluorescence probe measurement of the intralysosomal pH in living cells and perturbation of pH by various agents. Proc Natl Acad Sci USA 75: 3327–3331

97. Decker RS and Fuseler JW (1984) Methylated amino acids and lysosomal function in cultured heart cells. Exp Cell Res 154: 304–309

98. Wibo M and Poole B (1974) Protein degradation in cultured cells. II: The uptake of chloroquine by rat fibroblasts and the inhibition of cellular protein degradation and cathepsin B. J Cell Biol 63: 430–440

99. Wildenthal K and Crie SJ (1980) The role of lysosomal enzymes in cardiac protein turnover. Fed Proc 39: 37–41

100. Chien KR, Abrams J, Pfau RG and Farber JL (1977) Prevention by chlorpromazine of ischemic liver cell death. Am J Pathol 88: 539–558

101. Farber JL, Chien KR and Mittnacht JR (1981) The pathogenesis of irreversible cell injury in ischemia. Am J Pathol 102: 271–281

102. Chien KR, Pfau RG and Farber JL (1980) Ischemic myocardial cell injury. Prevention by chlorpromazine of accelerated phospholipid degradation and associated membrane dysfunction. Am J Pathol 97: 505–529

103. Ruth RC, Owens K and Weglicki WB (1980) Inhibition of lysosomal lipases by chlorpromazine: a possible mechanism of stabilization. J Pharmacol Exp Ther 212: 361–367

104. Beckman JK, Owens K, Knauer TE and Weglicki WB (1982) Hydrolysis of sarcolemma by lysosomal lipases and inhibition by chlorpromazine. Am J Physiol 242: H652–656

105. Weglicki WB (1980) Degradation of phospholipids of myocardial membranes. In: K Wildenthal (ed) Degradative Processes in Heart and Skeletal Muscle. Elsevier-North Holland Publ Co, Amsterdam pp 377–388

106. Chien KR, Abrams J, Seironi A, Martin JT and Farber JL (1978) Accelerated phospholipid degradation and associated membrane dysfunction in irreversible ischemic liver cell injury. J Biol Chem 252: 4809–4817

107. Chien KR, Han A, Sen A, Buja LM and Willerson JT (1984) Accumulation of unrestrified arachidonic acid in ischemic canine myocardium. Circ Res 54: 313–322

108. Burton KP, Hagler HK, Willerson JT and Buja LM (1981) Abnormal lanthanum accumulation due to ischemia in isolated myocardium: effect of chlorpromazine. Am J Physiol 241: H714–723

109. Weglicki WB and Lowe MG (1987) Phospholipases of myocardium. Basic Res Cardiol 82 (Suppl 1): 107–112

110. Chien KR, Crie JS, Decker RS and Wildenthal K (1983) Influence of chlorpromazine on lysosomal alterations during myocardial ischemia. Cardiovasc Res 17: 407–414

111. Welman E (1979) Stabilization of lysosomes in anoxic myocardium by propranolol. Brit J Pharm 65: 479–482

112. Victor T, la Cock C, Lochner A (1984) Myocardial tissue free fatty acids. J Mol Cell Cardiol 16: 709–721

113. Trotz M, Jellison EJ and Hostetler KY (1987) Propranolol inhibition of neutral phospholipase A of rat heart mitochondria and cytosol. Biochem Pharmacol 36: 4251–4256

114. Chiariello M, Ambrosio E, Capelli-Bigazzi M, Persone-Filardi P, Tritto I, Marone G and Condroelli M (1985) Mepindolol reduces myocardial necrosis in rats with coronary artery occlusion. J Cardiovasc Pharm 7 : 225–231

115. Okamatsu S and Lefer AM (1983) The protective effects of nifadipine in isolated cat heart. J Surg Res 35: 35–40
116. Ichihara K, Haneda T, Onodera S and Abiko Y (1987) Inhibition of ischemia induced subcellular redistribution of lysosomal enzymes in the perfused rat heart by the calcium entry blocker, diltiazem. J Pharmacol Exp Ther 242: 1109–1113
117. Ogletree ML and Lefer AM (1978) Prostaglandin induced preservation of the ischemic myocardium. Circ Res 42: 218–224
118. Lefer AM, Ogletree ML, Smith JB, Silver MJ, Nicolaou KC, Barnette WE and Gasic GD (1978) Prostacyclin: a potentially valuable agent for preserving myocardial tissue in acute myocardial ischemia. Science 200: 52–54
119. Tsuchida K, Aichara H, Isogai K, Hanada K and Shibota N (1986) Degradation of myocardial structural proteins in myocardial infarcted dogs is reduced by Ep 459, a cysteine proteinase inhibitor. Biol Chem Hoppe/Seyler 367: 39–45
120. Tolnai S and Korecky B (1986) Calcium dependent proteolysis and its inhibition in the ischemic rat myocardium. Can J Cardiol 2: 42–47
121. Jennings RB, Ganote CE and Reimer KA (1975) Ischemic tissue injury. Am J Pathol 81: 179–198
122. Decker RS and Wildenthal K (1980) Lysosomal alterations in hypoxic and reoxygenated hearts. II. Immunohistochemical and biochemical changes. Am J Pathol 98: 425–444
123. Mueller EA, Griffin WST and Wildenthal K (1977) Isoproterenol-induced cardiomyopathy: changes in cardiac enzymes and protection by methylprednisolone. J Mol Cell Cardiol 9: 565–578
124. Hearse DJ and Humphrey SM (1975) Enzyme release during myocardial anoxia: a study of metabolic protection. J Mol Cell Cardiol 7: 463–482
125. Ingwall JS, DeLuca M, Sybers HD and Wildenthal K (1975) Fetal mouse hearts: A model for studying ischemia. Proc Natl Acad Sci USA 72: 2809–2813
126. Sybers HD, Ingwall J and DeLuca M (1979) Autophagic response to sublethal injury in cardiac myocytes. J Mol Cell Cardio 11: 331–338
127. Wildenthal K and Crie SJ (1980) Lysosomes and cardiac protein catabolism. In: K Wildenthal (ed) Degradative Processes in Heart and Sekeltal Muscle. Elsevier-North Holland Biomed Press, Amsterdam pp 113–129
128. Ridout RM, Decker RS and Wildenthal K (1978) Modification by colchicine of autophagic vacuole formation in cultured fetal mouse hearts recovering from anoxia. J Cell Biol 79: 212
129. Hoffstein S, Goldstein IM and Weissmann G (1977) Role of microtubule assembly in lysosomal enzyme secretion from human polymorphonuclear leukocytes: A reevaluation. J Cell Biol 73: 242–256
130. Hensen PM (1976)[1] Secretion of lysosomal enzymes induced by immune complexes and complement. In: JT Dingle and RT Dean (eds) Lysosomes in Biology and Pathology, Vol 5. North Holland Publ. Co, Amsterdam pp 99–126
131. Kloner RA, Fishbein MC, Lew H, Maroko PR and Braunwald E (1978) Mummification of the infarcted myocardium by high dose corticosteroids. Circ 57: 56–63
132. Steenbergen CJ, Hill ML and Jennings RB (1987) Cytoskeletal damage during myocardial ischemia: changes in vinculin immunofluorescence staining during total in vitro ischemia in canine heart. Circ Res 60: 478–486
133. Ganote CE and Vander Heide RS (1987) Cytoskeletal lesions in anoxic myocardial injury. Am J Pathol 129: 327–344
134. Weglicki WB, Dickens BF and Mak IT (1984) Enhanced lysosomal phospholipid degradation and lysophospholipid production due to free radicals. Biochem Biophys Res Comm 124: 229–235
135. Mak IT and Weglicki WB (1988) Free radical and iron-mediated injury in lysosomes. In: PK Singal (ed) Oxygen Radicals in the Pathophysiology of Heart Disease. Kluwer Academic Publ, Boston pp 41–53

PART IV

The role of lipids

Detrimental effects of fatty acids and their derivatives in ischemic and reperfused myocardium

A. JAMES LIEDTKE and EARL SHRAGO

The Section of Cardiology, Department of Medicine and Department of Nutritional Sciences, University of Wisconsin, Madison, Wisconsin, USA

Introduction

In 1850, Richard Quain reported in a series of 83 autopsied patients, some of whom in life were troubled by chest and arm pains, shortness of breath, syncopy and fits of coma, a peculiar patchy, pale dirty brown appearance to the surface of the heart on morbid anatomical inspection [1]. This change in color and consistency, which was accompanied by surface or interstitial fat, like 'oil globules of milk bound in an albuminous envelope', in a setting of friable muscle fibers 'appeared to be connected with the causes on which the disease condition depend(ed) – *such as obstruction of the coronary arteries*'. Rokitansky and Virchow, both of whom thought (erroneously) that atherosclerosis and myocardial fibrosis were due to inflammation, felt this interlarding or fatty metamorphosis of cardiac muscle was an actual conversion of muscle fibrils to molecular fat [2, 3]. Virchow specifically advised that this formation of adipose tissue from connective tissue and parenchyma affected a derangement in motor power [4] or myomalacia cordes, a term that survived into the early twentieth century. From these rudimentary concepts evolved our modern understanding of myocardial ischemia, injury, and infarction and their interdependent relationships with fatty acids and altered lipid metabolism in heart muscle.

After a considerable period of neglect the topic was revived in the late 1960's and early 1970's when a series of reports were published describing the apparent harmful effects of excess fatty acids on cardiac function. Hoak *et al.* [5, 6], who had been studying the interesting causal association between long chain, saturated fatty acids and thrombus formation, noted in dogs, ducks, and geese infused with stearate or glucagon that, even when thrombosis was prevented, heart failure, shock and sudden death occurred with high preva-

H.M. Piper (ed.) Pathophysiology of severe ischemic myocardial injury, 149–166.

lence. Electron microscopy revealed acute myocardial degeneration and necrosis with fat droplet formation and destructive lesions of myofibrils and mitochondria together with mitochondrial inclusions. Henderson and workers [7, 8] further demonstrated that increasing the free fatty acid/albumin molar ratios with linoleate and octanoate depressed contractility at normoxic and hypoxic conditions in both isolated perfused rat hearts and rat papillary muscles. The report by Oliver *et al.* [9] importantly raised these observations from the laboratory esoteric to the clinically relevant when they documented in patients suffering acute myocardial infarction a key association between those experiencing the most complications (cardiogenic shock, serious arrhythmias including advanced heart block, ventricular tachycardia and fibrillation, and early and late deaths) and elevated levels of serum free fatty acids. This association was confirmed in part in alternate clinical studies (causality not implied) by Gupta and Rutenberg and colleagues [10, 11] and introduced the debate over the role of fatty acids on cardiac structure and function which persists up to the present time. The purpose of this article is to review the pros and cons of this debate and to specifically focus on its central hypothesis: *are fatty acids a causal factor for ischemic/hypoxic and reperfusion injury?* This review will be separately divided into sections dealing with myocardial ischemia and myocardial reperfusion following ischemic injury.

Myocardial ischemia

A spate of descriptive reports, almost all in animal models, has been developed in support of the notion of adverse lipid burden in ischemic heart muscle. Elevating coronary perfusate levels of fatty acids promoted left ventricular decompensation and heart failure in both aerobic and ischemic myocardium [12–14]. Conversely lowering fatty acids, the fatty acid/albumin ratio or fatty acid intermediates in either perfusate or myocardium appeared to lower the ischemic injury as estimated by surface ECG mapping [15–18], to lessen power failure [19] and to preserve mechanical function [20, 21]. Drugs and strategies used to accomplish this lowering included lipid-free albumin; b-pyridyl-carbinol to inhibit lypolysis [15, 16, 19]; p-chlorophenoxyisobutyrate, nicotinic acid and salicylates in part to depress free fatty acid extraction [22]; and oxfenicine and 2-tetradecylglycidic acid to intracellularly inhibit fatty acid transfer at the mitochondrial membrane [20, 21]. We employed a protocol in intact working pig hearts to shift intramyocardial levels of fatty acid amphiphiles with either oxfenicine or 4-bromocrotonic acid [23]. In ischemic myocardium, lowering amphiphiles improved mechanical function while increasing amphiphiles accomplished the reverse.

Similarly, excess fatty acids have been implicated in cardiac arrhythmogenesis. In addition to the early clinical descriptions of Oliver [9] and Gupta *et al.* [10], Rowe and workers [24] reported in 81 patients suffering acute infarction that a nicotinic acid analogue, if applied within five hours of the onset of symptoms, lowered plasma free fatty acids and brought a reduction in ventricular tachycardia and R-on-T ventricular premature beats. These observations were confirmed and extended in animal studies. Opie and colleagues [25] noted in a small series of dogs with coronary ligation that excess fatty acids exaggerated ectopic activity, but only in the presence of adrenalin infusions. In a comparable canine ligation model Kurien *et al.* [26] disputed this with data indicating that elevated fatty acids were arrhythmogenic independent of catecholamine activity. Similar findings were reported in perfused rat hearts [27]. Moschos *et al.* [28] in a chronic canine infarction model described a lower incidence of arrhythmias in the first week of follow-up, if treated with aspirin, which blocked plasma fatty acid elevations. Efforts to explain these events were developed in isolated animal systems. Early data suggested pronounced alterations in ventricular action potential morphology and functional refractory periods which could lead to spontaneous or electrically provoked fibrillation [29, 32]. Conversely, the ventricular fibrillation threshold in aerobic and ischemic myocardium has not been shown to vary as a result of excess fatty acids *per se* [33].

Regulation of fatty acid metabolism in aerobic heart muscle is less complex than in liver where it is intimately related to the gluconeogenic and lipogenic activities as well as synthesis of lipid compounds of the organ. Fatty acid oxidation in heart is primarily dependent on the free fatty acid concentration of plasma but also on the energy demand of the tissue [34]. Under normal conditions, energy demand is the major physiological mechanism for regulating myocardial metabolism. In particular, a lower energy demand leads to an increase of NADH and acetyl CoA and a decrease in free CoA which thereby inhibits pyruvate dehydrogenase, a key reaction in the tricarboxylic cycle, as well as 3-hydroxy acyl CoA dehydrogenase and 3-keto acyl CoA thiolase. These latter reactions explain the rate limiting steps in β-oxidation of fatty acids [34].

A variety of metabolic mechanisms have been offered to explain the impairments of fatty acids and their derivatives on cardiac structure and function in ischemia. Old notions of fatty acids as nonspecific detergents [8] have been updated to include detailed considerations of phospholipid hydrolysis in membranes, enhanced activation of a variety of phospholipases which occurs in ischemia, and altered lipid-gel distributions in membrane biolipid which in turn displace calcium and alter protein function [35, 36]. Old notions of fatty acids as antagonists to mitochondrial function and respiration [37–42] have been expanded to include a number of suborganelles, membranes, and enzyme systems (Table 1). *In vitro* the uncoupling effects of fatty acids on mitochondrial oxidative phosphorylation have been recognized for many years [37, 39]. The uncoupling ability has been attributed to the stimulation of latent ATPase [39], ionophore [57] and general detergent-like effects [35]. It has been proposed that the F_o component of the ATPase which serves as a proton conductor is dissipated by the fatty acid [48]. Whereas, at low concentrations fatty acids act as uncoupling agents with NAD-linked

Table 1. Enzymatic activities affected by amphiphiles.

Activity	Amphiphile	Effect	References
Sarcolemmal Ca^{++} ATPase	Fatty acid acyl carnitine	Inhibits	43, 44
Sarcolemmal (Na, K) ATPase	Fatty acid acyl carnitine	Inhibits	45
Plasma membrane (Na, K) ATPase (Kidney)	Acyl CoA	Stimulates	46
Mitochondrial NADH dehydrogenase	Fatty acid	Inhibits	47
Mitochondrial F_0 component of the ATP synthetase	Fatty acid	Uncouples or dissipates proton conductance	37, 39, 48
Mitochondrial adenine nucleotide translocase	Acyl CoA	Inhibits	49–54
Cytosolic triglyceride lipase	Fatty acids Acyl CoA Acyl carnitine	Inhibits	55, 56

substrates and succinate, at higher concentrations they are inhibitors of respiration. These results indicate a major effect of the fatty acids on NADH dehydrogenase [47].

Fatty acids and their derivatives all have general amphiphilic effects by interdicting themselves into membranes and thereby disrupting function such as displacing Ca^{++} from negatively charged binding sites on phospholipids [35]. It has been proposed that the predominant requirement of a membrane perturbant is simply that the perturbing molecule partition strongly into the membrane [58]. This perturbation increases with increasing chain length of the amphiphile [37, 39]. Using the anion transport protein of the erythrocyte membrane as a model system, Gruber and Low [59] reported that fatty acid action exhibited a graded preference for shorter alkyl chains which may in fact be a common feature among many transport proteins. Further analysis suggested a mechanism by which each additional CH$_2$ favors transfer away from sites on the protein towards the bulk lipid matrix [60]. The lipid hypothesis, by which the amphiphile modifies the lipid phase near the protein, thereby creating the perturbation, has now been modified to postulate the lipid as a competitor rather than a mediator of transport function [59, 60].

Heart and skeletal muscle of mammals contains approximately 4–6% of cytosolic fatty acid binding protein (FABP) [61, 62]. The role of FABPs in different cell types, and particularly heart, remains to be established. A majority of experiments addressing this question has been carried out in liver. Based on these results, it has been proposed that FABP in heart as in liver may provide protection by buffering against excess fatty acids and long chain acyl CoA and acylcarnitine esters that accumulate during ischemia and hypoxia [61, 62]. In liver, the primary role of the FABP may be to direct fatty acid flow to the microsomes for subsequent acylation rather than to mitochondria for β-oxidation [63, 64]. The opposite may be true for the heart protein [65, 66]. In fact, the FABPs in liver and heart are separate proteins which do not crossreact with antibodies to the opposite protein [67]. Their separate genes have now been cloned. More recently, Burrier and co-workers [64] have shown that rat heart FABP does not bind acyl CoA nor does it modulate the amount of acyl CoA formed as occurs in liver. Also, lysolecithin binds to liver but not to heart FABP. It thus seems apparent that if myocardial membranes exposed to the cytosol are to be protected from amphiphiles, they must be by proteins other than FABP.

Accumulations of amphiphile constituents between fatty acyl CoA and carnitine redistribute abnormally across mitochondrial membrane in myocardial ischemia [68]. We have shown physiologically that these esters further impair contractility in ischemic myocardium [69]. Amphiphiles can also significantly depress activity of ATP-dependent calcium transport in sarcoplasmic reticulum [43, 44] and (Na, K)-ATPase in sarcolemma, possibly through free radical-induced lipid peroxidation [45]. Fatty acids and acyl CoA esters also have the properties to depress enzyme systems in mitochondria, sarcoplasma reticulum and sarcolemma [70] as well as generate free-radical production [71]. In the cytosol, they have been found to inhibit triglyceride lipase [55, 56]. Lysophospholipids, break-down products of phospholipids which accumulate in membranes during ischemia, can cause arrhythmias, rapid myocyte contracture, and coronary artery constriction, even at subcritical micelle concentrations [72–74].

The contribution of peroxisomes to overall β-oxidation in heart muscle has not been completely elucidated. Recently an acyl CoA oxidase enzyme has been identified with a rather wide substrate specificity varying between C6 and C16 [75]. Overall, *in vitro* rates of palmitate oxidation (mitochondrial + peroxisomal) are reported to be 400–900 nmol/min/gram of heart tissue while isolated peroxisomal activity in rat heart was reported to be approximately 6 nmol/min/gram tissue [75]. This suggests a low activity of the peroxisomes in heart compared to liver. However, the peroxisomal acyl CoA oxidase pathway transfers electrons directly to O_2 to form H_2O_2. This pathway may play a more significant role in the ischemic myocardium and particularly during reperfusion with the generation of large amounts of H_2O_2 [76].

Neely and Morgan [77] described the profound decreases in fatty acid utilization in ischemic heart muscle, the rate limiting steps of fatty acid oxidation (see Table 2 [70]) and the consequent loss of energy production from this preferred substrate. Using clinical imaging techniques, this reduced utilization is perceived as a decreased clearance and uptake of iodinated or positron emitting isotopes of fatty acid analogues in ischemic or infarcted

Table 2. Specifics of long-chain fatty acid oxidation.

Major rate-regulating steps	Substrates	Products	Chief regulating mechanism[a]	Changes in flux with oxygen deficiency[b]
Cellular uptake by plasma membrane binding sites and anatomic channels	FFA, triacyl-glycerols	FFA	Plasma FFA concentrations, FFA: albumin molar ratio, FA properties, metabolic activity of cell, hormones	Decreased
Cytosolic activation by acyl-CoA synthetases	FAA, coen-zyme-A, ATP	Acyl-CoA, AMP, Pi	Product inhibition; coenzyme-A availability	Decreased
Cytosol-mitochondrial transfer by carnitine acyl transferase-translocase	Acyl-CoA, coenzyme-A, acyl-carnitine, carnitine	Acyl-CoA, coenzyme-A, acyl-carnitine, carnitine	Ratio of substrates to products	Decreased
β-oxidation	Acyl-CoA, FAD^+, NAD^+	Remaining acyl-CoA (–2 carbons), acetyl-CoA, $FADH_2$, NADH	Metabolic activity of cell, oxygen availability, flux through citric acid cycle	Profoundly decreased, chief inhibited step

* Exclusive of nonoxidative pathways to neutral and polar lipids.

[a] Signifies under aerobic physiologic conditions.

[b] Includes both anoxia and ischemia. FFA means free long-chain fatty acids bound to albumin or intracellular proteins.

tissue [78, 79]. As stated above, this loss of metabolic activity in fatty acid utilization leads to build-up of long-chain acyl esters of CoA and carnitine [68, 77, 80], *de novo* synthesis of free fatty acids [81, 82] possibly due to the action of lysosomes [83], and formation of micro- and macrodroplets of neutral lipid beginning at 3–6 hours of coronary occlusion [84, 85]. The accumulations of amphiphiles have been associated with the abnormal structural formation of intramitochondrial amorphous densities [86, 87]. These fatty acid derivatives together with increased triacylglycerols in turn result in mechanical dysfunction [68, 80, 88]. Conversely the *de novo* synthesis of fatty acids apparently occurs too late to explain mechanical decompensation [81].

The above survey of available literature incriminating fatty acids is not without its critics, and some investigators have either found no positive correlations between fatty acid excess and myocardial dysfunction or offer a third determinant as explaining both. Most *et al.* [89] reported no further worsening of ST-T changes on precordial mapping in a pig infarct model receiving lipid infusions. The same group, however, did show less tension development and less recovery in rat papillary muscles receiving fatty acids subjected to hypoxia and reoxygenation [90]. Rutenberg *et al.* [11] in early clinical trials of arrhythmogenesis did note a correlation between cardiac complications and elevated plasma free fatty acids in infarct patients but cautioned that both were probably due to cathecholamines. Moreover, some of the changes in mechanical function associated with excess fatty acids in ischemia has been only moderate [20, 69] and capable of being almost completely masked at more profound levels of ischemia [91]. Not withstanding the above, the weight of available evidence strongly implicates fatty acid/lipid derivatives as an adverse consequence of myocardial ischemia. Evolving research is beginning to point to structural alterations in biolipid membrane and function as the most attractive mechanism to explain these results.

An example of this is the biochemical effects of intracellular fatty acids and carnitine esters on adenine nucleotide translocase. A site specific interaction of long chain acyl CoA esters with the mitochondrial ADP/ATP carrier has been described [49]. The K_i for the acyl CoA is well below its critical micelle concentration. Competitive inhibition with adenine nucleotides on the cytosolic side of the inner mitochondrial membrane and the reversal of this inhibition by removal of the acyl CoA are properties which have been submitted as evidence to support the concept that long chain acyl CoA esters modulated the carrier and thereby exert an influence on the bioenergetics of the cell [50]. Under ischemic and hypoxic conditions mitochondrial adenine nucleotide transport is decreased [51]. However, the mechanism has been attributed to factors other than increased levels of acyl CoA. In particular, matrix adenine nucleotides are inordinately low and tend to impair the counter exchange of cytosolic ADP for matrix ATP [52]. In one study the compartmentation of long chain acyl CoA in the heart was found to be almost entirely restricted to the mitochondrial fraction [68]. Thus there remains some discrepancy as to whether the ADP/ATP carrier can be inhibited by long chain acyl CoA from the matrix side of the inner mitochondrial membrane. Conversely, effects of acyl CoA on the purified ADP/ATP carrier reconstituted into a liposome system identical to those in isolated mitochondria [53] together with recent evidence [54] on covalent binding of the carrier with an acyl CoA derivative photolabel provides evidence for a site specific interaction between the acyl CoA and the ADP/ATP carrier. This has been attributed to a receptor on the protein which recognizes the adenine moiety on the CoA molecule and is able to compete for ADP and ATP. While it is generally inferred that inhibition of the carrier by acyl CoA is deleterious, the ligand may, in fact, act as a normal metabolic regulator. Consistent with this hypothesis is the report [92] suggesting that inhibition of the translocase during ischemia or hypoxia is a protective mechanism to prevent the increased oxygen consumption stimulated by fatty acids. Of related interest was the study by Huang and co-workers [46] showing that at suboptimal concentrations of ATP, acyl CoA esters activated the kidney (Na, K)-ATPase by lowering the K_d for ATP.

Myocardial reperfusion

The two most prominent features of myocardial reperfusion following reversible ischemia are mechanical stunning and reperfusion arrhythmias. Both have been extensively described and a variety of mechanisms offered to explain the events. In the case of mechanical stunning, as first reported by Heyndrickx, Theroux, Braunwald, Bush and workers [93–97], these explanations remain at the present time associative rather than causative. Furthermore, none are truly rate-limiting since under a variety of therapeutic strategies stunning can be reversed. Reperfusion arrhythmias are likewise explained by several associative mechanisms and can be modulated nonspecifically with commonly used antiarrhythmics. Our first task in this section will be to provide a brief survey of these events and review their chief biochemical findings and second, to tie these in where applicable to any added influences introduced by excess fatty acids. The author has previously discussed the topic of stunning and will draw on this material [98].

Mechanical stunning can be looked on as a defect or delay in metabolic or anatomical recovery which prevents early return of muscle mechanics and function following reperfusion. Possible loci of metabolic impairments include: mitochondrial dysfunction either in the use of substrates and oxygen or the biosynthesis of ATP; abnormalities of transfer and transformation of this ATP out of the mitochondria and into the cytosol as creatine phosphate via the adenine nucleotide translocase and mito-creatine kinase (CK) enzyme systems; and decreased use of high energy phosphates by the myofibril either by depressed cytosolic or myofibrillar CK activity, ADP substrate availability, or local environmental accumulations of calcium, metabolic intermediates, or oxygen free radicals. Ultrastructural changes, presumably reversible, have also been described [99].

Mitochondria are injured in proportion to the severity of the ischemic stress preceding reperfusion and data are available showing depressed respiration, decreased efficiency of oxidative phosphorylation and P/O ratios, and oxygen wastage as a result [100–102]. On the other hand, injury may be less severe in transient ischemia and in fact mitochondria appear more resilient than other suborganelles to short-term oxygen deprivation [103]. Studies of autolysing tissue of > 1 hr have shown mitochondrial inner membranes well able to hold their potential change over this time course with little decay or leakiness [104]. In working pig or rat hearts we have similarly shown no mitochondrial dysfunction in terms of altered substrate preference during recovery (fatty acids $>$ propionate $>$ glucose $>$ pyruvate). Indeed, rates of fatty acid oxidation were increased in our hearts over aerobic levels [91, 105–107]. Regardless of the above differences in mitochondrial integrity and function following ischemia, most investigators agree that ATP resynthesis is delayed or impaired in reperfused hearts. Reibel and Rovetto [108] and DeBoer and Kloner et al. [109, 110] initially felt that this impairment was the sole explanation for stunning but this hypothesis has since been challenged [111].

All enzymes of energy transfer appear impaired during early reflow and reports are available showing decreased activities or velocities of reaction in adenine nucleotide translocase [112], mitochondrial CK [113], total CK [102], and MM CK [114]. The latter report also noted the free cytosolic ADP concentrations to be less than the Km for MM CK suggesting a limitation in substrate availability. With this formidable cascade of depressed activities, it is surprising that together they do not provide a rate limiting explanation for the stunning phenomenon.

Free radical formation has also received much recent emphasis as a mechanism of stunning and perhaps infarct extension. Available measuring techniques suggest a burst of oxy-radicals from heart muscle which peak in the first several seconds following reperfusion and which then continue to form at a lesser rate for several hours thereafter [115]. Debate remains as to how and by what process free radicals impair contractility, which cell line is responsible for the majority of oxygen metabolites generated, i.e., leukocytes or vascular endothelium since species devoid of xanthine oxidase in cardiomyocytes can still benefit from antioxidant therapy [116], and whether more animal data are required before initiating clinical trials to test the free radical hypothesis in man (one of the species without much xanthine oxidase in heart muscle) [117, 118]. Nevertheless, opinion is growing that free radical scavengers, if applied before reperfusion, can benefit mechanical recovery. This is but one of a host of such efficacious interventions, i.e., reactive hyperemia [119, 120], diltiazem [121], dopamine, epinephrine or postextrasystolic potentiation [122–124], and an acid pH in perfusate to lessen calcium influx or compete for intracellular calcium binding sites at reperfusion [125]. All of these enhance contractile reserve but provide little insight into a unified hypothesis for understanding at the present time.

Finally, to complete the stunning survey, ultrastructural data using scanning electron microscopy showed profound changes in extracellular collagen matrix with deletion, uncoiling and roughening of collagen cables and breakage of myocyte-to-myocyte struts [99]. This loss of cellular tethering and altered compliance could clearly attenuate regional shortening and promote bulging in otherwise viable tissue. Rates of collagen resynthesis and repair from this defect are at present unknown.

Manning and Hearst [126] credit Tennant and Wiggers [127] as first describing reperfusion arrhythmias in dogs. These arrhythmias attracted little research attention until the development and expanding clinical application of thrombolytic and revascularization protocols recently. Corr and Witkowski [128] proposed that with such treatments, these arrhythmias, which represent a heterogeneity of recovery of excitability in otherwise viable tissue, might prove a reliable marker of salvage in reversibly damaged myocardium. The careful review of both groups compiled and categorized material of theirs and others to provide new insights into the disorder. They observed that: 1) the rhythms were life threatening and included ventricular tachycardia and fibrillation; 2) the rhythms could be grouped according to onset after reperfusion and included immediate (sec-min), intermediate (min-hr), and delayed (days-weeks); 3) the immediate and intermediate dysrhythmias were probably caused by different mechanisms i.e., heterogenic re-entry and enhanced automaticity, respectively; and 4) these in turn were postulated to result from a plethora of derangements including the duration of ischemia, the rate of initiation of reflow, free radical formation, intracellular loss of potassium and magnesium ions, calcium overload, rapid shifts in PCO_2, abnormalities of lipid metabolism and increased cAMP. The dysrhythmias were particularly responsive to the application of α_1, α_2 and calcium channel blocking drugs, low dose glucose and mannitol [129, 130].

Excess fatty acids and abnormal lipid metabolism can sometimes be closely tied to the above hypotheses. While fatty acid uptake and oxidation are rapidly restored in reoxygenated or reperfused cardiac tissue [91, 131, 132], other aspects of fatty acid metabolism remain altered for relatively long periods of time. Miller et al. [133] reported enhanced activity of a radioiodinated, non-β-oxidized, long chain fatty acid analogue in reperfused myocardium, probably reflecting increased turn-over in triacylglycerols. Schwaiger et al. [134], showed in a three hour occlusion, four week reperfusion protocol in dogs that ^{11}C-clearances of positron emitting palmitic acid were depressed for one week in reversibly injured and reperfused tissue. Long-chain esters of CoA and carnitine which are elevated in ischemic hearts tend to fall during reflow but do not reach pre-ischemic levels. Ichihara and Neely [135] noted no correlation between myocardial levels of amphiphiles whereas others have. Lopaschuk and workers [136] described a 6-fold increase in long-chain acid carnitine and a lesser increase in acyl CoA in rat hearts treated with excess fatty acids which were observed to undergo a further deterioration in mechanical function during recovery. Excess fatty acids in dog hearts prevented reductions in acyl CoA during recovery which impaired mitochondrial respiration after reperfusion [137]. Amphiphiles added to a free radical-generating system in a suborganelle preparation (highly enriched sarcolemmal membranes) accelerated rates of peroxidation and decreased activity of sarcolemmal (Na, K)-ATPase [45].

Indeed the whole story of oxidative injury in reperfusion is connected in some way with tissue fatty acids and lipids and membrane phospholipids. Kajiyama and workers studied glutathione peroxidase in mitochondrial membranes from reperfused hearts [138]. This enzyme system is designed to protect membrane integrity from peroxidative events during detoxification of oxygen free radicals after reflow. Its activation shifts the levels of glutathione (GSH) toward oxidation and the formation of glutathione disulfide (GSSG) which inhibits sulfhydryl-sensitive proteins. One such enzyme is acyl CoA lysophosphatide acyltransferase which participates in reacylation of phospholipid breakdown products, believed to be accelarated by activation of phospholipase A_2 in ischemia and reflow, and protects against the net production of lysophospholipids. A host of information is available to indicate that lysophosphatidylcholine and lysophosphatidylethanolamine are capable of distorting action potentials in Purkinje fibers sufficient to potentate re-entry arrhythmias [139–142]. Thus in reperfusion we have evidence of two reactions designed to protect membrane function operating at cross purposes and in essence adversely affecting one another. This occurs under conditions where free radical mediated injury is clearly occurring [143] and which is increased in the presence of excess fatty acids, particularly in mixtures containing unsaturated fatty acids [71]. In a physiological study using Langendorff-perfused rat hearts, Bricknell and Opie [144] showed that palmitate-perfused hearts suffered the most severe arrhythmias during reperfusion which was reversed by glucose perfusion.

In conclusion, the authors feel that the fatty acid hypothesis as a causal factor for explaining certain events of ischemic and reperfusion injury remains viable and testable. The evidence to date is largely circumstantial and descriptive but of sufficient merit to establish trends of indictment. Specific biochemical effects of fatty acids and their acyl derivatives as well as more generalized detergent or amphiphilic effects have been described *in vitro* in heart tissue under both normal and ischemic or hypoxic conditions. Moreover, accumulation of these amphiphiles has been associated with impaired metabolic and mechanical function of the myocardium. Ultimate proof will derive from molecular characterizations of membranes and other lipid pools which are dynamically adjusting to the stress of ischemia and reflow.

Acknowledgements

This work was supported in part by PHS Grants HL 21209 and GM-14033, the Rennebohm Foundation of Wisconsin, and the Oscar Mayer Cardiovascular Research Fund.

References

1. Quain R (1850) On fatty disease of the heart. In: Medico Chirurgical Transactions. Published by The Royal Medical and Chirurgical Society Vol 33. London: Longman, Brown, Green and Longmans pp 121–196
2. Snellen HA (1984) History of cardiology. A brief outline of the 350 years' prelude to an explosive growth. Rotterdam: Donker Academic Publishers, 154–170
3. Rokitansky C (Translated by WE Swaine) (1854) Chapter 9. Anomalies of texture: Fat textures. In: A Manual of General Pathological Anatomy. London: Printed for the Sydenham Society, Sydenham Society Publications, Vol 1: 195–201
4. Virchow R (Translated by F Chance) (1860) Lecture 16. A more precise account of fatty metamorphosis. In: Cellular Pathology as based upon Physiological and Pathological Histology. Twenty Lectures Delivered in the Pathological Institute of Berlin During the Months of February, March, and April 1858. New York: Robert M De Witt, Publisher 383–408
5. Hoak JC, Connor WE, Eckstein JW, Warner ED (1964) Fatty acid-induced thrombosis and death: Mechanisms and prevention. J Lab Clin Med 63: 791–800
6. Hoak JC, Connor WE, Warner ED (1968) Toxic effects of glucagon-induced acute lipid mobilization in geese. J Clin Invest 47: 2701–2710
7. Henderson AH, Craig RJ, Gorlin R, Sonnenblick EH (1970) Free fatty acids and myocardial function in perfused rat hearts. Cardiovasc Res 4: 466–471
8. Henderson AC, Most AS, Parmley WW, Gorlin R, Sonnenblick EH (1970) Depression of myocardial contractility in rats by free fatty acids during hypoxia. Circ Res 26: 439–449

9. Oliver MF, Kurien VA, Greenwood TW (1968) Relation between serum-free-fatty-acids and arrhythmias and death after acute myocardial infarction. Lancet 1 (Jan-Jun): 710–715

10. Gupta DK, Jewitt DE, Young R, Hartog M, Opie LW (1969) Increased plasma-free-fatty-acid concentrations and their significance in patients with acute myocardial infarction. Lancet 2 (Jul-Dec): 1209–1213

11. Rutenberg HL, Pamintuan JC, Soloff LA (1969) Serum-free-fatty-acids and their relation to complications after acute myocardial infarction. Lancet 2 (Jul-Dec): 559–564

12. Severeid L, Connor WE, Long JP (1969) The depressant effect of fatty acids on the isolated rabbit heart. Proc Soc Exp Biol Med 131: 1239–1243

13. Kjekshus JK, Mjos OD (1972) Effect of free fatty acids on myocardial function and metabolism in the ischemic dog heart. J Clin Invest 51: 1767–1776

14. Russo JV, Margolis S (1972) Hemodynamic effects of free fatty acid augmentation following myocardial infarction. Circ 45–46 (Suppl II): II–215

15. Kjekshus JK, Mjos OD (1973) Effect of inhibition of lipolysis on infarct size after experimental coronary artery occlusion. J Clin Invest 52: 1770–1778

16. Mjos OD, Kjekshus JK, Lekven J (1974) Importance of free fatty acids as a determinant of myocardial oxygen consumption and myocardial ischemic injury during norepinephrine infusion in dogs. J Clin Invest 53: 1290–1299

17. Mjos OD, Miller NE, Riemersma RA, Oliver MF (1976) Effects of P-chlorophenoxyisobutyrate on myocardial free fatty acid extraction, ventricular blood flow, and epicardial ST-T segment elevation during coronary occlusion in dogs. Circ 53: 494–500

18. Miller NE, Mjos OD, Oliver MF (1976) Relationship of epicardial ST segment elevation to the plasma free fatty acids/albumin ratio during coronary occlusion in dogs. Clin Sci Mol Med 51: 209–213

19. Kjekshus JK (1974) Effect of inhibition of lipolysis on heart failure following acute coronary occlusion in the dog. Cardiovasc Res 8: 73–80

20. Liedtke AJ, Nellis SH, Mjos OD (1984) Effects of reducing fatty acid metabolism on mechanical function in regionally ischemic hearts. Am J Physiol 247 (Heart Circ Physiol 16): H378–H394

21. Miller WP, Liedtke AJ, Nellis SH (1986) Effects of 2-tetradecylglycidic acid on myocardial function in swine hearts. Am J Physiol 251 (Heart Circ Physiol 20): H547–H553

22. Vik-mo H, Riemersma RA, Mjos OD, Oliver MF (1979) Effect of myocardial ischaemia and antilipolytic agents on lipolysis and fatty acid metabolism in the *in situ* dog heart. Scand J Clin Lab Invest 39: 559–568

23. Molaparast-Saless F, Liedtke AJ, Nellis SH (1987) Effects of the fatty acid blocking agents, oxfenicine and 4-bromocrotonic acid, on performance in aerobic and ischemic myocardium. J Mol Cell Cardiol 19: 509–520

24. Rowe MJ, Neilson JMM, Oliver MF (1975) Control of ventricular arrhythmias during myocardial infarction by antilipolytic treatment using a nicotonic-acid analog. Lancet 1 (Jan-Jun): 295–300

25. Opie LH, Thomas M, Owen P, Norris RM, Holland AJ, Van Noorden S (1971) Failure of high concentrations of circulating free fatty acids to provoke arrhythmias in experimental myocardial infarction. Lancet 1: 818–822

26. Kurien VA, Yates PA, Oliver MF (1971) The role of free fatty acids in the production of ventricular arrhythmias after acute coronary artery occlusion. Europ J Clin Invest 1: 225–241

27. Willebrands AF, Ter Welle HF, Tasseron SJA (1973) The effect of high molar FFA/albumin ratio in the perfusion medium on rhythm and contractility of the isolated rat heart. J Mol Cell Cardiol 5: 259–273

28. Moschos CB, Haider B, Dela Cruz C, Lyons MM, Regan TJ (1978) Antiarrhythmic effects of aspirin during nonthrombotic coronary occlusion. Circ 57: 681–684

29. Cowan JC, Vaughan Williams EM (1977) The effects of palmitate on intracellular potentials recorded from Langendorff-perfused guinea-pig hearts in normoxia and hypoxia, and during

perfusion at reduced rate of flow. J Mol Cell Cardiol 9: 327–342

30. Cowan JC, Vaughan Williams EM (1980) The effects of various fatty acids on action potential shortening during sequential periods of ischaemia and reperfusion. J Mol Cell Cardiol 12: 347–369

31. Harada H, Azuma J, Hasegawa H, Ohta H, Yamauchi K, Ogura K, Awata N, Sawamura A, Sperelakis N, Kishimoto S (1984) Enhanced suppression of myocardial slow action potentials during hypoxia by free fatty acids. J Mol Cell Cardiol 16: 261–276

32. Wasilewska-Dziubinska E (1975) Are free fatty acids arrhythmogenic? Effects on cellular cardiac action potentials. J Mol Cell Cardiol 7: 153–154

33. Kostis JB, Mavrogeoregis EA, Horstmann E, Gotzoyannis S (1973) Effect of high concentrations of free fatty acids on the ventricular fibrillation threshold of normal dogs and dogs with acute myocardial infarction. Cardiology 58: 89–98

34. Schulz H (1985) Oxidation of fatty acids. In: Vance DE and Vance JE (eds) Biochemistry of Lipids and Membranes. Penlow Park, CA: Benjamin Cummings pp 116–142

35. Katz AM, Messineo FC (1981) Lipid-membrane interactions and the pathogenesis of ischemic damage in the myocardium. Circ Res 48: 1–16

36. Katz AM (1982) Membrane-derived lipids in the pathogenesis of ischemic myocardial damage. J Mol Cell Cardiol 14: 627–632

37. Borst P, Loos JA, Christ EJ, Slater EC (1962) Uncoupling activity of long-chain fatty acids. Biochim Biophys Acta 62: 509–518

38. Hulsmann WC, Elliot WB, Slater EC (1960) The nature and mechanisms of action of uncoupling agents present in mitochrome preparations. Biochim Biophys Acta 39: 267–276

39. Pressman BC, Lardy HA (1956) Effect of surface active agents on the latent ATPase of mitochondria. Biochim Biophys Acta 21: 458–466

40. Wojtczak L, Wojtczak AB (1960) Uncoupling of oxidative phosphorylation and inhibition of ATP-Pi exchange by a substance from insect mitochondria. Biochim Biophys Acta 39: 277–286

41. Lochner A, Kotze JCN, Gevers W (1976) Mitochondrial oxidative phosphorylation in myocardial anoxia: Effects of albumin. J Mol Cell Cardiol 8: 465–480

42. Lochner A, Kotze JCN, Benade AJS, Gevers W (1978) Mitochondrial oxidative phosphorylation in low-flow hypoxia: Role of free fatty acids. J Mol Cell Cardiol 10: 857–875

43. Lopaschuk GD, Tahiliani AG, Vadlaumudi RVSV, Katz S, McNeill JH (1983) Cardiac sarcoplasmic reticulum function in insulin or carnitine-treated diabetic hearts. Am J Physiol 245 (Heart Circ Physiol 14): H969–H976

44. Pitts BJR, Tate CA, Vanwinkle WB, Wood JM, Entman ML (1978) Palmitoyl carnitine inhibition of the calcium pump in cardiac and sarcoplasmic reticulum: A possible role in myocardial ischemia. Life Sci 23: 391–402

45. Mak IT, Kramer JH, Weglicki WB (1986) Potentiation of free radical-induced lipid peroxidative injury to sarcolemmal membranes by lipid amphiphiles. J Biol Chem 261: 1153–1157

46. Huang WH, Kakar SAS, Askari A (1986) Activation of Na^+K^+ATPase by long chain fatty acids and fatty acyl Co-enzymes A. Biochem Inter Nat 12: 521–528

47. Batayneh N, Kopacz SJ, Lee CP (1986) The modes of action of long chain alkyl compounds on the respiratory chain-linked energy transducing system in submitochondrial particles. Arch Biochem Biophys 250: 476–478

48. Rottenberg H, Hashimoto K (1986) Fatty acid uncoupling of oxidative phosphorylation in rat liver mitochondria. Biochemistry 25: 1747–1755

49. Shrago E (1978) The effect of long chain fatty acyl CoA esters on the adenine nucleotide translocase in myocardial metabolism. Life Sci 22: 1–6

50. Chua BH, Shrago E (1977) Reversible inhibition of adenine nucleotide translocation by long chain acyl CoA esters in bovine heart mitochondria and inverted submitochondrial particles. J Biol Chem 252: 6711–6714

51. Shrago E, Shug AL, Sul H, Bittar N, Folts JD (1976) Control of energy production in myocardial ischemia. Circ Res Suppl 1 (38): I–75–I–79

52. Lanoue KF, Watts JA, Koch CD (1981) Adenine nucleotide transport during cardiac ischemia. Am J Physiol 241: H663–H671
53. Woldegiorgis G, Shrago E, Kipp J, Yatvin M (1981) Fatty acyl Co-enzyme A sensitive adenine nucleotide transport in a reconstituted liposome system. J Biol Chem 256: 12297–12300
54. Ruoho AE, Woldegiorgis G, Kobayashi C, Shrago E (1989) Specific labeling of beef heart mitochondrial ADP/ATP carrier with ACT-CoA, a newly synthesized [125I] Co-enzyme A derivative photolabel. J Biol Chem 264: 4168–4172
55. Severson DL, Hurley B (1982) Regulation of rat heart triacylglycerol ester hydrolases by free fatty acids, fatty acyl CoA and fatty acyl carnitine. J Mol Cell Cardiol 14: 467–474
56. McDonough KH, Neely JR (1988) Inhibition of myocardial lipase by palmitoyl CoA, J Mol Cell Cardiol 20 (Suppl 2): 31–39
57. Flatmark T, Pederson JI (1975) Brown adipose tissue mitochondria, Biochem Biophys Acta 416: 53–103
58. Miller KW, Paton WDM, Smith EB, Smith RA (1972) Physicochemical approaches to the mode of action of general anesthetics. Anesthesiology 36: 339–351
59. Gruber HJ, Low PS (1988) Interaction of amphiphiles with integral membrane proteins. I. Structural destabilization of the anion transport protein of the erythrocyte membrane by fatty acids, fatty alcohols, and fatty amines. Biochem Biophys Acta 944: 414–424
60. Gruber HJ (1988) Interaction of amphiphiles with integral membrane proteins. II. A simple minimal model for the non-specific interaction of amphiphiles with the anion exchanger of the arythrocyte membrane. Biochim Biophys Acta 944: 425–436
61. Glatz JFC, Veerkamp JH (1985) Intracellular fatty acid binding proteins. Int J Biochem 17: 13–22
62. Veerkamp JH, Paulussen RJA (1987) Fatty acid transport in muscle: The role of fatty acid binding proteins. Biochem Soc Trans 15: 331–336
63. Wu-Rideout MYC, Elson C, Shrago E (1976) The role of fatty acid binding protein on the metabolism of fatty acids in isolated rat hepatocytes. Biochem Biophys Res Commun 71: 809–816
64. Burrier RE, Manson CR, Brecher P (1987) Binding of acyl CoA to liver fatty acid binding protein: Affect on acyl CoA synthesis. Biochem Biophys Acta 919: 221–230
65. Fournier NC, Zuker M, Williams RE, Smith ICP (1983) Self association of the cardiac fatty acid binding protein. Influence on membrane bound fatty acid dependent enzymes. Biochemistry 22: 1863–1872
66. Fournier NC, Rahim M (1985) Control of energy production in the heart. A new function for fatty acid binding protein. Biochemistry 24: 2387–2396
67. Jagschies G. Reers M, Utenberg C, Spener F (1985) Bovine fatty acid binding proteins: Isolation and characterization of two cardiac fatty acid binding proteins that are distinct from corresponding hepatic proteins. Eur J Biochem 152: 537–545
68. Idell-Wenger JA, Grotyohann LW, Neely JR (1978) Coenzyme A and carnitine distribution in normal and ischemic hearts. J Biol Chem 253: 4310–4318
69. Liedtke AJ, Nellis S, Neely JR (1987) Effects of excess free fatty acids on mechanical and metabolic function in normal and ischemic myocardium in swine. Circ Res 43: 652–661
70. Liedtke AJ (1981) Alterations of carbohydrates and lipid metabolism in the acutely ischemic heart. Prog Cardiovasc Dis 23: 321–336
71. Liedtke AJ, Mahar CQ, Ytrehus K, Mjos OD (1984) Estimates of free-radical production in rat and swine hearts: Method and application of measuring malondialdehyde levels in fresh and frozen myocardium. Basic Res Cardiol 79: 513–518
72. Corr PB, Gross RW, Sobel BE (1982) Arrhythmogenic amphiphilic lipids and the myocardial cell membrane. J Mol Cell Cardiol 14: 619–626
73. Corr PB, Gross RW, Sobel BE (1984) Amphipathic metabolites and membrane dysfunction in ischemic myocardium. Circ Res 55: 135–154
74. Bergmann SR, Ferguson TB, Sobel BE (1981) Effect of amphiphiles on erythrocytes,

coronary arteries, and perfused hearts. Am J Physiol 240 (Heart Circ Physiol 9): H229–H237
75. Harrison EH, Walusimbi-Kisit U. Properties in subcellular localization of myocardial fatty acyl-Coenzyme A oxidase. Am J Physiol 225: (Heart Circ Physiol 24) H441–H445
76. Kang ES, Mirvis DM (1984) Reversible, highly localized alterations in fatty acid metabolism in the chronically ischemic canine myocardium. Am J Cardiol 54: 411–414
77. Neely JR, Morgan HE (1976) Relationship between carbohydrate and lipid metabolism and the energy balance of heart muscle. Ann Rev Physiol 36: 413–459
78. Schelbert HR, Henze E, Keen R, Schon HR, Hansen H, Selin C, Huang S-C, Barreo JR, Phelps ME (1983) C-11 palmitate for the noninvasive evaluation of regional myocardial fatty acid metabolism with positron-computed tomography. IV. In vivo evaluation of acute demand-induced ischemia in dog. Am Heart J 106: 736–785
79. Jansen DE, Pippin J, Hansen C, Henderson E, Kulkarni P, Ugolini V, Corbett JR (1987) Use of radioactive iodine-labeled fatty acids for myocardial imaging. Am J Cardiac Imaging 1: 132–144
80. Feuvray D, Idell-Wenger JA, Neely JR (1979) Effects of ischemia on rat myocardial function and metabolism in diabetes. Circ Res 44: 322–329
81. Prinzen FW, Van der Vusse GJ, Rots T, Roemen THM, Koumans WA, Reneman RS (1984) Accumulation of nonesterified fatty acids in ischemic canine myocardium. Am J Physiol 247 (Heart Circ Physiol 16): H264–H272
82. Gercken G, Trotz M (1983) Fatty acid synthesis in the arrested rabbit heart during ischemia. Pflugers Arch 398: 69–72
83. Victor T, la Cock C, Lochner A (1984) Myocardial tissue free fatty acids. J Mol Cell Cardiol 16: 709–721
84. Jodalen H, Stangeland L, Grong K, Vik-mo H, Lekven J (1985) Lipid accumulation in the myocardium during acute regional ischaemia in cats. J Mol Cell Cardiol 17: 973–980
85. Bilheimer D, Buja LM, Parkey RW, Bonte FJ, Willerson JT (1978) Fatty acid accumulation and abnormal lipid deposition in peripheral and border zones of experimental myocardial infarcts. J Nucl Med 19: 276–283
86. Feuvray D (1981) Structural, functional, and metabolic correlates in ischemic hearts. Effects of substrates. Am J Physiol 240 (Heart Circ Physiol 9): H391–H398
87. Feuvray D, Plouet J (1981) Relationship between structure and fatty acid metabolism in mitochondria isolated from ischemic rat hearts. Circ Res 48: 740–747
88. Fields LE, Daugherty A, Bergmann SR (1986) Effect of fatty acid on performance and lipid content of hearts from diabetic rabbits. Am J Physiol 250 (Heart Circ Physiol 19): H1079–H1085
89. Most AS, Capone RJ, Szydlik P, Bruno CA, DeVona TS (1974) Failure of free fatty acids to influence degree of myocardial injury following acute coronary artery occlusion in pigs. Cardiol 59: 201–212
90. Most AS, Szydlik PA, Sorem KR (1972) Effect of free fatty acid on myocardial function during hypoxia. Cardiol 57: 322–332
91. Liedtke AJ, DeMaison L, Eggleston AM, Cohen LM, Nellis SH (1988) Changes in substrate metabolism and effects of excess fatty acids in reperfused myocardium. Circ Res 62: 535–542
92. Pande SV, Goswami T, Parvin R (1984) Protective role of adenine nucleotide translocase in O$_2$ deficient hearts. Am J Physiol 247: H25–H34
93. Heyndrickx GR, Millard RW, McRitchie RJ, Maroko PR, Vatner SF (1975) Regional myocardial functional and electrophysiological alterations after brief coronary artery occlusion in conscious dogs. J Clin Invest 56: 978–985
94. Theroux P, Ross J, Franklin D, Kemper WS, Sasayama S (1976) Coronary artery reperfusion. III. Early and late effects on regional myocardial function and dimensions in conscious dogs. Am J Cardiol 38: 599–606
95. Braunwald E, Kloner RA (1982) The stunned myocardium: Prolonged, postischemic ventricular dysfunction. Circ 66: 1146–1149
96. Bush LR, Buja LM, Samowitz W, Rude RE, Wathen M, Tilton GD, Willerson JT (1983)

Recovery of left ventricular segmental function after long-term reperfusion following temporary coronary occlusion in conscious dogs. Comparison of 2- and 4- hour occlusions. Circ Res 53: 248–263

97. Braunwald E, Kloner RA (1985) Myocardial reperfusion: A double-edged sword? J Clin Invest 76: 1713–1719

98. Liedtke AJ, Demaison L, Nellis SH (1988) Effects of L-propionylcarnitine on mechanical recovery during reflow in intact hearts. Am J Physiol 255 (Heart, Circ, Physiol 24): H169–H176

99. Zhao M, Zhang H, Robinson TF, Factor SM, Sonnenblick EH, Eng C (1987) Profound structural alterations of the extracellular collagen matrix in postischemic dysfunctional ("stunned") but viable myocardium. J Am Coll Cardiol 10: 1322–1334

100. Jennings RB, Herdson PB, Sommers HM (1969) Structural and functional abnormalities in mitochondria isolated from ischemic dog myocardium. Lab Invest 20: 548–557

101. Schwartz A, Wood JM, Allen JC, Bornet EP, Entman ML, Goldstein MA, Sordahl LA, Suzuki M (1973) Biochemical and morphologic correlates of cardiac ischemia. 1 Membrane Systems. Am J Cardiol 32: 46–61

102. Neubauer S Hamman BL, Perry SB, Bittl JA, Ingwall JS (1988) Velocity of the creatine kinase reaction decreases in postischemic myocardium: A^{31}P-NMR magnetization transfer study of the isolated ferret heart. Circ Res 63: 1–15

103. McDonough KH, Spitzer JJ (1983) Effects of hypoxia and reoxygenation on adult rat heart cell metabolism. Proc Soc Exp Biol Med 173: 519–526

104. Rouslin W (1987) Persistence of mitochondrial competence during myocardial autolysis. Am J Physiol 252 (Heart Circ Physiol 21): H985–H989

105. Bolukoglu H, Nellis SH, Liedtke AJ: Effects of proprionate on mechanical and metabolic performance in aerobic rat hearts. Cardiovasc Drugs and Therapy (in press)

106. Renstrom B, Liedtke AJ, Whitesell LF, Kneeland LM, Eggleston AM, Nellis SH (1988) Pyruvate oxidation in reperfused myocardium. Circ 78 (Suppl II): II–343

107. Renstrom B, Liedtke AJ, Nellis SH (1989) Metabolic oxidation of glucose during early myocardial reperfusion. Circ Res 65: 1094–1101

108. Reibel DK, Rovetto MJ (1978) Myocardial ATP synthesis and mechanical function following oxygen deficiency. Am J Physiol 234 (Heart Circ Physiol 3): H620–H624

109. DeBoer LWV, Ingwall JS, Kloner RA, Braunwald E (1980) Prolonged derangements of canine myocardial purine metabolism after a brief coronary artery occlusion not associated with anatomical evidence of necrosis. Proc Natl Acad Sci USA 77: 5471–5475

110. Kloner RA, DeBoer LWV, Darsee JR, Ingwall JS, Hale S, Tumas J, Braunwald E (1981) Prolonged abnormalities of myocardium salvaged by reperfusion. Am J Physiol (Heart Circ Physiol 10): H591-H599

111. Neely JR, Grotyohann LW (1984) Role of glycolytic products in damage to ischemic myocardium: Dissociation of adenosine triphosphate levels and recovery of function of reperfused ischemic hearts. Circ Res 55: 816–824

112. Demaison L, Liedtke AJ, Shrago E, Nellis SH, Woldegiorgis G (1989) Changes in energy energy metabolism and mitochondrial function in the reperfused working swine heart. J Applied Cardiol 4: 431–440

113. Bittl JA, Weisfeld ML, Jacobus WE. Creatine kinase of heart mitochondria. The progressive loss of enzyme activity during in vivo ischemia and its correlation to depressed myocardial function. J Biol Chem 260: 208–214

114. Greenfield RA, Swain JL (1987) Disruption of myofibrillar energy use: Dual mechanisms that may contribute to postischemic dysfunction in stunned myocardium. Circ Res 60: 283–289

115. Bolli R, Patel BS, Jeroudi MO, Lai EK, McCay PB: Demonstration of free radical generation in "stunned" myocardium of intact dogs with the use of the spin trap alpha-phenyl-N-tert-butylnitrone. J Clin Invest (in press)

116. Ambrosio G, Weisfeldt ML, Jacobus WE, Flaherty JT (1987) Evidence for a reversible oxygen radical-mediated component of reperfusion injury: Reduction by recombinant human superoxide dismutase administered at the time of reflow. Circ 75: 282–291

117. Cohen MV (1989) Free radicals in ischemic and reperfusion myocardial injury: Is this the time for clinical trial? Axual Int Med 111: 918–991

118. Bolli R (1988) Oxygen-derived free radicals and postischemic myocardial dysfunction ("stunned myocardium"). J Am Coll Cardiol 12: 239–249

119. Bagani M, Vatner SF, Baig H, Braunwald E (1978) Initial myocardial adjustments to brief periods of ischemia and reperfusion in the conscious dog. Circ Res 43: 83–92

120. Stahl L. Aversano T, Becker LC (1987) Functional overshoot after brief coronary occlusions in stunned and normal myocardium. J Am Coll Cardiol 9: 94A

121. Knabb RM, Rosamond TL, Fox KAA, Sobel BE, Bergmann SR (1986) Enhancement of salvage of reperfused ischemic myocardium by diltiazem. J Am Coll Cardiol 8: 861–871

122. Mercier JC, Lando U, Kanmatsu SE, Ninomiya K, Meerbaum S, Fishbein MC, Swan HJC, Ganz W (1982) Divergent effects of inotropic stimulation on the ischemic and severely depressed reperfused myocardium. Circulation 66: 397–400

123. O'Neill PG, Charlat ML, Hartley CJ, Roberts R, Bowley R (1987) Non-uniform transmural response of the "stunned" myocardium to inotropic stimulation. J Am Coll Cardiol 9: 145A

124. Becker LC, Levine JH, DiPaula AF, Guarinieri T, Aversano T (1986) Reversal of dysfunction in postischemic stunned myocardium by epinephrine and postextrasystolic potentiation. J Am Coll Cardiol 7: 580–589

125. Kitakaze M, Weisfeldt ML, Marban E (1988) Acidosis during early reperfusion prevents myocardial stunning in perfused ferret hearts. J Clin Invest 82: 920–927

126. Manning AS, Hearse DJ (1984) Reperfusion-induced arrhythmias: Mechanisms and prevention. J Mol Cell Cardiol 16: 497–518

127. Tennant R, Wiggers CJ (1935) The effect of coronary occlusion on myocardial contraction. Am J Physiol 112: 351–361

128. Corr PB, Witkowski FX (1983) Potential electrophysiologic mechanisms responsible for dysrhythmias associated with reperfusion of ischemic myocardium. Circulation 68 (Suppl 1): 16–24

129. Bernier M, Hearse DJ (1988) Reperfusion-induced arrhythmias: Mechanisms of protection by glucose and mannitol. Am J Physiol 254 (Heart Circ Physiol 23): H862–H870

130. Carbonen P, Di Gennaro M, Valle R, Weisz AM (1981) Inhibitory effect of anoxia on reperfusion-and digitalis-induced ventricular tachyarrhythmias. Am J Physiol 240 (Heart Circ Physiol 9): H730–H731

131. Chatelan P, Papgeorgiou I, Luthy P, Melchior JP, Rutishauser W, Lerch R (1987) Free fatty acid metabolism in "stunned" myocardium. Basic Res Cardiol 82 (Suppl I): 169–176

132. Lerch R, Gorge G, Papgeorgiou I, Rutishauser W (1988) Myocardial fatty acid metabolism following reperfusion: Effect of different degrees of ischemic injury. Second International Symposium on lipid metabolism in the normoxic and ischemic heart: 76

133. Miller DD, Gill JB, Livni B, Elmaleh DR, Aretz T, Boucher CA, Strauss HW (1988) Fatty acid analogue accumulation: A marker of myocyte viability in ischemic-reperfused myocardium. Circ Res 63: 681–692

134. Schwaiger M, Schelbert Hr, Ellison D, Hansen H, Yeatman L, Venten-Johansen J, Selin C, Barrio J, Phelps ME (1985) Sustained regional abnormalities in cardiac metabolism after transient ischemia in the chronic dog model. J Am Coll Cardiol 6: 336–347

135. Ichihara K, Neely JR (1985) Recovery of ventricular function in reperfused ischemic rat hearts exposed to fatty acids. Am J Physiol 249 (Heart Circ Physiol 18): H492–H497

136. Lopaschuk GD, Wall SR, Olley OM, Davies NJ (1988) Etomoxir, a carnitine palmitoltransferase I inhibitor, protects hearts from fatty acid-induced ischemic injury independent of changes in long-chain acylcarnitine. Circ Res 63: 1036–1043

137. Kotaka K, Miyazaki Y, Ogawa K, Satake T, Sugiyama S, Ozawa T (1982) Reversal of ischemia-induced mitochondrial dysfunction after coronary reperfusion. J Mol Cell Cardiol 14: 223–231

138. Kajiyama K, Pauly DF, Hughes H, Yoon SB, Entman ML, McMillian-Wood JB (1987) Protection by verapamil of mitochondrial glutathione equilibrium and phospholipid changes during reperfusion of ischemic canine myocardium. Circ Res 61: 301–310

139. Sobel BE, Corr PB. Robison AK, Goldstein RA, Witkowski FX, Klein MS (1978) Accumulation of lysophosphoglycerides with arrythmogenic properties in ischemic myocardium. J Clin Invest 62: 546–552

140. Corr PB, Cain ME, Witkowski FX, Price DA, Sobel BE (1979) Potential arrhythmogenic electrophysiological derangements in canine Purkinge fibers induced by lysophosphoglycerides. Circ Res 44: 822–832

141. Snyder DW, Crafford WA, Glashow JL, Rankin D, Sobel BE, Corr PB (1981) Lysophosphoglycerides in ischemic myocardium effluents and potentiation of their arrhythmogenic effects. Am J Physiol 241 (Heart Circ Physiol 10): H700–H707

142. Corr PB, Snyder DW, Lee BI, Gross RW, Keim CR, Sobel BE (1982) Pathophysiological concentrations of lysophosphatides and their slow response. Am J Physiol 243 (Heart Circ Physiol 12): H187–H195

143. Romaschin AD, Rebeyka I, Wilson GJ, Mickle DAG (1987) Conjugated dienes in ischemic and reperfused myocardium: An *in vivo* chemical signature of oxygen free-radical injury. J Mol Cell Cardiol 19: 289–302

144. Bricknell OL, Opie LH (1978) Effects of substrates on tissue metabolic changes in the isolated rat heart during underperfusion and on release of lactate dehydrogenase and arrhythmias during reperfusion. Circ Res 43: 102–114

Hydrolysis of phospholipids and cellular integrity

GER J. VAN DER VUSSE, MARC VAN BILSEN, TRUDI
SONDERKAMP and ROBERT S. RENEMAN
Department of Physiology, University of Limburg, Maastricht, The Netherlands

Key words: heart, myocardium, ischemia, reperfusion, sarcolemma,
phospholipids, fatty acids, arachidonic acid, phospholipases, oxygen free
radicals, calcium, osmotic load, ATP, cell death, necrosis

Abstract

Like all living cells, myocytes are enclosed in a plasma membrane (plasmalemma) which is composed of phospholipids, cholesterol and proteins. The
phospholipids form a lipid bilayer. Disruption of the plasmalemma has been
postulated to be a proximate cause of irreversible injury inflicted on the cell
by ischemia and/or reperfusion. Depletion of phospholipids, by either enhanced enzymatic hydrolysis or impaired resynthesis of the phospholipid
molecules, has been proposed as a mechanism underlying ischemia and
reperfusion-induced rupturing of the plasmalemma. Acidification of the
tissue, enhanced cytosolic Ca^{2+} levels, physico-chemical changes in the membrane, release of hydrolytic enzymes from endogenous stores, and too low
ATP contents may trigger the hydrolysis of membrane phospholipids during
the ischemic insult. In addition, lipid peroxidation, rapidly occurring after
reinstallation of blood flow and, hence, the supply of oxygen to the previously
ischemic cells, has been suggested to make phospholipids in the membrane
more susceptible to phospholipase-mediated hydrolysis.

According to an alternative theory, physical forces, like osmotic load and
mechanical stress, are the cause of fracturing of the sarcolemma. Prior to
disruption, the cell membrane is most likely labilized by a variety of events.
Impaired anchoring of the lipid bilayer to the cytoskeleton might result in
increased membrane fragility. In addition, internal reorganization of the lipid
bilayer, as reflected by the loss of phospholipid asymmetry, formation of
multilamellar vesicles and aggregation of membrane proteins due to phase
separation, might destabilize the plasmalemma. As a consequence of membrane disruption by physical forces, the cell dies and the remnants, including
the phospholipid-containing membranes, are digested by endogenous hydrolytic enzymes. In this respect, hydrolysis of phospholipids has to be considered as a feature of the healing process occurring after irreversible damage of
the cardiac cell and aiming at removal of cell debris by chemical means. When
the latter theory is correct, then it is unlikely that phospholipid hydrolysis

H.M. Piper (ed.) Pathophysiology of severe ischemic myocardial injury, 167–193.
© 1990 Kluwer Academic Publishers, Dordrecht –

plays a key role in the process involved in the transition from reversible to irreversible injury in ischemic and reperfused cardiac tissue.

To date, there is no conclusive evidence as to which of the two theoretical concepts is correct.

Introduction

Reduced blood supply to myocardial cells, a situation commonly called 'ischemia', results in a shortage of molecular oxygen required to maintain oxidative energy delivery. Furthermore, the removal of waste products of cellular metabolism is also impaired [56]. Reduced blood flow is associated with a rapid impairment of mechanical function [59]. Contractile failure is probably related to increased levels of H^+ ions and inorganic phosphate in the cardiac muscle cells [2]. Tissue creatine phosphate levels are rapidly depleted. The mitochondrial production of ATP is reduced or completely abolished, depending on the residual amount of oxygen supplied to the cell. The amount of anaerobically produced ATP in the glycolytic pathway is transiently enhanced. Due to acidification of the tissue and accumulation of lactate the glycolytic flux becomes depressed during prolonged ischemia [52]. The cellular content of ATP slowly declines with a concomitant accumulation of AMP and other degradation products, such as adenosine, inosine, and, to a lesser extent, hypoxanthine [40]. The ability to maintain cellular electrolyte balance is seriously challenged. Part of the intracellular potassium is released into the interstitial space and the cytosolic content of free Ca^{2+} is increased [72].

Prolongation of the time interval of ischemia ultimately results in lethal cell injury [40]. Electron microscopic studies have revealed disorganization of mitochondria and myofibrills [61], and fractured cell membranes [40]. Loss of intracellular macromolecules, such as cytosolic enzymes, and free diffusion of extracellular substances into the intracellular space readily occur. The mechanism underlying the transition of reversible to irreversible (lethal) cellular injury during ischemia is not completely understood [56]. This is also true of the injury inflicted on previously ischemic cells after restoration of flow. Although disagreements exist about the extent to which reperfusion *per se* causes additional damage to the affected cells, the mechanism involved in reperfusion-induced injury is generally thought to be different from that in oxygen deprived cells.

Since an intact cell membrane is essential for normal cell function, disruption of the plasmalemma has been considered as a proximate cause of lethal cell injury during ischemia and/or reperfusion. Basically, two different theories emerge from the literature with respect to the mechanism underlying the loss of plasmalemmal integrity. The first one assumes that phospholipid turnover in the cell becomes impaired by either enhanced phospholipid degradation or inhibition of resynthesis. On the one hand, this might result in the accumulation of degradation products, such as lysophospholipids and fatty acids, in the membrane structures, which, in turn, greatly enhances the vulnerability of the membrane. On the other hand, the number of phospholipids will be substantially reduced, which most likely results in loss of membrane function and, possibly, in fracturing of the membrane. Second, opposing the (bio) chemical theory, physical forces have been held responsible for the loss of cell membrane integrity. According to Jennings and co-workers [41], increased cellular osmolarity of the ischemic cells causes a shift of extracellular water into the interior of the cell and, hence, cell swelling. This event will impose considerable stress on the sarcolemma, ultimately resulting in disruption of the membrane.

In this chapter, the potentially detrimental role of the perturbed phospholipid homeostasis in flow deprived and reperfused cardiac tissue will be discussed.

Phospholipid homeostasis in normal cardiac cells

Phospholipid species and membrane composition

Myocytes are enclosed in a plasmalemma whereas internal membranes surround the organelles localized inside the cell. Phospholipids and cholesterol are the main lipid constituents of the membranes. Phospholipids are present in a variety of species. Phospholipids contain a hydrophobic tail and a hyrophilic head group. The hydrophobic tail is composed of two long-chain fatty acids, covalently bound to the first (Sn_1) and second (Sn_2) carbon atom of the glycerol backbone of the phospholipid molecule (Fig. 1). The hydrophilic head group, determining the phospholipid species, is an alcohol molecule bound to the third (Sn_3) carbon atom of the glycerol backbone via a phosphate group (Fig. 1). The most common alcohol moieties of phospholipids are choline, ethanolamine, serine, inositol and glycerol. The number of carbon atoms in the aliphatic chain is even and varies from 14 to 24. The number of unsaturated bonds varies as well. In fatty acids with very long chain lengths, up to 6 unsaturated bonds can be found. The relative composition of the fatty acyl moieties greatly differs from one phospholipid species to another. In most animal species, up to 40% of the total phospholipid pool in cardiac myocytes is present in the plasmalogen form. In these phospholipids the connection of the aliphatic chain with the first carbon atom of the glycerol backbone is a vinyl ether linkage instead of an ester bond. It should be noted that considerable differences in animal species with respect to the proportion of plasmalogens in cardiac tissue have been reported [34, 66, 81]. In addition to phospholipids, sphingomyelin, the backbone of which is a sphingosine molecule, is present in cardiac tissue.

The membranes are composed of two leaflets. In the case of the plasmalemma, the hydrophilic head groups of the outer leaflet of the lipid bilayer

170

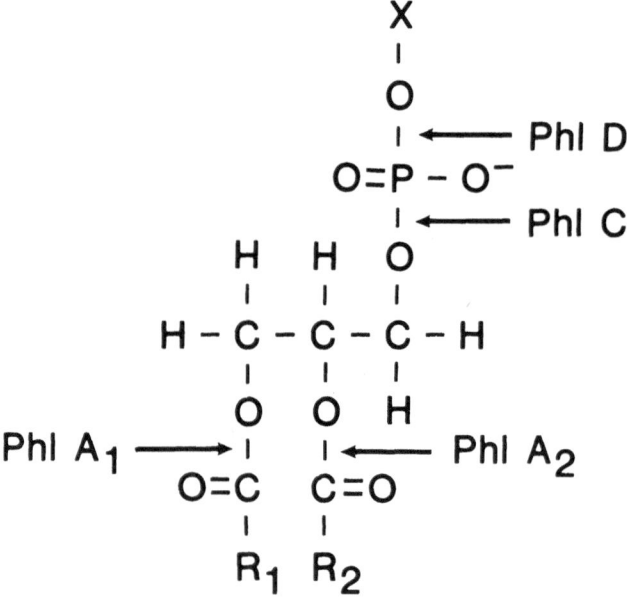

Fig. 1. Chemical structure of phospholipids and site of action of phospholipases. R_1 refers to the aliphatic tail of saturated fatty acids, such as palmitic and stearic acid, or monounsaturated fatty acids, such as oleic acid, which are covalently linked to the first carbon atom of the glycerol backbone. Polyunsaturated fatty acids, such as arachidonic acid, are generally bound to the middle carbon atom of glycerol. The tail of this fatty acid is denoted by R_2. In the case of plasmalogens, the first aliphatic tail is connected to glycerol via a vinyl ether linkage. The two aliphatic chains represent the hydrophobic part of the phospholipid molecule. The species of the phospholipid is determined by the nature of the X-group, which is linked via a phosphate-ester to the third carbon atom of glycerol. X is generally choline, ethanolamine, serine or inositol. The glycerol-phosphate-X part of the phospholipid molecule represents the hydrophylic head group. The specific site of action of the various phospholipases is indicated by an arrow. Reprinted from Van der Vusse *et al.* [87] with permission.

point toward the extracellular and those of the inner leaflet towards the intracellular space. The hydrophobic fatty acid tails are buried in the inner part of the lipid bilayer. The distribution of phospholipids over the two leaflets is asymmetric. The outer leaflet of the sarcolemma is relatively enriched in phosphatidylcholine and sphingomyelin. The inner leaflet contains phosphatidylethanolamine, phosphatidylserine, phosphatidylinositol and phosphatidylcholine [58]. To compensate for differences in fluidity between the two leaflets of the bilayer, more cholesterol is incorporated in the outer than in the inner leaflet [25].

Proper functioning of the membranes is required to ensure normal cellular performance. Membranes enable the cells and organelles to maintain an internal microenvironment with optimal conditions for their specific metabolic processes. Membranes are barriers for macromolecules and the majority of polar substances. Proteins are localized in the lipid bilayer to regulate, among others, the transport of molecules across the membrane. Approximately 50% of the plasmalemmal surface is occupied by proteins.

Phospholipid turnover

The phospholipids composing the lipid bilayers are subjected to a continuous turnover process. This cycle enables the cell to synthetize any required phospholipid, to regulate the composition and, to a certain extent, the properties of its membranes. There are several routes for the degradation and resynthesis of phospholipids in the cardiac cell (Fig. 2). The enzymes which initiate the turnover of phospholipids are phospholipases. Cardiac cells contain a variety of different phospholipases. These enzymes are named after the localization and nature of the chemical bond in the phospholipid molecule hydrolyzed by their action (Fig. 1). Phospholipase A_1 cleaves the Sn_1 glycerol acylester linkage, phospholipase A_2 hydrolyzes the Sn_2 glycerol acylester bond, phospholipase C cleaves the bond between the phosphate group of the polar head group and the third carbon atom of the glycerol backbone, and phospholipase D breaks the alcohol-phosphate bond of the polar head group.

Lysophospholipase (Fig. 2) removes the remaining fatty acyl chain in lysophospholipids, the products of phospholipase A_1 or A_2 action [33, 35, 51, 65]. Specific hydrolytic enzymes for the degradation of plasmalogens (plasmalogenases and plasmalogen specific phospholipase A_2) and sphingomyelin (sphingomyelinases) have been identified in cardiac tissue [3, 4, 50, 100]. Phospholipid hydrolyzing enzymes are localized in almost all compartments and membrane structures of the myocyte. Phospholipase A_1 and A_2 activity is present in the cytosol [10, 50, 51, 100]. The pH optimum varies from 7 in bovine heart to 8.4 in rat hearts. Phospholipase C has been detected in the cytosolic compartment and lysosomes of the heart [28, 63, 100]. In a variety of species phospholipase A_2 activity is present in the sarcolemma [26, 94]. The pH optimum varies from 6 to 9. Mitochondrial membranes host both phospholipase A_1 and A_2 activity with a mildly alkaline pH optimum [4, 30, 50, 55, 93]. The microsomal fraction, mainly consisting of fragmented sarcoplasmatic reticulum, shows phospholipase A_1 and A_2 activity [30, 93, 100]. Lysosomes contain phospholipase A_1 and A_2, both active at low pH, i.e. in the order of pH 4–5 [27, 50]. Lysophospholipase activity has been monitored in the cytosol [32, 50] and to a lesser extent in mitochondria, sarcoplasmic reticulum and lysosomes [50].

Resynthesis of phospholipids is most likely confined to the sarcoplasmic reticulum. Considering the synthesis of phosphatidylcholine (Fig. 2) several anabolic routes are potentially operative. First, when lysophosphatidylcholine is present as substrate, incorporation of the second fatty acyl chain is accomplished by action of lysophosphatidylcholine acyl transferase [31]. Alternatively, de novo phosphatidylcholine synthesis is regulated by the

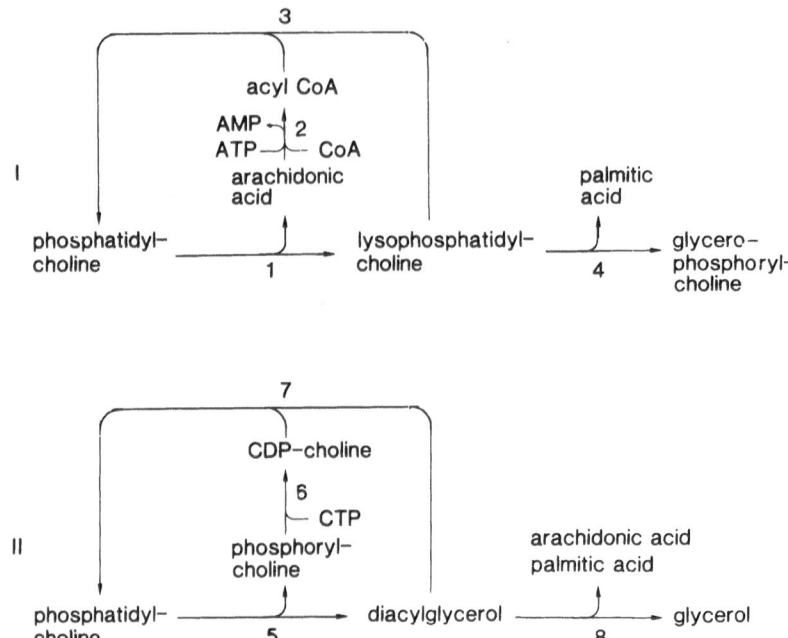

Fig. 2. Enzymatic turnover and degradation of phosphatidylcholine. Pathway I describes the deacylation-reacylation pathway of phosphatidylcholine. In this example palmitic acid and arachidonic acid are bound to the first and second carbon atom of the glycerol backbone, respectively. 1, 2, 3 and 4 refer to phospholipase A_2, acylCoA synthetase, lysophosphatidylcholine acyltransferase and lysophospholipase, respectively. Note: AMP is a potent inhibitor of acylCoA synthetase activity. Pathway II describes the turnover of phosphorylcholine, the hydrophylic head group in phosphatidylcholine. 5, 6, 7 and 8 refer to phospholipase C, phosphorylcholine cytidylyltransferase, phosphocholine transferase and diacylglycerol + monoacylglycerol lipase, respectively. CTP refers to cytidine triphosphate. Reprinted from Van der Vusse *et al.* [87] with permission.

action of choline-phosphotransferase, catalyzing the condensation of 1,2 diacylglycerol and CDP-choline (Fig. 2). Likewise, the synthesis of phosphatidylethanolamine takes place in mammalian cells. The *de novo* synthesis of phosphatidylserine and inositol starts with the formation of CDP-diacylglycerol from cytidine triphosphate and phosphatidic acid. CDP-diacylglycerol reacts with serine and inositol to produce phosphatidylserine and phosphatidylinositol, respectively. The newly synthesized phospholipids are transported by specific phospholipid binding proteins through the cytosol to the membranes [99]. The fatty acyl moieties to be incorporated into the phospholipid molecule have to be activated by acylCoA synthetase yielding acylCoA. The latter enzyme is localized at the outer mitochondrial membrane and in the sarcoplasmic reticulum.

Under regulated conditions, resynthesis of phospholipids has to keep pace with degradation in order to prevent net loss of phospholipid material.

Detailed knowledge of the turnover rate of the phospholipid pool in myocytes is lacking. *In vitro* measurements of phospholipase A in cardiac homogenates revealed a maximal activity of this enzyme of about 3 μmol phospholipids per hour per gram tissue [78]. Taking into account a total phosphatidylcholine and phosphatidylethanolamine pool of 20 μmol per gram tissue, this value indicates that in normal cells, complete turnover of the fatty acid moieties is accomplished in about 7 hours. Since it is unlikely that all phospholipases operate at their maximal activity, the estimated value must be considered as the minimal time period needed to hydrolyse the total phospholipid pool. It is possible that each phospholipid species in each subcellular compartment is subjected to a different rate of digestion and resynthesis [49]. It is not yet known whether the cycle characterized by hydrolysis of the fatty acyl moiety by action of phospholipase A and subsequent reacylation of the glycerol backbone is quantitatively more important than the cycle initiated by the phospholipase C-mediated removal of the hydrophylic head group (Fig. 2). Furthermore, the site of phospholipid degradation in normal cardiac tissue has not been completely elucidated. On the one hand, the ubiquitous phospholipase activity suggests that degradation starts at the site of localization, i.e. in the membrane itself. On the other hand, membrane fragments might be transported to the lysosomes in the interior of which digestion of the phospholipid constituents occurs.

Regulation of hydrolysis

There is a definite lack of information on the factors regulating the rate of the phospholipid turnover cycles. Although most phospholipase enzymes are surrounded by an overwhelming number of substrates, the activity of the enzyme is apparently well controlled [82]. It has been suggested that a variety of factors regulate the hydrolysis of phospholipids.

1. Ca^{2+} ions. Some phospholipases, like those localized in the mitochondria, are strongly Ca^{2+} dependent in their action [93]. The influence of Ca^{2+} is probably mediated by calmodulin. In contrast, lysosomal phospholipases have been found to be Ca^{2+} insensitive [50]. It is believed that changes in the internal Ca^{2+} distribution and/or rises in the cytosolic Ca^{2+} concentration are associated with increased hydrolysis of phospholipids.

2. Substrate availability. Subtle changes in the microenvironment of the membrane-bound phospholipases may render more phospholipid molecules available as substrate for the hydrolyzing enzymes. These changes might be caused by internal reorganization of the lipid structures in the inner and outer leaflets of the membrane. In this respect, the possible role of the cytoskeleton is worth mentioning. Certain proteins, being an integral part of the internal structure called cytoskeleton, are believed to be anchored to membrane proteins and/or phospholipids in the inner leaflet of the plasmalemma. Changes in the interaction between cytoskeleton and plasmalemma might

eventually result in changes in hydrolytic activity of membrane bound phospholipase.

3. Specific intracellular phospholipase inhibitors. The activity of cellular phospholipases might be regulated by endogenous compounds displaying an inhibitory action on the enzymes. Recent studies have shown the existence of proteins with phospholipase A_2 inhibiting properties and a relatively low molecular weight in a variety of mammalian cells including monocytes, neutrophils and renal medullary cells [92]. These proteins are collectively called lipocortins. It is tempting to state that cardiac myocytes also contain lipocortin-like phospholipase A_2 modulators.

Phospholipid hydrolysis in ischemic and reperfused cardiac tissue

Perturbations in myocardial phospholipid homeostasis

Cellular and intracellular membranes play a pivotal role in maintaining the integrity of the cell and its subcellular organelles. Since membranes are composed of phospholipids, cholesterol and proteins, perturbations in phospholipid homeostasis might be a decisive link in the chain of events leading to cell death. Hydrolysis of phospholipids, of either the polar headgroup or one or both fatty acyl moieties, might be such a perturbation.

During the past two decades, a substantial number of experimental findings have been in favor of the notion that hydrolysis of phospholipids plays an important role in the pathogenesis of ischemia and/or reperfusion induced myocardial cell injury. Firstly, the content of phospholipids declines and degradation products, such as arachidonic acid and lysophospholipids, accumulate in the affected tissue [14, 18, 68, 84, 95]. Restoration of flow appears to promote further the net degradation of phospholipids in the previously flow-deprived tissue [9, 20, 81]. Secondly, exposure of cardiac cells and cellular organelles to exogenous phospholipase A or phospholipase C results in changes in the lipid content associated with impairment of function closely resembling the effect of ischemia on cardiac structures. Thirdly, drugs with putative phospholipase A inhibiting properties attenuate the deleterious effect of ischemia in the heart. Fourthly, alternative experimental models, such as isolated myocytes poisoned with metabolic blockers, show a close relationship between release of endogenous arachidonic acid and the loss of cellular function.

Changes in tissue content of phospholipids and degradation products

Several investigators have reported alterations in the content of phospholipids and degradation products in ischemic myocardial tissue. The pioneering study of Weglicki and associates [95] has shown a significant production of linoleic acid and arachidonic acid in isolated blood perfused canine hearts, made ischemic for 30 minutes. Arachidonic acid, a fatty acid preferentially incorporated at the Sn_2 position of phospholipids, accumulates predominantly in the subendocardial regions of the ischemic dog heart [59, 84]. In these regions, blood flow is most severely depressed during the ischemic insult. Arachidonic acid starts to accumulate after a time delay of approximately 30 minutes following the onset of ischemia [14, 81]. In ischemic myocardium increased levels of lysophospholipids have been reported by a substantial number of investigators [18, 19, 46, 66, 68, 70]. The phospholipid pool in ischemic cardiac tissue has been reported to be diminished as well [11, 13, 47, 63, 70]. Loss of phospholipids from ischemic myocytes seems to be specifically confined to phosphatidylcholine and phosphatidylethanolamine. Schwertz and co-workers [63] observed a significant increase in the content of phosphatidylinositol in ischemic rat heart. Others reported increased levels of cardiolipin in flow-deprived tissue [13, 47]. Epps and co-workers [23] reported the presence of phosphatidyl-N-acyl-ethanolamine in infarcted myocardial tissue. This phospholipid species is not detectable in the normal heart.

Many researchers have studied the effect of ischemia on the lipid content of subcellular fractions isolated from ischemic cardiac tissue. Yanagishita and associates [101] and Kajiyama and colleagues [42] detected small losses of phospholipids from mitochondria obtained from dog hearts, made regionally ischemic for 30 and 60 minutes, respectively. The former researchers did detect degradation of phosphatidylcholine and cardiolipin, while the content of phosphatidylethanolamine remained virtually unaffected. Earlier studies [91] indicated a slight increase in the mitochondrial content of sphingomyelin associated with changes in the acyl composition of phosphatidylethanolamine and phosphatidylinositol during the ischemic insult. Victor and colleagues [91] failed to observe a diminution of the phospholipid content in mitochondria isolated from ischemic cardiac tissue. The content of both phosphatidylcholine and phosphatidylethanolamine decreases in the sarcoplasmic reticulum isolated from ischemic dog heart [101]. Suyatna and co-workers [75] reported unchanged levels of phospholipids and lysophospholipids in sarcolemmal preparations harvested from rat hearts that were kept under ischemic conditions for up to 60 minutes.

Reperfusion after a period of total or partial ischemia seems to lead to an increased degradation of phospholipids in the affected myocardium. Das and colleagues [20] and Burton and co-workers [9] reported substantial reductions in the tissue content of various phospholipids after restoration of flow. The latter observed that the myocardial content of arachidonic acid remained elevated in reperfused hearts. Studies from our laboratory conducted on dog hearts *in situ* and isolated rat hearts indicated that accumulation of arachidonic acid proceeds during reperfusion [81, 85]. Accumulation of arachidonic acid in reperfused rat hearts appears to correlate quite well with the amount of lactate dehydrogenase released by the heart after reinstallation of flow (Fig. 3).

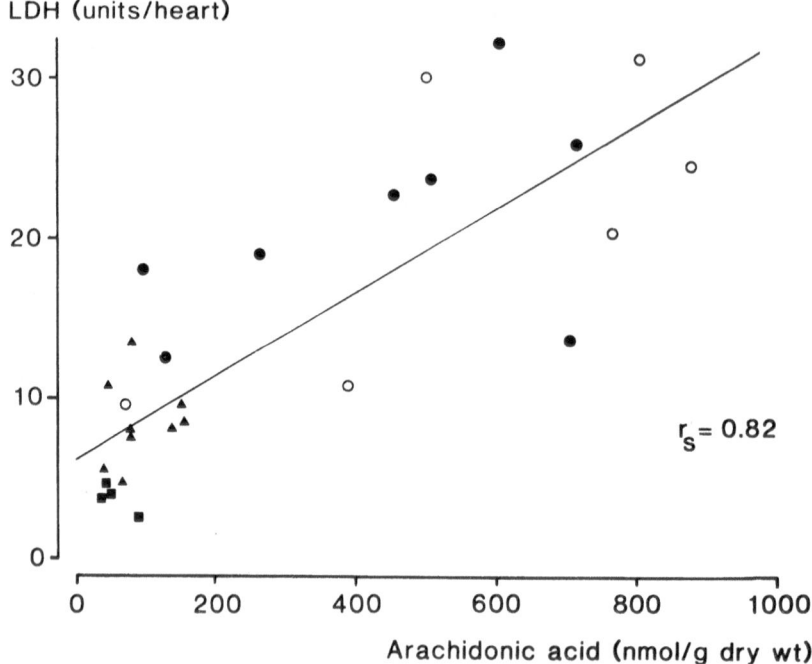

Fig. 3. Relationship between the content of arachidonic acid of reperfused hearts and the cumulative release of lactate dehydrogenase (LHD) during 30 minutes of reperfusion. The symbols refer to individual hearts previously subjected to 30 (■), 45▲, and 60 minutes of ischemia (● and ○ for electrically recovering and fibrillating hearts), respectively. r_s refers to the Spearman correlation coefficient. The matching regression equation was calculated to be $y = 0.026 \chi + 6.509$.

Bester and Lochner [8] failed to observe a significant change in the phospholipid content of sarcolemma obtained from isolated rat hearts made ischemic for 60 minutes and subsequently reperfused for 30 minutes. Hattori and colleagues [37] harvested mitochondria from canine hearts subjected to 15 minutes of ischemia followed by 5 minutes of reperfusion. The mitochondrial phospholipid content decreased by 30% in hearts which started to fibrillate after restoration of flow. No such decline could be detected in hearts which resumed normal electrical activity upon reperfusion.

Treatment of myocardial structures with phospholipase

The fact that myocardial structures are highly sensitive to exogenous phospholipase is commonly used as evidence that phospholipid degradation plays an important role in the pathogenesis of myocardial infarction. Isolated cardiac mitochondria were found to be highly sensitive to both exogenous phospholipase A_2 and phospholipase C [48]. Phospholipase treatment results in impairment of mitochondrial function and concomitant accumulation of degradation products of phospholipids. Similar studies conducted with isolated cardiac sarcoplasmic reticulum reveal that both phospholipase A_2 and phospholipase C evoke degradation of phospholipid constituents and impairment of membrane function [101]. Since the pattern of degradation products of phospholipase C treated microsomes closely resembles the composition of the lipid material accumulating in ischemic tissue, the authors concluded that phospholipase C, rather than phospholipase A_2, is involved in enhanced phospholipid degradation in flow deprived hearts.

Phospholipids in isolated sarcolemmal preparations are readily hydrolyzed by exogenous phospholipase A_2 and phospholipase C [1, 16, 73, 97]. The *in vitro* findings indicate that treatment with phospholipase A_2 results in the production of unsaturated fatty acids and lysophospholipids [16, 73], whereas phospholipase C provokes the release of both saturated and unsaturated fatty acids [73]. Phospholipases from lysosomes are a very effective means of hydrolyzing sarcolemmal phospholipids [6, 97, 98].

Intact isolated myocytes appear to be resistant against the attack of exogenous phospholipase A_2. In contrast, equal amounts of phospholipase C in the incubation medium caused considerable lysis of the myocytes as indicated by the loss of lactate dehydrogenase from the cytosolic compartment. At high intracellular ATP levels, the resistance of the myocytes to exogenous phospholipase C was found to be greatly enhanced [38].

Phospholipase inhibitors

The third kind of experimental data in favor of the notion that phospholipid hydrolysis is a key event in ischemia-induced cardiac injury is the protective effect of putative phospholipase inhibiting drugs against ischemia. An increasing number of pharmaceutical compounds, such as propranolol, amiodarone, verapamil, Q_{10}, chloroquine, chlorpromazine, mepacrine, diltiazem, commonly applied to reduce ischemia-induced damage in the heart in experimental studies, have been shown to possess phospholipase-inhibiting properties [12, 20, 39, 53, 67, 74, 76, 79, 80].

Alternative models of cellular injury

Experimental models, in which sarcolemmal disruption can be induced in a controlled and reproducible manner, have been used to delineate in more detail the possible causal relationship between phospholipid degradation and loss of sarcolemmal integrity. Chien and co-workers [15, 36, 64] applied a model in which the ATP content of cultured neonatal myocardial cells was depleted by metabolic blockade rather than ischemia or anoxia. The progressive release of arachidonic acid from endogenous phospholipids is closely related to the development of sarcolemmal membrane defects, electrolyte derangements, including calcium accumulation, and the associated loss of cell viability. This model suggests that hydrolysis of membrane phospholipids and loss of cellular integrity are causally related. The investigators intervened in the process leading to cell damage with U 26,384, a presumed specific phospholipase A_2 inhibitor. The drug blocked the degradation of phosphatidylcholine and the accumulation of arachidonic acid during ATP depletion. Concomitantly, the drug prevented sarcolemmal membrane defects and the release of creatine kinase from the cultured myocytes.

Putative mechanisms of action

Phospholipid hydrolysis

Proponents of the theory that hydrolysis of phospholipids and loss of cellular integrity are causally related have proposed a variety of mechanisms of action to explain net degradation of phospholipid molecules in ischemic myocytes.

Enhanced phospholipid hydrolysis might result from increased enzymatic activity of intracellular phospholipase A and/or phospholipase C. Theoretically, increased enzymatic activity can be caused by transition of the enzyme from an inactive into an active form by phosphorylation or dephosphorylation of the protein or by transformation of the enzyme molecule from a biological inactive pro-enzyme into the biological active form. With respect to cardiac phospholipases, such processes are unlikely to occur.

Increased intracellular levels of stimulating cations, such as Ca^{2+}, and changes in acidity are also candidates for stimulation of endogenous phospholipid hydrolysis. Part of the phospholipases A present in the heart is Ca^{2+} dependent and, in particular, lysosomal phospholipases show their maximal activity at low pH. Acidification of cardiac tissue during the ischemic attack is a well-known phenomenon and recent observations of Steenbergen and colleagues [72] indicate that the cytosolic free Ca^{2+} content increases rapidly after the onset of ischemia.

Ischemia-induced fracture of lysosomal membranes will promote the release of phospholipid hydrolyzing enzymes into the cytosolic compartment of the myocyte [29]. Alternatively, physico-chemical changes in the sarcolemma and intracellular membranes might increase the accessibility of phospholipids to the phospholipase enzymes. Phase transition of the phospholipids, potentially resulting in lipid domains devoid of proteins, multilammellar vesicles and extrusion of membrane material (the so-called 'blebs'), occurs in flow-deprived cardiac tissue (see below). These membrane changes might allow phospholipases to attack more vigorously the phospholipid constituents of the affected membranes.

Weglicki and colleagues [96, 98] have proposed that oxygen free radicals promote phospholipid hydrolysis. According to the 'free radical-triggered lipolysis by phospholipases theory', the bilayer is first peroxidized by an oxygen free radical mediated process to alter the acyl chain of some phospholipids and, hence, the physical characteristics of the membrane. In this theory, in the micro-environment of initial peroxidation, unchanged phospholipids would then become more preferred substrates for phospholipase attack, either by phospholipase A or phospholipase C [98]. Recent studies have shown that oxygen free radicals promote the release of hydrolytic enzymes from the interior of the lysosomes [22]. Although these oxygen free radical mediated processes are more likely to be operative in cardiac tissue after reinstallation of flow and, hence, renewed supply of molecular oxygen, it cannot be excluded that oxygen free radicals are also generated in ischemic cells since residual supply of oxygen is generally present, as has been argued by Kako and Kato [43].

It should be stressed that none of these possible mechanisms underlying enhanced phospholipid hydrolysis have been definitively proven to occur in the ischemic myocyte. Interestingly, several authors have reported a decline rather than an increase in the activity of cardiac phospholipases isolated from ischemic or hypoxic cardiac cells [7, 35]. It is tempting to state that (partial) inhibition of phospholipase activity in ischemic and hypoxic tissue is an intrinsic measure of the cardiac cells to protect their membranes against the attack of phospholipid hydrolyzing enzymes. Both mitochondrial, lysosomal and cytosolic phospholipases respond in this way. This inhibition might be caused by lysophospholipids and acyl carnitine [7] or by structural changes in the enzyme molecule. Since cytosolic phospholipase A_1 appears to contain sulfhydryl groups [5], the activity of this particular enzyme might be highly vulnerable to oxidative stress caused by oxygen free radicals. In contrast, microsomal phospholipase A activity appears to be enhanced rather than depressed in ischemic pig hearts [20, 54].

In vitro studies indicate that the activity of phospholipase C is enhanced under acidic conditions [29]. However, no conclusive evidence has been provided to conclude that the activity of this enzyme is stimulated in the ischemic heart. On the contrary, Schwertz and colleagues [63] reported depressed activity of (phosphatidylinositol-specific) phospholipase C in flow-restricted rat hearts. Higgins and colleagues [38] have shown a link between the energy state of the myocyte and reduced resistance of the membrane phospholipids to the attack of exogenous phospholipase C. They suggested that the increased vulnerability could result from failure of an ATP-dependent protective mechanism like phosphorylation-dephosphorylation of membrane components, as found in erythrocytes. However, it remains to be established whether this mechanism is also responsible for the ischemia-induced degradation of myocyte phospholipids by endogenous hydrolytic enzymes.

Impaired phospholipid resynthesis

Impaired resynthesis of phospholipids associated with an unchanged rate of hydrolysis also results in net loss of phospholipids. Reacylation of lysophospholipids in order to resynthesize phospholipids requires the catalyzing activity of acylCoA synthetase and lysophosphatidyl acyltransferase (Fig. 2). The acylCoA synthetase mediated conversion of fatty acids, such as arachidonic acid, into acylCoA is dependent on ATP and is hampered by high cytosolic levels of AMP and adenosine [21]. It has recently been demonstrated that the decline in tissue ATP levels precedes arachidonic acid accumulation during the ischemic insult [81]. Arachidonic acid starts to accumulate significantly when ATP levels are lower than 8 to 10 $\mu mol.g^{-1}$ dry weight (Fig. 4). Since these ATP levels are substantially above the affinity constant of acylCoA synthetase for ATP (0.8 mM or about 4 $\mu mol/g$ dry weight of tissue), ATP is probably less likely to be responsible for the diminished reincorporation of arachidonic acid into phospholipids during the initial stage of ischemia. In the same study [81], it was shown that the increase in tissue AMP and adenosine paralleled in time the accumulation of arachidonic acid during the ischemic insult (Fig. 4). In ischemic cardiac tissue, the level of AMP easily exceeds 2 $\mu mol.g^{-1}$ dry weight. Since *in vitro* studies have shown that the activity of acylCoA synthetase is inhibited by AMP with an inhibition constant of 0.2 mM or 1.0 $\mu mol/g$ dry weight, a modulatory action of AMP should be considered. In addition, studies performed on ischemic pig hearts revealed a reduction of lysophosphatidylcholine acyltransferase activity [20]. Since the activity of this enzyme was assayed *in vitro* in a subcellular fraction of the previously flow-deprived pig heart, the latter observation suggests that the enzyme is either permanently blocked by an endogenous inhibitor or the configuration of the enzyme molecule is changed.

Reperfusion-induced loss of phospholipids

Various mechanisms have been proposed to explain the enhanced loss of phospholipids from cardiac structures after restoration of flow. Reperfusion of ischemic cardiac tissue is associated with a rapid and substantial influx of Ca^{2+} ions into the affected cells [40, 56]. These Ca^{2+} ions might cause myofibrillar contracture, but they also activate Ca^{2+}−dependent phospholipases. According to an alternative hypothesis, phospholipids might become more prone to the hydrolytic activity of either phospholipase A or phospholipase C after peroxidative injury of the membrane [43, 98]. Recent studies have indicated that increased supply of molecular oxygen in association with reperfusion of previously ischemic myocardial tissue results in an outburst of oxygen free radicals. The biologically active oxygen species avidly attack the unsaturated bonds of the fatty acyl moieties incorporated in the phosphilipids.

Direct stimulation of phospholipase A_2 must also be considered. This

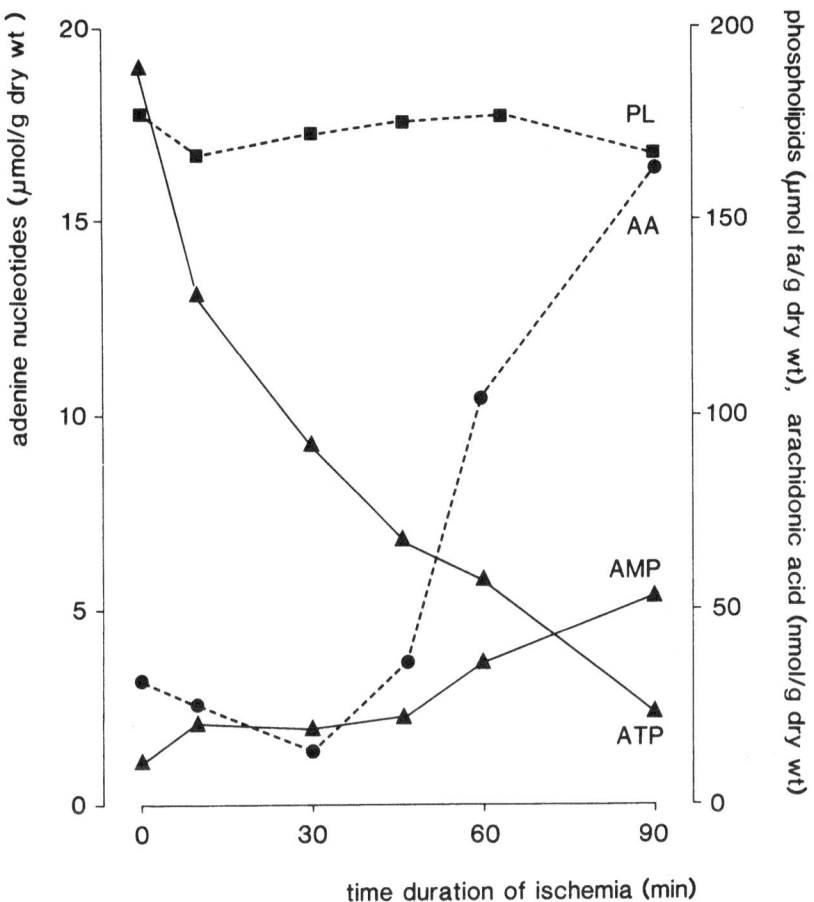

Fig. 4. Time course of changes in the content of ATP, AMP, phospholipids and arachidonic acid in ischemic, isolated rat hearts. PL and AA refers to total phospholipids and arachidonic acid, respectively. Note the 1000 fold difference in scale of the units of tissue PL and AA content. No significant change in the total phospholipid pool is observed during 90 minutes of ischemia. The steep increase in tissue arachidonic acid levels coincides with the second rise in the tissue AMP level. Reprinted from Van der Vusse *et al.* [87] with permission.

enzyme showed a permanently enhanced activity when monitored in the microsomal fraction harvested from reperfused pig myocardium [20].

The possibility that impaired resynthesis of phospholipids contributes to the reported net loss of phospholipids in reperfused cardiac tissue cannot be ruled out. Loss of ATP or essential substrates for rebuilding of phospholipid molecules might be responsible for depressed resynthesis. Inhibition of acyl-CoA synthetase by AMP and/or adenosine is unlikely in reperfused tissue since the tissue content of these two degradation products of ATP rapidly returns to normal values upon restoration of flow [81]. Kajiyama and colleagues [42] have suggested that oxidation of glutathione to glutathione disulfide during ischemia sets the stage for the dysfunction of the sulfhydryl-sensitive lysophosphatidyl acyltransferase during the subsequent period of reperfusion. The reduced ability to resynthesize phospholipids might be the cause of the specific loss of phosphatidylethanolamine from mitochondria, as observed after restoration of flow [42]. Reduced lysophosphatidyl acyltransferase activity was also observed by Das and colleagues [20] in reperfused pig myocardium.

Effect of phospholipid degradation products on membrane function

Phospholipase-mediated hydrolysis of phospholipids results in the production of amphiphiles, such as lysophospholipids and fatty acids. When these products accumulate in membranes, a vicious circle, resulting in severe perturbation of the sarcolemma and intracellular membranes, might be initiated. The effect of elevated contents of amphiphiles on membrane function appears to be complex. As extensively reviewed by Katz and Messineo [44], low concentrations of amphiphiles probably exert a 'stabilizing' effect on the membrane whereas high amphiphile concentrations have 'detergent-like' actions on membranes.

The majority of studies on the effects of amphiphiles on membranes have been conducted on erythrocytes. Incorporation of low concentrations of fatty acids in erythrocyte membranes causes a disproportionate change in the membrane surface area. This effect suggests that amphiphiles cause phase transition in the lipid bilayer. Incorporation of amphiphiles in membranes may also displace Ca^{2+} ions from negatively charged binding sites on phospholipids and, hence, alter the physico-chemical properties of the bilayer. As found in studies with isolated sarcoplasmic reticulum, incorporation of low concentrations of amphiphiles also induces changes in the biological activity of membrane proteins, probably by acting on the phospholipid environment around the hydrophobic region of the protein [44].

Incorporation of high concentrations of amphiphiles into membranes may cause the lipid bilayer to disintegrate into mixed micelles composed of endogenous phospholipids and amphiphile material. Consequently, the integrity of the biological membrane will be destroyed. The membrane will lose its ability to function as a barrier and extracellular ions, such as Ca^{2+}, are then allowed to enter freely into the cell interior [45].

Lysophospholipids, in particular, have been found to influence the electrical behavior of cardiac cells and are proposed to be one of the main arrhythmogenic compounds, accumulating in both ischemic and reperfused cardiac tissue [17, 18]. However, Katz [45] has pointed out that the well-known effects of amphiphiles on normal membranes may not reflect the situation in the ischemic myocardium since the effects of exogenous lysophospholipids and fatty acids may be considerably different from the effects evoked when these amphiphiles are generated within the membrane by phospholipase-mediated degradation of endogenous phospholipids. Moreover, hardly any information is available on the precise cellular site of accumulation of the degradation products of phospholipids during the ischemic insult. In this respect, the experimental findings of Suyatna and colleagues [75] are worthy to mention. They reported that sarcolemmal preparations isolated from rat hearts and kept under ischemic condition for a maximum of 60 minutes did not show enhanced levels of lysophospholipids, despite severe structural defects of the sarcolemma, as assessed with electron microscopy.

These above, mentioned considerations make it difficult to conclude that endogenously produced amphiphiles enforce the deleterious effect of ischemia and/or reperfusion on the integrity of cardiac membranes.

Arguments against a crucial role of phospholipid hydrolysis

Time course of lipid changes

Opponents of the notion that phospholipid hydrolysis plays a pivotal role in ischemia and/or reperfusion induced damage have suggested that the time course of changes in the tissue content of lipids does not run parallel with morphological alterations, known to reflect loss of cell membrane integrity [41, 70, 75]. In isolated pieces of dog heart, kept under anoxic conditions, Steenbergen and Jennings [70] have shown that fragmentation of the sarcolemma precedes the accumulation of lysophospholipids and depletion of phospholipids in the affected tissue. Suyatna and colleagues [75] studied the chemical composition of sarcolemmal vesicles isolated from ischemic rat hearts and found no change in the sarcolemmal content of phospholipids and lysophospholipids, despite electron microscopically visible ruptures in the sarcolemma. Although these findings are quite suggestive, some points of concern have to be raised. It is uncertain whether net production of lysophospholipids is a reliable index for phospholipid hydrolysis. The presence of lysophospholipase in the cardiac cells [32, 50] might promote degradation of newly produced lysophospholipids. Further degradation of lysophospholipids could well explain the observed rise of saturated and mono-unsaturated fatty acids during ischemia [14, 59, 81, 84, 95], as lysophospholipids are highly enriched with these fatty acids. Because of the high content of phospholipids in the cell and the technical difficulties of measuring these lipids with a high degree of accuracy, small changes to the order of a few percent will easily be missed. In contrast, the determination of arachidonic acid has to be considered as a very sensitive technique to monitor slight changes in cardiac phospholipid homeostasis, since in the normal heart the content of free arachidonic acid is extremely low [84]. Unfortunately, Steenbergen and Jennings [70] and Suyatna and colleagues [75] did not measure the changes in arachidonic acid content in their experimental models.

The effect of the addition of phospholipases

The high vulnerability of cardiac cells, isolated membranes and cellular organelles to added (either exogenous or endogenous) phospholipases, as discussed above, only supports, but does not prove conclusively the hypothesis that similar processes are responsible for the loss of membrane integrity during ischemia and reperfusion. In addition, Soons and co-workers [69] have reported that the cardiotoxic effect of snake venom phospholipase A_2 is due to a non-enzymatic action. In this study, the damage inflicted upon heart tissue appeared to be unrelated to hydrolysis of phospholipids.

Phospholipase inhibitors

A serious concern with studies applying phospholipase inhibitors is the fact that these compounds lack specificity. Most of the drugs used exhibit strong negative inotropic effects, are well-established calcium entry blockers or classified as ß-adrenoceptor antagonists. Therefore, it is uncertain whether the drugs employed do directly interfere with the hydrolysis of phospholipids by enzymatic action or mitigate the ischemic insult in another way. In case phospholipid degradation is the effect rather than the cause of irreversible cellular injury (see below) these anti-ischemic drugs will also attenuate the hydrolysis of phospholipids, albeit in an indirect manner. The fact that most of these compounds have been shown to inhibit the activity of phospholipases, purified from the heart, cannot be taken as proof that they directly affect the phospholipases *in situ*. In most cases, the concentration required to block *in vitro* phospholipase activity is rather high. It remains to be established whether high concentrations of the drugs are reached in the intact heart.

Alternative experimental models

Extrapolation of results obtained in alternative experimental models, in which the relationship between sarcolemmal damage and hydrolysis of phospholipids has been studied, should be done with care. The conditions of neonatal isolated myocyte cultures, the ATP production of which is blocked by metabolic inhibitors, are likely to be different from those in myocardial tissue deprived of oxygen and limited in its ability to remove waste products generated by enhanced anaerobic glycolysis and impaired oxidative processes.

Another popular model used to study the loss of sarcolemmal integrity is the isolated heart subjected to the calcium paradox [102]. In this model, cellular Ca^{2+} overload, thought also to occur during ischemia and/or reperfusion, is a key event resulting in the loss of cellular integrity. Readmission of Ca^{2+} ions to the heart after a period of calcium-free perfusion results in a sudden release of proteins from the cytosolic compartment into the extracellular space. Release of over 50% of the total cytosolic content is accomplished within 2 minutes after readmission of Ca^{2+}. Due to the high degree of reproducibility this model has been adapted to study detrimental changes assumed to occur at a slower rate in ischemic myocytes. Analysis of the tissue content of the various phospholipid classes and arachidonic acid just prior to and at 90 seconds and at 10 minutes, respectively, after readmission of Ca^{2+} ions reveals that the lipid content is not measurably changed within 90 seconds of Ca^{2+} repletion, notwithstanding the fact that a substantial part of cytosolic lactate dehydrogenase activity was lost from the heart [86]. This indicates severe damage of the sarcolemma without significant degradation of the phospholipid pool of the heart. Ten minutes after repletion of calcium ions, the tissue content of arachidonic acid was found to be considerably increased, most likely reflecting post-mortem hydrolysis of cellular phospholipids. These results strongly suggest that phospholipase-mediated hydrolysis of membrane phospholipids does not play a significant role in the chain of events leading to loss of integrity of the plasmalemma during the calcium paradox.

Alternative theories explaining disruption of cardiac membranes

Physical stresses imposed on the cell membrane

Jennings and associates [41] have hypothesized that physical forces are the cause of sarcolemmal rupture of ischemic cardiac cells. According to their hypothesis, hydrolysis of membrane phospholipids is of minor importance during the initial phase of ischemia and is not involved in the transition of reversible to irreversible damage of the flow deprived myocyte. The nature of the physical force, to which ischemic myocytes are subjected, is an increased osmotic load. Due to intracellular accumulation of low-molecular weight substances, such as lactate and inorganic phosphate, a shift of water from the extracellular to the intracellular space results in enhanced osmotic forces on the plasmalemma. Furthermore, mechanical stress as imposed on the plasmalemma of the flow-deprived cells by adjacent non-ischemic, contracting myocytes in the case of regional ischemia, or mechnaical stress due to contracture of the ischemic cells themselves, might have a detrimental effect on the plasmalemma of the ischemia-enfeebled myocyte.

Since the membranes of normal myocytes can withstand quite high physical forces, the plasmalemma of the ischemic cell has to be weakened prior to rupture due to enhanced physical stress [41]. The nature of the process leading to membrane labilization in the ischemic myocyte has not been precisely elucidated.

Recent studies have revealed a variety of changes in the sarcolemma of ischemic and/or reperfused cardiac cells that might be important links in the chain of events leading to destabilization of the cell membrane. The stability of the sarcolemma is determined, among others, by the asymmetric distribution of phospholipids and cholesterol across the inner and outer leaflet of the lipid bilayer, the composition of the fatty acyl chains in the phospholipid molecules and the presence of membrane proteins. Specific interactions between the cytoskeleton or membrane skeleton in the cell interior and the inner leaflet of the sarcolemma also influence the stability of the membrane.

Physical changes of lipids in the membrane

It is tempting to state that changes in the physical state of the lipid bilayers render the cell more vulnerable to stresses imposed upon the sarcolemma during the ischemic insult. Lateral diffusion of amphiphiles in the plasmalemma is greatly enhanced in anoxic, isolated cardiac myocytes [24]. The authors hypothesized that under normal conditions the lateral diffusion is hindered by the division of the cell membrane into a patchwork of more or less isolated domains by lateral and longitudinal barriers of spectrin, a component of the cytoskeleton. The network of spectrin probably undergoes rearrangements under anoxic circumstances which permits lipid material in the plasmalemma a greater freedom of movement.

Changes in protein material of the cytoskeleton have been observed in canine cardiac tissue, kept anoxic *in vitro* for 60 minutes [71]. The intracellular localization of vinculin, a protein probably involved in anchoring sarcolemmal phospholipids to the cytoskeleton, dramatically changes during the ischemic insult. In addition, calcium-dependent proteases might be responsible for hydrolysis of cytoskeletal components, which, in turn, impairs the interaction of the plasmalemma with vinculin. Degradation of cytoskeletal proteins by endogenous proteases might consequently evoke the loss of membrane phospholipid asymmetry. A strict correlation between these two events seems to be present in activated platelets [103].

Reorganization of cell surface phospholipids probably occurs in ischemic myocytes. Studies employing lactoperoxidase catalyzed radioiodination of phospholipids suggest an increased transfer of phosphatidylethanolamine from the inner to the outer leaflet in the ischemic myocyte [89]. This effect seems to be specific to this phospholipid species since exposure to the extracellular environment of phosphatidylserine and phosphatidylinositol, abundantly present in the inner leaflet of the plasmalemma of normal cardiac myocytes, does not increase during ischemia. Takahashi and Kako [77] have reported that ischemia followed by reperfusion affects sarcolemmal phosphatidylethanolamine in two different ways. Firstly, the total phosphatidylethanolamine content of the sarcolemma decreases. Secondly, their findings suggest a shift of this phospholipid species from the inner to the outer leaflet of the sarcolemma.

It is uncertain whether detachment of the cytoskeleton from the cellular membrane results in extrusion of lipid material from the membrane. These morphological changes of the sarcolemma certainly reflect alterations in the physical state of membrane lipids. The changed morphological features comprise clustering of membrane proteins associated with lipid areas in the sarcolemma devoid of protein material [5, 57, 90], formation of multilamellar vesicles in sarcolemmal and intracellular membranes and extrusion of lipid material from the membranes, i.e. formation of the so-called 'blebs'. The trigger causing these morphological changes in the cell membranes might be Ca^{2+} and H^+ ions accumulating in the ischemic myocytes. These ions are found to be capable of causing phase transition (from liquid-crystalline to gel phase) in model membranes containing phospholipids [90].

Loss of cholesterol from the sarcolemma is likely to seriously influence the physical state of the membrane. Reduced sarcolemmal contents of cholesterol associated with increased levels in mitochondria have been observed in ischemic cardiac tissue [60]. These findings indicate that impaired cholesterol homeostasis in the ischemic myocyte might also play a role in the destabilization of palsmalemma [83]. Alternatively, intercalation of high concentrations of amphiphiles in the sarcolemma severely reduces the stability of this membrane [44].

Phospholipid degradation following irreversible damage

As discussed above, no decisive data are available to conclude whether hydrolysis of phospholipids by endogenous phospholipase actually does precede morphological changes in the sarcolemma. Recent studies performed by Schrijvers and colleagues [62] revealed a temporal relationship between the accumulation of arachidonic acid and the occurrence of multilamellar vesicles in the sarcolemma of ischemic rabbit hearts. It is not known whether these two events are causally related. It cannot be excluded that accumulation of arachidonic acid, being a very sensitive sign of phospholipid degradation, occurs in a small subpopulation of myocytes in which the transition from reversible to irreversible injury has already taken place [81]. In that case, phospholipid degradation has to be considered as part of the healing process following irreversible cellular injury. After cell death, the cell debris has to be removed [87]. This can be accomplished via phagocytosis by circulating cells and by hydrolytic enzymes present in the remnants of the dead cells. The latter process is undeniably active after death of the cardiac cells. Recently performed experiments conducted on blood-free rat hearts, deliberately damaged by freezing and thawing prior to storage under anoxic conditions [88], indicate that cellular phospholipids are rapidly degradated at a rate of about 0.2 μmol per minute per gram wet weight. It should be stressed, however, that these findings do not exclude the fact that phospholipid degradation also occurs prior to the transition from reversible to irreversible damage.

Concluding remarks

In this chapter, the possible involvement of the hydrolysis of membrane phospholipids in the mechanism underlying irreversible loss of cellular function during ischemia and/or reperfusion has been evaluated. The content of arachidonic acid and lysophospholipids increases in the flow-deprived myocardium. Putative phospholipase A inhibitors, such as chlorpromazine and mepacrine, prevent the depletion of phospholipids in the ischemic heart cells and reduce ischemia-provoked cellular damage. However, currently available data do not allow the definite conclusion that hydrolysis of phospholipids is the proximate cause of irreversible injury inflicted upon the cardiac cell by ischemia and/or reperfusion. The specificity of the phospholipase-inhibiting drugs is uncertain and the great cell to cell variation in susceptibility to the ischemic insults hampers the establishment of a clear-cut causal relationship between the hydrolysis of phospholipids and the loss of integrity of cardiac membranes. Furthermore, most of the studies published on this subject produce conflicting results.

In recent years, physical alterations in the sarcolemma of the ischemic and reperfused myocyte have been reported. This includes separation of lipid and protein material in the membrane, partial loss of the asymmetric distribution of phosphatidylethanolamine in the lipid bilayer, the formation of multilamellar vesicles and extrusion of lipid material from the cellular membranes. Such changes might render the membrane more susceptible to the physical stress imposed on the membrane during the ischemic insult. In the latter case, phospholipid hydrolysis might occur after irreversible damage of the cell and consequently reflects post-mortem clearance of cell debris.

Physical alterations in the membranes of the flow-deprived myocytes and biochemical changes, including hydrolysis of phospholipids, might occur concomitantly in the ischemic and/or reperfused heart prior to irreversible injury. It remains to be seen whether these processes are causally related.

Acknowledgements

The authors are greatly indebted to Lucienne de Boer and Emmy van Roosmalen for their skilful help in preparing the manuscript.

Supported by Medigon/NWO (grant nr 900–516–091).

References

1. Ajioka M, Nagai S, Ogawa K, Satake T, Sugiyama S and Ozawa T (1986) The role of phospholipase in the genesis of reperfusion arrhythmia. J Electrocardiol 19: 1065–1172
2. Allen DG and Orchard CH (1987) Myocardial contractile function during ischemia and hypoxia. Circ Res 60: 153–168

3. Arthur G, Covic L. Wientzek M and Choy PC (1985) Plasmalogenase in hamster heart. Biochim Biophys Acta 833: 189–195
4. Arthur G, Page L, Mock T and Choy PC (1986) The catabolism of plasmenylcholine in guiena pig heart. Biochem J. 236: 475–480
5. Ashraf M, and Halverson CA (1977) Structural changes in the freeze-fractured sarcolemma of ischemic myocardium. Am J Pathol 88: 583–588
6. Beckman JK, Owens K, Knauer TE and Weglicki WB (1982) Hydrolysis of sarcolemma by lysosomal lipases and inhibition by chlorpromazine. Am J Physiol 242: H652–H656
7. Bentham JM, Higgens AJ and Woodward B (1987) The effect of ischaemia, lysophosphatidylcholine and palmitoylcarnitine on rat heart phospholipase A₂ activity. Basic Res Cardiol 82 (suppl II): 127–137
8. Bester R. and Lochner A (1988) Sarcolemmal phospholipid fatty acid composition and permeability. Biochim Biophys Acta 941: 176–186
9. Burton KP, Buja LM, Sen A, Willerson JT and Chien KR (1986) Accumulation of arachidonate in triacylglycerols and unesterified fatty acids during ischemia and reflow in the isolated rat heart. Am J Pathol 124: 238–245
10. Cao YA, Tam SW, Arthur G, Chen H and Choy PC (1987) The purification and characterization of a phospholipase A in hamster heart cytosol for the hydrolysis of phosphatidylcholine. J Biol Chem 262: 16927–16935
11. Chiariello M, Ambrosio G, Cappelli-Bigazzi M, Nevol E, Perrone-Filardi P, Manone G and Condorelli M (1987) Inhibition of ischemia induced phospholipase activation by quinacrine protects jeopardized myocardium in rats with coronary artery occlusion. J Pharmacol Exp Ther 241: 560–568
12. Chien KR, Pfau RG and Farber JL (1979) Ischemic myocardial cell injury. Prevention by chlorpromazine of an accelerated phospholipid degradation and associated membrane dysfunction. Am J Pathol 97: 505–529
13. Chien KR, Reeves JP, Buja LM, Parkey RW and Willerson JT (1981) Phospholipid alterations in canine ischemic myocardium. Circ Res 48: 711–719
14. Chien KR, Han A, Sen A, Buja LM and Willerson JT (1984) Accumulation of unesterified arachidonic acid in ischemic canine myocardium. Circ Res 54: 313–322
15. Chien KR, Sen A, Reynolds R, Chang A, Kun Y, Gunn MD, Buja LM and Willerson JT (1985) Release of arachidonate from membrane phospholipids in cultured neonatal rat myocardial cells during ATP-depletion. J Clin Invest 75: 1770–1780
16. Colvin RA (1987) Deinhibition of cardiac sodium-potassium ATPase after exposure to exogenous phospholipase A₂. Am J Physiol 252: H32–H39
17. Corr PB, Gross RW and Sobel BE (1982) Arrythmogenic amphiphilic lipids and the myocardial cell membrane. J Mol Cell Cardiol 14: 619–626
18. Corr PB, Gross RW and Sobel BE (1984) Amphiphatic metabolites and membrane dysfunction in ischemic myocardium. Circ Res 55: 135–154
19. Corr PB, Yamada KA, Creer MH, Sharma AD and Sobel BE (1987) Lysophosphoglycerides and ventricular fibrillation early after onset of ischemia. J Mol Cell Cardiol 14 (suppl. V): 45–53
20. Das DK, Engelman RM, Rousou JA, Breyer RH, Otani H and Lemeshow S (1986) Role of membrane phospholipids in myocardial injury induced by ischemia and reperfusion. Am J Physiol 251: H71–H78
21. De Jong JW and Hülsmann WC (1970) Effects of Nagarse, adenosine and hexokinase on palmitate activation and oxidation. Biochim Biophys Acta 210: 499–501
22. Dickens BF, Mak IT and Weglicki WB (1988) Lysosomal lipolytic enzymes, lipid peroxidation, and injury. Mol Cell Biochem 82: 119–123
23. Epps DE, Natarjan V, Schmid PC and Schmid HHO (1980) Accumulation of N-acylethanolamine glycerophospholipids in infarcted myocardium. Biochim Biophys Acta 618: 420–430
24. Finch SAE, Piper HM. Spieckermann PG and Stier A (1985) Anoxia influences the lateral

diffusion of a lipid probe in the plasma membrane of isolated cardiac myocytes. Basic Res Cardiol 80 (suppl 1): 149–152

25. Fisher KA (1976)   Analysis of membrane halves: cholesterol. Proc Natl Acad Sci USA 73: 173–177
26. Franson RC, Pang DC, Towle PW and Weglicki WB (1978)   Phospholipase A activity of highly enriched preparations of cardiac sarcolemma from hamster and dog. J Mol Cell Cardiol 10: 921–930
27. Franson RC, Waite M and Weglicki W (1972)   Phospholipase A activity of lysosomes of rat myocardial tissue. Biochemistry 11: 472–476
28. Franson R, Gamache D, Blackwell W, Eisen D and Hess ML (1986)   Sarcoplasmic reticulum dysfunction: phospholipid alterations induced by lysosomal phospholipase C. Am J Physiol 254: H1017–H1023
29. Gamache DA, Hess ML and Franson RC (1987)   Phospholipid alterations in canine cardiac sarcoplasmic reticulum induced by an acid-active phospholipase C. Basic Res Cardiol 82 (suppl 1): 107–112
30. Gross RW and Sobel BE (1979)   Augmentation of cardiac phospholipase activity induced with negative liposomes. Trans Ass Am Phys 92: 136–174
31. Gross RW and Sobel BE (1982)   Lysophosphatidylcholine metabolism in the rabbit heart. Characterization of metabolic pathways and partial purification of myocardial lysophospholipase-transacylase. J Biol Chem 257: 6702–6708
32. Gross RW and Sobel BE (1983)   Rabbit myocardial cytosolic lysophospholipase. Purification, characterization, and competitive inhibition by L-palmitoyl carnitine. J Biol Chem 258: 5221–5226
33. Gross RW, Ahumada GG and Sobel BE (1984)   Cytosolic lysophospholipase in cardiac myocytes and its inhibition by L-palmitoyl carnitine. Am J Physiol 15: C266–C270
34. Gross RW (1985)   Identification of plasmalogen as the major phospholipid constituent of cardiac sarcoplasmic reticulum. Biochemistry 24: 1662–1668
35. Grynberg A, Nalbone G, Degois M, Leonardi J, Althias P and Lafont H (1988)   Activities of some enzymes of phospholipid metabolism in cultured rat ventricular myocytes in normoxic and hypoxic conditions. Biochim Biophys Acta 958: 24–30
36. Gunn MG, Sen A, Chang A, Willerson JT, Buja LM and Chien KR (1985)   Mechanisms of accumulation of arachidonic acid in cultured myocardial cells during ATP depletion. Am J Physiol 249: H1188–H1194
37. Hattori M, Ogawa K, Satake T, Sugiyama S and Ozawa T (1985)   Depletion of membrane phospholipid and mitochondrial dysfunction associated with coronary reperfusion. Basic Res Cardiol 80: 241–250
38. Higgins TJC, Bailey PJ and Allsopp D (1981)   The influence of ATP depletion on the action of phospholipase C on cardiac myocyte membrane phospholipids. J Mol Cell Cardiol 13: 1027–1030
39. Hostetler KY and Jellison EJ (1989)   Role of phospholipases in myocardial ischemia, effect of cardioprotective agents on the phospholipases A of heart cytosol and sarcoplasmic reticulum in vitro. Mol Cell Biochem 88: 77–82
40. Jennings RB and Reimer KA (1981)   Lethal myocardial ischemic injury. Am J Pathol 102: 241–255
41. Jennings RB, Reimer KA and Steenbergen C (1986).   Myocardial ischemia revisited. The osmolar load, membrane damage, and reperfusion. J Mol Cell Cardiol 18: 769–780
42. Kajiyama K, Pauly DF, Hughes H, Yoon SB, Entman ML and McMillin-Wood JB (1987)   Protection by verapamil of mitochondrial glutathione equilibrium and phospholipid changes during reperfusion of ischemic canine myocardium. Circ Res 61: 301–310
43. Kako KJ and Kato M (1987)   Phospholipid metabolism in heart membranes. Dev Cardiovasc Med (Myocard Ischemia) 67: 99–112
44. Katz AM and Messineo FC (1981)   Lipid-membrane interactions and the pathogenesis of ischemic damage in the myocardium. Circ Res 48: 1–16

45. Katz AM (1982) Membrane derived lipids and the pathogenesis of ischemic myocardial damage. J Mol Cell Cardiol 14: 627–632
46. Kinnaird AAA, Choy PC and Man RYK (1988) Lysophosphatidylcholine accumulation in the ischemic canine heart. Lipids 23: 32–35
47. Man RYK, Slater TL, Pelletier MP and Choy PC (1983) Alterations of phospholipids in ischemic canine myocardium during acute arrhythmia. Lipids 18: 677–681
48. Miyazaki Y, Nagai S, Ogawa K, Satake T, Sugiyama S and Ozawa T (1984) The role of phospholipase in mitochondrial dysfunction after coronary reperfusion in the canine myocardium. Jpn Circ J 48: 498–507
49. Miyazaki Y, Gross RW, Sobel BE and Saffitz JE (1987) Biochemical and subcellular distribution of arachidonic acid in rat myocardium. Am J Physiol 253: C846–C853
50. Nalbone G and Hostetler KY (1985) Subcellular localisation of the phospholipase A of rat hearts. Evidence for a cytosolic phospholipase A_1. J Lip Res 26: 104–114
51. Nalbone G, Hostetler KY, Leonardi J, Trotz M and Lafont H (1986) Partial characterization of rat heart cytosolic phospholipase A_1 and demonstration of essential sufhydryl groups. Biochim Biophys Acta 877: 88–95
52. Opie LH (1976) Effects of regional ischemia on metabolism of glucose and fatty acids. Circ Res 38 (suppl 1): 52–68
53. Otani H, Engelman RM, Breyer RH, Rousou JA, Lemeshow S and Das DK (1986) Mepacrine a phospholipase inhibitor. J Thorac Cardiovasc Surg 92: 247–254
54. Otani H, Engelman RM, Rousou JA, Breyer RH, Lemeshow S and Das DK (1987) The mechanism of myocardial reperfusion injury in neonates. Circulation 76 (suppl V): 161–167
55. Palmer JW, Schmid PC, Pfeiffer DR and Schmid HHO (1981) Lipids and lipolytic enzyme activities of rat heart mitochondria. Arch Biochem Biophys 211: 674–682
56. Poole-Wilson, PA (1984) What causes cell death? In: Hearse DJ and Yellon DM (eds) Therapeutic approach to myocardial infarct size limitation, Raven Press, New York, pp 43–60
57. Post JA, Leunissen-Bijlevelt J, Ruigrok TJC and Verkley AJ (1985) Ultrastructural changes of sarcolemma and mitochondria in the isolated rabbit heart during ischemia and reperfusion. Biochim Biophys Acta 845: 119–123
58. Post JA, Langer GA, Op den Kamp JAF and Verkley AJ (1988). Phospholipid asymmetry in cardiac sarcolemma. Analysis of intact cells and gas-dissected membranes. Biochim Biophys Acta 943: 256–266
59. Prinzen FW, Van der Vusse GJ, Arts T, Roemen THM, Coumans WA and Reneman RS (1984) Accumulation of nonesterified fatty acids in ischemic canine myocardium. Am J Physiol 247: H264–H272
60. Rouslin W, MacGee J, Gupte S, Wesselman A and Epp DE (1982) Mitochondrial cholesterol content and membrane properties in porcine myocardial ischemia. Am J Physiol 242: H254–H259
61. Schaper J, Mulch J, Winkler B and Schaper W (1979) Ultrastructural, functional, and biochemical criteria for estimation of reversibility of ischemic injury: a study on the effects of global ischemia on the isolated dog heart. J Mol Cell Cardiol 11: 521–541
62. Schrijvers AHGJ, Frederik PM, Heijnen VVTh and Reneman RS (1988) Increased number of multilamellar extrusions after prolonged ischemia and reperfusion in rabbit myocardium. J Mol Cell Cardiol 20 (suppl V): 531
63. Schwertz D, Halverson J, Isaacson T, Feinberg H and Palmer JW (1987) Alterations in phospholipid metabolism in the globally ischemic rat heart: emphasis on phosphoinositide specific phospholipase C activity. J Mol Cell Cardiol 19: 685–697
64. Sen A, Miller JC, Reynolds R, Willerson JT, Buja LM and Chien KR (1988) Inhibition of the release of arachidonic acid prevents the development of sarcolemmal membrane defects in cultured rat myocardial cells during adenosine triphosphate depletion. J Clin Invest 82: 1333–1338
65. Severson, DL and Fletcher T (1985) Regulation of lysophosphatidylcholine-metabolizing enzymes in isolated myocardial cells from rat heart. Canad J Physiol Pharmacol 63: 944–952

66. Shaikh NA and Downar E (1981) Time course of changes in porcine myocardial phospho-lipid levels during ischemia. Circ Res 49: 316–325

67. Shaikh NA and Downar E (1987) Effects of chronic amiodarone treatment on cat myocardial phospholipid content and on *in vitro* catabolism. Mol Cell Biochem 78: 17–25

68. Sobel BE, Corr PB, Robison AK, Goldstein RA, Witkowski FX and Klein MS (1978) Accumulation of lysophosphoglycerides with arrhythmogenic properties in ischemic myocardium. J Clin Invest 62: 546–553

69. Soons KR, Yang CC and Rosenberg P (1984) Binding of phospholipase A_2 to isolated heart muscle. Biochem Pharmacol 33: 3914–3917

70. Steenbergen C and Jennings RB (1984) Relationship between lysophospholipid accumula-tion and plasmamembrane injury during total *in vitro* ischemia in dog heart. J Mol Cell Cardiol 16: 605–621

71. Steenbergen C, Hill ML and Jennings RB (1987) Cytoskeletal damage during myocardial ischemia: changes in vinculin immunofluorescence staining during total *in vitro* ischemia in canine heart. Circ Res 60: 476–486

72. Steenbergen C, Murphy E, Levy L and London RE (1987) Elevation of cytosolic free calcium concentration early in myocardial ischemia in perfused rat heart. Circ Res 60: 700–707

73. Sugiyama S, Hattori M, Miyazaki Y, Nagai S and Ozawa T (1985) The effect of verapamil on reperfusion arrhythmia in canine heart. Jpn Circ J 49: 1235–1242

74. Sugiyama S, Hattori M, Nagai S, Takamura and Ozawa T (1985) The effect of co-enzyme Q_{10} on the action of phospholipase. Arzneim Forsch 36: 187–189

75. Suyatna FD, Van Veldhoven PP, Borgers M and Mannaerts GP (1988) Phospholipid composition and amphiphile content of isolated sarcolemma from normal and autolytic rat myocardium. J Mol Cell Cardiol 20: 47–62

76. Takahashi K and Kako KJ (1984) Ischemia induced changes in sarcolemmal sodium-potassium ATP-ase, potassium-pNPPase, sialic acid, and phospholipid in the dog and effects of the nisoldipine and chlorpromazine treatment. Biochem Med 31: 271–286

77. Takahashi K and Kako KJ (1986) The effects of myocardial ischemia and nisoldipine pretreatment on the assymmetric distribution of phosphatidylethanolamine in a canine heart sarcolemmal preparation. Biochem Med 31: 308–321

78. Terminé E, Léonardi J, Lafont H and Nalbone G (1987) Intracellular phospholipase activity in rat heart. Comparison between endogenous and exogenous substrates. Biochemie 69: 245–248

79. Trotz M, Jellison E and Hostetler KY (1987) Propanolol inhibition of the neutral phospho-lipases of rat heart mitochondria, sarcoplasmic reticulum and cytosol. Biochem Pharmacol 144: 83–90

80. Van Bilsen M (1988) The significance of myocardial non-esterified fatty acid accumulation during ischemia and reperfusion. Thesis. University of Limburg, Maastricht, The Netherlands

81. Van Bilsen M, Van der Vusse GJ, Willemsen PHM, Coumans WA, Roemen THM and Reneman RS (1989) Lipid alterations in isolated, working rat hearts during ischemia and reperfusion: Its relation to myocardial damage. Circ Res 64: 304–314

82. Van den Bosch H (1980) Intracellular phospholipases A. Biochim Biophys Acta 604: 191–246

83. Van der Laarse A (1987) Cholesterol and myocardial membrane function. Basic Res Cardiol 82 (Suppl 1): 137–145

84. Van der Vusse GJ, Roemen THM, Coumans WA and Reneman RS (1982) Uptake and tissue content of fatty acids in dog myocardium under normoxic and ischemic conditions. Circ Res 50: 538–546

85. Van der Vusse GJ, Prinzen FW and Reneman RS (1987) Disturbances in myocardial lipid homeostasis during ischemia and reperfusion. In: S Sideman. R Beyar (eds) Activation, metabolism and perfusion of the heart. Martinus Nijhoff Publ, Dordrecht-New-York pp 665–681

86. Van der Vusse GJ, Van Bilsen M, Willemsen P and Reneman RS (1988) The myocardial

content of fatty acids and phospholipids during the calcium paradox. J Mol Cell Cardiol 20: 617–623

87. Van der Vusse GJ, Van Bilsen M and Reneman RS (1989) Is phospholipid degradation a critical event in ischemia and reperfusion induced damage? News Physiol Sci 4: 49–53

88. Van der Vusse GJ, De Groot MJM, Willemsen P, Van Bilsen M and Reneman RS (1989) Degradation of phospholipids and triacylglycerol, and accumulation of fatty acids in anoxic myocardial tissues disrupted by freeze-thawing. Mol Cell Biochem 88: 83–90

89. Vemuri R, Meresel M, Heller M and Pinson A (1988) Studies on oxygen and volume restriction in cultured cardiac cell: possible rearrangement of sarcolemmal lipid moieties during anoxia and ischemia-like states. Mol Cell Biochem 79: 39–46

90. Verkley AJ and Post JA (1987) Physico-chemical properties and organization of lipids in membranes: their possible role in myocardial injury. Basic Res Cardiol 82 (Suppl 1): 85–91

91. Victor T, Van der Merwe N, Benade AJS, La Cock C and Lochner A (1985) Mitochondrial phospholipid composition and microviscosity in myocardial ischemia. Biohim Biophys Acta 834: 215–223

92. Wallner BP, Mattaliano RJ, Hession C, Cate RL, Tizard R, Sinclair LK, Foeller C, Chow EP, Browning JL, Ramachandran KL and Pepinsky RB (1986) Cloning and expression of human lipocortin, a phospholipase A$_2$ inhibitor with potential anti-inflammatory activity. Nature 320: 77–81

93. Weglicki WB, Waite M, Sisson P and Shohet P (1971) Myocardial phospholipase A with a microsomal and mitochondrial fractions. Biochim Biophys Acta 231: 512–519

94. Weglicki WB, Waite BM and Stam AC (1972) Association of phospholipase A with a myocardial membrane preparation containing the $(NA^+-K^+)-Mg^{2+}-ATPase$. J Mol Cell Cardiol 4: 195–201

95. Weglicki WB, Owens K, Urschel CW, Serur JR and Sonnenblick EH (1973) Hydrolysis of myocardial lipids during acidosis and ischemia. Rec Adv Stud Cardiac Struct Metab 3: 781–793

96. Weglicki BW, Dickens BF and Mak IT (1984) Enhanced lysosomal phospholipid degradation and lysophospholipid production due to free radicals. Biochem Biophys Res Comm 124: 229–235

97. Weglicki WB, Kramer JH, Franson RC, Pang DC and Owens K (1985) Perturbations of sarcolemma by lipases and amphiphiles. Dev Cardiovasc Res (Pathobiol Cardiovasc Inj) 49: 258–272

98. Weglicki WB and Low MG (1987) Phospholipases of the myocardium. Basic Res Cardiol 87 (suppl 1): 107–112

99. Wirtz KWA (1982) Phospholipid transfer proteins. In: PC Jost and OK Griffith (eds) Lipid-protein interactions. Wiley Interscience, New York vol 1 pp 152–231

100. Wolf RA and Gross RW (1985) Identification of neutral active phospholipase C which hydrolyses choline glycerophospholipids and plasmalogen selective phospholipase A$_2$ in canine myocardium. J Biol Chem 260: 7295–7303

101. Yanagishita T, Konno N, Goshi E and Katagiri T (1987) Alterations in phospholipids in acute ischemic myocardium. Jpn Circ J 5: 41–50

102. Zimmerman ANE and Hülsmann WC (1966) Paradoxical influence of calcium ions on the permeability of the cell membrane of the isolated rat heart. Nature 211: 646–647

103. Zwaal RFA, Bevers EM, Comfurius P, Rosing J, Tilly RHJ and Verhallen PFJ (1989) Loss of membrane phospholipid asymmetry during activation of blood platelets and sickled red cells: mechanisms and physiological significance. Mol Cell Biochem, in press

Eicosanoids and the ischemic myocardium

K. SCHRÖR and T. HOHLFELD

Institut für Pharmakologie der Heinrich-Heine-Universität Düsseldorf, Moorenstr 5, D-4000 Düsseldorf 1, FRG

Summary

Arachidonic acid (AA) accumulation in the ischemic myocardial tissue, its release and subsequent metabolization into several classes of eicosanoids and lipid peroxides occurs simultaneously with the development of myocardial ischemic injury. This situation differs fundamentally from the controlled release and quantitative conversion of AA into eicosanoids under physiological conditions. The profile of eicosanoid release during ischemia and reperfusion differs both quantitatively and qualitatively from that seen under non-ischemic conditions. This is at least partially due to the presence of stimulated inflammatory cells and platelets with a considerable activity of AA-metabolizing enzymes. Thus, cardiac eicosanoid release in non-ischemic conditions is primarily beneficial, resulting in more effective adaptation of its function to the needs of circulation. Eicosanoid release in acute ischemia is primarily deleterious and enhances inflammatory-type reactions and functional disturbances of the myocardium.

Eicosanoids are intimately involved in several pathophysiologic alterations, typical for the reperfused ischemic heart: Arrhythmias (TXA_2), platelet- (TXA_2) and PMN-activation (LTB_4) fatty acid peroxides), vasospasm and 'cyclical reductions in coronary flow' (TXA_2), peptide leukotrienes, fatty acid peroxides) and aggravation of the ischemic injury and edema formation by chemotactic properties (LTB_4) fatty acid peroxides).

There are some positive reports that agents selectively inhibit the formation and/or action of these compounds in animal experiments but as insufficient experience with these compounds in man. Prostacyclin (and iloprost) have been proved to be potent cardioprotective agents in animal experiments yet to be ineffective in man. This discrepancy might be explained by a lower dosage of the compounds which can safely be administered to man and a pre-existing vascular pathology (atherosclerosis) which is usually absent in acute myocardial ischemia in laboratory animals. Prostacyclins appear to have a unique position because of their 'cytoprotective' activity, whose underlying mechanism is, however, still poorly understood.

H.M. Piper (ed.) Pathophysiology of severe ischemic myocardial injury, 195–217.
© *1990 Kluwer Academic Publishers, Dordrecht –*

Formation of eicosanoids in myocardial ischemia

Regulation of arachidonic acid release in the ischemic and non-ischemic heart

Formation of eicosanoids, i.e. prostaglandins, prostacyclin, thromboxanes, leukotrienes and numerous other metabolites of polyunsaturated fatty acids, is generally considered to occur as a local process in response to local cell stimulation. The rate-limiting step is the availability of the free precursor, i.e. arachidonic acid (AA). Stimulation of cellular activity, i.e. generation of a Ca^{++} signal, by chemical mediators or membrane depolarization, is usually accompanied by activation of phospholipases and AA release from its binding sites, mainly in the ß-position of membrane phosphoglycerides. In these physiological situations, AA probably exerts no important actions on its own but rather modulates cellular activity via the generation of its metabolites, the eicosanoids. This is reflected by the cell-specific profile of AA-metabolites which usually also act locally on the synthesizing cell or cells in the vicinity and are rapidly inactivated after entering the blood stream.

This situation differs fundamentally from that found in tissue injury, i.e. myocardial ischemia and infarction. In this situation, AA liberation appears to be closely related to cell membrane destruction and is accompanied by release of other fatty acids. Since fatty acids, including AA, are constituents of all cell membranes, the amount liberated depends upon the intensity and duration of the noxious stimulus that determines the extent of membrane disruption. This AA release is 'uncontrolled' and the free fatty acid is no longer quantitatively converted into eicosanoids but may also accumulate and exert actions on its own. This includes detergent activity and becoming substrate for enzymatic or non-enzymatic peroxidation. Furthermore, the local accumulation of inflammatory cells and platelets as well as interactions between them, including 'precursor exchange', allow for the biosynthesis of AA metabolites which are not formed in the non-ischemic heart and merely consist of compounds that aggravate cell injury. Thus, AA metabolites which physiologically act as modulators of cell activity may become a major detrimental factor under conditions of cell injury. Table 1 summarizes these differences in availability, metabolism and function of AA in ischemic and non-ischemic hearts.

Metabolic pathways and cellular sources of eicosanoid formation

Principally, AA and its metabolites are released from all cells and tissues that become activated or injured during the process of myocardial ischemia and/or reperfusion, i.e. endothelium, myocytes, platelets and polymorphonuclear leukocytes. These compounds may trigger further cell-specific reactions, such as release of serotonin from platelets or lysosomal enzymes from PMN.

Table 1. Differences in availability, metabolism and function of arachidonic acid (AA) in non-ischemic and ischemic hearts.

Parameter	Non-ischemic	Ischemic
AA release controlled	yes	no
Free AA available	traces	huge amounts
Other PUFA's available	traces	huge amounts
Major AA metabolites	PGI_2	TXA_2, PGI_2, LT's
Major site of synthesis myocardial	endothelium	all injured myocardial tissue, white cells
Cells		platelets
Precursor exchange	small if any	significant

Figure 1 and Table 2 summarize major sites of formation and biological activities of those eicosanoids which appear to be particularly relevant to myocardial ischemia: Thromboxanes, leukotrienes, fatty acid peroxides (exemplified with 12-H(P)ETEλ) and prostacyclin (PGI_2 [1].

Studies in cultured cardiac myocytes subjected to high-energy phosphate depletion have shown that AA release occurs simultaneously with the development of severe cellular and sarcolemmal damage [2]. Similar results were obtained in hypoxic myocytes: CK-release, a biochemical marker of muscle cell membrane injury, was a primary event, followed by secondary release of PGE_2 and LTC_4 into the culture medium [3] (Fig. 2). Similar results were obtained in the isolated *in situ* pig heart [4], where myocardial ischemia resulted in a significant phospholidpid breakdown which could be inhibited by

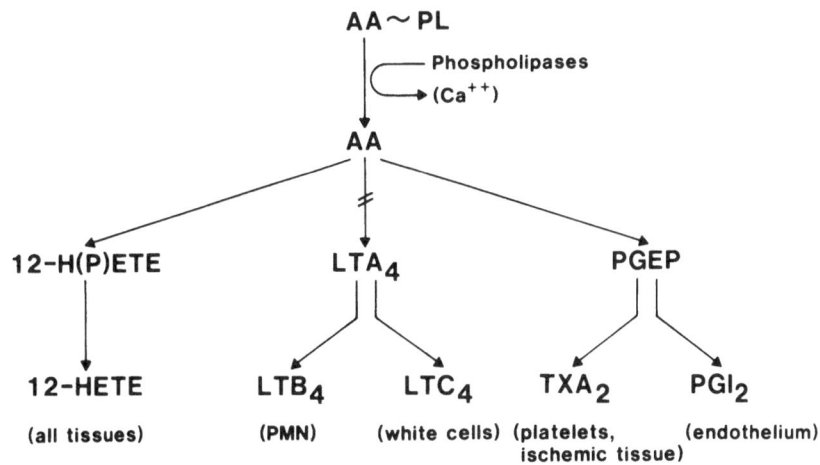

Fig. 1. Principal pathways of arachidonic acid (AA) metabolism in various tissues. PL: Phospholipid, HPETE: Hydroperoxy eicosatetraenoic acid, HETE: Hydroxy eicosatetraenoic acid, LT: leukotriene, PG: prostaglandin, TX: thromboxane.

Table 2. Selected arachidonic acid metabolites and their major biological functions.

Metabolite	Formed by	Action on	Type of action
PGI$_2$	endothelium	platelets	inhibition
		vascular smooth muscle	relaxation
		macrophages	inhibition
TXA$_2$	platelet	platelet	stimulation
		vascular smooth muscle	contraction
12-H(P)ETE	platelet	leukocytes	stimulation
	endothelium		
	vasculature		
	myocytes	vascular smooth muscle	contraction
LBT$_4$	granulocyte	granulocytes	stimulation
		vascular permeability	increase
LTC$_4$, LTD$_4$	leukocytes	vascular permeability	increase
		vascular smooth muscle	contraction

mepacrine, an inhibitor of phospholipases. These data and other investigations [1, 5–6] suggest that ischemia induced phospholipase activation is a primary step, providing free AA as substrate for peroxidation resulting in cell-specific generation of eicosanoids. Interestingly, high levels of AA have also been found in the heart muscle of men dying from sudden cardiac death [7].

Eicosanoid overflow during ischemia

In vivo, myocardial ischemia is associated with significant release ('overflow') of eicosanoids into the coronary effluent. In animal experiments, it was shown that this eicosanoid release comes from the ischemic tissue [8] and is most prominent during initial reperfusion. All major classes of eicosanoids have been detected in the effluent of ischemic or hypoxic hearts, in particular thromboxane A$_2$ [8], leukotrienes [9, 10], fatty acid peroxides, such as 12-H(P)ETE [11, 12], 5- and 15-H(P)ETE [12] and prostacyclin [8]. This 'overflow' of eicosanoids probably represents the 'successful' metabolism of AA, accumulated in the ischemic area as discussed above. Additionally, AA is released from membrane phospholipids during initial reperfusion. Moreover, activated polymorphonuclear cells (PMN) and platelets are now available at the site of AA release which form increasing amounts of noxious metabolites, such as TXA$_2$ (platelets) and leukotrienes (white cells).

Thromboxane

A number of early studies have indicated that myocardial ischemia is associated with significant thromboxane formation [1, 13]. It was also shown that severe myocardial ischemia could be produced in rabbits after injection of a thromboxane-generating system [14–16]. From these and other data it was

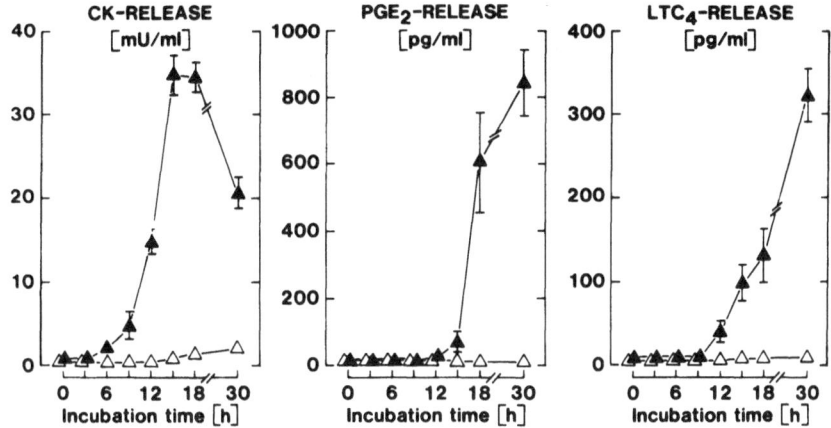

Fig. 2. The time course of release of creatine kinase (CK), PGE_2 and LTC_4 from cultured heart cells to the medium under hypoxic (95% N_2 and 5% CO_2, closed marks) and aerobic conditions (95% air and 5% CO_2, open marks). Modified after [3].

concluded that TXA_2, released from activated platelets might be a major detrimental factor in the aggravation or even production of myocardial ischemia. Furthermore, platelet-derived AA-metabolites, such as TXA_2 or 12-HETE, might promote local leukocyte accumulation in the vicinity of the ischemic myocardium [17]. A close correlation has been shown between infarct size and local 12-HETE or thromboxane accumulation in the ischemic area of the myocardium [12].

Interestingly, platelets are not the only source of thromboxane formation during ischemia. Ischemic vessel walls and/or the ischemic myocardium have been found to be important sources for TX generation [12, 18].

Similar results have been obtained with myocardial infarction in man. Enhanced excretion of thromboxane metabolites in the urine has been detected [19] and was found to persist for at least seven days after myocardial infarction [20]. Recent evidence suggests enhanced TXA_2 formation shortly after successful lysis by streptokinase in man [21, 22]. A significant transcardiac gradient of thromboxane was found during stress-induced angina in aspirin-treated patients [23]. This, together with the animal data cited above, would further suggest additional sources for TX generation than the platelet alone. This is important for the pharmacological design of thromboxane antagonists (see below) which was primarily done by using the simple platelet model.

Leukotrienes and fatty acid peroxides
In comparison with the detection of thromboxane release in myocardial ischemia, the first descriptions of leukotriene formation by ischemic coronary vessels and myocardial tissue [9, 10, 24] appeared rather late. As already seen with thromboxane, leukotrienes are not endogenous eicosanoids that are

released into the coronary effluent in any significant amount in non-ischemic conditions. It is probable that white cells are the most important cell type for leukotriene production. Consequently, the release of leukotrienes should be at its maximum at early reperfusion, i.e. after significant accumulation of inflammatory white cells has occurred [25, 26].

Enhanced tissue levels of 12-H(P)ETE in the injured myocardium have been repeatedly described [11, 12, 28]. 12-HETE formation is related to the degree of leukocyte infiltration in the ischemic dog heart [12] and the maximum tissue levels in this species appear to coincide with the maximum leukocyte infiltration, i.e. about 1 day after coronary artery ligation [11]. In contrast to most species, including man, the dog PMN primarily metabolizes AA to 12-HETE and not to 5-HETE and leukotrienes [27]. Thus, PMN are probably a less important source for 12-HETE formation in other species where platelets and ischemic tissue dominate as putative sources [1]. Because of its chemotactic properties [28] and generalized formation, 12-HETE is an important eicosanoid to be considered as a detrimental factor.

Prostacyclin

In contrast to the elevated generation of thromboxane, leukotrienes and fatty acid peroxides during myocardial ischemia, the increase in PGI_2 formation is apparently less pronounced or even absent and definitely fails to reach levels which exert a beneficial effect [1]. There is evidence for some increase in PGI_2 after myocardial injury in dogs [8] and man [22]. This PGI_2 release appears to occur secondary to tissue injury and, therefore might reflect the stimulation of undamaged endothelium by products released from the injured tissue. Green *et al.* [29] have recently reported that 6/20 patients suffering an acute myocardial infarction failed to increase their PGI_2 production. Interestingly, PGI_2 is the only inhibitory eicosanoid released during myocardial ischemia, whereas all other compounds stimulate cell function. Thus, an imbalance between inhibitory and stimulatory eicosanoids will occur and is the rationale for the use of prostacyclin mimetics [5], agents which stimulate the endogenous prostacyclin release [30] and thromboxane- and leuko-triene-inhibitory [31] agents in myocardial ischemia.

Actions of eicosanoids on the ischemic heart

Because of the broad spectrum of eicosanoids released during myocardial ischemia, it is difficult to ascribe a certain effect to a certain compound. Additionally, most of the active eicosanoids released from the injured myo-cardium are short-lived compounds and, therefore, difficult to study. Investi-gations on the biological properties of eicosanoids in myocardial ischemia tried to overcome this problem by two different types of protocols: (a) use of selective antagonists of certain eicosanoids; (b) use of specific mimetics, in particular of thromboxane A_2 (e.g. carbocyclic thromboxane A_2 (CTA_2)) or chemically stable prostacyclin analogs (e.g. iloprost).

This section discusses the involvement of selected classes of eicosanoids in the pathophysiology of ischemia and major actions exerted by them on myocardial and coronary function, platelets and white cells.

Prostacycline and PGE₁

Animal studies

In the late 1970s, the first studies were published demonstrating beneficial effects of PGE_1 [32] and PGI_2 [33] in acute myocardial ischemia *in vivo* and *in vitro* [34]. This was confirmed in numerous later investigations [35, 36]. After the detection of more stable analogs, in particular iloprost, these results were also extended to the synthetic compounds [37].

These beneficial effects of prostacyclin, its analogs and PGE_1 were usually determined by chemical indices of myocardial injury, such as loss of cytosolic enzymes (CK, LDH, SOD) or demonstration of reduced infarct size [38, 39]. Furthermore, antiarrhythmic effects of prostacyclin have been demonstrated, including reduced ventricular fibrillation and improved survival [49]. It is also important to note that early administration of prostacyclin, in contrast to anti-inflammatory steroids [41, 42], does not interfere with scar formation, i.e. the healing process [43].

Clinical studies

Because of these exciting data in animal experiments, several studies have employed prostacyclins in human myocardial ischemia. Unfortunately, all published data report negative results [19, 44–47] and no beneficial effect was seen with iloprost [48, 49] either. Interestingly, PGE_1 was found to be protective in unstable angina pectoris [50] and in acute infarction, if applied together with streptokinase [51].

One major difference between animal experiments and the clinical situation is the dose of prostacyclins which can be safely administered without a greater fall in blood pressure. In fact, doses can be 100–200 times higher (weight for weight) in cats and dogs without large changes in blood pressure. Therefore, the full potential of prostacyclins might not be available for clinical benefit [52]. Furthermore, most of the published animal experiments have used healthy animals and were designed to study the acute event, whereas in the clinics the vast majority of patients will suffer from atherosclerosis. Nor are the consequences of long-term treatment yet known. A significant reduction of prostacyclin receptors was reported by Jaschonek *et al.* for patients suffering from acute infarction [53]. Therefore, platelets of these patients and, eventually, other cells might be less sensitive to these compounds than experimental animals. There is clinical evidence for this [54, 55].

Taken together, these data suggest that supply with exogenous PGI_2 tends to improve the outcome of the reperfused ischemic myocardium. However, the doses necessary cannot be used in the clinics because of extremely severe side effects.

Major sites of action

Cardiac myocytes and energy stores. Prostacyclins beneficially influence all major pathophysiological variables of the reperfused ischemic myocardium in acute ischemia and improve tissue preservation [1, 34, 56]. These actions can be demonstrated in the absence of changes in blood perfusion and in the absence of formed elements of the blood. Several studies have shown that prostacyclins improve the resistance of the cell membrane, resulting in less 'leakage' of large cytosolic molecules, such as CK and SOD (Table 3). Prostacyclins reduce the phospholipid breakdown ([5], Table 4) and diminish the release of marker fatty acids from membrane phospholipids during ischemia by a membrane stabilizing action [56].

One important consequence of this membrane stabilization is an improved antioxidative potential of the myocardium. In particular, the reduced loss of cytosolic superoxide dismutase (SOD), the enzyme which catalyses the transformation of O_2- into H_2O_2, by iloprost, also results in the preservation of SOD activity within the ischemic myocardium, probably by inhibition of washout as a consequence of improved membrane preservation [56, 57].

Ventricular performance is related to tissue ATP metabolism. Thus, loss of adenine nucleotides during oxygen deficiency may impair subsequent aerobic re-synthesis of ATP and, possibly, mechanical function. Several studies have shown that PGI_2 and PGI_2 mimetics retard or reduce the loss of energy-rich nucleotides from the ischemic myocardium, prevent the accumulation of lactate and pyruvate and considerably attenuate glykogenolysis [58–60]. In contrast to calcium antagonists, this action of cardioprotective eicosanoids is not associated with any negative inotropic action on the non-ischemic myocardium.

Brief periods of coronary occlusion for 5–20 minutes do not generally result in necrosis but may lead to a severe state of regional dyskinesia during reperfusion. This myocardial 'stunning' might persist for hours or even days and is associated with typical alterations in myocardial energy stores: reduced tissue ATP at enhanced tissue creatine phosphate, suggesting a defect in energy utilization.

Two recent studies in the pig [61] and dog [62] have shown that iloprost improves regional functional recovery of the jeopardized myocardium. Interestingly, this effect can still be observed even if the treatment is started at the onset of reperfusion [62].

A number of investigations have shown that ischemia is associated with a considerable 'overflow' of cardiac noradrenaline into the extraneuronal space (see [38]). Extraneuronal noradrenaline, accumulating in the ischemic myo-

Table 3. SOD- and CK-specific activities in ischemic (MI) and non-ischemic (NMI) areas of left ventricular myocardium of cats subjected to 3 h of LAD occlusion + 2 h of reperfusion (OP). Animals were treated with vehicle (VEH) or iloprost (ILO), starting 30 min after LAD occlusion and compared with sham-operated (SOP) controls. The data are mean + SEM of n experiments.

Group	n	CK [IU/mg protein]		n	SOD [IU/mg protein]	
		MI	NMI		MI	NMI
OP-VEH	8	16.3 ± 3.9*	67.3 ± 4.2	7	8.3 ± 1.0*	16.8 ± 2.0
OP-ILO	7	41.7 ± 6.0	63.8 ± 3.8	6	14.5 ± 2.8	20.3 ± 1.3
SOP	5	66.7 ± 5.8	69.3 ± 4.0	9	16.9 ± 2.1	18.6 ± 2.3

*): $P < 0.05$ (OP vs. SOP)

Table 4. Phospholipid concentration [nmoles Pi/mg protein] in ischemic (MI) and non-ischemic (NMI) areas of rat hearts subjected to 6h of LAD occlusion and treatment with iloprost (ILO) or vehicle (VEH).

Group	n	Total PL		PC		PE	
		MI	NMI	MI	NMI	MI	NMI
OP-VEH	7	256±13*	286±12	99±4*	113±4	86±4*	96±4
OP-ILO	8	300±7	289±4	112±2	116±3	103±2	104±2

*): $P < 0.05$ (MI vs. NMI)
Treatment with iloprost (100 ng/kg × min, iv) was started 20 min after LAD occlusion (Darius *et al.*, 1987 [5]).

cardium, will increase myocardial energy metabolism, i.e. oxygen requirement, which is particularly deleterious under conditions of restricted coronary flow and aggravates myocardial injury [63] as well as the incidence of arrhythmias [64]. This ischemia induced redistribution of myocardial catecholamines is antagonized by postacyclins, even if applied at 30 minutes of ischemia [65–67]. This results in an improved contractile function, including a considerable reduction in the increase in left ventricular end diastolic pressure [63]. Probably the most convincing finding to support the functional significance of catecholamine redistribution was the complete prevention of ischemia induced cAMP elevations in the myocardium by PGI_2 [68]. Inhibition of local cAMP accumulation would also contribute to the antiarhythmic actions of these compounds.

Thus, cytoprotective actions of prostacyclins might be considered as a common denominator to explain the inhibition of catecholamine overflow and ischemia-induced changes in myocardial energy metabolism and myocardial contractile function [69]. Interestingly, stimulation of endogenous PGI_2 formation by defibrotide results in significant cardioprotection comparable to the effects seen with prostacyclins [70–72].

Coronary perfusion. Prostacyclin, its mimetics and PGE_1 are vasodilators. One might, therefore, expect them to improve the metabolic situation of the ischemic myocardium by enhancing the perfusion of ischemic areas, for example by improving collateral perfusion. However, most of the available studies, using prostacyclin at a non-blood pressure lowering dose failed to demonstrate any significant improvement of blood supply to the ischemic area under conditions where blood supply to the non-ischemic myocardium was significantly elevated [73–75]. *In vitro*, iloprost protects frog ventricular strip preparations (Rana ridibunda) from hypoxic injury in the absence of coronary vessels [76] and was also reported to protect isolated, globally ischemic hearts from reperfusion injury at concentrations which did not dilate coronary vessels [56, 63]. Thus, the cardioprotective actions of prostacyclins do not appear to involve selective coronary vasodilation as an essential factor. Additionally, there is also evidence for a reduced responsiveness of coronary vessels against prostacyclins in the presence of vasoconstrictor compounds such as TXA_2, catecholamines or serotonin [77, 78] and the number of PGI_2 receptors (on platelets) is reduced during myocardial ischemia [53]. Thus, while prostacyclins are coronary dilating agents, the high local concentrations necessary to produce this effect may not be obtained at conditions of local vasospastic mediator release. Consequently, increasing the dose in man has been reported to produce hypotension and reflectory increases in heart rate due to increased sympathetic tone. This might result in additional vasoconstrictor and platelet stimulating effects or even cause acute myocardial dysfunction, due to a 'coronary-steal'-like phenomenon [79]. Similarly neither PGI_2 [80] nor iloprost [81] were able to increase the exercise tolerance in patients with angina pectoris at doses which reduced the coronary vascular resistance.

Platelet function. Cardioprotective eicosanoids such as prostacyclin and PGE1 are not only arterial vasodilators but also antiplatelet agents. There is clear evidence from animal studies that prostacyclin not only prevents ischemia induced platelet activation [82] but also redissolves preformed circulating platelet aggregates [37]. However, for a number of reasons, antiplatelet effects of prostacyclins cannot be considered to be the only or even the most important factor in explaining their beneficial effects in acute myocardial ischemia. Removal of platelets by an antiplatelet serum did not contribute much to the outcome of the ischemic process [83], beneficial effects have been obtained with prostacyclins in platelet-free perfused *in vitro* systems [34, 56, 63, 66] and a prostacyclin analog without antiplatelet activity was found to be protective in myocardial ischemia *in vivo* [84]. Iloprost administration to man with stable angina consistently reduced platelet aggregation. This, however, did not correlate with its effects on exercise capacity [49]. It has also been shown that prevention of platelet-associated TXA_2 release did not influence the reperfusion injury under conditions when iloprost was active [85].

Leukocytes and reactive oxygen species. Much interest has been centered on the role of polymorphonuclear leukocytes as putative sources of lytic enzymes and reactive oxygen species [26]. In particular, during reperfusion of previously ischemic areas known to have a reduced antioxidative potential [86], local accumulation of these cells has been demonstrated. Depletion of blood leukocyte count by antileukocyte serum was found to reduce the extent of ischemic injury [25]. Cardioprotective eicosanoids, such as iloprost, antagonise leukocyte accumulation at the borderzone of the developing infarct and were found to exhibit antineutrophil activities *ex vivo* [39, 87–89]. However, prostacyclins also prevent reperfusion injury of the ischemic myocardium *in vitro*, i.e. in absence of neutrophils [34, 56, 63, 66]. Furthermore, neutrophil-inhibitory prostaglandins, such as PGE_2, were ineffective in experimental ischemia [35, 90] and the molar concentrations of prostacyclins necessary to inhibit neutrophil function (> 10 μM) [91] are probably not obtained *in vivo*. Finally, PGE_1, although possessing a clear antineutrophil potential in experimental myocardial ischemia *in vivo* [92, 93] failed to directly inhibit neutrophil function [93]. This suggests that direct antineutrophil activities of prostacyclins are not necessary to explain the beneficial actions of the agents. In fact, the explanation for inhibition of ischemia induced leukocytosis and neutrophil accumulation in the ischemic areas by prostacyclins is probably improved tissue preservation, resulting in less release of chemotactic compounds, such as 12-HETE and other fatty acid peroxides.

Thromboxanes

Animal data

The biologically active thromboxane A_2 (TXA_2) has many properties which make the compound a major deleterious factor in myocardial ischemia. TXA_2 is a potent constrictor of coronary vessels [94, 95] and a powerful platelet-stimulating agent [96]. Additionally, TXA_2 exerts a labilizing effect on cell membranes, including those of lysosomes, eventually resulting in release of cytolytic enzymes [96, 97]. All of these properties might be relevant to ischemia-induced arrhythmias [40].

Administration of synthetic thromboxane A_2 [96], TXA_2-mimetics, such as carbocyclic thromboxane A_2 (CTA_2) [98] or thromboxane generating systems, such as stimulated platelets [15, 16] results in deleterious effects on the non-ischemic myocardium and enhances tissue damage in ischemia. This includes release of cytosolic enzymes, enhanced incidence of arrhythmias and membrane labilization [97].

Interest therefore, centers on compounds which selectively inhibit thromboxane generation or action. In animal experiments, TX-synthetase inhibitors have been proved to be effective against biochemical and ECG alterations of acute myocardial ischemia [99–102]. Similar beneficial effects have been reported for selective inhibitors of thromboxane receptors [103–107].

Clinical data

There are only a few clinical studies designed to investigate the consequences of selective antagonism of thromboxanes for the outcome of the ischemic myocardium [108–109]. Thaulow *et al.* [109] reported beneficial effects of the thromboxane synthetase inhibitor dazoxiben (reduced lactate release into the coronary sinus, reduced ST-depression) in man. A major problem for clinical use of these compounds is the short half-life and the competitive type of inhibition – in contrast to the irreversible blockage of platelet-derived thromboxane formation by aspirin [110].

Major sites of action

Cardiac myocytes. There is little information available on direct actions of thromboxane or thromboxane mimetics on cardiac myocytes. Lefer *et al.* [97] have shown that CTA_2 labilizes cell membranes and it is generally thought that TXA_2 might enhance the C^{++}-influx into the platelet. Certainly, any deterioration of cell membrane structure would facilitate the generation of functional disturbances, such as arrhythmias. Alternatively, thromboxane synthetase inhibitors and receptor antagonists in general protect myocardial tissue from the loss of cytosolic enzymes, such as CK, disruption of lysosomal membranes and proteolysis [39, 97, 103–106, 111].

Coronary perfusion. Normally, coronary flow and myocardial function are dependent on each other. Reduced coronary perfusion during ischemia will result in depressed myocardial function. After the original work of Folts *et al.* [112], TXA_2 released from activated platelets has been generally considered as a major cause of coronary flow reductions. This was confirmed in later investigations, when it was shown that cyclical reductions in coronary flow occurring after critical stenosis of a coronary artery can be prevented by thromboxane antagonists and are probably due to platelet deposition at the surface of ischemically injured vessels [18]. However, it is not clear whether the detrimental effects of TXA_2 in myocardial ischemia are critically determined by the vasoconstrictor properties of the compound. For example, natural TXA_2 was found to exert highly variable effects on coronary vessel tone [96] and vasoconstrictor activities required concentrations which were considerably higher than those necessary for platelet activation. These data suggest that limitations in coronary perfusion by TXA_2 might contribute to its detrimental effects on the ischemic myocardium but they are by no means the sole explanation.

Platelet function. In addition to causing mechanical obstruction of coronary vessels, platelet activation during ischemia is also associated with release of vasospastic mediators, such as serotonin and TXA_2. Thromboxane A_2 stimulates platelet activation and secretion, eventually contributing to the 'no-reflow' phenomenon. In addition to their direct vasoconstrictory property, thromboxanes will promote mechanical obstruction of coronary vessels by the formation of platelet clumps [112]. Additionally, TXA_2 might trigger the release of vasospastic mediators from platelets (serotonin) [113] or white cells (leukotrienes) [17].

However, for a number of reasons, platelet-antagonistic properties of thromboxane antagonists cannot be considered to be the sole or even the most important factor in explaining their beneficial effects in acute myocardial injury. Removal of platelets by an antiplatelet serum contributed little to the outcome of the ischemic process [83]. It has also been shown that prevention of platelet-associated TXA_2 release did not influence the reperfusion injury under conditions when prostacyclin was active [85]. Application of the thromboxane receptor antagonist 13-azaprostanoic acid was not very effective in acute myocardial ischemia at antiplatelet doses [114]. Administration of the thromboxane synthetase inhibitor dazoxiben to isolated, saline-perfused ischemic Langendorff-hearts resulted in considerable tissue protection without any platelet being present [115]. In conclusion, the majority of available data suggests that inhibition of platelet function by thromboxane antagonists is a useful and even selective mechanism [116] in preventing myocardial ischemic injury but does not fully explain the beneficial actions of the compounds.

Leukocytes and reactive oxygen species. Polymorphonuclear leukocytes produce little if any thromboxane A_2, neither are they stimulated significantly by exogenous thromboxane mimetics [107]. In addition to the work of Bednar *et al.* [17], Wargovich *et al.*. [117] have found that inhibition of the thromboxane synthetase results in inhibition of myocardial neutrophil accumulation and postulated a complex interaction between platelets, leukocytes and endothelium which might be amplified by TXA_2. Corresponding with this, thromboxane antagonists prevent the ischemia induced leukocytosis [107] (Fig. 3) and leukocyte activation in the ischemic myocardium (Smith, personal communication). Thus, it is myocardial tissue injury, associated with neutrophil infiltration in early reperfusion [118], that is beneficially influenced by thromboxane antagonists rather than any direct action of the compounds on thromboxane pathways in polymorphonuclear cells. Mullane and Fornabaio [119] have recently shown that the beneficial actions of thromboxane synthetase inhibition on ischemia induced myocardial injury disappear if the animals are platelet depleted by a specific antiserum. This would suggest that it is not the removal of TXA_2 which protects the myocardium but the generation of other eicosanoids, such as PGD_2 or PGI_2 from platelet-derived endoperoxides which accounts for myocardial protection.

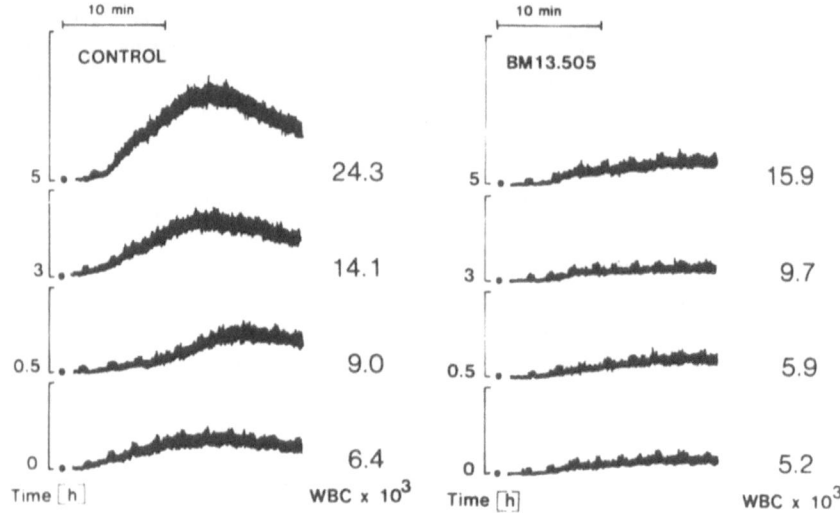

Fig. 3. Time-dependent alterations in the myeloperoxidase (MPO) activity of
zymosan-stimulated blood *ex vivo* from cats subjected to 3 h of coronary artery occlusion
followed by 2 h of reperfusion [3]. The figure compares one original registration of a vehicle
treated cat (control) with that of one treated with the thromboxane receptor antagonist
daltroban (BM 13.505). Note the considerable attenuation of the release of MPO and the
reduction in white blood cell count (WBC) by daltroban treatment.

Leukotrienes and fatty acid peroxides

Animal studies

Fatty acid peroxides [120] are potent constrictions of coronary vessels (Fig.
4). Fatty acid peroxides and leukotrienes increase membrane permeability
and have potent chemotactic effects [28, 121]. Thus, these AA-metabolites
will also contribute to membrane injury of the ischemic myocardium and may
be particularly relevant to edema formation and late increase in coronary
vascular resistance [122].

There is currently little information on the activity of leukotriene antagonists in myocardial infarction [123–126]. Clearly, glucocorticoids have an
acute beneficial effect in myocardial ischemia and will also inhibit leukotriene
formation – however these compounds have no value in myocardial infarction
in man because of their deleterious effects on wound healing and scar
formation [41].

An inhibition of lipid peroxidation might be expected from treatment with
antioxidative substances, such as vitamin E, nafazatrom or chemical agents
that improve the metabolism of deleterious oxygen free radicals, such as the
superoxide anion, into less toxic metabolites, including superoxide dismutase
and catalase.

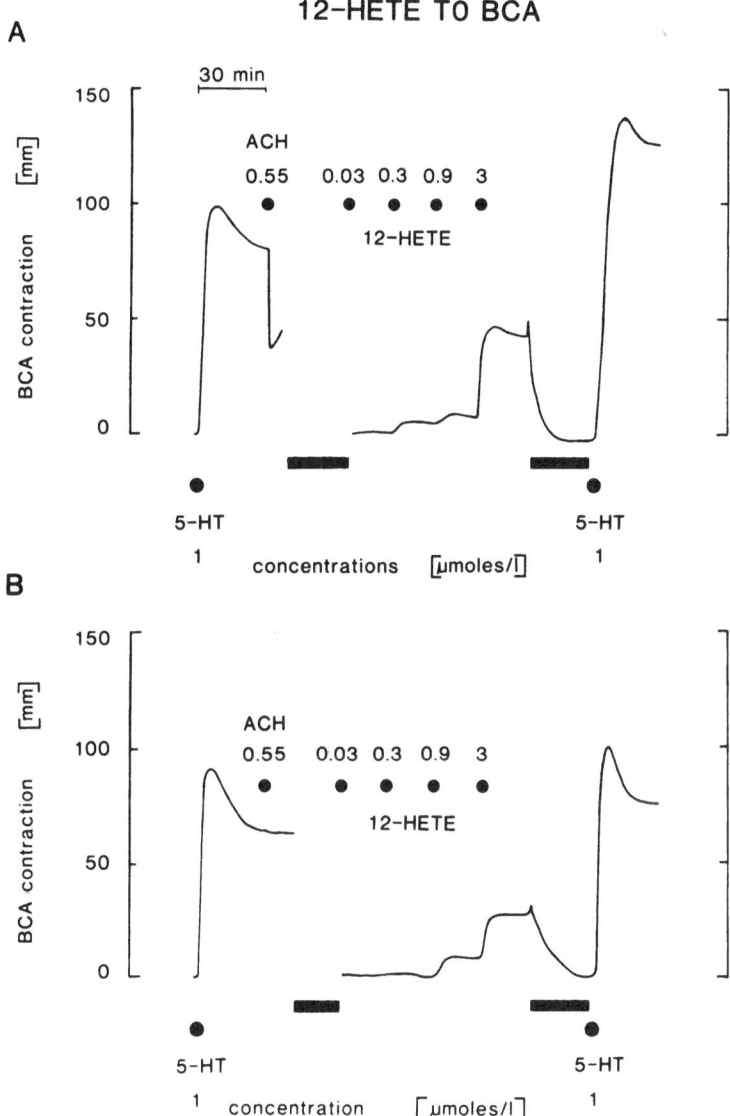

Fig. 4. Changes in coronary vessel tone after cumulative addition of 12-HETE in presence (A) and absence (b) of endothelium. Endothelial function was determined by addition of acetylcholine (ACH).
(●) addition, (▬) washout. (From: Schrör K, Verheggen R (1987) Platelets, eicosanoids and coronary vasospasm. In: Prostaglandins in clinical research. H Sinzinger, K Schrör (eds.), Alan R Liss, New York, p. 167.)

Major sites of action

Myocyte. Only limited information is available on direct action of leukotrienes on cardiac myocytes. Hypoxia is associated with leukotriene release [3] and several studies have reported negative inotropic actions of peptide leukotrienes [127–130]. However, the majority of investigators now believes that this is an indirect effect, caused by regional ischemia due to coronary vasoconstriction [127].

Coronary flow. In anaphylactic guinea pig hearts, peptide leukotrienes such as LTC4 cause coronary vasoconstriction which can be separated from the early coronary vasoconstriction, mediated by vasoactive cyclooxygenase products, such as TXA2 [122]. Peptide leukotrienes, such as LTC4 and LTD4, released from coronary vessels [131] or the injured myocardium [24] are potent coronary vasoconstrictors [27, 128–130] and might considerably aggravate the severity of the ischemic injury. This will also reduce myocardial contractile force (see above), although LTD4 (and thromboxane) induced constriction of myocardial resistance vessels is not considered to be a likely complication of acute thrombotic coronary occlusion [132]. Nevertheless, any limitations in coronary flow will lead to higher local levels of accumulated products, such as unmetabolized arachidonic acid of lysophospholipids, because of reduced wash-out.

Leukocytes and reactive oxygen species. Leukocytes are not only a major site of leukotriene formation but also a major target of leukotriene action [26]. Prevention of leukocyte accumulation in the injured myocardium and/or inhibition of leukotriene-synthesizing pathways by appropriate drugs, such as the dual inhibitor BW 755c [125, 126] was found to result in a reduced infarct size. Interestingly, Klein and associates [126] have demonstrated in the pig heart that significant reduction in infarct size is detectable at 4 hours but there is no significant change at 2 weeks of reperfusion of the ischemic myocardium. Thus, the evaluation of lipoxygenase product-associated alterations in AA metabolism requires further study.

Acknowledgements

This work was supported by a grant of the Deutsche Forschungsgemeinschaft (SFB 242)

References

1. Schrör K (1987) Lipid metabolism in the normoxic and ischaemic heart. Bas Res Cardiol 82, Suppl 1: 235–243
2. Chien KR, Sen A, Reynolds R, Chang A, Kim Y, Gunn MD, Buja M, Willerson JT (1985) Release of arachidonate from membrane phospholipids in cultured neonatal rat myocardial cells during adenosine triphosphate depletion. Correlation with the progression of cell injury. J Clin Invest 75: 1770–1780
3. Ikeda U, Toyooka T, Arisaka H, Hosoda S (1987) Stimulated synthesis of prostaglandin E_2 or

leukotriene C_4 from myocardial cells is not a cause but a result of their injury under hypoxia. J Mol Cell Cardiol 19: 523–526

4. Das DK, Engelman RM, Rousou JA, Breyer RH, Otani H, Lemeshow S (1986) Role of membrane phospholipids in myocardial injury induced by ischemia and reperfusion. Am J Physiol 251: H71–H79

5. Darius H, Osborne JA, Reibel DK, Lefer AM (1987) Protective actions of a stable prostacyclin analog in ischemia induced membrane damage in rat myocardium. J Mol Cell Cardiol 19: 243–250

6. Yanagishita T, Konno N, Geshi E, Katagiri T (1987) Alterations in phospholipids in acute ischemic myocardium. Jap Circ J 51: 41–50

7. Gudbjarnason S, Hallgrimsson J (1976) Prostaglandins and polyunsaturated fatty acids in heart muscle. Acta Biol Med Germ 35: 1069–1080

8. Coker SJ, Parratt JR, Ledingham IMcA, Zeitlin IJ (1981) Thromboxane and prostacyclin release from ischaemic myocardium in relation to arrhythmias. Nature 291: 323–324

9. Evers AS, Murphree S, Saffiz JE, Jakschik BA, Needleman P (1985) Effects of endogenously produced leukotrienes, thromboxane and prostaglandins on coronary vascular resistance in rabbit myocardial infarction. J Clin Invest 75: 992–999

10. Barst S, Mullane K (1985) The release of a leukotriene D_4 like substance following myocardial infarction in rabbits. Eur J Pharmacol 114: 383–387

11. McCluskey ER, Murphree S. Saffitz JE, Morrisson AR, Needleman P (1985) Temporal changes in 12-HETE formation in two models of canine myocardial infarction. Prostaglandins 29: 387–403

12. Kuzuya T, Hoshida S, Nishida M, Kim Y, Takenobu K, Tada M (1987) Increased production of arachidonate metabolites in an occlusion-reperfusion model of canine myocardial infarction. Cardiovasc Res 21: 551–558

13. Hirsh PD, Hillis LD, Campbell WB, Firth BG, Willerson JT (1981) Release of prostaglandin and thromboxanes into the coronary circulation in patients with ischemic heart disease. N Engl J Med 304: 686–691

14. Morooka S, Kobayashi M, Takayashi T, Takashima Y, Sakamoto M, Shimamoto T (1979) Experimental ischemic heart disease – effects of synthetic thromboxane A_2. Exptl Mol Pathol 30: 449–257

15. Shimamoto T, Takahashi T, Takashima Y, Motomiya F, Numano F, Kobayashi M (1977) Prevention by phtalazinol of thromboxane A_2 induced myocardial infarction in rabbits. Proc Jap Acad Series B 53: 43

16. Numano F, Yajima M. Nishiyama K, Shimakoda K, Numano F, Sasagawa S, Moriya K (1982) Effects of thromboxane A_2 injection on the rabbit coronary artery. II. The production of infarcts in cholesterol-fed animals. Exptl Mol Pathol 37: 118–132

17. Bednar M, Smit B, Punto A, Mullane KM (1985) Neutrophil depletion suppresses 111-In-labeled platelet accumulation in infarcted myocardium. J Cardiovasc Pharmacol 7: 906–912

18. Schmitz JM, Apprill PG, Buja LM, Willerson JT, Campbell WB (1985) Vascular prostaglandin and thromboxane production in a canine model of myocardial ischemia. Circ Res 57: 223–231

19. Henriksson P, Wennmalm A, Edhag O, Vesterqvist O, Green K (1986) In vivo production of prostacyclin and thromboxane in patients with acute myocardial infarction. Br Heart J 55: 543–548

20. Friedrich T, Lichey J, Nigam S, Priesnitz M, Wegscheider K (1985) Follow-up of prostaglandin plasma levels after acute myocardial infarction. Am Heart J 109: 218–222

21. Walinski P, Smith BJ, Lefer AM, Lebenthal M, Urban P, Greenspon A, Goldberg S (1984) Thromboxane A_2 in acute myocardial infarction. Am Heart J 108: 868–872

22. FitzGerald DJ, Catella F, Roy L, FitzGerald GA (1988) Marked platelet activation in vivo after intravenous streptokinase in patients with acute myocardial infarction. Circulation 77: 142:150

23. Neri-Serneri GG, Prisco D, Rogasi PG, Casolo GC, Castellani S (1985) Cardiac prostaglandin synthesis in spontaneous and in effort angina. Adv Prostaglandin Thrombox Leukotr Res 13: 59–70

24. Evers AS, Needleman P (1984) Endogenously produced leukotrienes cause vasoconstriction in infarcted rabbit hearts. Anaesthesiology 61: A88
25. Romson JL, Hook BG, Kunkel SL, Abrams GD, Schork MA, Lucchesi BR (1983) Reduction of the extent of ischemic myocardial injury by neutrophil depletion in the dog. Circulation 67: 1016–1023
26. Lucchesi BR, Mullane KM (1986) Leukocytes and ischemia-induced myocardial injury. Ann Rev Pharmacol Tox 26: 201–224
27. Mullane KM, Read N, Salmon JA, Moncada S (1984) Role of leukocytes in acute myocardial infarction in anaesthetized dogs: Relationship to myocardial salvage by anti-inflammatory drugs. J Pharmol Exp Ther 228: 510–522
28. Goetzl EJ, Woods JM, Gorman RR (1977) Stimulation of human eosinophil and neutrophil polymorphonuclear leukocyte chemotaxis and random migration by 12-L-hydroxy-5, 8, 10, 14-eicosatetraenoic acid. J Clin Invest 59: 179–183
29. Green K, Vesterqvist O, Rassmanis G, Edhag O, Henriksson P (1987) Deficient prostacyclin formation after acute myocardial infarction. Lancet 1: 1037–1038
30. Niada R, Mantovani M, Prino G, Pescador R, Berti F, Omini C, Folco GC (1981) Antithrombotic activity of a polydeoxyribonucleotide substance extracted from mammalian organs: A possible link with prostacyclin. Thromb Res 23: 233–246
31. Lefer AM (1986) Leukotrienes as mediators of ischemia and shock. Biochem Pharmacol 35: 123–127
32. Takano T, Vyden JK, Rose HB, Corday E, Swan HJC (1977) Beneficial effects of PGE_1 in acute myocardial infarction. Am J Cardiol 39: 297
33. Ogletree ML, Lefer AM, Smith JB, Nicolaou KC (1979) Studies on the protective effect of prostacyclin in acute myocardial ischemia. Eur J Pharmacol 56: 95–103
34. Araki H, Lefer AM (1980) Role of prostacyclin in the preservation of ischemic myocardial tissue in the perfused cat heart. Circ Res 47: 757–763
35. Jugdutt BI, Hutchins GM, Bulkley BH, Becker LC (1981) Dissimilar effects of prostacyclin, prostaglandin E_1 and prostaglandin E_2 on myocardial infarct size after coronary occlusion in conscious dogs. Circ Res 49: 685–700
36. Ribeiro LG, Brandon TA, Hopkins DG, Reduto LA, Taylor AA, Miller RR (1981) Prostacyclin in experimental myocardial ischemia: Effects on hemodynamics, regional myocardial blood flow, infarct size and mortality. Am J Cardiol 47: 835–840
37. Schrör K, Ohlendorf R, Darius H (1981) Beneficial effects of a new prostacyclin derivative, ZK 36374, in acute myocardial ischemia. J Pharmacol Exp Ther 219: 243–249
38. Schrör K (1987) Actions of prostaglandins on the heart. In: RJ Gryglewski and G Stock (eds) Prostacyclin and its stable analog iloprost. Springer Verlag, Berlin-Heidelberg pp 159–178
39. Schrör K, Smith EF III, Lefer AM (1988) The cat as an *in vivo* model for myocardial ischemia and infarction. Progr Pharmacol 6: 31–91
40. Parratt JR, Coker SJ, Wainwright CL (1987) Eicosanoids and susceptibility to ventricular arrhythmias during myocardial ischemia and reperfusion. J Mol Cell Cardiol 19, Suppl V: 55–66
41. Mannisi JA, Weisman HF, Bush DE, Dudeck P, Healy B (1987) Steroid administration after myocardial infarction promotes early infarct extension. J Clin Invest 79: 1431–1439
42. Hammerman H, Kloner RA, Schoen FJ, Brown EJ Jr, Hale S, Braunwald E (1984) Indomethacin-induced scar thinning following experimental infarction. Circulation 69: 611–617
43. Jugdutt, BI (1985) Delayed effects of early infarct-limiting therapies on healing after myocardial infarction. Circulation 72: 907–914
44. Grose R, Greenberg M, Strain J, Mueller H (1985) Intracoronary prostacyclin in evolving acute myocardial infarction. Am J Cardiol 55: 1625–1626
45. Kiernan FJ, Kluger J, Regnier JC, Rutkowski M, Fieldman A (1986) Epoprostenol sodium (prostacyclin) infusion in acute myocardial infarction. Br Heart J 56: 428–432
46. Henriksson P, Edhag O, Wennmalm A (1985) Prostacyclin infusion in patients with acute myocardial infarction. Br Heart J 53: 173–179

47. Armstrong PW, Langevin LM, Watts DG (1988) Randomized trial of prostacyclin infusion in acute myocardial infarction. Am J Cardiol 61: 455–457

48. Swedberg K, Held P, Wadenvik H, Kutti J (1987) Central haemodynamic and antiplatelet effects of iloprost – a new prostacyclin analogue – in acute myocardial infarction in man. Eur Heart J 8: 362–368

49. DeCaterina R, Pelosi G, Carpeggiani C, Bernini W, Gianessi D, Lazzerini G, L'Abbate A (1986) Iloprost in Prinzmetal's angina. Am J Cardiol 58: 553–554

50. Siegel RJ, Shah FK, Nathan M, Rodriguez L (1984) Prostaglandin E_1 infusion in unstable angina: Effects on anginal frequency and cardiac function. Am Heart J 108: 863–868

51. Sharma B, Wyeth RP, Gimenez HJ, Franciosa JA (1986) Intracoronary prostaglandin E1 plus streptokinase in acute myocardial infarction. Am J Cardiol 58: 1161–1166

52. Darius H, Hossmann V, Schrör K (1986) Antiplatelet effects of intravenous iloprost in patients with peripheral arterial obliterative disease. Klin Wochenschr 64: 545–551

53. Jaschonek K, Karsch KR, Weisenberger H, Tidow S, Faul C, Renn W (1986) Platelet prostacyclin binding in coronary artery disease. J Am Coll Cardiol 8: 259–266

54. Mueller HS, Rao PS, Greenberg MA, Buttrick PM, Sussman II, Levite HA, Grose RM, Perez-Davila V, Strain JE, Spaet TH (1985) Systemic and transcardiac platelet activity in acute myocardial infarction in man: resistance to prostacyclin. Circulation 72: 1336–1345

55. Sinzinger H, Kaliman J, Widhalm K, Pachinger O, Probst P (1981) Value of platelet sensitivity to antiaggregatory prostaglandins (PGI_2, PGE_1, PGD_2) in 30 patients with myocardial infarction at young age. Prostaglandins Med 7: 125–132

56. Smith EF III, Kloster G, Stöcklin G, Schrör K (1984) Effect of iloprost on membrane integrity in ischemic rabbit hearts. Biomed Biochem Acta 43: S155–S158

57. Thiemermann C, Steinhagen-Thiessen E, Schrör K (1984) Inhibition of oxygen-centered free radical formation by the stable prostacyclin mimetic iloprost (ZK 36374) in acute myocardial ischemia. J Cardiovasc Pharmacol 6: 365–366

58. Gercken G, Gallenkämper W, Schrör K, Trotz M (1982) Effects of ciloprost on myocardial metabolism during acute ischemia and heart arrest. Pflüger's Arch 394, Suppl: R-14

59. Van Gilst WH, Boonstra PW, Terpstra JA, Wildevuur CRM, de Langen CDJ (1985) Improved recovery of cardiac function after 24 h of hypothermic arrest in the isolated rat heart: Comparison of a prostacyclin analogue (ZK 36374) and a calcium entry blocker (diltiazem). J Cardiovasc Pharmacol 7: 520–524

60. Pissarek M, Goos H, Nöhring J, Graff J, Buller G, Beyerdörfer I, Mest H-J, Lindenau KF, Krause H-G (1987) Prostacyclin and iloprost: Equal efficiency in preservation of high energy phosphates in the dog heart following coronary artery ligation. Basic Res Cardiol 82: 566–575

61. van der Giessen WJ, Schoutsen B, Tijsen JGP, Verdouw PD (1986) Iloprost (ZK 36374) enhances recovery of regional myocardial function during reperfusion after coronary artery occlusion in the pig. Br J Pharmacol 87: 23–27

62. Farber NE, Pieper GM, Thomas JP, Gross GJ (1988) Beneficial effects of iloprost in the stunned canine myocardium. Circ Res 62: 204–215

63. Schrör K, Funke K (1985) Prostaglandins and myocardial noradrenaline overflow after sympathetic nerve stimulation during ischemia and reperfusion. J Cardiovasc Pharmacol 7, Suppl 5: S50–S54

64. Opie LH (1978) Myocardial metabolism and heart disease. Jap Circ J 42: 1223–1247

65. Schrör K, Addicks K, Darius H, Ohlendorf R, Rösen P (1981) PGI_2 inhibits ischemia-induced platelet activation and prevents myocardial damage by inhibition of catecholamine release. Evidence for cAMP as a common denominator. Thromb Res 21: 175–180

66. Schrör K, Darius H, Addicks K, Köster R, Smith EF III (1982) PGI_2 prevents ischaemia-induced alterations in cardiac catecholamines without influencing nerve-stimulation induced catecholamine release in non-ischaemic conditions. J Cardiovasc Pharmacol 4: 741–748

67. Zylka V, Addicks K, Deutsch H-J, Friedrich R, Griebenow G, Hirche H-J (1981) The antiarythmic effect of prostacyclin (PGI_2) in severe myocardial ischemia of pig heart. [abstract] Pflüger's Arch 389, Suppl: R-1

68. Rösen R, Rösen P, Ohlendorf R, Schrör K (1981) Prostacyclin prevents ischemia-induced

214

increase of lactate and cyclic AMP in ischemic myocardium. Eur J Pharmacol 69: 489–491

69. Schrör K (1989) Cytoprotection by prostacyclines in myocardial ischemia. In: Tor U, Naor Z, Danon A (eds.) New Trends Lipid Mediators Res. Vol. 3, Kargel-Basel

70. Niada R, Porta R, Pescador R, Mantovani M, Prino G (1985) Cardioprotective effects of defibrotide in acute myocardial ischemia in the cat. Thromb Res 38: 71–81

71. Thiemermann C, Löbel P, Schrör K (1985) Usefulness of defibrotide in protecting ischemic myocardium from early reperfusion damage. Am J Cardiol 56: 978–982

72. Hohlfeld T, Thiemermann C, Schrör K (1989) Protection from myocardial ischemic injury in cats and pigs by defibrotide – different mode of action? In: K. Schrör, H. Sinzinger (eds.) Prostaglandins in Clinical Research. Alan R Liss, New York pp 137–141

73. Einzig S, Sotomova R, Rao GHR, Gerrard JM, Foker E, White JG (1980) Effect of low-dose prostacyclin infusion on blood flow in acutely ischemic canine myocardium. Prostaglandins Med 5: 209–219

74. Coker SJ, Parratt JR (1981) Prostacyclin-induced changes in coronary blood flow and oxygen handling in the normal and acutely ischemic canine myocardium. Bas Res Cardiol 76: 457–462

75. Smith EF III, Gallenkämper W, Beckmann R, Thomsen T, Mannesmann G, Schrör K (1984) Early and late administration of a PGI_2-analogue, ZK 36374 (iloprost): Effects on myocardial preservation, collateral blood flow and infarct size. Cardiovasc Res 28: 163–173

76. Aksulu HE, Türker RK (1986) Protection by iloprost of the myocardial contractility and rhythmicity in frog ventricular strips. Experientia 42: 297–298

77. Dusting GJ, Angus JA (1984) Interactions of epoprostenol (PGI_2) with vasoconstrictors on diameter of large coronary arteries of the dog. J Cardiovasc Pharmacol 6: 20–27

78. Schrör K, Verheggen R (1986) Prostacyclins are only weak antagonists of coronary vasoconstriction induced by authentic thromboxane A_2 and serotonin. J Cardiovasc Pharmacol 8: 483–490

79. Bugiardini R, Galvani M, Ferrini D, Gridelli C, Tollemeto D, Macri N, Puddu P, Lenzi S (1987) Myocardial ischemia during intravenous prostacyclin administration: Hemodynamic findings and precautionary measures. Am Heart J 113: 234–240

80. Ganz P, Gaspar J, Colucci S, Barry WH, Mudge GH, Alexander RW (1984) Effects of prostacyclin on coronary hemodynamics at rest and in response to cold pressure testing in patients with angina pectoris. Am J Cardiol 53: 1500–1504

81. Bugiardini R, Galvani M, Ferrini D, Gridelli C, Mari L, Puddu P, Lenzi S (1986) Effects of iloprost, a stable prostacyclin analog, on exercise capacity and platelet aggregation in stable angina pectoris. Am J Cardiol 58: 453–459

82. Ohlendorf R, Perzborn E, Schrör K (1980) Prevention of infarction-induced decrease in circulating platelet count by prostacyclin. Thrombosis Res 19, 447–453

83. Mullane KM, McGiff JC (1985) Platelet depletion and infarct size in an occlusion-reperfusion model of myocardial ischemia in anesthetized dogs. J Cardiovasc Pharmacol 7: 733–737

84. Schrör K, Darius H, Ohlendorf R, Matzky R, Klaus W (1982) Dissociation of antiplatelet effects from myocardial cytoprotective activity during acute myocardial ischemia in cats by a new carbacyclin derivative (ZK 36375). J Cardiovasc Pharmacol 4: 554–561

85. Thiemermann C, Schrör K (1984) Comparison of the thromboxane synthetase inhibitor dazoxiben and the prostacyclin mimetic iloprost in an animal model of acute ischemia and reperfusion. Biomed Biochim Acta 43: S151–S154

86. Meerson FZ, Kagan VE, Kozlov YP, Belkin LM, Arkhipenko YV (1982) The role of lipid peroxidation in pathogenesis of ischemic damage and the antioxidant protection of the heart. Bas Res Cardiol 77: 465–485

87 Arnold G. Thiemermann C, Heymans L, Schrör K (1985) Morphological analysis of the iloprost effects on reperfused ischemic myocardium. In: K Schrör (ed.) Prostoglandins and Other Eicosanoids in the Cardiovascular System. Kargel Basel, pp 254–258

88. Simpson PJ, Mickelson J, Fantone JC, Gallagher KP, Lucchesi BR: (1987) Iloprost inhibits neutrophil function in vitro and in vivo and limits experimental infarct size in canine heart. Circ Res 60: 666–673

89. Simpson PJ, Mitsos SE, Ventura A, Gallagher AP, Fantone JC, Abrams GD, Schork MA, Lucchesi BR (1987) Prostacyclin protects ischemic reperfused myocardium in the dog by inhibition of neutrophil activation. Am Heart J 113: 129–137

90. Darius H, Thomsen T, Schrör K (1987) Cardiovascular actions *in vitro* and cardioprotective effects *in vivo* of nileprost – a mixed-type PGI_2/PGE_2 agonist. J Cardiovasc Pharmacol 10: 144–152

91. Ney P, Schrör K (1989) E-type prostaglandins but not iloprost inhibit platelet activating factor induced generation of leukotriene B_4 by human polymorphonuclear leukocytes. Br J Pharmacol 96: 186–192

92. Simpson PJ, Mickelson J, Fantone JC, Gallagher KP, Lucchesi BR (1988) Reduction of experimental canine cardiac infarct size with prostaglandin E1 – Inhibition of neutrophil migration and activation. J Pharmacol Exp Ther 244: 619–624

93. Schrör K, Thiemermann C, Ney P (1988) Protection of the ischemic myocardium from reperfusion injury by prostaglandin E_1 – inhibition of ischemia induced neutrophil activation. Naunyn-Schmiedeberg's Arch Pharmacol 338: 268–274

94. Terashita Z-I, Fukui H, Nishikawa K, Hirata M, Kikuchi S (1978) Coronary vasospastic action of thromboxane A_2 in isolated, working guinea pig hearts. Eur J Pharmacol 53: 49–56

95. Svensson J, Hamberg M (1976) Thromboxane A_2 and prostaglandin H_2 potent stimulators of the swine coronary artery. Prostaglandins 12: 943–950.

96. Holzgrefe HH, Buchanan LV, Bunting S (1987) *In vivo* characterization of synthetic thromboxane A_2 in canine myocardium. Circ Res 60: 290–296

97. Lefer AM (1987) Beneficial effects of thromboxane receptor antagonists in acute cardiovascular crises. In: H Sinzinger, K Schrör (eds.) Prostaglandins in Clinical Research. Alan R Liss, New York pp 221–228

98. Smith EF III, Lefer AM, Aharony D, Smith BJ, Magolda RL, Claremon D, Nicolaou KC (1981) Carbocyclic thromboxane A_2: Aggravation of myocardial ischemia by a new synthetic thromboxane A_2 analog. Prostaglandins 21: 443–456

99. Burke SE, Lefer AM, Smith GM, Smith JB (1983) Prevention of extension of ischemic damage following acute myocardial ischemia by dazoxiben, a new thromboxane synthetase inhibitor. Br J Clin Pharmacol 15: 97–101

100. Burke SE, DiCola G, Lefer AM (1983) Protection of ischemic cat myocardium by CGS-13080, a selective potent thromboxane A_2 synthesis inhibitor. J Cardiovasc Pharmacol 5: 842–847

101. Austin JC, Berrizbeitia LD, Schoen FJ, Kauffman RP, Hechtman HB, Cohn LH (1988) Thromboxane synthetase inhibition reduces ventricular irritability after coronary occlusion and reperfusion. Am Heart J 115: 505–509

102. O'Connor KM, Friehling TD, Kelliher GJ, MacNab MW, Wetstein L, Kowey PR (1986) Effect of thromboxane synthetase inhibition on vulnerability to ventricular arhythmia following coronary occlusion. Am Heart J 111: 683–688

103. Schrör K, Smith EF III, Bickerton M, Smith JB, Nicolaou KC, Magolda R, Lefer AM (1980) Preservation of the ischemic myocardium by pinane thromboxane A_2. Am J Physiol 238: H87–H92

104. Brezinski ME, Yanagisawa A, Darius H, Lefer AM (1985) Anti-ischemic actions of a new thromboxane receptor antagonist during acute myocardial ischemia in cats. Am Heart J 110: 1161–1167

105. Schrör K, Thiemermann C (1986) Treatment of acute myocardial ischemia with a selective antagonist of thromboxane receptors (BM 13.177) Br J Pharmacol 87: 631–637

106. Brezinski ME, Yanagisawa A, Lefer AM (1987) Cardioprotective actions of a specific thromboxane receptor antagonist in acute myocardial ischemia. J Cardiovasc Pharmacol 9: 65–71

107. Thiemermann C, Ney P, Schrör K (1988) The thromboxane receptor antagonist daltroban protects the myocardium from ischemic injury resulting in suppression of leukocytosis. Eur J Pharmacol 155: 57–67

108. Hutton I, Tweddel AC, Rankin AC, Walker ID, Davidson JF (1983) Effects of dazoxiben

on transcardial thromboxane levels and haemodynamics in coronary heart disease. Br J Clin Pharmacol 15 (Suppl 1): 79S–82S

109. Thaulow E, Dale J, Myhre E (1984) Effects of a selective thromboxane synthetase inhibitor, dazoxiben, and of acetylsalicylic acid on myocardial ischemia in patients with coronary artery disease. Am J Cardiol 53: 1255–1258

110. Oates JA, FitzGerald GA, Branch RA, Jackson EK, Knapp HR, Roberts LJ (1988) Clinical implications of prostaglandin and thromboxane A_2 formation. I. N Engl J Med 319: 689–698

111. Brezinski ME, Osborne JA, Yanagisawa A, Lefer AM (1987) Beneficial action of the thromboxane receptor antagonist AH-23,848, in acute myocardial ischemia. Meth Find Exptl Clin Pharmacol 9: 703–709

112. Folts JD, Crowell EB, Rowe GG (1976) Platelet aggregation in partially obstructed vessels and its elimination with aspirin. Circulation 54: 365–370

113. Verheggen R, Schrör K (1986) The modification of platelet-induced coronary vasoconstriction by a thromboxane receptor antagonist. J Cardiovasc Pharmacol 8: 483–490

114. Burke SE, Roth DM, Lefer AM (1983) Antagonism of platelet aggregation by 13-azaprostanoic acid in acute myocardial ischemia and sudden death. Thromb Res 29: 473–488

115. Lefer AM, Messenger M, Okamatsu S (1982) Salutary action of thromboxane inhibition during global myocardial ischemia. Naunyn-Schmiedeberg's Arch Pharmacol 321: 130–134

116. Grover GJ, Schumacher WA (1988) Effect of the thromboxane receptor antagonist SQ 29,548 on myocardial infarct size in dogs. J Cardiovasc Pharmacol 11: 29–35

117. Wargovich TJ, Mehta J, Nichols WM, Ward MB, Lawson D, Franzini D, Conti CR (1987) Reduction in myocardial neutrophil accumulation and infarct size following administration of thromboxane inhibitor U-63,557 A. Am Heart J 114: 1078–1085

118. Smith EF III, Egan JW, Bugelski PJ, Hillegass LM, Hill DE, Griswold DE (1988) Temporal relation between neutrophil accumulation and myocardial reperfusion injury. Am J Physiol 255: 1060–1068

119. Mullane KM, Fornabaio D (1988) Thromboxane synthetase inhibitors reduce infarct size by a platelet-dependent, aspirin-sensitive mechanism. Circ Res 62: 668–678

120. Aharony D, Smith JB, Smith EF III, Lefer AM (1981) Effects of arachidonic acid hydroperoxides on vascular and non-vascular smooth muscle. Prostaglandins Med 7: 527–535

121. Palmer RMJ, Stepney RJ, Higgs GA, Eakins KE (1980) Chemotactic activity of arachidonic acid lipoygenase products on leukocytes of different species. Prostaglandis 20: 411–418

122. Weinerowski P, Wittmann G, Aehringhaus U, Peskar BA (1985) Pharmacological modification of leukotriene release and coronary constrictor effect in cardiac anaphylaxis. Adv Prostaglandin Thrombox Leukotriene Res 13: 47–50

123. Lepran I, Lefer AM (1985) Protective actions of propyl gallate, a lipoxygenase inhibitor, on the ischemic myocardium. Circ Shock 15: 79–88

124. Mullane K, Hatala MA, Kraemer R, Sessa W, Westlin W (1987) Myocardial salvage by REV-5901: An inhibitor and antagonist of leukotrienes. J Cardiovasc Pharmacol 10: 398–406

125. Mullane KM, Moncada S (1982) The salvage of ischaemic myocardium by BW 755c in anaesthetized dogs. Prostaglandins 24: 255–265

126. Klein HH, Pich S, Bohle RM, Lindert S, Nebendahl K, Buchwald A, Schuff-Werner P, Kreuzer H (1988) Antiinflammatory agent BW 755c in ischemic reperfused porcine hearts. J Cardiovasc Pharmacol 12: 338–344

127. Bittl JA, Pfeffer MA, Lewis RA, Mehrotra MM, Corey EJ, Austen F (1985) Mechanism of the negative inotropic action of leukotrienes C_4 and D_4 on isolated rat heart. Cardiovasc Res 19: 426–432

128. Michelassi F, Lauda L, Hill RD, Lowenstein E, Watkins WD, Petkan AJ, Zapol WM (1982) Leukotriene D_4: A potent coronary artery vasoconstrictor associated with impaired ventricular contraction. Science 217: 841–843

129. Panzenbeck MJ, Kaley G (1983)   Leukotriene D_4 reduces coronary blood flow in the anaesthetized dog. Prostaglandins 25: 661–670

130. Ertl G, Fiedler V, Abram TS, Kochsiek K (1986)   Effects of nifedipine and indomethacin on leukotriene C_4 and D_4 induced coronary constriction at normal and reduced coronary perfusion in dogs. J Cardiovasc Pharmacol 8: 1078–1085

131. Piper PJ, Letts LG, Galton SA (1983)   Generation of a leukotriene-like substance from porcine vascular and other tissues. Prostaglandins 25: 591–599

132. Laurindo FRM, Finton CK, Ezra D, Czaja JF, Feuerstein GZ, Goldstein RE (1988)   Inhibition of eicosanoid-mediated coronary constriction during myocardial ischemia. FASEB J 2: 2479–2486

PART V

The role of oxygen radicals

Importance of free radicals generated by endothelial and myocardial cells in ischemia and reperfusion

R. FERRARI, S. CURELLO, A. CARGNONI, E. CONDORELLI,
L. COMINI, S. GHIELMI and C. CECONI
Chair of Cardiology, University of Brescia, Brescia, Italy

Introduction

In recent years, the effects of oxygen free radicals and their metabolites on biologic systems have received much attention because they are known to play an important role in many biochemical reactions which maintain normal cell functions. In the myocardium, for example, molecular oxygen is particularly important as the final acceptor of electrons in the mitochondrial electron transport system and generate free radicals.

At the same time, increasing evidence indicates that oxygen free radicals are also very important mediators of several forms of tissue damage, such as injury associated with inflammatory responses [1–3], ischemic injuries to different organs and tissues [4–6] and injuries resulting from intracellular metabolism of chemical and physical agents, such as drugs and radiation [7–10].

More specifically, over the past 3–5 years there has been an incredible growth of interest in the concept that oxygen free radicals play a role in the pathogenesis of myocardial ischemia and infarction. The majority of studies in this field have dealt with reperfusion models, since with coronary reperfusion following myocardial ischemia, oxygen is reintroduced into the system. It follows, then, that the concept of an oxygen free radicals-mediated cardiotoxicity has important clinical implications in the situation of myocardial ischemia followed by reperfusion. Interventions such as streptokinase, tissue plasminogen activator and percutaneous transluminal angioplasty are commonly used to re-establish coronary flow in patients with myocardial infarction. In addition, ischemia and reperfusion sequences occur in patients with vasospastic angina, or during coronary angioplasty or cardiopulmonary bypass.

Interestingly, it is known that reperfusion is not always accompanied by a recovery of myocardial function and may often cause further negative consequences, directly influencing the occurrence of cell death. It is obvious that if oxygen free radicals are a factor in these circumstances, then their neutralization could be very important from the therapeutical point of view.

H.M. Piper (ed.) Pathophysiology of severe ischemic myocardial injury, 221–238.
© *1990 Kluwer Academic Publishers, Dordrecht*

The relative importance of free radical production to irreversible injury of the animal and particularly of the human heart, however, is far from clear. Equally unclear and certainly contradictory is the value of therapeutic approaches of limiting the free-radical mediated component of reperfusion injury.

Thus several controversies exist regarding the role of oxygen radicals in the setting of myocardial ischemia and reperfusion. Perhaps one of the most important and much debated questions is the objective of this chapter: are oxygen free radicals abnormally produced within the myocytes during ischemia and reperfusion? If so, from which sources? We have therefore tried to review current knowledge relating to these problems and we have deliberately ignored the role of neutrophils, as it is specifically addressed in another chapter in this book.

As will become obvious upon reading, not all the controversies have been resolved and it is likely that work in this field will continue for several years to come.

Chemistry

A free radical is any chemical species that has one or more unpaired electrons.

Molecular oxygen is relatively non-reactive because of its unusual structure including two unpaired electrons with parallel electron spin. The majority of organic compounds which might react with oxygen contain paired electrons. The simultaneous insertion of two such paired electrons into a molecule of oxygen would violate the rules of quantum mechanics [11]. This restriction explains why ordinary molecular oxygen is relatively non-reactive.

Incoming electrons prefer to enter the orbitals one at a time, thus leading to the formation of reduced oxygen intermediates or oxygen free radicals.

The reduction of oxygen to water in the myocardium proceeds by two pathways. The mitochondrial cytochrome oxidase reduces 95% of oxygen to water by tetravalent reduction without the production of any intermediates. The remaining 5% of oxygen proceeds by univalent pathway in which several intermediates are produced.

When molecular oxygen (O_2) accepts an electron from a quite unstable species, the primary product generated is the superoxide (O_2^-) anion [12]. In aqueous environments, O_2^- is in equilibrium with its protonated form, $^{\cdot}HO_2$. Since the pKa for this equilibrium reaction is 4.8, O_2^- is the dominant species at neutral pH. However, relatively high concentrations of $^{\cdot}HO_2$ are favoured in acidic environments (such as during ischemia).

Although O_2^- is relatively non-reactive, several of its derivative compounds (including $^{\cdot}HO_2$) are capable of oxidizing organic molecules such as polyunsaturated fatty acids of membrane phospholipids to form alkoxy radicals ($RO^{\cdot}$). This reaction, however, is prevented by dismutation to hydrogen peroxide. When the reduced form of molecular oxygen (O_2^-) and the protonated form of the superoxide anion ($^.HO_2$) approach equal molar concentrations, spontaneous dismutation occurs, and H_2O_2 is generated as a direct dismutation product. H_2O_2 can also form as a direct result of a double reduction of molecular oxygen [11, 12] or by an enzyme-catalyzed dismutation of O_2^-. Superoxide dismutase (SOD) is present in varying concentrations in eukaryotic and prokaryotic cells and is capable of dismutating O_2^- to form hydrogen peroxide and oxygen.

Even hydrogen peroxide could be toxic, but only at high concentrations. The major danger of increased tissue concentration of hydrogen peroxide is the production of hydroxyl radical ($^.OH$) by the Haber Weiss or Fenton reaction [11, 12]. The hydroxyl radical is very reactive and unstable and reacts with a large variety of compounds and membranes. Particularly, under pathological circumstances, this radical attacks unsaturated fatty acid side chains by subtracting hydrogen and leaving a carbon radical. The lipid radical so formed, in turn, produces a conjugated diene and, in the presence of oxygen, results in the formation of organic oxygen radicals. These again, can abstract hydrogen from additional fatty acid side chains resulting in a chain reaction with the production of lipid peroxidation, greatly increased by the presence of iron or copper. In addition to lipid peroxidations, all these radicals are capable of various toxic effects such as inactivation of enzymes by oxidation of sulphydryl bounds, cross-linking of protein and DNA breakdown [13–15].

Additional oxygen-derived reactive metabolites that have been identified or predicted to exist in biological systems include singlet oxygen [12], hypohalous acids and a variety of n-chloramine compounds.

Myocardial sources of oxygen free radicals under normal conditions

It is interesting to note that even in the normal aerobic myocardium there is continuous production of oxygen free radicals. Superoxide anions are normally produced in the electron transport systems as by-products of various enzyme-substrate reactions (xanthine oxidase) and by auto-oxidations of a variety of low-molecular-weight molecules. Hydrogen peroxide may be produced as a direct product or as an enzyme-catalyzed (SOD) dismutation product of each of these sources of O_2^-.

Undoubtedly, the mitochondrial electron transport system is the most important site of free radical production under physiological conditions. 2% of the oxygen utilized by intact, aerobic mitochondria is partially reduced by electrons which escape from electron carriers in the respiratory chain [16]. The primary production sites of O_2^- by cardiac mitochondria, responsible for 75% of the superoxide generation, are the region between quinones and cytochrome b, on the internal mitochondrial membrane. Superoxide anions are formed by auto-oxidation of semiquinones rather than as a direct catalytic product [17]. In addition, several other auto-oxidizable electron carriers exist in the inner mitochondrial membrane such as NADH dehydrogenase which are responsible for the remainder of the radical generation [18].

Since mitochondria are rich in superoxide dismutase, it appears that the majority of O_2^- generated as a consequence of mitochondrial electron transport is enzymatically dismutated to H_2O_2 and O_2. Hydroxyl radicals can, therefore, be formed within the mitochondria because of the interactions between O_2^- and H_2O_2 via the mechanisms described above. Electron transport mechanisms which operate within the endoplasmic reticulum and within the nuclear membranes of eukaryotic cells may also generate O_2^- and H_2O_2. It should be mentioned that mixed-function oxidases such as cytochromes P450 and b5 or flavin-containing oxidases and flavoproteins that contain cytochrome reductases have been identified in cell membranes, and all these compounds are capable of generating O_2^- and H_2O_2. Peroxisomes also exist, and contain oxidases which can generate H_2O_2 directly, without superoxide anion intermediates [19]. Up to 40% of the H_2O_2 generated in peroxisomes can diffuse in the cytoplasm and result in injury to the cytosolic components.

Superoxide anions in the myocardium can also be the final product of the reaction between xanthine and xanthine-oxidase, an enzyme localized in the vascular endothelium [20, 21]. It should be specified that the native form of the enzyme is a dehydrogenase which cannot reduce molecular oxygen and, therefore, cannot produce superoxide. However, it appears that healthy tissues contain approximately 10% of their total enzyme in the oxidase form [22].

In addition, studies on the distribution of xanthine-oxidase among various tissues and species provide evidence that enzyme activity varies widely and, indeed, certain organs in certain species sometimes show no activity. Relevant to the following discussion is the discovery that the rabbit, pig, and human heart have little, if any, xanthine-oxidase activity [22–25].

Antioxidant mechanisms

The aerobic myocardium is able to handle and survive continuous oxygen free radical production because of the delicate balance between cellular systems which generate the various oxidants and those that maintain the antioxidant defence mechanism.

In the heart, these defence mechanisms include the enzymes superoxide dismutase, catalase and glutathione peroxidase plus other endogenous antioxidants such as vitamin E, ascorbic acid and cysteine [26, 27]. The primary mechanism for clearance of superoxide anions is the superoxide dismutase. This enzyme, which was isolated in 1969 by McCord and Fridovich, catalyzes the dismutation of superoxide anions to H_2O_2 and O_2 [28].

The reaction can also proceed spontaneously, but superoxide dismutase is able to increase the rate of intracellular dismutation by a factor of 10^9. At least three separate forms of SOD have been characterized. One contains copper and zinc and is present in the cytosol. Another contains manganese and is present in the mitochondria. The third contains iron and is associated with the cytoplasm of *Escherichia coli*.

Two enzyme systems are important in the metabolism of H_2O_2 produced by the univalent reduction of superoxide anion [29, 30]. The first is catalase, an enzyme, mainly present in cytosol, which catalyzes the reduction of H_2O_2 to water. Catalase, however, is only present at very low concentrations in the myocardium, whilst the second enzyme, glutathione peroxidase (a selenium-dependent enzyme) is present at significant concentrations in the cytosol of the heart [31].

The hexose monophosphate shunt produces through glucose-6-phosphate oxidation the reducing equivalents (NADPH) for the action of glutathione reductase. Reduced glutathione (GSH) is then utilized by GSH peroxidase to form oxidized glutathione (GSSG), but it is also in dynamic equilibrium with all cellular sylphydryl groups. In fact, glutathione mixed disulfides with proteins constitute an important part of the total cellular glutathione pool and the entire equilibrium is regulated by thiol transferases.

There is much evidence to suggest that glutathione plays an important role in myocardial metabolism [32]. In the heart, glutathione predominantly occurs intracellularly in concentrations of 1.1 µM. More than 95% of cardiac glutathione is in the form of GSH, GSH/GSSG ratio of aerobic myocardium being over 50 [32]. Among other functions, glutathione is a key factor in the detoxification of electrophilic metabolites and reactive oxygen intermediates. As the determinant of the sulphydryl disulfide ratio [33], glutathione modulates the activity of a number of enzymes and is also involved in the transport of amino acids across cell membranes [32]. Furthermore, GSH as a co-substrate of glutathione peroxidase provides essential protection against oxygen free radicals and prevents peroxidation of membrane lipids, the activity of superoxide dismutase in the heart being nearly four times less than in the liver, and catalase activity being extremely low [33]. This protective mechanism results in an increased formation of intracellular oxidized glutathione (GSSG). It follows that the changes of glutathione status provide important information in the cellular oxidative events, and tissue accumulation and/or release of GSSG in the coronary effluent is a sensitive and accurate index of oxidative stress [34-40]. In addition, an antioxidant which has long been known of biologic systems is alpha-tocopherol (vitamin E). Vitamin E has been identified at significant concentrations in both myocardial cytosolic and mitochondrial membrane [41-43]. *In vitro* studies have shown alpha-tocopherol to function as a free radical scavenger and to protect heart membrane from lipid peroxidation by free radicals [44-46]. Vitamin E functions synergically with ascorbic acid (vitamin C) which can react with vitamin E radicals to regenerate vitamin E. Vitamin C radicals, in turn, can be reduced by NADH reductase [47].

In the light of its lipophilic nature, vitamin E is likely to act as an antioxidant within membranes, while vitamin C, as a water-soluble electron-transport system, acts in the cytosol or in extracellular fluid. It should be emphasized, however, that although there is sufficient *in vitro* and *in vivo* evidence to support vitamin E as an important antioxidant, a protective role for this compound at physiologic concentration in humans has not been well documented.

Ischemia and reperfusion injury

With this information as background, we shall now consider the potential role of the myocardial oxygen free radicals in the pathogenesis of ischemic and reperfusion injury.

The subject is quite complex, as there is still a fair amount of debate concerning the existence of additive, reflow-induced damage. It is in fact known that reperfusion is essential for the mechanical recovery of the ischemic myocardium as, without reperfusion, no recovery is possible at all [48, 49]. There is experimental and clinical evidence that early coronary reperfusion reduces acute myocardial infarct size and mortality [50–56] and, with the exception of rhythm disturbances [57, 58], has no negative effects. With increasing duration of ischemia prior to reperfusion, the degree of recovery is less pronounced and, in many circumstances, there is no recovery at all with a further exacerbation of the biochemical, mechanical and ultrastructural disarrangements induced by ischemia [48, 49, 59–61].

This evidence from experimental and clinical studies supports the concept of a reperfusion component to the myocardial damage observed following protracted ischemia and, in our opinion, justifies the use of the term 'reperfusion injury', although it has different meanings for different investigators. We believe that it should strictly refer to the injury due to the act of reperfusion itself, in which cells, reversibly injured at the end of ischemia, become irreversibly injured upon reperfusion. There are studies utilizing *in vitro* models of myocardial ischemia and reperfusion which have demonstrated that reperfusion injury exists, is susceptible to treatment and is, in part at least, mediated by the readmission of calcium [62, 63]. In the same models, however, reperfusion damage was also associated with the occurrence of oxidative stress, suggesting that the reintroduction of molecular oxygen might be deleterious [27, 32, 33, 39, 64]. In addition, studies with *in vivo* models showed that, when oxygen radical scavengers were given during reperfusion alone, there was a reduction of myocardial infarct size, presumably by preventing reperfusion injury [65, 66]. However, not all studies assessing myocardial infarct size in occlusion-reperfusion models, in which agents against oxygen radicals were given, have been positive [67, 68].

Thus several controversies exist regarding the role of oxygen free radicals in mediating myocardial damage during ischemia and particularly during reperfusion.

To date, the majority of evidence of toxic effects of oxygen free radicals is indirect and it is derived from studies in which substances known to eliminate or reduce these toxic species have resulted in evidence of less severe myocardial injury in the setting of ischemia and reperfusion. However, we cannot ignore that some of these studies have been negative, that oxygen radical scavengers might have other complementary, pharmacological or hemodynamic effects, apart from reducing oxygen toxicity. Furthermore, it is not clear if their positive effects are permanent or merely a delay in the development of necrosis [69].

There are then, several fundamental questions which must be addressed before accepting the thesis that oxygen radicals are important mediators of ischemia and reperfusion injury. First, what evidence is there that they are produced in ischemic and reperfusion injury above the neutralizing capacity of the myocardium, and what are the potential sources of production? What are the effects of ischemia and reperfusion on the defence mechanisms against oxygen free radicals? In addition, what are the critical intracellular targets leading to irreversible myocardial injury and how might this process be interrupted?

Demonstration of oxygen free radical production during ischemia and reperfusion

Direct measurement of free radical species has been limited primarily by the instability of these oxygen metabolites. One primary technique has been used: electron paramagnetic resonance (EPR) spectroscopy, a system employed for many years to identify and characterize free radicals in simple chemical systems with or without the use of spin trap agents. Conflicting results, however, have been obtained.

Zweier et al. [70] identified a spectral signal similar to superoxide oxygen centered free radicals which increased significantly during ten minutes of ischemia and even more significantly during the first ten seconds of reperfusion. However, Luber and associates [71] using the same EPR technique in a similar model of ischemia and reperfusion failed to confirm the presence of such oxygen derived free radical species and doubted the importance of free radical generation during post-ischemic reperfusion.

Following the original report of Zweier et al. [70] many other authors using different spin trap agents have reported that superoxide or its derivative radicals can be demonstrated in the reperfused isolated hearts [72–74] or in in vivo animals as much as 3 hours after reperfusion [75]. However, electron spin resonance spectra reported by other investigators did not produce the same conclusion [76, 77]. Additionally, Nakazawa et al. [78] performing experiments with either isolated, perfused rat and rabbit hearts or open-chest canine hearts subjected to ischemia and reperfusion have pointed out that electron-spin resonance results need to be analysed with caution, since artifictual radicals are misleading problems common to this method. In particular, the superoxide and nitrogen-centered radicals commonly detected have been shown to be artifictually produced by pulverization of the frozen samples. Interestingly, these authors identified the radicals native to the myocardium as coenzyme Q_{10}, suggesting that the mitochondria might be an important site of production of these radicals. Therefore, the studies employing EPR technique seem to suggest that free radicals are produced in significant amounts during aerobic reperfusion. The presence of blood in the system is not a prerequisite for oxygen free radical production, suggesting a possible direct myocardial formation of these toxic species. At the moment, however, it is not possible to determine which radicals are produced under these circumstances.

Indirect evidence of oxygen free radical production also comes from experiments in which the occurrence of oxidative stress has been measured. Oxidative stress is a condition in which oxidant metabolites can exert their toxic effect because of increased production, or because of an altered cellular mechanism of protection [37, 79, 80].

In previous studies, we have demonstrated that in the isolated and perfused rabbit hearts ischemia induces a progressive reduction of tissue content of reduced glutathione (GSH) with a concomitant decline of the GSH/GSSG ratio [27, 32, 35, 36]. Reperfusion after a short period of ischemia normalizes the myocardial glutathione status, whilst reperfusion after a prolonged period of ischemia results in a release of GSH from the myocardium with a further depauperation of the tissue content [37]. At the same time, an important accumulation and release of oxidized glutathione occurs, causing a further reduction of GSH/GSSG ratio and a shift of cellular thiol redox state towards oxidation. Thus, during reperfusion after prolonged ischemia, the glutathione system, which represents an important mechanism of defence against oxygen toxicity, is under stress, and the reduced availability of cellular GSH becomes a rate limiting factor for detoxification of oxygen metabolites, probably hydrogen peroxide and lipid peroxides.

Interestingly, the occurrence of an oxidative stress has also been demonstrated in a group of coronary artery disease patients subjected to different periods of global ischemia followed by reperfusion during coronary artery by-pass grafting [39, 81, 82]. Oxidative stress was measured by determining the arterial and coronary sinus difference of GSH and GSSG. When the period of clamping (ischemia) was contained within 30 minutes, reperfusion resulted in only a small and transient rise of GSH and GSSG in the coronary sinus which, probably, represents a wash-out process. Reperfusion reinstated after 60 minutes of ischemia led to important release of GSH and GSSG in the coronary sinus which was still continuing at the end of the procedure, suggesting the occurrence of oxidative damage. Furthermore, there was an inverse correlation between the degree of oxidative stress and the recovery of hemodynamic function after surgery [82]. It is relevant to note here that these studies [37, 81, 82], together with that of Ferreira et al. [83], are the only evidence that oxygen free radicals might be involved in reperfusion damage in man.

Sources of oxygen radicals in ischemic and reperfusion myocardium

By definition, myocardial ischemia is a condition which exists when oxygen delivery to the myocardium is insufficient to meet the needs of mitochondrial oxidation [84]. The fact that there is a lack of oxygen available during ischemia, however, does not necessarily mean that oxygen free radicals cannot be formed. On the contrary, the metabolical disarrangements which occur during ischemia might predispose the formation of free radicals from the residual molecular oxygen. Five main possible sources have been theoretically identified for the production of active oxygen species: the altered mitochondrial electron transport system, the enzyme xanthine oxidase, the activation of phospholipase, the auto-oxidation of catecholamines and the activated polymorphonuclear leukocytes. As already mentioned, this latter possibility is specifically analyzed in another section of this book and is therefore not considered in the following discussion.

Altered mitochondrial electron transport system

It is well accepted that during ischemia, the adenine nucleotide pool is partially degraded, thus leaving the mitochondrial carriers in a more fully reduced state [85, 86]. This condition results in a higher increase of electron leakage from the respiratory chain which, in turn, reacts with the residual molecular oxygen entrapped within the inner mitochondrial membrane, thus leading to the formation of superoxide radicals. It seems probable that, in the early phase of ischemia, the increased oxygen free radical production from the mitochondria is neutralized by the normal functioning of the defence mechanisms against oxygen toxicity, mainly the mitochondrial superoxide dismutase. Increasing the duration or the severity of ischemia leads to a progressive decline of mitochondrial superoxide dismutase [27, 40, 43], leaving the mitochondria less well-equipped to deal with the increased radical influx.

Reintroduction of oxygen with reperfusion will re-energize the mitochondria, but electron egress through cytocrome oxidase will be reduced because of the lack of ADP. As a result, the percentage of electron leakage will further increase and there will be ample molecular oxygen to react to. Interestingly, reperfusion after prolonged periods of ischemia does not restore mitochondrial superoxide dismutase activity [40].

If ischemia and reperfusion lead to an increase in mitochondrial radical production with a decrease in radical scavenging capability, it is possible to suppose a self-induced progression of mitochondrial injury with further deterioration of normal electron flow which will cause further production of oxygen free radicals.

If the above postulated sequence of events is correct, it should be possible to measure an increased oxygen free radicals production of mitochondria isolated from ischemic and reperfused myocardium. Surprisingly, only a few studies have been undertaken in this direction and they have shown an increased production of reduced oxygen intermediates after ischemia and, particularly, after reperfusion from submitochondrial particles [14, 15, 87]. Otani et al. [88] studied the effects of oxygen on ATP production by mitochondria isolated from globally ischemic rabbit heart. Incubation of the mitochondria with superoxide dismutase and catalase enhanced ATP production and supressed the appearance of hydroxyl radical signal detected with electron spin resonance. Guarnieri et al. [89] found that in vitro formation of free radicals (generated by xanthine-xanthine-oxidase) resulted in an increase of malondialdehyde formation and reduced mitochondrial respiration, while Ceconi et al. [90] showed that iron-induced lipid peroxidation of myocardial mitochondria results in impaired calcium transporting capacities and oxidative phosphorylation, effects that could be inhibited by additional superoxide dismutase and catalase. A similar decrease in calcium uptake occurred after the exposure of oxygen radicals to isolated sarcoplasmic reticulum, the other organelle which might be involved in oxygen free radical formation [91, 92]. Interestingly, a loss of calcium sequestration by sarcoplasmic reticulum has been shown to occur after ischemia and reperfusion.

Xanthine oxidase

Sautgstad and Aesen [93] recognized that the increase of plasma hypoxantine during hypoxia and/or ischemia could, during reoxygenation and/or reperfusion, support the production of superoxide by xanthine oxidase. At the same time, the drug allopurinol, an inhibitor of xanthine dehydrogenase and oxidase, has been shown to exert protective effects against ischemia and reperfusion [94] or hemorrhagic shock [95].

For this reason xanthine oxidase was a prime candidate for oxygen free radical production [96]. The enzyme is localized not in the myocytes, but in the vascular endothelial cell. During ischemia, xanthine dehydrogenase is converted, probably by an increase of cytosolic calcium [97] or by limited proteolysis, or by the oxidation of thiol groups [98, 99], to the oxidase form [100]. At the same time, adenosine triphosphate is degraded to hypoxanthine which accumulates in ischemic tissue [95]. On reperfusion, with the readmission of large quantities of molecular oxygen, in the presence of high concentrations of hypoxanthine, the other substrate for xanthine oxidase, there may be a burst of O_2^- production. Following this hypothesis, many investigators have provided evidence that inactivation of xanthine oxidase, either with allopurinol [101–110] or with tungsten [111, 112], results in protection of the ischemic and reperfused myocardium, suggesting that generation of super-oxide by xanthine oxidase may play an important pathogenetic role in reperfusion injury.

This conclusion, although very challenging, is not, in our opinion, completely justified.

First of all, there is the possibility that allopurinol may reduce the severity of myocardial ischemic injury by mechanisms other than an inhibition of xanthine oxidase activity [107–109]. Secondly, not all the studies are positive. Authors using very similar experimental models provided entirely different results [67, 113–115], suggesting that careful analysis of the interpretation of positive results and of experimental conditions is warranted. In addition, in the positive studies cited above, the protection produced by allopurinol was quite remarkable, i.e. up to 87% decrease in CPK release during reoxygena-tion of the isolated rat heart or more than 70% reduction of infarct size in the occluded canine myocardium. These findings suggest that the generation of superoxide by xanthine oxidase may account for most of the injury [86]. This conclusion, however, cannot be accepted. As reported earlier, the distribu-tion of xanthine oxidase among tissues and species varies widely, the rabbit, pig and human myocardium having essentially no activity and, yet, these species are not immune to reperfusion injury. Finally, it is important to realise that one of the first studies [93] to suggest that production of super-oxide by xanthine oxidase might be a problem for reoxygenated myocardium was carried out in pigs, which were later shown to have no xanthine oxidase activity.

Metabolism of arachidonic acid and catecholamines

Arachidonic acid is released and subsequently metabolized to prostaglandins and leukotrienes during ischemia [116–118]. These metabolic pathways gen-erate electrons which can initiate the formation of free radicals [119, 120]. Kontos [121] found that application of arachidonate to the brain resulted in vascular endothelial lesions which were similar to those seen in ischemic, traumatic or hypertensive injuries: these lesions were reduced if superoxide dismutase, catalase or the cyclooxygenase inhibitor indometacin were added simultaneously with arachidonate. In addition, it has been suggested that the ischemia and reperfusion induced calcium overload would activate phospho-lipases [122, 123], which, in turn, may degrade cell membrane phospholipids, releasing arachidonic acid. Studies with isolated myocytes [124] have shown that lipid peroxidation can be activated by increasing calcium concentration. Furthermore, even the phenomenon of 'calcium paradox' has been associated with enhanced free radical production [125] although the occurrence of oxidative damage during the event of the calcium paradox has been doubted [126]. At present, however, the role of arachidonic acid metabolism as a source of free radicals in the setting of myocardial ischemia and reperfusion is still not completely known. Finally, the auto-oxidation of catecholamines which are abundantly released from the ischemic myocardium could provide, through the formation of adrenochrome, oxygen free radicals [127, 128]. Vitamin E has been shown to protect against isoprenaline-induced myocardial damage, whereas depletion of the vitamin exacerbates the damage [129]. However, as in the case of arachidonic acid metabolism, the precise role of catecholamines in oxygen free radicals production is not yet known [119, 120].

Conclusions

In this chapter, the results, conclusions and criticisms from different experiments have been brought together to consider the possibility that oxygen derived free radicals are generated from the myocardium during ischemia and reperfusion above the neutralizing capacity of the myocytes.

This possibility is by no means proven. There is, however, evidence that prolonged ischemia reduces the defence mechanism against oxygen toxicity, thus making the myocardium more vulnerable to the damaging effects of oxygen free radicals. On the other hand, there is also evidence, albeit preliminary, that the formation of these toxic species is enhanced after ischemia and, particularly, after reperfusion. At the moment, it is not possible to discriminate which radicals are produced under these circumstances and from which sources. It seems that the presence of blood is not a prerequisite for oxygen free radical formation, and that mitochondria are likely to be an important source of production.

Finally, several controversies exist regarding the meaning of the studies in which agents known to eliminate or reduce oxygen free radical species have provided protection against ischemia and reperfusion. The pathophysiological conclusions derived from such studies should be considered with some caution.

References

1. Kuehl, FA, Humes J, Torchiana ML (1979) Oxygen-centered radicals in inflammatory processes. Adv Inflam Res 1: 419–430
2. Samuelsson B (1983) Leukotrienes: Mediators of immediate hypersensitivity reactions and imflammation. Science 220: 568–575
3. Pryor WA (1982) Free radical biology: xenobioties, cancer and aging. Ann NY Acad Sci 393: 1–22
4. Fridovich I (1983) Superoxide radical: an endogenous toxicant. Ann Rev Pharmacol Toxicol 23: 239–257
5. Fridovich I (1978) The biology of oxygen radicals. Science 201: 875–888
6. Mc Cord JM, Roy RS (1982) The pathophysiology of superoxide: Roles in inflammation and ischemia. Can J Physiol Pharmacol 60: 1345–1352
7. Estabrook RW, Werringloer J (1977) Cytochrome P-450: its role in oxygen activation for drug

metabolism. In: Gould RF (ed) Drug Metabolism Concepts. Washington DC, American Chemical Society, pp 1–26

8. Thayer WS (1977) Adryamicin stimulated superoxide formation in submitochondrial particles. Chem Biol Interact 19: 256–278

9. Lefer AM, Araki H, Okamatsu S (1981) Beneficial actions of a free radical scavenger in traumatic shock and myocardial ischemia. Circ Shock 8: 273–282

10. Hutchinson F (1966) The molecular basis for radiation effects on cells. Cancer Res 26: 2045–2052

11. Thompson JA, Hess ML (1986) The oxygen free radical system: a fundamental mechanism in the production of myocardial necrosis. Progress in Cardiovascular Diseases 6: 449–462

12. Fee JA, Valentine JS (1977) Chemical and physical properties of superoxide. In: Michelson AM, McCord JM (eds) Superoxide and superoxide dismutase Fridovich. New York Academic Press Inc., pp 19–66

13. Tappel AL (1973) Lipid peroxidation damage to cell components. Fed Proc 32: 1870–1874

14. Turner JF, Boveris A (1980) Generation of superoxide anion by NADH dehydrogenase of bovine heart mitochondria. Biochem J 191: 421–430

15. Ferrari R, Bongrani S, Cucchini F, Di Lisa F, Guarnieri C, Visioli O (1982) Effects of molecular oxygen and calcium on heart metabolism during reperfusion. In: Bertrand ME (ed) Coronary arterial spasm. pp 46–59

16. Boveris A. Chance B (1973) The mitochondrial generation of hydrogen peroxide: general properties and effect of hyperbaric oxygen. Biochem J 134: 707–716

17. Boveris A, Cadenas E (1975) Mitochondrial production of superoxide anion and its relationship to the antimicyn-insensitive respiration. FEBS Lett 54: 311–314

18. Turrens JF, Boveris A (1980) Generation of superoxide anion by the NADH dehydrogenase of bovine heart mitochondria. Biochem J 191: 421–427

19. Masters C, Holmes R (1977) Peroxisomes: New aspects of cell physiology and biochemistry. Physiol Rev 57: 816–888

20. Braunwald E, Kloner RA (1985) Myocardial reperfusion: a double edged sword? J Clin Invest 76: 1713–1719

21. Mc Cord JM (1985) Oxygen-derived free radicals in post-ischaemic tissue injury. N Engl J Med 312: 159–163

22. Roy RS, McCord JM (1983) Superoxide and ischemia: Conversion of xanthine dehydrogenase to xanthine oxidase. In: Greenwald R, Cohen G (eds) Oxy radicals and their scavenger systems: Vol II, cellular and molecular aspects. New York, Elsevier Science, pp 145–153

23. Al-Khalidi UAS, Chaglassian TH (1965) The species distribution of xanthine oxidase. Biochem J 97: 318–320

24. Downey J, Chambers D, Miura T, Yellon D, Jones D (1986) Allopurinol fails to limit infarct size in a xanthine oxidase-deficient species. Circulation 74 (Suppl. II): 372

25. Eddy L, Stewart J, Jones H, Yellon D, Mc Cord JM, Downey J (1986) Xanthine oxidase is detected in ischemic rat heart but no human hearts. Physiologist 29: 166

26. Diplock AT, Lucy JA (1974) The biochemical model of action of vitamin E and selenium: a hypothesis. Febs Letters 29: 205–212

27. Ferrari R, Ceconi C, Curello S, Cargnoni A, Agnoletti G, Boffa GM, Visioli O (1986) Intracellular effects of myocardial ischaemia and reperfusion: role of calcium and oxygen. Eur Heart J 7: 3–12

28. Mc Cord JM, Fridovich I (1969) Superoxide dismutase: an enzymatic function for erythrocuprein (hemocuprein). J Biol Chem 244: 6049–6055

29. Roos D, Weening RS, Wyss SR (1980) Protection of human neutrophils by endogenous catalase: studies with cells from catalase-deficient individuals. J Clin Invest 65: 1515–1522

30. Chance B, Sies H, Boveris A (1979) Hydroperoxide metabolism in mammalian organs. Physiol Rev 59: 527–605

31. Lawrence RA, Burk RF (1978) Species, tissue, and subcellular distribution of selenium dependent glutathione peroxidase activity. J Nutr 108: 211–215

32. Ferrari R, Curello S, Ceconi C, Cargnoni A, Condorelli E, Albertini A (1988) Alterations of

glutathione status during myocardial ischaemia and reperfusion. In: Singel PK (ed) Oxygen Radicals in the Pathophysiology of Heart Disease. Kluwer Ac Publ, pp 145–160

33. Ferrari R, Ceconi C, Curello S, Cargnoni A, Albertini A, Visioli O (1986) Oxygen utilization and toxicity at myocardial level. In: Benzi G, Packer L, Siliprandi N (eds) Biochemical aspects of physical exercise. Amsterdam, Elsevier

34. Ferrari R, Ceconi C, Curello S, Cargnoni A, Medici D (1986) Oxygen free radicals and reperfusion injury; the effects of ischaemia and reperfusion on the cellular ability to neutralize oxygen toxicity. J Mol Cell Cardiol 18: 67–69

35. Ferrari R, Ceconi C, Curello S, Cargnoni A, Albertini A, Visioli O (1987) Molecular events occurring during post-ischaemic reperfusion. In: Dhalla NS, Innes IR, Beanish RE (eds) Myocardial ischaemia. Boston, Nijhoff Publishing, pp 67–85

36. Ferrari R, Ceconi C, Curello S, Cargnoni A, Albertini A, Visioli O (1986) Myocardial protection against oxygen free radicals. In: Benzi G, Packer L, Siliprandi N (eds) Biochemical aspects of physical exercise. Amsterdam, Elsevier

37. Curello S, Ceconi C, Cargnoni A, Ferrari R, Albertini A (1987) Improved procedure for determining glutathione plasma as an index of myocardial oxidative stress. Clinical Chemistry 33/8: 1448–1449

38. Curello S, Ceconi C, Bigoli C, Ferrari R, Albertini A, Guarnieri C (1985) Change in the cardiac glutathione status after ischaemia and reperfusion. Experientia 41: 42–43

39. Curello S, Ceconi C, Medici D, Ferrari R (1986) Oxidative stress during myocardial ischaemia and reperfusion: experimental and clinical evidences. J Appl Cardiol 1: 311–327

40. Ferrari R, Ceconi C, Curello S, Guarnieri C, Caldarera CM, Albertini A, Visioli O (1985) Oxygen-mediated myocardial damage during ischaemia and reperfusion: role of the cellular defences against oxygen toxicity. J Mol Cell Cardiol 17: 937–945

41. Ferrari R, Visioli O, Caldarera CM, Nayler WG (1982) Vitamin E and the heart: possible role as antioxidants. Acta Vitamin et Enzymol 5: 11–22

42. Guarnieri C, Ferrari R, Visioli O, Caldarera CM, Nayler WG (1978) Effect of alpha-tocopherol on hypoxic reperfused and reoxygenated rabbit. J Mol Cell Cardiol 10: 893–906

43. Ferrari R, Cargnoni A, Ceconi C, Curello S, Albertini A, Visioli O (1987) Role of oxygen in myocardial ischaemic and reperfusion damage: protective effects of vitamin E. In: Hayaishi O, Mino M (eds) Clinical and Nutritional Aspects of Vitamin E. Amsterdam, Elsevier

44. Lucy JA (1972) Functional and structural aspects of biological membranes: A suggested structural role of vitamin E in the control for membrane permeability and stability. Ann NY Acade Sci 203: 4–11

45. Guarnieri C, Flamigni F, Rossoni-Caldarera C, Ferrari R (1982) Myocardial mitochondrial function in alpha-tocopherol deficient and refed rabbits. Advances in Myocardiology, Plenum Publishing Corporation 3: 621–627

46. Ferrari R, Cargnoni A, Ceconi C, Curello S, Albertini A, Visioli O (1987) Role of oxygen in myocardial ischemic and reperfusion damage: protective effects of Vitamin E. In: Hayaishi O, Mino M (eds) Clinical and Biochemical Aspects of Vitamin E. Amsterdam, Elsevier

47. Packer JE, Slater TF, Willson RL (1979) Direct observation of a free radical interaction between vitamin E and vitamin C. Nature 278: 737–738

48. Ferrari R, Curello S, Cargnoni A, Condorelli E, Belloli S, Albertini A, Visioli O (1988) Metabolic changes during post-ischaemic reperfusion. J Mol Cell Cardiol 20: 119–133

49. Ferrari R, Niccoli L, Visioli O, Harris P (1987) Myocardial metabolism during intracoronary thrombolysis. Two illustrative cases. Inter J Cardiol 15: 293–299

50. Patel B, Kloner RA (1987) Analysis of reported randomized trials of streptokinase therapy for acute myocardial infarction in the 1980s. Am J Cardiol 59: 501–504

51. TIMI Study Group (1985) The thrombolysis in myocardial infarction (TIMI) trial: phase I findings. N Engl J Med 312: 932–936

52. Gruppo Italiano per lo Studio della streptochinasi nell'infarto miocardico (GISSI) (1986) Effectiveness of intravenous thrombolytic treatment in acute myocardial infarction. Lancet 22: 397–401

53. Reimer KA, Lowe JE, Rasmussen MM, Jennings RB (1987) The wavefront phenomenon of

ischemic cell death. Myocardial infarct size vs duration of coronary occlusion in dogs. Circulation 56: 786–793

54. Ellis SG, Wynne J, Braunwald E, Henschke CI, Sandor T, Kloner RA (1984) Response of reperfusion salvaged stunned myocardium to inotropic stimulation. Am Heart J 107: 13–19

55. Barry WH, Als AV, Paulin S, Grossman W, Braunwald E (1981) Myocardial salvage after intracoronary thrombolysis with streptokinase in acute myocardial infarction. N Engl J Med 305: 777–782

56. Tennant R, Wiggers CJ (1985) The effect of coronary occlusion on myocardial contraction. Am J Physiol 112: 351–361

57. Corr PB, Witkowski FX (1983) Potential electrophysiologic mechanisms responsible for dysrhythmias associated with reperfusion of ischaemic myocardium. Circulation 68 (Suppl 1): 16–24

58. Manning AS, Hearse DJ (1984) Reperfusion-induced arrhythmias: Mechanism and prevention. J Mol Cell Cardiol 16: 497–518

59. Valente M, Klugman S, Niccoli L, Ferrari R, Terrosu' P, Camerini F, Ibba GV, Visioli O, Bellandi M, Contini GM, Ettori F, Franceschino V, Leonzi O, Salvi A (1988) Importance of early recanalization of the occluded coronary artery in acute myocardial infarction for preservation of left ventricular function. J Mol Cell Cardiol 20: 145–154

60. Jennings RB, Reimer KA (1987) Lethal myocardial ischaemic injury. Am J Pathol 92: 187–214

61. Hearse DJ (1977) Reperfusion of ischaemic myocardium. J Mol Cell Cardiol 9: 607–616

62. Ferrari R, Curello S, Ceconi C, Di Lisa F, Raddino R, Visioli O (1986) Myocardial recovery during post-ischaemic reperfusion: effects of nifedipine, calcium and magnesium. J Mol Cell Cardiol 18: 487–488

63. Shine KI, Douglas AM (1983) Low calcium reperfusion of ischaemic myocardium. J Mol Cell Cardiol 15: 251–260

64. Hearse DJ, Hymphrey SM, Bullock GR (1978) The oxygen paradox and the calcium paradox. Two facets of the same problem? J Mol Cell Cardiol 10: 641–668

65. Jolly SR, Kane WJ, Baile MB, Abrams GD, Lucchesi BR (1984) Canine myocardial reperfusion injury. Its reduction by the combined administration of superoxide dismutase and catalase. Circ Res 54: 277–285

66. Ambrosio G, Becker LC, Hutchins GM, Weisman HF, Weisfeldt ML (1986) Reduction in experimental infarct size by recombinant human superoxide dismutase: insights into the pathophysiology of reperfusion injury. Circulation 74: 1424–1433

67. Reimer KA, Jennings RB (1985) Failure of xanthine oxidase inhibitor allopurinol to limit infarct size after ischemia and reperfusion in dogs. Circulation 71: 1069–1075

68. Gallagher KP, Buda AJ, Pace D, Gerren RA, Shlafer M (1986) Failure of superoxide dismutase and catalase to alter size of infarction in conscious dogs after 3 hours of occlusion followed by reperfusion. Circulation 73: 1065–1076

69. Zweier JL, Rayburn BK, Flaherty JT, Weisfeldt ML (1987) Recombinant superoxide dismutase reduces oxygen free radical concentrations in reperfused myocardium. J Clin Invest 80: 1728–1734

70. Zweier JL, Flaherty JT, Weisfeldt ML (1987) Direct measurement of free radical generation following reperfusion of ischemic myocardium. Proc Natl Acad Sci USA 84: 1404–1407

71. Luber JM, Rao PS, Crowder MS: Identification of free radicals produced during myocardial ischemia and reperfusion using electron paramagnetic resonance spectroscopy and high precision liquid chromatography. J Thorac Cardiovasc Surg, in press

72. Arroyo CM, Kramer JH, Dickens BF, Weglicki WB (1987) Identification of free radicals in myocardial ischemia/reperfusion by spin trapping with nitron DMPO. FEBS Lett 221: 101–104

73. Arroyo CM, Kramer JH, Leiboff RH, Mergner GW, Dickens BF, Weglicki WB (1987) Spin trapping of oxygen and carbon-centered free radicals in ischaemic canine myocardium. Free Radical Biology and Medicine 3: 313–316

74. Garlick PB, Davies MJ, Hearse DJ, Slater TF (1987) Direct detection of free radicals in the reperfused rat heart using electron spin resonance spectroscopy. Circ Res 61: 757–760

75. Bolli, R, Patel BS, Jeroudi MO, Lai EK, McCay PB (1988) Demonstration of free radical generation in "stunned" myocardium of intact dogs with use of the spin trap alpha-phenyl n-ter-butyl nitrone. J Clin Invest 82: 476–485
76. Limm W, Mugiishi M, Piette LH, McNamara JJ (1987) Quantitative assessment of free radical generation during ischemia and reperfusion in the isolated rabbit heart (Abstract). Proc Fourth Int Cong Oxygen Radicals. La Jolla, CA, pp 123–125
77. Nakazawa H, Ban K, Okino H, Masuda T, Aoki N, Hori S, Yoshino H (1986) The quantification of free radicals in myocardium obtained by super rapid sampling and freezing. Circulation 74 (Suppl): 433
78. Nakazawa H, Ichimori K, Shinozaki Y, Okino H, Hori S (1988) Is superoxide demonstration by electro-spin resonance spectroscopy really superoxide? Am J Physiol 255: H213–215
79. Adams JD, Lauterburg BM, Mitchell JR (1983) Plasma glutathione and glutathione disulfide in the rat: regulation and response to oxidative stress. J Pharmacol Exp Ther 227: 749–754
80. Ishikawa H, Sies H (1984) Cardiac transport of glutathione disulfide and S-conjugate. J Biol Chem 259: 383–392
81. Curello S, Ceconi C, Cargnoni A, Medici D, Condorelli E, Ferrari R (1987) Evidence of myocardial oxidative stress in human during ischaemia and reperfusion. In: Benzi G (ed) Advances in myochemistry. Libbey Eurotext Ltd., pp 365–367
82. Ferrari R, Alfieri O, Curello S, Ceconi C, Cargnoni A, Marzollo P, Pardini A, Caradonna E, Visioli O: The occurrence of oxidative stress during reperfusion of the human heart. Circulation, in press
83. Ferreira R, Llesuy S, Milei S, Scordo D, Hourquebie H, Molteni L, De Palma C, Boveris A (1988) Assessment of myocardial oxidative stress in patients after myocardial revascularization. Am Heart J 115: 307–312
84. Jennings RB (1970) Myocardial ischaemia: observations, definitions and speculation. J Mol Cell Cardiol 1: 345–349
85. Freeman BA, Crapo JD (1982) Biology of disease. Free radicals and tissue injury. Lab Invest 47: 412–426
86. Mc Cord JM (1988) Free radicals and myocardial ischaemia: overview and outlook. Free Radical Biology and Medicine 4: 9–14
87. Nohl H (1982) The biochemical mechanism of the formation of reactive oxygen species in heart mitochondria. In: Caldarera CM, Harris P (eds) Advances in studies on heart metabolism. Bologna Cooperative Libraria Universitaria Editrice Bologna, pp 413–421
88. Otani H, Tanaka H, Inove T, Umemoto M, Omoto K, Tanaka K, Sato T, Osako T, Masuda A, Nonoyama A, Kagawa T (1984) In vitro studies on contribution of oxidative metabolism of isolated rabbit heart mitochondria to myocardial reperfusion injury. Circ Res 55: 168–172
89. Guarnieri C, Ceconi C, Muscari C, Flamigni F (1982) Influence of oxygen radicals on heart metabolism. In: Caldarera CM, Harris P (eds) Advances in studies on heart metabolism. Bologna, CLUEB, 423–431
90. Ceconi C, Curello S, Albertini A, Ferrari R (1988) Effect of lipid peroxidation on heart mitochondria oxygen consuming and calcium transporting capacities. Molecul and Cellul Biochem 81: 131–135
91. Krause SM, Hess ML (1984) Characterization of canine sarcoplasmic reticulum function during short term, normothermic global ischaemia. Circ Res 55: 176–184
92. Hess ML, Okabe E, Ash P, Kontos HA (1984) Free radical mediation of the effects of acidosis on calcium transport by cardiac sarcoplasmic reticulum in whole heart homogenates. Cardiovasc Res 18: 149–157
93. Saugstad OD, Aasen AO (1980) Plasma hypoxanthine concentrations in pigs a prognostic aid in hypoxia. Eur Surg Res 12: 123–129
94. De Wall RA, Vasko KA, Stanley EL, Kezdi P (1971) Responses of the ischemic myocardium to allopurinol. Am Heart J 82: 362–370
95. Jones CE, Crowell JW, Smith EE (1968) Significance of increased blood uric acid following extensive hemorrhage. Am J Physiol 214: 1374–1377

96. Granger DN, Rutilio G, Mc Cord JM (1981) Superoxide radicals in feline intestinal ischaemia. Gastroenterology 81: 22–29

97. Roy RS, Mc Cord JM (1983) Superoxide and ischaemia: Conversion of xanthine dehydrogenase to xanthine oxidase. In: Greenwald RA, Cohen G (eds) Radicals and their scavenger systems. Amsterdam, Elsevier Science, pp 145–153

98. Battelli MG, Della Corte E, Stirpe F (1972) Xanthine oxidase type D (dehydrogenase) in the intestine and other organs of the rat. Biochem 126: 747–749

99. Della Corte E, Stirpe F (1972) The regulation of rat liver xanthine oxidase: involvement of thiol groups in the conversion of the enzyme activity from dehydrogenase (type D) into oxidase (type O) and purification of the enzyme. Biochem 126: 736–745

100. Mc Cord JM (1984) Are free radicals a major culprit? In: Hearse DJ, Yellon DM (eds) Therapeutic approaches to myocardial infarct size limitation. New York, Raven Press, pp 209–218

101. Grisham MB, Russell WJ, Roy RS, Mc Cord JM (1986) Reoxygenation injury in the isolated perfused working rat heart: roles of xanthine oxidase and transferrin. In: Rotilio G (ed) Superoxide and superoxide dismutase in chemistry, biology and medicine. Amsterdam, Elsevier, pp 571–575

102. Chambers DE, Parks DA, Patterson G, Roy RS, Mc Cord JM, Yoshida S, Parmley L, Downey JM (1985) Xanthine oxidase as a source of free radical in myocardial ischaemia. J Mol Cell Cardiol 17: 145–152

103. McCord JM, Roy RS, Schaffer SW (1985) Free radicals and myocardial ischaemia. The role of xanthine oxidase. Adv Myocardiol 5: 183–189

104. Werns SW, Shea MJ, Mitsos SE, Dysko RC, Fantone JC, Schork MA, Abrams GD, Pitt B, Lucchesi BR (1986) Reduction of the size of infarction by allopurinol in the ischaemic-reperfused canine heart. Circulation 73: 518–524

105. Manning AS, Coltart DJ, Hearse DJ (1984) Ischaemia and reperfusion-induced arrhythmias in the rat. Effect of xanthine oxidase inhibition with allopurinol. Circ Res 55: 545–548

106. Kloner RA (1988) Introduction to the role of oxygen radicals in myocardial ischaemia and infarction. Free Radical Biology and Medicine 4: 5–7

107. Adachi H, Motomatsu K, Yara I (1979) Effect of allopurinol on patients undergoing open-heart surgery. Japanese Circ J 43: 395–401

108. Arnold WL, DeWall RH, Keydi P, Eward HH (1985) The effect of allopurinol on the degree of early myocardial ischaemia. Am Heart J 99: 614–624

109. Wexler BC, McMurty JP (1981) Allopurinol amelioration of the pathophysiology of acute myocardial infarction in rats. Atherosclerosis 39: 71–87

110. Downey JM, Hearse DJ, Yellon DM (1988) The role of xanthine oxidase during myocardial ischaemia in several species including man. J Mol Cell Cardiol 20 (Suppl II): 55–63

111. Johnson JL, Rajagopalan KV, Cohen HJ (1974) Molecular basis of the biological function of molybdenum: effect of tungsten on xanthine oxidase and sulfite oxidase in the rat. J Biol Chem 249: 859–866

112. Johnson JL, Waud WR, Cohen HJ, Rajagopalan KV (1974) Molecular basis of the biological function of molybdenum: molybdenum-free xanthine oxidase from livers of tungstentreated rats. J Biol Chem 249: 5056–5061

113. Parratt JR, Wainwright CL (1987) Failure of allopurinol and a spin-trapping agent N-t-alpha-phenyl nitrone to modify significantly ischaemia and reperfusion-induced arrhythmias. Brit J Pharmacol 91: 49–59

114. Podzuweit J, Braun W, Müller A, Schaper W (1986) Arrhythmias and infarction in the ischemic pig heart are not mediated by xanthine-derived free oxygen radicals. Circulation 74 (Suppl II): II–346

115. Kehrer JP, Piper H, Sies H (1987) Xanthine oxidase is not responsible for reoxygenation injury in isolated-perfused rat heart. Free Rad Res Commun 3: 69–78

116. Coker SJ, Parratt JR, Ledingham IM, Zeitlin IJ (1981) Thromboxane and prostacyclin release from ischaemic myocardium in relation to arrhythmias. Nature 29: 323–324

238

117. Daa UN (1981) Prostaglandins and cardiac arrhythmias – a new concept. IRCS Med Sci BIBR Compend 9: 385–387
118. Hsueh W, Needleman P (1978) Sites of lipase activation and Prostaglandin synthesis in isolated perfused rabbit hearts and hydronephrotic kidneys. Prostaglandins 16: 661–681
119. Demopoulos HB, Flamm ES, Pietronigro DD, Selingman ML (1980) The free radical pathology and the microcirculation in the major central nervous system disorders. Acta Physiol Scand 492 (Suppl): 91–120
120. Hammond B, Kontos HA, Hess ML (1985) Oxygen radicals in the adult respiratory distress syndrome, in myocardial ischaemia and reperfusion injury, and in cerebral vascular damage. Can J Physiol Pharmacol 63: 173–187
121. Kontos HA, Wei EP, Povlishock JT (1983) Cerebral arteriolar damage by arachidonic acid and prostaglandin G_2. Science 209: 156–169
122. Reimersma RA (1982) Myocardial catecholamine release in acute myocardial ischaemia: relationship to cardiac arrhythmias. In: Parratt JR (ed) Early arrhythmias resulting from myocardial ischaemia. London, Macmillan, pp 125–138
123. Schomig A, Dart DM, Dietz R, Mayer E, Kubler W (1984) Release of endogenous catecholamines in the ischaemic myocardium of the rat. Circ Res 55: 689–710
124. Singal PK, Beamish RE, Dhalla NS (1983) Potential oxidative pathways of catecholamines in the formation of lipid peroxides and genesis of heart disease. Adv Exp Med Biol 161: 391–401
125. Julicher R, Sterrenberg L, Koomen J, Bast A, Noordhoek J (1984) Evidence for lipid peroxidation during the calcium paradox in vitamin E-deficient rat heart. Archives of Pharmacology 326: 87–89
126. Ferrari R, Ceconi C, Cargnoni A, Curello S, Ruigrok T: No evidence of oxidative stress during calcium paradox. Basic Res Cardiol, in press
127. Blackwell GJ, Flower RJ (1983) Inhibition of phospholipase. Br Med Bull 39: 260–264
128. Wolf RA, Gross RW (1985) Identification of a neutral phospholipase C which hydrolyzes choline glycerophospholipids and plasmalogen selective phospholipase A_2 in canine myocardium. J Biol Chem 260: 7295–7303
129. Kagan VE, Savov VM, Didenko VV, Arkhypenko Yu V, Meerson FZ (1983) Calcium and lipid peroxidation in mitochondrial and microsomal membranes of the heart. Biull Eksp Biol Med 95: 458–461

The role of leukocytes in ischemic damage, reperfusion injury and repair of the myocardium

KEVIN M. MULLANE[1] and C. WAYNE SMITH[2]

[1] Gensia Pharmaceuticals, Inc., San Diego, California 92121 and [2]Department of Pediatrics, Leukocyte Biology Section, Baylor College of Medicine, Houston, Texas 77054, USA

Introduction

> "It was six men of Indostan
> To learning much inclined.
> Who went to see the Elephant
> (though all of them were blind);
> That each by observation
> Might satisfy his mind."

> John Godfrey Saxe (1816–1887)[1]
> "The Blind Men and the Elephant"

The response to occlusion of a coronary artery in dogs was first described by Chirac in 1698 [2], thereby preceding the clinical recognition of myocardial infarction. Although it is acknowledged that the treatment of any pathologic process can be carried out intelligently and scientifically only when it is based on a thorough understanding of how the lesion develops and resolves, and the speed with which these processes occur [3], almost 300 years later the process and events involved in defining the ultimate extent of myocardial injury remain poorly understood. Yet the histologic changes in acute myocardial infarction develop relatively slowly [4], and have been documented extensively (see references [5–7] for review). Moreover, as ischemic heart disease is a major cause of premature morbidity and mortality in the western world, there have been a multitude of studies on the pathogenesis of myocellular necrosis and how it can be influenced by a variety of different interventions, leading Braunwald [8] to conclude,

> "Just because myocardial tissue lies within the distribution of a recently occluded coronary artery, does not mean that it is necessarily condemned to cell death."

The time for clinically evaluating interventions to reduce infarct size was said to have come [9]. So why is it that despite a wealth of experimental and clinical information, no single therapeutic agent has gained widespread acceptance as an effective treatment for the ischemic heart? Clearly, one reason is

H.M. Piper (ed.) Pathophysiology of severe ischemic myocardial injury, 239–267.

that ischemia-induced myocardial damage represents a complex interplay of multiple events from which it is difficult to define a singular mechanism which can be uniformly targeted. Contributing to this uncertainty are the problems of performing clinical trials in patients with primary myocardial infarction at an early stage, and identifying meaningful end-points to define the therapeutic benefits, other than mortality [10]. Perhaps another reason is that as invesitgators we remain 'blinded' by our preconceived ideas, and interpret and design studies based on concepts proposed 20 to 50 years ago.

The purpose of this chapter is to review the evidence implicating polymorphonuclear leukocytes (PMNs) as one of the determinants of myocardial damage. The perceived role of PMNs in myocardial infarction has evolved from that of a passive respondent to an active contributor to a process whereby the infarct is resolved and repaired [3, 11, 12]. More recently, PMNs have been suggested to exacerbate the damage induced by myocardial ischemia, and mediate some of the deleterious consequences of restoring flow to an ischemic tissue [13–18]. Epidemiologic evidence has proposed circulating PMNs as a major independent risk factor for the initiation of acute myocardial infarction [19–23], the immediate and long-term prognosis after an infarct [24–26], and in predicting the incidence of reinfarction [27, 28]. Perhaps these different components, like the six blind men describing different parts of the elephant [1], each provide a limited perspective of a more complex, interrelated pathophysiologic event, which should not be considered independently.

It is important to recognize also the interactions between events which occur in ischemic injury, which are depicted in a simplified form in Fig. 1. In this scenario, it is the summation of multiple components of injury which then exceed the threshold for irreversibility or cellular destruction. Thus, leukocytes alone may not be responsible for myocellular necrosis, but when coupled with other components of injury, the cumulative effect is overwhelming. This multiple component theory of tissue injury also has been proposed by McCord [29]. Another feature of this model is that elimination of any single component reduces the total level of injury below the threshold of irreversibility. Consequently, a variety of pharmacologic interventions acting upon different mechanisms can result in similar degrees of protection from tissue damage. The residual components may be sufficient to cause functional derangements and/or localized injury.

It is appropriate to define terms 'injury' and 'damage' as they are used in the context of this review. Injury is a general term for loss or impairment, and implies compromise of both functional and structural aspects of the myocardium, including reversible derangements such as the stunned myocardium. Damage is reserved for overt destruction, synonymous with cell lysis and tissue necrosis. The reason for the distinction is that ischemic injury in the clinical setting can be subtle and varied, and may often be manifested as functional derangements without obvious structural counterparts.

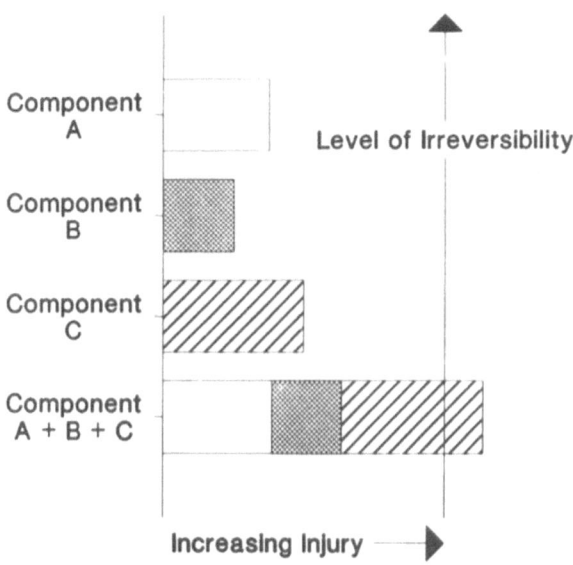

Fig. 1. A diagrammatic representation of multiple components of tissue injury. Three representative components are depicted and the sum of the individual components exceeds the threshold for irreversible damage.

The first blind man: PMN influx is a response to tissue injury

The infiltration of leukocytes into an experimental myocardial infarct was first described by Baumgarten in 1899 [30]. A more elaborate description of the histopathologic changes of myocardial infarction was published by Karsner and Dwyer [31] who observed interstitial edema, congestion and mild hemorrhage occurring within 30 minutes of occluding a coronary artery, with necrosis and PMN infiltration evident after 12 hours. The recognition of PMN infiltration as a hall-mark of acute myocardial infarction in the clinic was provided by the seminal study of autopsy material by Mallory and colleagues [3], who stated:

> As a *result* of the necrosis of muscle, polymorphonuclear leukocytes are attracted and soon begin to infiltrate around and into the necrotic muscle.

PMN infiltration into the damaged tissue was observed within the first 24 hours and increased over the ensuing 4 days, with the authors concluding that tissue necrosis and the influx of PMNs were the most important histopathologic features of acute myocardial infarction in the first week [3].

Subsequent experimental and clinical studies confirmed these observations [32, 33, 4, 10]. However, Sommers and Jennings [4] observed dilation of blood vessels and early margination of PMNs at the periphery of the infarct four hours after occluding the coronary artery of dogs, while Mullane and colleagues [13] reported PMNs, adhesion to the endothelium and trans-endothelial migration in vessels within the ischemic zone after just one hour of ischemia. These studies indicated that PMN activation and accumulation not only commenced much earlier than previously recognized, but occurred while the process of tissue damage was ongoing. In addition, Mallory and colleagues [3] observed that leukocytes rarely penetrate the central core of the infarct, and removal of the necrotic debris at the edges of the infarct did not provoke a secondary influx of PMNs to the inner portion. These observations suggest that the infiltration of neutrophils may not merely be a response to myocellular necrosis.

The second blind man: PMNs contribute to ischemic injury

Evidence implicating the inflammatory response as one determinant of the ultimate extent of myocellular necrosis arose from studies in the mid to late 1970's in which various interventions directed against 'heterolytic' processes were shown to reduce infarct size [34]. The cardioprotection afforded by the glucocorticoids, hydrocortisone or methylprednisolone, was originally attributed to stabilization of lysosomal membranes within the myocardium, thereby preventing the release of hydrolytic enzymes [35–39]. However, the steroid-induced reduction in infarct size was associated with a diminution in the influx of neutrophils, leading to the suggestion that the well-known anti-inflammatory actions of these compounds contributed to their efficacy [40, 41]. Subsequently, the non-steroidal anti-inflammatory drug ibuprofen was also found to limit ischemic damage [42, 43], although this was not a general finding with this class of compound [44].

Hill and Ward [45] proposed a phlogistic role for the complement system in acute myocardial infarction, with the generation of leukotactic complement fragments. Patients suffering a myocardial infarct show consumption of complement components in serum [46] and deposition of the cytolytic terminal C5b-9 complex in infarcted areas at autopsy [47]. Constituents of human heart subcellular (particularly mitochondrial) membranes can activate complement by both classical and alternative pathways [46, 48], while mitochondrial proteins released during ischemia bind human C1q to also trigger the complement cascade [49]. PMNs selectively accumulate at sites of complement activation [50]. Complement depletion with cobra venom factor attenuates the release of chemotactic activity from the ischemic myocardium [51], prevents complement deposition [52] and PMN accumulation [45, 51, 53, 54] in the damaged region, and reduces the size of the necrotic area [52–54]. The apparent association between cobra venom factor induced suppression of both the PMN influx and ischemic injury prompted Hartmann and colleagues [51] to try to evaluate the effect of severe neutropenia on infarct size, but they were unable to maintain neutropenic animals for 24 hours after coronary ligitation.

Consequently, a number of studies were linking pharmacological manipulation of the leukocytes with protection of the ischemic myocardium. By 1977 these observations caused Hillis and Braunwald [55] to conclude,

> All patients with acute infarction, regardless of their hemodynamic state, may benefit from an anti-inflammatory agent, ...

However, there were significant gaps in the studies implicating PMNs as the prime suspect of the inflammatory component of ischemic injury. The evidence could only be regarded as circumstantial at best, being based on 'guilt by association' rather than any direct evidence. One major limitation was the failure to demonstrate PMNs within the ischemic myocardium in a time-frame compatible with the development of tissue damage. There were at least two experimental problems which contributed to this limitation. Attempts to detect the inflammatory response using indium-111-labeled PMNs and non-invasive cardiac imaging [56, 57] were limited by the need for blood pools of radio-activity to subside as the radiolabeled PMNs were cleared, before images of the heart could be taken without interference from blood in the left ventricle. Thus the earliest time point which could be obtained was the 24 hours and was already the time of maximal epicardial PMN accumulation, while the peak of endocardial PMN accumulation occurred at 48 hours [57]. Consequently, these studies could not determine when PMN influx began, although Thakur *et al.* [57] made the important observation that the maximal PMN accumulation occurred in the regions of lowest flow, prompting an association between cell influx and vascular perfusion.

The second limitation to defining the start of PMN sequestration in the ischemic myocardium was related to cell accumulation first occurring at intravascular sites, with attachment to the endothelium, and entrapment within capillaries [13, 16, 58]. The importance of the intravascular PMNs has only recently been appreciated where these cells reduce subendocardial perfusion and may contribute to the progressive vasoconstriction which occurs during ischemia [58–60]. The significance of this observation of intravascular cells is that the presence of PMNs within blood vessels of histological sections of the heart can be easily overlooked. To quantitate accurately this accumulation of leukocytes requires extensive and laborious post-mortem histological analysis [58] or direct 'real-time' imaging of myocardial capillaries, using a microscope linked to a video camera, for example [61]. The application of such techniques has led to the recognition that PMN margination, rolling and attachment occurs within 20 to 60 minutes of ischemia [13, 58, 62–64], which is compatible with the development of tissue injury. The relative importance of intravascular vs. extravascular PMNs in the process of myocardial injury has yet to be defined. The contribution of PMNs to ischemic damage was established further when selective neutropenia with either antiserum or busulfan was demonstrated to decrease infarct size at 6 hours after a permanent occlusion [65]. Moreover, the cardioprotection afforded by ibuprofen or the 5-lipoxygenase inhibitor AA-861 in models of permanent occlusion was attributed to suppression of PMN activation and accumulation [43, 66].

Unfortunately, these observations were made at a time when other experimental and clinical studies indicated that steroidal and non-steroidal anti-inflammatory agents may inhibit the healing of an infarct [67–69], thereby increasing the risk of ventricular rupture or aneurysm [70, 71]. Because this was attributed to interruption of the inflammatory response and the leukocyte-mediated repair process (see following section) there were concerns that inhibition of PMN influx was not a viable target for therapeutic intervention. Moreover, although a variety of pharmacologic agents were demonstrated to reduce infarct size in models of permanent occlusion [34], it was generally agreed that without the restoration of flow these drugs would only delay the ultimate destruction of the tissue [72]. Recognition that the timely restoration of flow will, of itself, limit myocardial damage [73–77] shifted attention to models of ischemia and reperfusion where the further addition of a pharmacologic agent may lead to a sustained reduction in infarct size.

The third blind man: PMNs represent the first stage of a repair process

PMN infiltration is a cardinal feature of all acute inflammatory events [78]. Tissue damage leads to the formation of chemotactic factors which subsequently recruit PMNs to the site of injury [78]. Consequently, it was envisioned that PMN accumulation was the result of myocardial necrosis and represented the first stage of a healing process in which a fibrous scar tissue of great tensile strength is deposited to replace the nonfunctional necrotic tissue [3]. The PMNs are replaced by mononuclear cells which remove the cellular debris, then proliferating fibroblasts deposit the collagen-rich scar tissue.

The concept that the acute inflammatory response may be beneficial to the repair of the infarcted myocardium was supported by clinical observations with glucocorticoids [70, 71]. Reduction of infarct size in experimental animal models by hydrocortisone [35, 38] and methylprednisolone [38] led to their use in patients with acute myocardial injury. However, therapy was associated with an increased incidence of ventricular aneurysm and rupture; effects attributed to inadequate repair of the infarct [70, 71]. Experimental studies confirmed these observations [67–69]. High doses of methylprednisolone, which suppressed the inflammatory response induced by myocardial injury, slowed the removal of damaged myocytes resulting in the necrotic mass becoming surrounded by a fibrous capsule that prevented healing [40], and resulted in ventricular wall thinning [67]. That inhibition of the repair process was linked to the anti-inflammatory effects of the steroids was apparently underscored by the finding that a non-steroidal anti-inflammatory agent which suppressed the PMN influx, ibuprofen [43], also induced ventricular wall thinning [68]. Moreover, leukopenia produced by whole body

Table 1. Lack of a relationship between PMN inhibition and impaired healing of a myocardial infarct.

Agents	PMN suppression	Scar thinning	References
Methylprednisolone (single dose)	No	No	41, 38, 67
Methylprednisolone (multiple dose)	No	Yes	41, 38, 67
Ibuprofen	Yes	Yes	43, 100, 68
Indomethacin	No	Yes	13, 69
Aspirin	No	No	196, 68
Cobra Venom Factor	Yes	No	53, 54, 41
Superoxide Dismutase	Yes	No	197, 198

irradiation reduced collagen degradation, an index of proteolytic cellular digestion, in the infarct zone after 24 hours of coronary occlusion [79]. Thus, various pieces of evidence pointed to the white cells as an important component of myocardial repair.

However, there are at least two counter-arguments to the premise that interrupting the acute inflammatory response prevents resolution of the infarct. Long-term treatment with various drugs can provoke ventricular wall thinning, but this action does not correlate with the drug's ability to either reduce infarct size or inhibit the influx of PMNs (Table 1). Investigating the role of complement fragment C3 as a leukotactic agent in myocardial infarcts, Hill and Ward [45] remarked that:

> The exclusion of these cells (neutrophils) in the inflammatory reaction has not been associated with any obvious defect in the formation of granulation tissue in the infarcted heart. C3-depleted rats seem to lay down a dense fibrous scar in the infarcted tissue in the absence of neutrophils and C3, just as did the control rats.

PMNs are poor phagocytic cells for clearing cellular debris. This is generally regarded as a function of the mononuclear cells which accumulate in the infarcted myocardium after the PMNs [3, 10, 11, 33]. Roberts and co-workers [41] suggested that inhibition of mononuclear cell infiltration, rather than the PMN influx, was associated with wall thinning. Complement depletion with cobra venom factor selectively inhibited PMN accumulation [41, 54] and did not retard the healing process [41]. Chronic use of methylprednisolone suppressed both PMNs and mononuclear cells, and induced wall thinning [38, 41]. A corollary of this observation is that PMN infiltration can be interrupted without detriment, provided that the drug does not impair the chronic inflammatory response typified by the influx of mononuclear cells. Studies indicate that this is feasible by two different mechanisms. Either the PMNs can be selectively targeted [41], or a drug can be administered within a time-frame associated with the PMN influx and then withdrawn to allow for the accumulation of mononuclear cells and the normal repair process to develop. For example, methylprednisolone given for the first 24 hours is as effective as chronic treatment at diminishing myocellular necrosis [38], but does not provoke the wall thinning and ventricular dilatation seen with repeated administration [41].

> The art of medicine consists of amusing the patient
> while Nature cures the disease.
>
> Voltaire (1694–1788)

The fourth blind man: The concept of reperfusion injury

The extent of irreversible damage provoked by an ischemic insult depends upon both its duration and severity. The re-establishment of coronary flow represents the most obvious and straightforward means of limiting the progression of necrosis. A number of studies have shown that the early restoration of flow reduces infarct size when compared to sustained arterial occlusion, and that the benefits decline as the duration of ischemia is prolonged [73–77]. This experimental approach assumed that reperfusion stopped all damage, and that infarct size measurement after several hours of reperfusion merely reflected the extent of damage present at the end of the ischemic period.

However, while the benefits of restoring coronary blood flow are obvious, it is not without hazard [80]. Initially, the histological and morphological changes apparent in the reperfused myocardium – contraction-band necrosis, explosive cell swelling, edema, calcium deposits in mitochondria and the infiltration of PMNs – were thought to occur only within the region already deemed irreversibly injured [4, 81]. However, in recent years it has become recognized that reperfusion may also extend the area of damage [82, 83] and cause necrosis of cells which would be expected to be salvaged by reperfusion. Administration of pharmacologic agents such as BW755C [84], superoxide dismutase (SOD) plus catalase [85], SOD alone [86, 87], fluosol [88] or adenosine [89] at reperfusion results in a significant reduction in infarct size and implies that additional injury must result from reperfusion.

Collateral blood flow is a major determinant of the severity of ischemia resulting in an inverse correlation between infarct size and collateral flow [90]. An extension of this observation has been the understanding that it is the areas of highest collateral blood flow during ischemia (which are just insufficient for maintaining normal tissue viability) which are most readily protected by drugs that act to decrease the oxygen demands or improve the oxygen supply to the myocardium [8, 34]. In contrast, it is the regions with the lowest flow during ischemia which suffer the greatest amount of reperfusion injury, and gain the most from a therapeutic intervention, rather than those marginally compromised [87, 91]. Consequently, infarct size measurements in occlusion-reperfusion models represent ischemic injury plus additional damage elicited by reperfusion. Previous studies demonstrating a reduction in infarct size by reperfusion [73–77] may have overestimated the extent of damage resulting from coronary occlusion, and generally did not take reperfusion injury into consideration.

Reperfusion of the ischemic myocardium promotes a rapid influx of PMNs. Within 5 minutes of reflow the tissue PMN content has increased by 25% [59], and 60 minutes of reperfusion after a 90 minute period of ischemia results in a 5- to 7- fold increase in PMNs in the ischemic region when compared to a non-ischemic portion of the heart [92]. The rate and extent of the PMN accumulation is related to both the duration of the ischemic insult [92] and the length of reperfusion [18, 93, 94]. Longer periods of ischemia apparently increase the *rate* of the leukocyte influx [92], while the actual cell number peaks about 24 to 48 hours after reflow [57, 94]. The increased cellular infiltration after longer periods of ischemia may not simply reflect greater myocellular necrosis because the PMN influx is always greater in the reperfused heart when compared to one which is permanently ischemic [95]. However, in both the ischemia and the ischemia-reperfusion models of injury there is a direct correlation between the PMN influx and infarct size [18, 93, 94].

Evidence that PMNs contribute to myocardial injury and damage during reperfusion

The potential role of PMNs in ischemic reperfusion injury has been studied directly utilizing procedures that deplete animals of circulating leukocytes. Anti-neutrophil antibodies [96–98], and chemicals [13] or filters [60] which produce neutropenia have all been employed. A consistent finding has been that leukopenia is associated with a smaller infarct [13, 96–98] and improved myocardial blood flow [59, 60], although the duration of the ischemic insult may be a critical factor [95–97]. Though these studies generally support a pathogenic role for PMNs, it is difficult to unequivocally exclude the possibility that these experimental treatments influence important behaviors of other cells (e.g. platelets). However, when taken in the context of a broad array of studies, there is considerable evidence implicating PMNs as one component of the injurious processes initiated during reperfusion of ischemic tissues. This evidence can be broadly outlined as follows [18, 99]:

1. PMNs do not normally sequester in the heart, but respond to processes activated during ischemia and reoxygenation that lead to their accumulation [13, 16, 50].
2. PMNs are temporally, regionally, and quantitatively associated with the development of myocardial injury and damage [13, 93, 94].
3. PMNs possess a variety of effector mechanisms potentially deleterious to the heart which have been implicated in other forms of tissue injury [18, 99, 100].

4. Experimental manipulations which either prevent PMN activation or accumulation, or produce profound neutropenia are associated with reduced myocardial damage or injury, even when the pharmacologic agents or experimental maneuvers are affected solely at reperfusion [13, 59, 84, 88, 89, 96–99, 101–109].

Potential mechanisms for PMN accumulation in ischemic/reperfused tissue

The accumulation of inflammatory cells in ischemic-reperfused tissue may be attributed, in part, to the trapping of PMNs in vessels of small diameter [58]. To pass through capillaries the cell must deform. However, the cytoplasmic viscosity of PMNs is about 2000 times that of erythrocytes and when activated, PMNs become adherent, and their deformability decreases further [16]. Both responses work against the cells' movement within capillaries where surface contact with endothelial cells is quite large [16]. In addition to being entrapped in small vessels, PMNs migrate into the ischemic tissue. It is likely that the predominate mechanisms leading to emigration into ischemic tissue are those used by leukocytes to gain entry into other inflamed tissues.

Direct observations of blood vessels during the initiation of inflammation reveal characteristic behaviors of PMNs in veins and post capillary venules. Cells are seen rolling along the vessel wall, adhering to the endothelium and migrating through the vessel wall [110–112]. While much attention has been given to the response of PMNs to soluble chemotactic factors, recent studies *in vitro* have shown that both the PMN and the endothelial cell have the potential to play active roles in the processes of emigration. Stimulation of endothelial cells with thrombin, leukotriene (LT)C_4, LTD$_4$, H$_2$O$_2$, tumor necrosis factor alpha (TNFα), interleukin-1 (IL-1), TNFß and endotoxin result in increased adhesion of unstimulated PMNs to the apical surface of confluent endothelial monolayers [113–121]. Thrombin and H$_2$O$_2$ induce a rapid response that peaks within 20 minutes and is gone within 1 hour. LTC$_4$ and LTD$_4$ also induce a rapid response which exhibits a somewhat more prolonged duration. In contrast, stimulation of endothelial cells with cytokines does not lead to increased adhesion until about 1 hour, while peak adhesion occurs after 4 hours.

The molecular mechanisms involved in PMN-endothelial adhesion are now becoming clearer. Thrombin, LTC$_4$, LTD$_4$, and H$_2$O$_2$ stimulate synthesis of platelet activating factor (PAF) [117, 118, 121]. The newly synthesized PAF remains largely associated with the endothelial cells, and its presence is closely correlated with increased adhesion. A direct role for PAF in the adherence of PMNs is supported by the findings that PMNs desensitized to PAF adhere poorly to the stimulated endothelial cells, and specific PAF antagonists inhibit PMN adhesion to stimulated endothelial cells [117, 118, 120, 121]. While PAF appears to be involved in these short-term responses, the molecules responsible for intercellular attachment have not been identified.

Cytokine stimulation of endothelial cells produces a complex array of events. There is coincident expression of two newly defined molecules at the cell surface, endothelial-leukocyte adhesion molecule-1 (ELAM-1) [122–124] and intercellular adhesion molecule-1 (ICAM-1) [122, 125–127]. Both appear to be involved in the attachment of PMNs. Expression of ELAM-1 is transient, peaking at 4 hours and returning to very low levels by 8 hours. ICAM-1 peaks at 4 hours and continues to be expressed on the cell surface for more than 24 hours. PAF is also synthesized, and while most remains associated with the endothelial cell, a significant portion (20–30%) appears to be released [128]. The relative contributions of these factors to adhesion have been evaluated using monoclonal antibodies or specific PAF antagonists, and experimental protocols correlating expression of these factors with adhesion. The results to date clearly associate ELAM-1 and ICAM-1 with adhesion. The PMN surface determinant which interacts with ELAM-1 has not been defined, while the PMN determinant which interacts with ICAM-1 has been shown to be a leukocyte integrin, CD11a/CD18 (LFA-1) [127, 129]. An adhesive role for PAF following stimulation of the endothelial cells with cytokines is much less clear [130].

In addition, cytokine (TNFα and IL-1) stimulation of endothelial monolayers induces rapid transendothelial migration of adherent PMNs in the absence of exogenously added chemotactic factors [126, 131, 132]. While this phenomenon has not been explained in molecular terms, two observations are of potential importance. Unstimulated PMNs become activated (i.e. their membranes become ruffled, they assume a polarized shape and they begin to migrate) upon contacting the stimulated endothelial cells, and anti-ICAM-1 antibodies markedly inhibit migration [126]. The former observation indicates the presence of a chemotactic stimulus (e.g. PAF), and indeed, stimulated endothelial cells appear to produce more than one chemotactic factor [133–135]. Overall, these studies clearly show that endothelial cells have the potential to play an active role in leukocyte accumulation at sites of inflammation.

PMNs also appear capable of playing an active role in the adhesion process. Chemotactic factors such as C5a, LTB$_4$, PAF and N-formyl-methionyl peptides (e.g. f-Met-Leu-Phe) stimulate increased adhesion to endothelial cells and many non-cellular surfaces [126, 136, 137] and migration across confluent monolayers [138]. Recent studies address the molecular mechanisms involved. Chemotactic stimulation leads to activation of the leukocyte integrin CD11b/CD18 (also called Mo1, Mac-1 or CR3). The nature of this activation is currently not understood but appears to involve both qualitative and quantitative changes in this heterodimer at the cell surface [139–141]. The specific ligands for this integrin have not been defined, but experimental evidence indicates that CD11b/CD18 plays an important role in several chemotactic factor activated adhesive functions *in vitro* involving apparently different ligands – homotypic aggregation [139], adhesion to endothelial cells [115, 116, 120, 127] and some non-cellular surfaces [139], and migration of PMNs across surfaces [139, 142].

The extent to which any of the specific mechanisms leading to PMN-endothelial interactions *in vitro* play a role in the rapid accumulation of PMNs in reperfused myocardium is at present poorly understood. While the stimulants promoting these cellular interactions *in vitro* are likely to be present *in vivo* in reperfused tissue, their relative contribution *in vivo* remains to be determined. Some recent investigations provide potentially important information: a possible role for LTC_4/D_4 in the accumulation of PMNs is open to question. Detection of these leukotrienes has been most clearly obtained in *ex vivo* preparations of rabbit hearts stimulated with the chemotactic factor f-Met-Leu-Phe, 2 days after ischemia/reperfusion, and is correlated with the infiltration of macrophages [18, 143]. This suggests that the formation of these leukotrienes is not temporally associated with the recruitment of PMNs. However, one additional possible source which would put the formation and release of LTC_4/D_4 within the appropriate time frame are the cardiac mast cells which react to reoxygenation of isolated perfused hearts [144].

A possible role for H_2O_2 in the activation of PMN-endothelial cell adhesion is strengthened by several observations. PMNs [145] and vascular endothelial cells [146–148] *in vitro* appear to produce oxygen radicals upon reoxygenation. PMNs adherent to endothelial cells *in vitro* produce massive quantities of H_2O_2 when stimulated with chemotactic [149]. Oxygen-derived free radicals are generated in myocardial tissue when oxgen is restored to that tissue. This has been directly demonstrated by electron paramagnetic resonance spectroscopy [150–151]. Release occurs within the first few seconds of reperfusing an isolated, buffer-perfused heart after 10 to 30 minutes of ischemia, with micromolar quantities of free radicals produced. The potential for oxygen-derived free radicals to stimulate endothelial cells *in vivo* for increased adhesion [121] is clearly present, but this action remains to be determined. However, ischemia and reperfusion clearly evoke changes in endothelial function [183], including impaired relaxations, or even contractions, of epicardial coronary arteries *ex vivo* to agents which release endothelium-derived relaxing factor, including thrombin [154], acetylcholine [155], bradykinin [44], ergonovine [155], or the addition of platelets [156].

Chemotactic factors are also found in reperfused heart tissue (e.g. lipoxygenase products) [17, 18]. Immunoreactive LTB_4 was found to be generated by hypoxic rabbit myocardial tissue [157], and was assumed to be responsible for the accumulation of leukocytes in the ischemic tissue since two inhibitors of lipoxygenase, nordihydroguaiaretic acid and diethylcarbamazine, inhibited accumulation in isolated perfused hearts. Sasaki *et al.* [66] also found increased LTB_4 levels in ischemic myocardium *ex vivo* that preceded the accumulation of PMNs. Several lipoxygenase inhibitors, BW755C, nafazatrom, REV-5901 and AA-861, have been reported to reduce myocardial necrosis *in vivo*, an effect attributed to the suppression of PMN activation and/or accumulation [13, 84, 102, 103, 108]. While these pharmacologic studies may support the view that LTB$_4$ or other lipoxygenase metabolites amplify reperfusion injury by the recruitment of PMNs, the anti-oxidant properties of most of these agents make interpretation uncertain. Complement activation may generate C5a [49, 50]. C5a appears to be capable of directly activating granulocytes within the coronary circulation resulting in the accumulation of granulocytes within these vessels, and is associated with a reduction in coronary blood flow [158]. Another potential source of chemotactic activity was suggested by the finding of superoxide-dependent activation of PMN chemotactic activity in plasma [159]. The observation that oxygen-derived free radicals are generated upon reperfusion of ischemic myocardium suggests the potential for superoxide-dependent activation of chemotactic activity in ischemic/reperfused myocardium.

The leukocyte integrins (CD 18 family of glycoproteins) appear to be involved in reperfusion damage of the myocardium. A monoclonal antibody (60.3) against the common beta subunit of the leukocyte integrins reduces PMN accumulation in rabbit hearts following a 30 min occlusion and a 3 hr reperfusion [160]. Of interest in this study was the fact that antibody was applied to the ^{111}In-labeled PMNs *in vitro* [160]. Another monoclonal antibody (R3.3) against the common beta subunit was found to reduce infarct size after 5 hours of reperfusion in an ischemia/reperfusion model in rabbits when administered systemically 15 minutes before a 1 hour occlusion of the coronary artery [161]. A possible role for CD11b/CD18 had been addressed using a monoclonal antibody reactive with the alpha subunit of CD11b/CD18 in a canine ischemia/reperfusion model [162]. Systemic administration reduced infarct size with a 90 minute occlusion and up to 72 hours of reperfusion [163]. The prolonged protection of the myocardium occurred in the face of persistent normal blood PMN counts, and seems to indicate that this antibody did not simply delay reperfusion injury [164]. Persistent severe neutropenia appears to produce the same effect [165]. Additionally, accumulation of leukocytes or tissue damage has been found in other reperfusion models to involve the CD18 family of glycoproteins. In one model, hemorrhagic shock [166], rabbits subjected to a 1 hour shock exhibited a 29% survival rate after 5 days. In contrast, survival was 100% in animals treated with monoclonal antibody 60.3, and organ injury associated with hypovolemic shock was markedly reduced. The multiple organ injury and death in this model in both rabbits and rats [167] appears to be linked to PMN adhesion possibly leading to capillary obstruction. In another model, feline intestinal ischemia/reperfusion [168], neutropenia induced by anti-neutrophil antiserum significantly reduced the microvascular permeability observed during reperfusion. Monoclonal antibody 60.3, which markedly reduces the adherence of feline PMNs *in vitro*, also significantly reduced the microvascular permeability during reperfusion without altering the number of circulating PMNs.

Potential mechanisms for PMN-mediated injury in ischemic/reperfused myocardium

Once present in the reperfused tissue, the mechanisms by which PMNs contribute to tissue injury and damage appear to involve mechanical obstruction and specific secretory products [15–18, 99]. The failure of blood flow to be fully restored upon reperfusion and the impaired coronary reserve have been attributed in part to microvascular plugging by leukocytes [58, 169]. Though flow may be initially restored to all regions of the post-ischemic myocardium, some areas subsequently become blocked and prevent further perfusion [170]. This no-reflow phenomenon is observed principally after periods of ischemia sufficient to produce myocyte necrosis. Blockade of three or more adjacent capillaries can result in local ischemia thereby preventing potential salvage of affected myocytes [171].

The determinants controlling production and release of specific PMN secretory products are poorly understood. While chemotactic factors may play an important role in recruitment of PMNs to the ischemic tissue, the concentrations required to induce secretory responses *in vitro* are much higher than those required to induce cell adhesion or locomotion. Many early studies of effector mechanisms *in vitro* have utilized very high concentrations of agonists, non-physiologic stimulants (e.g. ionophores PMA) or non-physiologic accessory molecules (e.g. cytochalasin B). As a result the relationship of the phenomenon observed *in vitro* to cellular behaviors *in vivo* may be quite distant [17, 18]. More recent investigations of possible synergism between stimuli have brought the study of factors influencing PMN responses into a potentially physiologic context [17, 18]. Chemotactic factors alone are ineffectual stimulants of the respiratory burst and associated release of oxygen radicals, the release of granule contents, or the synthesis and release of lipid mediators (e.g. PAF or LTB_4). However, certain combinations of stimuli result in markedly heightened secretory responses to chemotactic stimulation. Some examples will illustrate this point. PMNs would appear to be a major source of LTB_4 and 20-OH LTB_4 as indicated by the large amounts of these mediators released *in vitro* upon stimulation with calcium ionophore. However, while the machinery to generate these products is clearly within the PMN, little is known about physiologic regulation of leukotriene synthesis. Chemotactic stimulation does not lead to measurable leukotriene generation from endogenous arachidonic acid (AA) although it leads to transient conversion of exogenous AA into leukotrienes. A 'priming' step appears to be required which apparently regulates necessary phospholipase(s) not activated by the chemotactic stimulus alone. This priming can be accomplished by granulocyte/macrophage colony-stimulating factor (GM-CSF) or endotoxin [172, 173]. A second example involves H_2O_2 production by stimulated (f-Met-Leu-Phe, TNFα, GM-CSF, G-CSF) PMNs. These stimuli alone are ineffectual. However, PMNs adherent to laminin or serum-coated plastic, or monolayers of endothelial cells produce H_2O_2 at a level near that of cells stimulated with PMA [149, 174]. Another example involves PMN-mediated injury to endothelial cells *in vitro* [175]. Neutrophils adherent to endothelial cells produce minimal injury even after stimulation with chemotactic factors (e.g. f-Met-Leu-Phe or C5a). In contrast, if adherent cells are primed by initial incubation with endotoxin, chemotactic stimulation results in substantial injury to the endothelium, a result apparently linked to the release of neutrophil elastase [175].

Another attractive hypothetical mechanism of PMN-mediated tissue injury involves an interaction between PMN-derived chlorinated oxidants and metalloproteinases. Enzymes such as collagenase and gelatinase are released from PMNs in latent forms and activated by HOCl or HOCl-derived products such as the N-chloroamines [176]. Moreover, tissues are generally shielded from the injurious effects of neutrophil elastase by an α_1-proteinase inhibitor present in plasma, but this inhibitor is inactivated by a metalloproteinase derived from the PMN which also requires chlorinated oxidants for expression of activity [177]. Thus, Weiss and his colleagues [176–178] have proposed that PMNs can transform the short-acting and relatively non-specific effects of oxygen metabolites into long-acting and relatively specific effects through oxidant-mediated regulation of endogenous proteolytic activity.

Overall, the factors controlling synthesis and release of potentially cytotoxic products from PMNs appear to be quite complex, precluding a direct assumption that events observed *in vitro* are of pathogenic significance *in vivo*. Direct investigations utilizing procedures to deplete animals of circulating leukocytes have supported the view that PMNs play a pathogenic role in reperfusion injury. The specific mechanisms remain to be identified.

The fifth blind man: Leukocytes provoke the onset of myocardial injury

Epidemiologic studies have shown a positive correlation between the circulating leukocyte count and the incidence of myocardial infarction [19–20]. The data from over 30,000 patients suggests that the incidence of myocardial infarction is ~2 to 4 times greater in patients with a peripheral white blood cell count of > 9 to 10,000/μl, when compared to subjects with a leukocyte count of < 4 to 6,000/μl [20, 22], with PMN counts showing the strongest association [22]. Apparently, Yemenite Jews, who are naturally leukopenic, rarely suffer an infarct [21]. In the Multiple Risk Factor Intervention Trial (MRFIT), the white blood cell count was predictive of non-fatal myocardial infarction and sudden cardiac death [27]. A reduction in circulating leukocytes during the trial was associated with a decrease in the risk of cardiac death, where a decrement of 1,000 WBC per μl lowered the risk by 14%, independent of other cardiac risk factors.

The circulating white cell count may not be predictive only of the incidence of myocardial infarction, but also the prognosis. Patients suffering an infarct had a four-fold greater risk of death within two months [24] and a five-fold increased incidence of ventricular fibrillation in the first 24 hours after admission to a hospital [25] if the leukocyte count exceeded 15,000/μl. Of 272 patients with a myocardial infarct, the 68 who died within twelve months had a significantly higher white cell count than the 204 survivors [26]. Moreover, while the short-term prognosis is poor in patients with myocardial infarction and elevated circulating leukocytes, the incidence of a recurrent infarction also correlated strongly with the total number of white cells [27, 28]. Patients with a count greater than 9000/μl had a 3.5-fold greater chance of reinfarction [28].

Clearly, such epidemiologic studies do not imply a causal relationship between the leukocytosis and myocardial infarction. The white cells could merely reflect other ongoing events which may be unrecognized, such as a viral infection or chronic inflammation, which could contribute to the risk of an ischemic event [179]. Alternatively, the leukocytes could play a role in the pathogenesis of myocardial infarction [180]. This could be due to exacerbation of a transient and relatively benign ischemic event into a larger readily apparent infarction by the variety of mechanisms already outlined, in particular, by interfering with coronary perfusion because of their physiodynamic properties [16, 180]. Moreover, PMN function is enhanced in patients with ischemic heart disease, as indicated by marked pseudopod formation, spontaneous clumping, increased chemotactic activity and LTB_4 generation [181]. Alternatively, the leukocytes could contribute to the development of atherosclerosis. The white blood cell count is predictive of the prevalence and severity of coronary artery disease [182, 183, 23], and rupture of an atherosclerotic plaque in a major coronary artery is a major initiating event for a myocardial infarct.

Finally, circulating leukocyte counts are increased by tobacco smoking [184–186, 20], a high cholesterol diet [187] or stress [180]. An increase in leukocyte counts or cell activation may represent a common mechanism for these cardiac risk factors. It is highly unlikely that autopsy studies would identify increased leukocytes as a causal feature of myocardial infarction. The leukocytes have rarely been quantitated, so no 'standard' exists. Leukocyte influx and efflux (or removal by mononuclear cells) is a dynamic process dependent upon the age of the infarct, and intravascular leukocytes which might provoke the onset of ischemia could be missed because the pathologist would expect to observe PMNs within the vessels. Differences in cell number within a vessel are probably not obvious and difficult to quantitate without laborious and specific procedures combined with simultaneous assessments of perfusion defects.

The sixth blind man: Dogmas, trends and bandwagons

Enthusiasm for the concept of 'anti-ischemic' drugs declined with the recognition that without reflow, drugs will only delay an inevitable process of necrosis, and do not reduce ultimate infarct size [72]; while the advent of thrombolytic therapy heralded a means to restore blood flow and alleviate the cellular damage [188]. Although the concept of reperfusion injury preceded the widespread use of thrombolytic agents [82, 83], the subsequent enthusiasm for reperfusion injury has rekindled interest in adjunctive pharmacological therapy to limit further the myocardial damage. Like most worthwhile ideas, it is provocative and controversial, and this has spawned some elegant and innovative studies. A role for PMNs in reperfusion injury is attractive because it is, perhaps, easier to envision PMNs gaining access to the injured myocardium with reflow. However, neutrophil-mediated tissue damage is *not* synonymous with reperfusion injury, and few studies have attempted to differentiate the extent to which the injurious processes of reperfusion differ from those responsible for ischemic damage. The first studies to link interruption of the inflammatory response with myocardial protection using agents such as cobra venom factor [53, 51], serine protease inhibitors like aprotinin [51, 189], steroidal and non-steroidal anti-inflammatory drugs [35, 38, 42], or allopurinol [190, 36], utilized permanent occlusion of a coronary artery to produce the infarct. Many of these studies which sought to interrupt the inflammatory response have been repeated in settings of occlusion-reperfusion because these models are currently in vogue, but with similar results and conclusions to those derived from models of permanent occlusion. It has been argued that PMNs cannot gain access to the ischemic myocardium; however, histological and biochemical studies demonstrate PMNs at the periphery of the infarct, an ideal location to extend the area of damage [3, 4, 92, 93].

Table 2 compares the results of various anti-inflammatory therapies in models of permanent or temporary coronary artery occlusion. Although drugs were frequently administered prior to temporary occlusion such that it is not possible to clearly differentiate effects on the ischemic or reflow periods, there is remarkable consistency in the results obtained. The benefits of these interventions during the occlusive phase or in the post-ischemic period should now be distinguished. Moreover, we should not be too dogmatic in ascribing the protective actions of these chemically diverse agents to their 'anti-inflammatory' or 'anti-leukocyte' properties until the mechanisms of leukocyte recruitment and induction of tissue injury are defined, and suppression of these events is related to the therapeutic intervention. Many anti-inflammatory drugs which suppress PMN activation are also antioxidants and may attenuate injury mediated by reactive oxygen metabolites [44, 99].

The ability of interventions directed against the leukocytes to reduce myocardial damage associated with either permanent occlusion or temporary ischemia does not imply that reperfusion injury does not occur. Functional derangements such as myocardial stunning [191–193] and the no-reflow phenomenon [194], and autopsy studies of contraction band necrosis of successfully revascularized areas in patients subjected to by-pass graft surgery [195] combined with the efficacy of drugs given at the time of reperfusion in

Table 2. Reduction in infarct size (IS) in models of permanent occlusion or ischemia-reperfusion.

Agent	Permanent occlusion IS	Temporary occlusion IS	References
Ibuprofen	↓	↓	42, 43, 101, 199
Nafazatrom	↓	↓	102, 200, 201
PGI$_2$/Iloprost	↓	↓	106, 107, 202–204
AA-861	↓	↓	66, 108
Corticosteriods	↓	→	35, 67, 13, 205
Neutrophil depletion	↓	↓	65, 96–98
Thromboxane synthase Inhibitors/receptor			196, 206–211
Antagonists	↓	↓	
Indomethacin	→/↑	→	13, 212
Aspirin	→	→	196, 213
Perfluorochemical	↓	↓	88, 208, 214
Allopurinol	↓	↓	36, 190, 215, 216

↓ = Decrease ↑ = Increase → = No change

reducing experimental infarct size [84–89] clearly demonstrate that some aspects of myocardial injury proceed beyond the period of ischemia. However, failure to recognize the contribution of neutrophils to *ischemic* injury may limit our understanding of mechanisms involved in neutrophil recruitment and tissue damage, and the time-course of these events, thereby preventing appropriate focus on viable targets for therapeutic intervention, perhaps prophylactically in patients with ischemic heart disease.

> And so these men of Indostan
>   Disputed loud and long,
> Each in his own opinion
>   Exceeding stiff and strong,
> Though each was partly in the right
>   And all were in the wrong!
>
> Moral
>
> So oft in theologic wars,
>   The disputants, I ween,
> Rail on in utter ignorance
>   Of what each of other mean,
> And prate about an Elephant
>   Not one of them has seen! [1]

Acknowledgements

The excellent seretarial assistance of Ms. Carmella P. Laspina is gratefully acknowledged.

References

1. Saxe JG (1985) 'The blind man and the elephant'. In: Oxford Book of Children's Verse in America pp 82–83
2. Chirac P (1698) De motu cordis. Adversaria Analytica, p 121
3. Mallory GK, White PD, Salcedo-Salgar J (1939) The speed of healing of myocardial infarction. A study of the pathologic anatomy in seventy-two cases. Am Heart J 18: 647–671
4. Sommers HM, Jennings RB (1964) Experimental acute myocardial infarction. Histologic and histochemical studies of early myocardial infarcts induced by temporary or permanent occlusion of a coronary artery. Lab Invest 13: 1491–1503
5. Jennings RB, and Ganote CE (1974) Structural changes in myocardium during acute ischemia. Circ Res 34–35 (Suppl. III): III–156–III–172
6. Jennings RB, Ganote CE and Reimer KA (1975) Ischemic tissue injury. Am J Pathol 81: 179–198
7. Jennings RB and Reimer KA (1981) Lethal myocardial ischemic injury. Am J Pathol 102: 241–255
8. Braunwald E (1974) Reduction of myocardial infarct size. N Engl J Med 291: 525–526
9. Braunwald E and Maroko PR (1974) The reduction of infarct size – an idea whose time (for testing) has come. Circulation 50: 206–209
10. Oliver M (1984) Has the study of infarct size limitation done any good? In: DJ Hearse and DM Yellon (eds) Therapeutic Approaches to Myocardial Infarct Size Limitation. Raven Press, NY, pp xiii–xvi
11. Fishbein MC, Maclean D and Maroko PR (1973). The histopathologic evolution of myocardial infarction. Chest 73: 843–849
12. McClusky ER, Corr PB, Lee BI, Saffitz JE and Needleman P (1982) The arachidonic acid metabolic capacity of canine myocardium is increased during healing of acute myocardial infarction. Circ Res 51: 743–750
13. Mullane KM, Read N, Salmon JA and Moncada S (1984) Role of leukocytes in acute myocardial infarction in anesthetized dogs: Relationship to myocardial salvage by anti-inflammatory drugs. J Pharmacol Exp Ther 228: 510–522
14. Lucchesi BR, Romson JL and Jolly SR (1984) Do leukocytes influence infarct size? In: DJ Hearse and DM Yellon (eds) Therapeutic Approaches to Myocardial Infarct Size Limitation. Raven Press, NY, pp 219–248
15. Lucchesi BR, and Mullane KM (1986) Leukocytes and ischemia-induced myocardial injury. Ann Rev Pharmacol Toxicol. 26: 201–224
16. Schmid-Schonbein GW and Engler RL (1986) Granulocytes as active participants in acute myocardial ischemia and infarction. Am J Cardiovasc Pathol 1: 15–30
17. Mullane KM (1988) Myocardial ischemia-reperfusion injury: Role of neutrophils and neutrophil derived mediators. In: G Marone, LM Lichtenstein, M Condorelli, AS Fauci (eds) Human Inflammatory Disease. Clinical Immunology vol 1. BC Decker Inc, Philadelphia PA, pp 143–159
18. Mullane KM, Westlin W and Kraemer R (1988) Activated neutrophils release mediators that may contribute to myocardial injury and dysfunction associated with ischemia and reperfusion. In: R Levi and RD Krell (eds) Biology of the Leukotrienes vol 524. Ann NY Acad Sci, pp 103–121
19. Friedman GD, Klatsky AL and Siegelaub AB (1974) The leukocyte count as a predictor of myocardial infarction. New Eng J Med 290: 1275–1278
20. Zalokar JB, Richard JL and Claude JR (1981) Leukocyte count, smoking, and myocardial infarction. N Eng J Med 304: 465–468
21. Shoenfeld PJ and Pinkhas J (1981) Leukopenia and low incidence of myocardial infarction. New Eng J Med 304: 1606
22. Prentice RL, Shimizu Y, Lin CH, Peterson AV, Kato H, Mason MW and Szatrowski TP (1982) Leukocyte counts and coronary heart disease in a Japanese cohort. Am J Epidemiol 116: 496–506

23. Grimm RH, Neaton JD and Ludwig W (1985) Prognostic importance of the white blood cell count for coronary, cancer and all-cause mortality. J Am Med Assoc 254: 1932–1937

24. Cole DR, Singian EB and Kate LN (1954) The long-term prognosis following myocardial infarction and some factors which affect it. Circulation 9: 321–334

25. Maisel AS, Gilpin A, LeWinter M, Henning H, Ross J Jr and Engler R (1985) Initial leukocyte count during acute myocardial infarction independently predicts early ventricular fibrillation. Circulation 72 (Suppl III): III414

26. Haines AP, Howarth D, North WR, Goldenbog E, Meade TW, Raftery EB and Millar CMW (1983) Haemostatic variables and the outcome of myocardial infarction. Thromb Haemost 50: 800–803

27. Schlant RC, Forman S, Stamler J and Lanner PL (1982) The natural history of coronary heart disease: Prognostic factors after recovery from myocardial infarction in 2789 men. Circulation 66: 401–414.

28. Lowe GDO, Machado SG, Krol WF, Barton BA and Fobres CD (1985) White blood cell count and hematocrit as predictors of coronary recurrence after myocardial infarction. Thromb Haemost 54: 700–703

29. McCord JM (1988) Free radicals and myocardial ischemia: Overview and outlook. Free Radical Biol Med 4: 9–14

30. Baumgarten W (1899) Infarction in the heart. Am J Physiol II: 245–265

31. Karsner HT and Dwyer JE Jr (1916) Studies in infarction IV: Experimental bland infarction of the myocardium, myocardial regeneration and cicatrization. J Med Res 76: 21–39

32. Lodge-Patch I (1951) The aging of cardiac infarcts and its influence on cardiac rupture. Br Heart J 13

33. Bing RJ, Castellanos A, Gradel E, Lupton C and Siegel A (1956) Experimental myocardial infarction: Circulatory biochemical and pathologic changes. Am J Med Sci 232: 533–554

34. Braunwald E and Maroko PR (1978) Limitation of infarct size. Current Problems Cardiol 3: 1–51

35. Libby P, Maroko PR, Bloor CM, Sobel BE and Braunwald E (1973) Reduction of experimental myocardial infarct size by corticosteroid administration. J Clin Invest 52: 599–607

36. Shatney CH, Mac Carter DJ and Lillehei RC (1976) Effects of allopurinol, propranolol and methylprednisolone on infarct size in experimental myocardial infarction. Am J Cardiol 37: 572–580

37. Fox AC, Hoffstein S and Weissmann G (1976) Lysosomal mechanisms in production of tissue damage during myocardial ischemia and the effects of treatment with steroids. Am Heart J 91: 394–397

38. Maclean D, Fishbein MC, Braunwald E and Maroko PR (1978) Long-term preservation of ischemic myocardium after experimental coronary artery occlusion. J Clin Invest 61: 541–551

39. Decker RS, Poole AR, Dingle JT and Wildenthal K (1978) Influence of methylprednisolone on the sequential redistribution of cathepsin D and other lysosomal enzymes during myocardial ischemia in rabbits. J Clin Invest 62: 797–804

40. Kloner RA, Fishbein MC, Lew H, Maroko PR and Braunwald E (1978) Mummification of the infarcted myocardium by high dose corticosteroids. Circulation 57: 56–63

41. Roberts CS, Maclean D, Maroko P and Kloner RA (1985) Relation of early mononuclear and polymorphonuclear cell infiltration to late scar thickness after experimentally induced myocardial infarction in the rat. Basic Res Cardiol 80: 202–209.

42. Lefer AM and Polansky EW (1979) Beneficial effects of ibuprofen in acute myocardial ischemia. Cardiology 64: 265–279

43. Flynn PJ, Becker WK, Vercellotti GM, Weisdorf DJ, Craddock PR, Hammerschmidt DE, Lillehei RC and Jacobs HS (1984) Ibuprofen inhibits granulocyte responses to inflammatory mediators: A proposed mechanism for reduction of experimental myocardial infarct size. Inflammation 8: 33–44

44. Mullane KM, Salmon JA, Kraemer R (1987) Leukocyte-derived metabolites of arachidonic acid in ischemia-induced myocardial injury. Fed Proc 46: 2422–2433

45. Hill JH and Ward PA (1971)   The phlogistic role of C3 leukotactic fragments in myocardial infarcts of rats. J Exp Med 133: 885–900
46. Pinckard RN, Olson MS, Giclas PC, Terry R, Boyer JT and O'Rourke A (1975)   Consumption of classical complement components by heart subcellular membranes in vitro and in patients after acute myocardial infarction. J Clin Invest 56: 740–750
47. Schafer H, Mathey D, Hugo F and Bhakdi S (1986)   Deposition of the terminal C5b-9 complement complex in infarcted areas of human myocardium. J Immunol 137: 1945–1949
48. Giclas PC, Pinckard RN and Olson MS (1979)   In vitro activation of complement by isolated human heart subcellular membranes. J Immunol 122: 146–151
49. Rossen RD, Michael LH, Kagiyama A, Savage HE, Hanson G, Reisberg MA, Moake JN, Kim SH, Self D, Weakley S, Giannini E and Entman ML (1988) Mechanism of complement activation after coronary artery occlusion: Evidence that myocardial ischemia in dogs causes release of constituents of myocardial subcellular origin that complex with human C1q in vivo. Circ Res 62: 572–584
50. Rossen RD, Swain JL, Michael LH, Weakley S, Giannini E and Entman ML (1985) Selective accumulation of the first component of complement and leukocytes in ischemic canine heart muscle. A possible initiator of an extra myocardial mechanism of ischemic injury. Circ Res 57: 119–130
51. Hartmann JR, Robinson JA and Gunnar RM (1977)   Chemotactic activity in the coronary sinus after experimental myocardial infarction: Effects ot pharmacologic interventions on ischemic injury. Am J Cardiol 40: 550–555
52. Pinckard RN, .O'Rourke RA, Crawford MH, Grover FS, McManus LM, Ghidoni JL, Storrs SB and Olson MS (1980) Complement localization and mediation of ischemic injury in baboon myocardium. J Clin Invest 66: 1050–1056
53. Maroko PR, Carpenter CB, Chiariello M, Fishbein MC, Radvany P, Knostman JD and Hale SL (1978) Reduction by cobra venom factor of myocardial necrosis after coronary artery occlusion. J Clin Invest 61: 661–670
54. Crawford MH, Grover FL, Kolb WP, McMahan CA, O'Rourke RA, McManus LM and Pinckard RN (1988) Complement and neutrophil activation in the pathogenesis of ischemic myocardial injury. Circulation 78: 1449–1458
55. Hillis LD and Braunwald E (1977)   Myocardial Ischemia. New Engl J Med 296: 1093–1096
56. Weiss ES, Ahmed SA, Thakur ML, Welch MJ, Coleman RE and Sobel BE (1977)   Imaging of the inflammatory response in ischemic canine myocardial with [111]indium-labeled leukocytes. Am J Cardiol 40: 195–199
57. Thakur ML, Gottschalk A, Zaret BL (1979)   Imaging experimental myocardial infarction with indium-111-labeled autologous leukocytes: Effects of infarct age and residual regional myocardial blood flow. Circulation 60: 297–305
58. Engler RL, Schmid-Schonbein GW and Pavelec RS (1983)   Leukocyte capillary plugging in myocardial ischemia and reperfusion in the dog. Am J Pathol 111: 98–111
59. Engler RL, Dahlgren MD, Peterson MA, Dobbs A and Schmid-Schonbein GW (1986) Accumulation of polymorphonuclear leukocytes during 3-h experimental myocardial ischemia. Am J Physiol 251: H93–H100
60. Engler RL, Dahlgren MD, Morris DD, Peterson MA and Schmid-Schonbein GW (1986) Role of leukocytes in response to acute myocardial ischemia and reflow in dogs. Am J Physiol 251: H314–H322
61. McDonagh PF, Niven AT and Roberts D (1984)   Direct visualization of the coronary microcirculation for pharmacologic and physiologic studies. Microvasc Res 28: 180–196
62. Tillmanns H and Kubler W (1984)   What happens in the microcirculation? In: DJ Hearse and DM Yellon (eds) Therapeutic Approaches to Myocardial Infarct Size Limitation. Raven Press, NY, pp. 107–124
63. McDonagh PF and Larsen JB (1985)   Myocardial ischemia-reperfusion, with or without leukocytes, causes a decrease in coronary microvascular perfusion. Circulation 72 (Suppl III): III 65

64. Reynolds JM, Weidow MJ, Rauzzino MJ and McDonagh PF (1988) Early in reperfusion after ischemia leukocytes not platelets exacerbate the no-reflow phenomenon and increase coronary resistance. FASEB J 2: A1684

65. Ksiezycka E, Hastie R. Maroko PR (1983) Reduction in myocardial damage after experimental coronary artery occlusion by two techniques which deplete neutrophils. Circulation 68 (Suppl III): 111–185

66. Sasaki K, Ueno A, Katori M and Kikawada R (1988) Detection of leukotrine B_4 in cardiac tissue and its role in infarct extension through leukocyte migration. Cardiovasc Res 22: 142–148

67. Hammerman H. Kloner RA, Hale S, Schoen FJ, Braunwald E (1983) Dose-dependent effects of short-time methylprednisolone on myocardial infarct exent, scar formation and ventricular function. Circulation 68: 446–452

68. Brown EJ Jr, Kloner RA, Schoen FJ, Hammerman H, Hale S and Braunwald E (1983) Scar thinning due to ibuprofen administration after experimental myocardial infarction. Am J Cardiol 5: 877–883

69. Hammerman H, Kloner RA, Schoen FJ, Brown EJ Jr, Hale S and Braunwald E (1983) Indomethacin-induced scar thinning after experimental myocardial infarction. Circulation 67: 1290–1295

70. Bulkley BH and Roberts WC (1974) Steroid therapy during acute myocardial infarction – a cause of delayed healing and of ventricular aneurysm. Am J Med 56: 244–250

71. Roberts R, Demello V and Sobel BE (1976) Deleterious effects of methylprednisolone in patients with myocardial infarction. Circulation 53 (Suppl I): I–204–I–207

72. Hearse DJ (1988) The protection of the ischemic myocardium: Surgical success vs. clinical failure? Prog Cardiovasc Dis 30: 381–402

73. Ginks WR, Sybers HD, Maroko PR, Covell JW, Sobel BE and Ross J Jr (1972) Coronary artery reperfusion. II. Reduction of myocardial infarct size at 1 week after the coronary occlusion. J Clin Invest 51: 2717–2723

74. Costantini C, Corday E, Lang T-W, Meerbaum S, Brasch J, Kaplan L, Rubins S, Gold H and Osher J (1975) Revascularization after 3 hours of coronary arterial occlusion: Effects on regional cardiac metabolic function and infarct size. Am J Cardiol 36: 368–384

75. Mathur VS, Guinn GA and Burris WH III (1975) Maximal revascularization (reperfusion) in intact conscious dogs after 2 to 5 hours of coronary occlusion. Am J Cardiol 36: 252–261

76. Baughma KL, Maroko PR and Vatner SF (1981) Effects of coronary artery reperfusion on myocardial infarct size and survival in conscious dogs. Circulation 63: 317–323

77. Murdock RH Jr, Chu A, Grubb M and Cobb FR (1985) Effects of reestablishing blood flow on extent of myocardial infarction in conscious dogs. Am J Physiol 249: H783–H791

78. Weissmann G, Zurier RB and Hoffstein S (1973) Leukocytes as secretory organs of inflammation. Agents Actions 3: 270–279

79. Cannon RO III, Butany JW, McManus BM, Speir E, Kravits AB, Bolli R and Ferrans VJ (1983) Early degradation of collagen after acute myocardial infarction in the rat. Am J Cardiol 52: 390–395

80. Braunwald E and Kloner RA (1985) Myocardial reperfusion: A double-edged sword? J Clin Invest 76: 1713–1719

81. Corday E and Meerbaum S (1983) Symposium on the present status of reperfusion of the acutely ischemic myocardium. Part 1. J Am Coll Cardiol 1: 1031–1036

82. Hearse DJ, Humphrey SM, Nayler WG, Slade A and Border D (1975) Ultrastructural damage associated with reoxygenation of the anoxic myocardium. J Mol Cell Cardiol 7: 315–324

83. Hearse DJ (1977) Reperfusion of the ischemic myocardium. J Mol Cell Cardiol 9: 605–616

84. Mullane KM and Moncada S (1982) The salvage of ischaemic myocardium by BW755C in anaesthetised dogs. Prostaglandins 24: 255–266

85. Jolly SR, Kane WJ, Bailie MB, Abrams GD and Lucchesi BR (1984) Canine myocardial reperfusion injury. Its reduction by the combined administration of superoxide dismutase and catalase. Circ Res 54: 277–285

86. Werns SW, Shea MJ, Driscoll EM, Cohen D, Abrams GD, Pitt B and Lucchesi BR (1985) The independent effects of oxygen radical scavengers on canine infarct size. Reduction by superoxide dismutase but not catalase. Circ Res 56: 895–898

87. Ambrosio G, Becker LC, Hutchins GM, Weisman HF and Weisfeldt ML (1986) Reduction in experimental infarct size by recombinant human superoxide dismutase: Insights into the pathophysiology of reperfusion injury. Circulation 74: 1424–1433

88. Forman MB, Bingham S, Kopelman HA, Wehr C, Sandler MP, Kolodgie F, Vaughan WK, Friesinger GC and Virmani R (1985) Reduction of infarct size with intracoronary perfluorochemical in a canine preparation of reperfusion. Circulation 71: 1060–1068

89. Olafsson B, Forman MB, Puett DW, Pou A, Cates CU, Friesinger GC and Virmani R (1987) Reduction of reperfusion injury in the canine preparation by intracoronary adenosine: Importance of the endothelium and the no-reflow phenomenon. Circulation 76: 1135–1145

90. Reimer KA, Jennings RB, Cobb FR, Murdock RH, Greenfield JC Jr, Becker LC, Bulkley BH, Hutchins GM, Schwartz RP, Bailey KR and Passamani ER (1985) Animal models for protecting ischemic myocardium: Results of the NHLBI cooperative study. Comparison of unconscious and conscious dog models. Circ Res 56: 651–665

91. Bolli R, Patel BS, Jeroudi MO, Lai EK and McCay PB (1988) Demonstration of free radical generation in 'stunned' myocardium of intact dogs with the use of the spin trap α-phenyl N-tert-butyl nitrone. J Clin Invest 82: 476–485

92. Go LO, Murry CE, Richard VJ, Weischedel GR, Jennings RB and Reimer KA (1988) Myocardial neutrophil accumulation during reperfusion after reversible or irreversible ischemic injury. Am J Physiol 255: H1188–H1198

93. Mullane KM, Kraemer R and Smith B (1985) Myeloperoxidase activity as a quantitative assessment of neutrophil infiltration into ischemic myocardium. J Pharmacol Methods 14: 157–167

94. Smith EF III, Egan JW, Bugelski PJ, Hillegass LM, Hill DE and Griswold DE (1988) Temporal relation between neutrophil accumulation and myocardial reperfusion injury. Am J Physiol 255: H1060–1068

95. Chatelain P, Latour J-G, Tran D, de Lorgeril M, Dupras G and Bourassa M (1987) Neutrophil accumulation in experimental myocardial infarcts: Relation with extent of injury and effect of reperfusion. Circulation 75: 1083–1090

96. Romson JL, Hook BG, Kunkel SL, Abrams GD, Schork A and Lucchesi BR (1983) Reduction of the extent of ischemic myocardial injury by neutrophil depletion in the dog. Circulation 67: 1061–1023

97. Jolly SR, Kane WJ, Hook BG, Abrams GD, Kunkel SL and Lucchesi BR (1986) Reduction of myocardial infarct size by neutrophil depletion: Effect of duration of occlusion. Am Heart J 112: 682–690

98. de Lorgeril M, Basmadjian A, Lavallee M, Clement R, Millette D, Rousseau G and Latour J-G (1989) Influence of leukopenia on collateral flow, reperfusion flow, reflow ventricular fibrillation, and infarct size in dogs. Am Heart J 117: 523–532

99. Mullane KM (1989) Oxygen-derived free radicals and reperfusion injury of the heart. In: E Sonnenblick, JH Laragh and M Lesch (eds) New Frontiers in Cardiovascular Therapy: focus on angiotensia converting enzyme inhibition. pp 234–270, Excerpta Medica, Princeton

100. Fantone JC and Ward PA (1982) Role of oxygen-derived free radicals and metabolites in leukocyte-dependent inflammatory reactions. Am J Pathol 107: 397–418

101. Romson JL, Hook BG, Rigot VH, Schork MA, Swanson DP and Lucchesi BR (1982) The effect of ibuprofen on accumulation of indium-111-labeled platelets and leukocytes in experimental myocardial infarction. Circulation 66: 1002–1011

102. Bednar M, Smith B, Pinto A and Mullane KM (1985) Nafazatrom-induced salvage of ischemic myocardium in anesthetized dogs is mediated through inhibition of neutrophil function. Circ Res 57: 131–141

103. Mullane K, Hatala M, Kraemer R, Sessa W and Westlin W (1987) Myocardial salvage induced by Rev-5901: an inhibitor and antagonist of the leukotrienes. J Cardiovasc Pharmacol 10: 398–406

104. Jolly SR and Lucchesi BR (1983) Effect of BW755C in an occlusion-reperfusion model of

ischemic myocardial injury. Am Heart J 106: 8–13

105. Klein HH, Pich S, Bohle RM, Lindert S, Nebendahl K, Buchwald A, Schuff-Werner P and Kreuzer H (1988) Antiinflammatory agent BW775C in ischemic reperfused porcine hearts. J Cardiovasc Pharmacol 12: 338–344

106. Simpson PJ, Mitsos SE, Ventura A, Gallagher KP, Fantone JC, Abrams GD, Schork MA and Lucchesi BR (1987) Prostacyclin protects ischemic reperfused myocardium in the dog by inhibition of neutrophil activation. Am Heart J 113: 129–137

107. Simpson PJ, Mickelson J, Fantone JC, Gallagher KP and Lucchesi BR (1987) Iloprost inhibits neutrophil function in vitro and in vivo and limits experimental infarct size in canine heart. Circ Res 60: 666–673

108. Toki Y, Hieda N, Torii T, Hashimoto H, Ito T, Ogawa K and Satake Y (1988) The effects of lipoxygenase inhibitor and peptidoleukotriene antagonist on myocardial injury in a canine coronary occlusion-reperfusion model. Prostaglandins 35: 555–571

109. Bajaj AK, Cobb MA, Virmani R, Gay JC, Light RT and Forman MB (1989) Limitation of myocardial reperfusion injury by intravenous perfluorochemicals: Role of neutrophil activation. Circulation 79: 645–656

110. Atherton A and Born GVR (1973) Relationship between the velocity of rolling granulocytes and that of the blood flow in venules. J Physiol 233: 157–165

111. House SD and Lipowsky HH (1987) Leukocyte-endothelium adhesion: microhemodynamics in mesentery of the cat. Microvasc Res 34: 363–379

112. Sekizuka E, Benoit JM, Grisham MB and Granger DN (1989) Dimethylsulfoxide prevents chemoattractant-induced leukocyte adherence. Am J Physiol 256: H594–H597

113. Harlan JM, Killen PD, Senecal FM, Schwartz BR, Yee EK, Taylor RF, Beatty PG, Price TH and Ochs HD (1985) The role of neutrophil membrane glycoprotein GP-150 in neutrophil adherence to endothelium in vitro. Blood 66: 167–178

114. Bevilacqua MP, Pober JS, Wheeler ME, Cotran RS and Gimbrone MA Jr (1985) Interleukin 1 acts on cultured human vascular endothelium to increase the adhesion of polymorphonuclear leukocytes, monocytes, and related leukocyte cell lines. J Clin Invest 76: 2003–2011

115. Gamble JR, Harlan JM, Klebnoff SJ and Vades MA (1985) Stimulation of the adherence of neutrophils to umbilical vein endothelium by human recombinant tumor necrosis factor. Proc Natl Acad Sci USA 82: 8667–8674

116. Pohlman TH, Stanness KA, Beatty PG, Ochs HD and Harlan JM (1986) An endothelial cell surface factor(s) induced in vitro by lipopolysaccharide, interleukin 1, and tumor necrosis factor-α increases neutrophil adherence by a CDw18-dependent mechanism. J Immunol 136: 4548–4553

117. Zimmerman GA, McIntyre, TM and Prescott SM (1986) Thrombin stimulates neutrophil adherence by an endothelial cell-dependent mechanism: characterization of the response and relationship to platelet-activating factor synthesis. Ann NY Acad Sci 485: 349–367

118. McIntyre TM, Zimmerman GA and Prescott SM (1986) Leukotrienes C_4 and D_4 stimulate human endothelial cells to synthesize platelet-activating factor and bind neutrophils. Proc Natl Acad Sci USA 83: 2204–2208

119. Pober JS, Lapierre LA, Stolpen AH, Brock TA, Springer TA, Fiers W, Bevilacqua MP, Mendrick DL and Gimbrone MA Jr (1987) Activation of cultured human endothelial cells by recombinant lymphotoxin: comparison with tumor necrosis factor and interleukin 1 species. J Immunol 138: 3319–3324

120. Zimmerman GA and McIntyre TM (1986) Neutrophil adherence to human endothelium in vitro occurs by CDw18 (Mol, MAC-1-/LFA-1/GP150, 95) glycoprotein-dependent mechanisms. J Clin Invest 81: 531–537

121. Lewis MS, Whatley RE, Cain P, McIntyre TM, Prescott SM and Zimmerman GA (1988) Hydrogen peroxide stimulates the synthesis of platelet-activiting factor by endothelium and induces endothelial cell-depedent neutrophil adhesion. J Clin Invest 82: 2045–2055

122. Pober JS, Gimbrone MA, Lapierre LA. Mendrick DL, Fiers W, Rothlein R and Springer TA (1986) Activation of human endothelium by lymphokines: overlapping patterns of anti-

genic modulation by interleukin 1, tumor necrosis factor and immune interferon. J Immunol 137: 1893–1896

123. Bevilacqua MP, Pober JS, Mendrick DL, Cotran RS and Gimbrone MA Jr (1987) Identification of an inducible endothelial-leukocyte adhesion molecule. Proc Natl Acad Sci USA 84: 9238–9242

124. Bevilacqua MP, Stengelin S, Gimbrone MA Jr, Seed B (1989) Endothelial leukocyte adhesion molecule. 1: An inducible receptor for neutrophils related to complement regulatory proteins and lectins. Science 243: 1160–1165

125. Rothlein R, Dustin ML, Marlin SD and Springer TA (1986) An intercellular adhesion molecule (ICAM-1) distinct from LFA-1. J Immunol 137: 1270–1275

126. Smith CW, Rothlein R, Hughes BJ, Mariscalco MM, Rudloff HE, Schmalstieg FC and Anderson DC (1988) Recognition of an endothelial determinant for CD18-dependent human neutrophil adherence and transendothelial migration. J Clin Invest 82: 1746–1756

127. Smith CW, Marlin SD, Rothlein R. Toman C and Anderson DC (1989) Cooperative interactions of LFA-1 and Mac-1 with ICAM-1 in facilitating adherence and transendothelial migration of human neutrophils in vitro,J Clin Invest 83: 2008–2017

128. Bussolino F, Camussi G and Baglioni C (1988) Synthesis and release of platelet-activating factor by human vascular endothelial cells treated with tumor necrosis factor or interleukin 1a*. J Biol Chem 263: 11856–11861

129. Marlin SD and Springer TA (1987) Purified intercellular adhesion molecule-1 (ICAM-1) is a ligand for lymphocyte function-associated angiten-1 (LFA-1). Cell 51: 813–819

130. Breviario F, Bertocchi F, Dejana E and Bussolino F (1988) IL-1-induced adhesion of polymorphonuclear leukocytes to cultured human endothelial cells: Role of platelet-activating factor. J Immunol 141: 3391–3397

131. Furie MB and McHugh DD (1987) Stimulation of neutrophil transendothelial migration by interleukin-1. J Cell Biol 105: 276A

132. Moser R, Schleiffenbaum B, Groscurth P and Fehr J (1989) Interleukin 1 and tumor necrosis factor stimulate human vascular endothelial cells to promote transendothelial neutrophil passage. J Clin Invest 83: 1–12

133. O'Brien RF, Seton MP, Makarski JS, Center DM and Rounds S (1984) Thiourea causes endothelial cells in tissue culture to produce neutrophil chemoattractant activity. Am Rev Respir Dis 130: 103–109

134. Mercandetti AJ, Lane TA and Colmerauer MEM (1984) Cultured human endothelial cells elaborate neutrophil chemoattractants. J Lab Clin Med 104: 370–377

135. Gudewicz PW, Odekon LE, DelVecchio PJ and Saba TM (1988) Generation of neutrophil chemotactic activity by phorbol ester-stimulated calf pulmonary artery endothelial cells. J Leukocyte Biol 440: 1–7

136. Gimbrone MA Jr, Brock AF and Schafer AI (1984) Leukotriene B_4 stimulates polymorphonuclear leukocyte adhesion to cultured vascular endothelial cells. J Clin Invest 74: 1552–1555

137. Tonnesen MG, Anderson DC, Springer TA, Knedler A, Avdi N and Henson PM (1989) Adherence of neutrophils to cultured human microvascular endothelial cells: stimulation by chemotactic peptides and lipid mediators and dependence upon the Mac-1, LFA-1, p 150, 95 glycoprotein family. J Clin Invest 83: 637–646

138. Furie MB, Naprstek BL and Silverstein SC (1987) Migration of neutrophils across monolayers of cultured microvascular endothelial cells. J Cell Sci 88: 161–175

139. Anderson DC, Miller LJ, Schmalstieg FC, Rothlein R and Springer TA (1986) Contributions of the Mac-1 glycoprotein family to adherence-dependent granulocyte functions: structure-function assessments employing subunit-specific monoclonal antibodies. J Immunol 137: 15–27

140. Detmers PA, Wright SD, Olsen E, Kimball B and Cohen ZA (1987) Aggregation of complement receptors on human neutrophils in the absence of ligand. J Cell Biol 105: 1137–1145

141. Altiere DC and Edgington TS (1988) The saturable high affinity association of Factor X to

ADP-stimulated monocytes defines a novel function of the Mac-1 receptor. J Biol Chem 263: 7007–7015

142. Schmalstieg FC, Rudolff HE, Hillman GR and Anderson DC (1986) Two dimensional and three dimensional movement of human polymorphonuclear leukocytes: two fundamentally different mechanisms of locomotion. J Leukocyte Biol 40: 677–708

143. Freed MS, Needleman P, Dunkel CG, Saffitz JE and Evers AS (1989) Role of invading leukocytes in enhanced atrial eicosanoid production following rabbit left ventricular myocardial infarction. J Clin Invest 83: 205–212

144. Keller AM, Clancy RM, Barr ML, Marboe CC and Cannon PJ (1988) Acute reoxygenation injury in the isolated rat heart: Role of resident cardiac mast cells. Circ Res 63: 1044–1052

145. Hallet MB, Shandall A and Young HL (1985) Mechanism of protection against 'reperfusion injury' by aprotinin. Roles of polymorphonuclear leukocytes and oxygen radicals. Biochem Pharmacol 34: 1757–1761

146. Ratych RE, Chuknyiska RS and Bulkley GB (1987) The primary localization of free radical generation after anoxia/reoxygenation in isolated endothelial cells. Surgery 102: 122–131

147. Zweier JL, Kuppusamy P and Lutty GA (1988) Measurement of endothelial cell free radical generation: evidence for a central mechanism of free radical injury in postischemic tissues. Proc Natl Acad Sci USA 85: 4050–4060

148. Schinetti ML, Sbarbati R and Scarlattini M (1989) Superoxide production by human umbilical vein endothelial cells in an anoxia-reoxygenation model. Cardiovasc Res 23: 76–80

149. Nathan CF (1987) Neutrophil activation on biological surfaces: massive secretion of hydrogen peroxide in response to products of macrophages and lymphocytes. J Clin Invest 80: 1550–1560

150. Zweier JL, Flaherty JT and Weisfeldt ML (1987) Direct measurement of free radical generation following reperfusion of ischemic myocardium. Proc Natl Acad Sci USA 84: 1404–1407

151. Zweier JL (1988) Measurement of superoxide-derived free radicals in the reperfused heart. J Biol Chem 263: 1353–1357

152. Arroyo CM, Kramer JH, Dickens BF and Weglicki WB (1987) Identification of free radicals in myocardial ischemia/reperfusion by spin trapping with nitrone DMPO. Fed Eur Biochem Soc 221: 101–104

153. Forman MB, Puett DW and Virmani R (1989) Endothelial and myocardial injury during ischemia and reperfusion: pathogenesis and therapeutic implications. J Am Coll Cardiol 13: 450–459

154. Ku DD (1982) Coronary vascular reactivity after acute myocardial ischemia. Science 218: 576–578

155. VanBenthuysen KM, McMurtry IF and Horwitz LD (1987) Reperfusion after acute coronary occlusion in dogs impairs endothelium-dependent relaxation to acetylcholine and augments contractile reactivity in vitro. J Clin Invest 79: 265–274

156. VanBenthuysen KM, Ashmore RC, Dauber IM, McMurtry IF and Horwitz LD (1988) Contractile hyperreactivity to aggregating platelets following ischemia and reperfusion. Clin Res 36: 325A

157. Gillespie MN, Kojima S, Owasoyo JO, Tai HH and Jay M (1987) Hypoxia provokes leukotriene-dependent neutrophil sequestration in perfused rabbit hearts. J Pharmacol Exp Ther 241: 812–816

158. Martin SE, Chenoweth DE, Engler RL, Roth DM and Longhurst JC (1988) C5a decreases regional coronary blood flow and myocardial function in pigs: implications for a granulocyte mechanism. Circ Res 63: 483–491

159. Petrone WF, English DK, Wong K and McCord JM (1980) Free radicals and inflammation: Superoxide-dependent activation of a neutrophil chemotactic factor in plasma. Proc Natl Acad Sci USA 77: 1159–1163

160. Williams FM, Collins PD, Nourshargh S and Williams TJ (1988) Suppression of ^{111}In-neutrophil accumulation in rabbit myocardium by MoAb 60.3 following ischemic injury. J Mol Cell Cardiol 20: S33

161. Seewaldt-Becker E, Rothlein R and Dammgen JW (1989) CDw18 dependent adhesion of leukocytes to endothelium and its relevance for cardiac reperfusion. In: TA Springer, DC Anderson, R Rothlein and AS Rosenthal (eds) Structure and Function of Molecules Involved in Leukocyte Adhesion. Srpinger-Verlag, NY

162. Simpson PJ, Todd RF III, Fantone JC, Mickelson JK, Griffin JD and Lucchesi BR (1988) Reduction of experimental canine myocardial reperfusion injury by a monoclonal antibody (anti-Mol, antiCD11b) that inhibits leukocyte adhesion. J Clin Invest 81: 624–629

163. Simpson PJ, Todd RF, Mickelson JK, Fantone JC, Gallagher KP, Tamura Y, Lee KA, Kitzen JM and Lucchei BR (1988) Sustained limitation of myocardial reperfusion injury by a monoclonal antibody that inhibits leukocyte adhesion. FASEB J 2: A1237

164. Todd RF III, Simpson PJ and Lucchesi BR (1989) The anti-inflammatory properties of monoclonal anti-Mol (CD11B/CD18) antibodies *in vitro* and *in vivo*. In: TA Springer, DC Anderson, R Rothlein and AS Rosenthal (eds) Structure and Function of Molecules Involved in Leukocyte Adhesion. Srpinger-Verlag, NY

165. Simpson PJ, Fantone JC, Mickelson JK, Gallagher KP and Lucchesi BR (1988) Identification of a time window for therapy to reduce experimental canine myocardial injury: Suppression of neutrophil activation during 72 hours of reperfusion. Circ Res 63: 1070–1079

166. Veder NB, Winn RK, Rice CL, Chi EY, Arfors KE and Harlan JM (1988) A monoclonal antibody to adherence-promoting leukocyte glycoprotein, CD18, reduces organ injury and improves survival from hemorrhagic shock and resuscitation in rabbits. J Clin Invest 81: 939–944

167. Barroso-Aranda J, Schmid-Schonbein GW, Zweifach BW and Engler RL (1988) Granulocytes and no-reflow phenomenon in irreversible hemorrhagic shock. Circ Res 63: 437–447

168. Hernandez LA, Grisham MB, Twohig B, Arfors KE, Harlan JM and Granger DN (1987) Role of neutrophils in ischemia-reperfusion-induced microvascular injury. Am J Physiol 238: H699–H703

169. Nichols WW, Mehta JL, Donnelly WH, Lawson D, Thompson L and ter Riet M (1988) Reduction in coronary vasodilator reserve following coronary occlusion and reperfusion in anesthetized dog: Role of endothelium-derived relaxing factor, myocardial neutrophil infiltration and prostaglandins. J Mol Cell Cardiol 20: 943–954

170. Ambrosio G, Weisman HF and Becker LC (1986) The 'no-reflow' phenomenon: A misnomer? Circulation 74 (Suppl II): II–260

171. Honig CR and Odoroff CL (1981) Calculated dispersion of capillary transit times: significance for oxygen exchange. Am J Physiol 240: H199–H208

172. Dahinden CA, Zingg J, Maly FE and Deweck AL (1988) Leukotriene production in human neutrophils primed by recombinant human granulocyte/macrophage colony-stimulating factor and stimulated with the complement component $c5$ and fmlp as second signals. J Exp Med 167: 1281–1295

173. Doerfler ME, Danner RL, Shelhamer JH and Parrillo JE (1989) Bacterial lipopolysaccharides prime human neutrophils for enhanced production of leukotriene B4. J Clin Invest 83: 970–977

174. Nathan CF (1989) Respiratory burst in adherent human neutrophils: triggering by colony-stimulating factors CSF-GM and CSF-G. Blood 73: 301–306

175. Smedley LA, Tonnesen MG, Sandhaus RA, Haslett C, Guthrie LA, Johnston RB Jr, Henson PM and Worthen GS (1986) Neutrophil-mediated injury to endothelial cells. Enhancement by endotoxin and essential role of neutrophil elastase. J Clin Invest 77: 1233–1243

176. Weiss SJ and Peppin GJ (1986) Collagenolytic metallo-enzymes of the human neutrophil. Characteristics, regulation and potential function *in vivo*. Biochem Pharmacol 35: 3189–3197

177. Desrochers PE and Weiss SJ (1988) Proteolytic inactivation of alpha-1-proteinase inhibitor by a neutrophil metalloproteinase. J Clin Invest 81: 1646–1650

178. Weiss SJ (1989) Tissue destruction by neutrophils. New Engl J Med 320: 365–376

179. Spodick DH (1985) Inflammation and the onset of myocardial infarction. Ann Intern Med 102: 699–702

180. Ernst E, Hammerschmidt DE, Bagge U, Matrai A and Dormandy JA (1987) Leukocytes

and the risk of ischemic diseases. JAMA 257: 2318–2324

181. Mehta J, Dinerman J, Mehta P, Saldeen TGP, Lawson D, Donnelly WH and Wallin R (1989) Neutrophil function in ischemic heart disease. Circulation 79: 549–556

182. Kostis JB, Turkevich D, Sharp J (1984) Association between leukocyte count and the presence and extent of coronary atherosclerosis as determined by coronary angiography. A J Cardiol 53: 997–999

183. Yarnell JWG, Sweetnam PM, Elwood PC, Eastham R, Gilmour RA, O'Brien JR and Ehterington MD (1985) Haemostatic factors and ischaemic heart disease: The Caerphilly study. Br Heart J 53: 483–487.

184. Howell RW (1970) Smoking habits and laboratory tests. Lancet 2: 152

185. Corre F, Lellouch J and Schwartz D (1971) Smoking and leukocyte counts. Lancet 2: 632–634

186. Banks DC (1971) Smoking and leukocytes counts. Lancet 2: 815

187. Feldman DL, Mogelesky TM, Liptak BF and Gerrity RG (1988) Leukocytes in cholesterol-fed rabbits. FASEB J 2: A1172

188. Braunwald E (1987) The path to myocardial salvage by thrombolytic therapy. Circulation 76 (Suppl II): II–2–II–7

189. Diaz PE, Fishbein MC, Davis MA, Askenazi J and Maroko PR (1977) Effect of the kallikrein inhibitor aprotinin on myocardial ischemic injury after coronary occlusion in the dog. Am J Cardiol 40: 541–549

190. DeWall RA, Vasko KA, Stanley EL and Kezdi P (1971) Responses of the ischemic myocardium to allopurinol. Am Heart J 82: 362–370

191. Heyndrickx GR, Millard RW, McRitchie RJ, Maroko PR and Vatner SF (1975) Regional myocardial functional and electrophysiological alterations after brief coronary artery occlusion in conscious dogs. J Clin Invest 56: 978–985

192. Weiner JM, Apstein CS, Arthur JH, Pirzada FA and Hood WB Jr (1976) Persistence of myocardial injury following brief periods of coronary occlusion. Cardiovasc Res 10: 678–686

193. Braunwald E and Kloner RA (1982) The stunned myocardium: Prolonged, postischemic ventricular dysfunction. Circulation 66: 1146–1149

194. Kloner RA, Ganote CE and Jennings RB (1974) The 'no-reflow' phenomenon after temporary coronary occlusion in the dog. J Clin Invest 54: 1496–1508

195. Bulkley BH and Hutchins GM (1977) Myocardial consequences of coronary artery bypass graft surgery: The paradox of necrosis in areas of revascularization. Circulation 56: 906–913

196. Mullane KM and Fornabaio D (1988) Thromboxane synthetase inhibitors reduce infarct size by a platelet-dependent, aspirin-sensitive mechanism. Circ Res 62: 668–678

197. Werns SW, Simpson PJ, Mickelson JK, Shea MJ, Pitt J and Lucchesi BR (1988) Sustained limitation by superoxide dismutase of canine myocardial injury due to regional ischemia followed by reperfusion. J Cardiovasc Pharmacol 11: 36–44

198. Werns SW, Shea MJ, Vaporciyan A, Phan S, Abrams GD, Buda AJ, Pitt B and Lucchesi BR (1987) Superoxide dismutase does not cause scar thinning after myocardial infarction. J Am Coll Cardiol 9: 898–902

199. Jugdutt BI, Hutchins GM, Bulkly BG and Becker LC (1980) Salvage of ischemic myocardium by ibuprofen during infarction in the conscious dog. Am J Cardiol 46: 74–82

200. Fiedler VB (1984) Reduction of acute myocardial ischemia in rabbit hearts by nafazatrom. J Cardiovasc Pharmacol 6: 318–324

201. Shea MJ, Murtagh JJ, Jolly SR, Abrams GD, Pitt B and Lucchesi BR (1984) Beneficial effects of nafazatrom on ischemic reperfused myocardium. Eur J Pharmacol 102: 63–70

202. Ribeiro LTG, Brandon TA, Hopkins DG, Reduto LA, Taylor AA and Miller RR (1981) Prostacyclin in experimental myocardial ischemia: Effects on hemodynamics, regional myocardial blood flow, infarct size and mortality. Am J Cardiol 17: 835–840

203. Lefer AM, Ogletree MC, Smith JB, Silver MJ, Nicolaou KC, Barnette WE and Gasic GP (1978) Prostacyclin: A potentially valuable agent for preserving myocardial tissue in acute myocardial ischemia. Science 200: 52–54

204. Schror K, Ohlendorf R, Darius H (1981) Beneficial effects of a new carbacyclin derivative, ZK36374, in acute myocardial ischemia. J Pharmacol Exp Ther 219: 243–249
205. Vogel WM, Zannori VG, Abrams GD and Lucchesi BR (1977) Inability of methylprednisoline sodium succinate to decrease infarct size or preserve enzyme activity measured 24 hrs after coronary occlusion in the dog. Circulation 55: 588–595
206. Wargovich TJ, Mehta J, Nichols WW, Ward MB, Lawson D, Franzini D and Conti CR (1987) Reduction in myocardial neutrophil accumulation and infarct size following administration of thromoboxane inhibitor U-63, 557A. Am Heart J 114: 1078–1085
207. Grover GJ and Schumacher WA (1989) Effect of the thromboxane A_2 receptor antagonist SQ 30,741 on ultimate myocardial infarct size, reperfusion injury and coronary flow reserve. J Pharmacol Exp Ther 248: 484–491
208. Smith EF III, Lefer AM and Smith JB (1980) Influence of thromboxane inhibition on the severity of myocardial ischemia in cats. Can J Physiol Pharmacol 15: 294–300
209. Brezinski ME, Yangisawa A and Lefer AM (1987) Cardio-protective actions of specific thromboxane receptor antagonists in acute myocardial ischemia. Eur J Pharmacol 9: 65–71
210. Burke SE, Dicola G and Lefer AM (1983) Protection of ischemic cat myocardium by CGS 13080, a selective inhibition. J Cardiovasc Pharmacol 5: 842–847
211. Egan JW, Griswold DE, Hillegass LM and Smith EF III (1988) Reduction of ischemic damage and polymorphonuclear leukocyte infiltration in myocardium following coronary artery occlusion and reperfusion by the thromboxane receptor antagonist BM 13,505. FASEB 2: A919
212. Jugdutt BI, Hutchins GM, Bulkley BH, Pitt B and Becker LC (1979) . Effect of indomethacin on collateral blood flow and infarct size in the conscious dog. Circulation 59: 734–743
213. Bonow RO, Lipson LC, Sheehan LC, Capurro NL, Isner JM, Roberts WC, Goldstein RE and Epstein SC (1981) Lack of effect of aspirin on myocardial infarct size in the dog. Am J Cardiol 47: 258–264
214. Glogar DH, Kloner RA, Muller J, DeBoer LVW, Braunwald E and Clark LC (1981) Fluorocarbons reduce myocardial ischemic damage after coronary occlusion. Science 211: 1439
215. Akizuki S, Yoshida S, Chambers DE, Eddy L, Parmley L, Yellon DM and Downey JM (1985) Infarct size limitation by the xanthine oxidase inhibitor, allopurinol, in closed check dogs with small infarcts. Cardiovasc Res 19: 686–692
216. Werns SW, Shea MJ, Mitsos SE, Dysko RC, Fantone JC, Schork A, Abrams GD, Pitt B and Lucchesi BR (1986) Reduction of the size of infarction by allopurinol in the ischemic-reperfused canine heart. Circulation 73: 518–524

Problems associated with reperfusion of ischemic myocardium

WOLFGANG SCHAPER and JUTTA SCHAPER

Max-Planck-Institute for Physiological and Clinical Research, Department of Experimental Cardiology, Bad Nauheim, FRG

Summary

We have analyzed the evidence for the existence of reperfusion injury and found it inconclusive. Experimental therapeutic studies designed to change the outcome of reperfusion either remain contradictory (SOD ibuprofen) or lack a biochemical basis (no xanthine oxidase in the hearts of humans, pigs and rabbits).

Our own studies emphasize the beneficial effects of reperfusion. The only universally accepted sign of reperfusion injury (fully reversible when treated, easy to prevent by gentle reperfusion) is ventricular fibrillation.

Introduction

Around 1970, when the danger of coronary heart disease became known to its full extent and when no pathophysiologically based treatment was in sight, the NIH decided to invite and fund projects dedicated to the experimental therapy of ischemic myocardium in experimental animals [1]. Alongside these efforts, projects were set up to develop better quantitative diagnostic methods and research aiming at a better understanding of processes leading to cell death. Although these efforts initially concentrated more on the ischemic myocardium than on the diseased coronary arteries, many interesting therapeutic principles were established, notably the treatment with beta-blockers and calcium-antagonists.

An important development of that early phase in the battle against myocardial infarction was the precise measurement of the size of an infarct in relation to the area at risk of infarction [2–4]. This was the basis on which the efficacy of interventions aimed at reduction of infarct size (or better: aimed at preventing ischemic myocardium from becoming completely infarcted) could be judged.

The establishment of objective and more precise methods of measuring infarct size also exerted a sobering effect: many of the previously tested and

H.M. Piper (ed.) Pathophysiology of severe ischemic myocardial injury, 269–280.
© *1990 Kluwer Academic Publishers, Dordrecht –*

apparently active drugs or principles were found to be inactive [5] with one notable exception: reperfusion of ischemic myocardium.

This was, however, only valid if carried out within a time window that could be shifted by variations in MVO_2 [6] and by the level of existing residual perfusion (i.e. collateral flow).

The discovery that ischemic damage and the effects of reperfusion are time dependent [7, 8] became the pathophysiological basis for the important second stage in the battle against infarction:

Reperfusion of the human myocardium by thrombolytic agents

The clinical practice of intracoronary or intravenous thrombolysis and its results have proved that the promise of the pathophysiological concept is correct: the best results were achieved by those groups which reached the patient soon after the onset of symptoms and where treatment started during or even before transport to hospital [9].

However, most clinicians have had unexplained and unexpected failures of thrombolytic therapy in that the occluded blood vessel became patent but the myocardium could not be resuscitated. Based on the personal experience of therapy failure, the newly developed concept of reperfusion damage may have become more credible. Coupled with the evidence (strong or otherwise) of reperfusion injury in experimental animals and in isolated hearts was the desire to treat it and several principles are awaiting clinical testing within the context of post-thrombolytic reperfusion. The intention is to minimize reperfusion damage which might be expected during reflow following thrombolysis by giving the experimental drug together with the thrombolytic compound.

Possible mechanisms of reperfusion injury

Definition of reperfusion injury

1. The classical definition.

Before reperfusion injury became an issue, reperfusion itself was the discriminator between life and death in experiments dealing with questions of whether ischemic damage was reversible or irreversible. In our own experiments [6] and in those of Reimer and Jennings [2], short coronary occlusions of up to 20 minutes when followed by reperfusion did not lead to lasting structural damage and reperfusion was beneficial. With occlusions lasting 40–45 minutes, subendocardial necrosis developed upon reperfusion. Depending on the availability of collateral flow (i.e. in the dog but not in pigs, rats and rabbits, potentially present – but not always-in man) present even longer occlusions (90 minutes, 3 hours and more) can be tolerated without large infarctions (dogs when MVO_2 was low) but usually infarcts become transmural and maximal in the pigs or with high MVO_2 or in the absence of collateral flow.

Because of this clear relationship between the time progression of the ischemic damage and the reverse relationship between the decreasing benefit of reperfusion with time, the classical definition stated that irreversible ischemic damage is assumed when the myocardial structure did not recover on reperfusion.

The damage visible on reperfusion was believed to be the damage inflicted by ischemia – not by reperfusion.

Although reasonably straightforward and based on factual evidence, this definition had a few weak points:

a. The criteria of judging whether a cell is still living or is already dead are sometimes not as discriminatory as they might be. Sometimes the criteria are arbitrarily chosen (such as 'critical' ATP-levels).

b. When reperfusion comes too late, reperfused tissue does indeed look worse than non-reperfused tissue: the edema, tissue bleeding and general tissue destruction are visible with the naked eye. When coming closer to the point-of-no-return these changes become less severe, but an uncertainty remains as to whether severely but sublethally damaged myocytes may not have been pushed over the brink by reperfusion.

c. It cannot be denied that reperfusion causes severe and potentially lethal changes in myocytes that are only mildly injured: reperfusion under the full arterial pressure following a period of only 15 minutes of ischemia usually causes ventricular fibrillation. This can be completely avoided by reperfusion over a pressure-flow-limiting stenosis or at pressure lower than the full arterial pressure.

2. Present definition.

The prevailing view in today's literature is that reperfusion is regarded as a double-edged sword: while it clearly has potentially beneficial actions it may also have damaging effects, especially if administered relatively late. The hypothesis here is that myocytes that might still be viable at the end of the ischemic period might enter an irreversible state of damage when reperfused. The difficulty with this hypothesis is that it is almost untestable: with reperfusion the myocyte might die from reperfusion damage, without reperfusion it certainly dies from ischemia, i.e. cell death alone is not an accurate indicator.

An interesting definition of reperfusion injury comes from Buckberg (cited by Reimer, [10]), initially developed only for the surgical setting but in my (and Reimer's [10]) view also applicable to regional ischemia: reperfusion injury refers to 'those metabolic functional and structural consequences of restoring coronary flow that can be avoided or reversed by modification of the conditions of reperfusion'. This definition also clarifies why so much emphasis is placed on experimental therapy in ischemia-reperfusion experiments: successful treatment is the only proof that reperfusion injury exists.

B. Possible mechanisms of cell death in reperfusion

1. The classical view of cell death states that if the energy level of the cell falls below a critical level the cell dies because the activation energy for vital processes is lacking, and even the re-introduction of oxygen cannot change that condition. Failure of the ion pumps coupled with anaerobic metabolism which converts large-molecular glycogen into small-molecular lactate, which results in an osmolar load (increased by the breakdown of high energy phosphates), lead to intracellular edema. A certain level of energy is needed to pump out cell water and difficulties arise when that level cannot be maintained.

This theory puts the emphasis on ischemic damage and largely ignores reperfusion damage for the simple reason that an additional factor does not seem necessary.

2. Additional working hypotheses to explain cell death.

Almost from the conception of the myocardial salvage theory, several investigators felt that the lack (or severe reduction) of ATP is insufficient to explain cell death. Additional hypotheses were formulated because lack of energy alone does not explain the destruction of a cell. These additional hypotheses were:
- release of catecholamines in ischemic tissue and resulting adrenergic overstimulation;
- activation (or labilization) of lysosomes and cellular suicide;
- calcium overload by failure of the calcium pumps;
- premature attack by leucocytes;
- damage by oxygen free radicals.
These working hypotheses are believed to be applicable in ischemic as well as in reperfusion injury.

Although interesting observations were put forward in favor of each of these hypotheses, the situation remained inconclusive because strong counter-arguments were also presented.

Beta-adrenergic blocking agents failed to modify cell death in coronary occlusion experiments [11] and it has so far not been established whether abnormal calcium influx occurs in myocytes before they are irreversibly damaged. Recent evidence shows that the intracellular calcium concentration may increase in reversibly damaged isolated myocytes but that reoxygenation reverses this process [12]. Studies with radioactively labelled calcium in intact dog hearts showed no increase in reversibly damaged myocytes [13].

Leucocytes are known to destroy dead myocytes but the premature attack by leucocytes of only reversibly injured myocytes remains highly controversial. We were among the first [14] to report early invasion of leucocytes into ischemic tissue, but leucocytes in our experiments always migrated towards irreversibly damaged leucocytes. We do not recall a single instant where a leucocyte was found in the interstital space attached to a reversibly damaged myocytes.

Reimer and Jennings [15] were unable to reproduce the experiments of the Lucchesi group [16, 17] and treatment of hearts with agents reported to limit leucocyte invasion was often ineffective [5, 18, 19].

The possible role of oxygen free radicals

Oxygen free radicals have been implicated in reperfusion damage because reperfusion also means the re-introduction of oxygen and re-oxygenation was described by Hearse [20] as toxic (especially when done sometime after ischemia and called the 'oxygen-paradox'). Hearse and his colleagues [21] believed that free radicals were involved in the molecular mechanisms of the oxygen paradox and they claimed that xanthine oxidase is the radical generating enzyme system. Ischemic conditions lead to the conversion of xanthine de-hydrogenase into xanthine oxidase and so ideal conditions may exist at the onset of reperfusion: the enzyme as well as the substrate (=hypoxanthine from ATP breakdown) are present and radicals are produced together with urate.

Subsequently, Hearse and colleagues and others showed that inhibition of xanthine oxidase with allopurinol suppressed reperfusion related arrhythmias in rat hearts and reduced infarct size in rats, rabbits and dogs [21–23].

Free radicals once generated can be neutralized by super-oxide dismutase (SOD) plus catalase and recombinant SOD (as well as endotoxin contaminated SOD from animal sources) were found to be active in reducing reperfusion damage [24, 25]. However, all investigators had difficulties in explaining how an injected protein (SOD) leaves the circulation, enters the myocyte and crosses the mitochondrial membrane. Other investigators could not reproduce the beneficial effects of SOD in dogs [26] and pigs [19] and the SOD-part of the free radical hypothesis is still in doubt.

There is no doubt, however, of the part played by xanthine oxidase: it is rejected as irrelevant because it may only be applicable (if at all) in the rat. Downey et al. [27] were unable to demonstrate urate production in human patients and human myocardial tissue is devoid of xanthine oxidase activity. Podzuweit [28] was able to reproduce Downey's result in man and showed furthermore that pig myocardium is also devoid of xanthine oxidase. Muxfeldt [29] confirmed Podzuweit's findings in the pig and showed furthermore that the rabbit heart also has no xanthine oxidase activity, thereby confirming Downey's result in that species. Since all these species devoid of xanthine oxidase develop large infarcts quickly after coronary occlusion and reperfusion, the contribution of xanthine oxidase-generated free radicals is nil. Even in rat heart, which produces urate in ischemia, free radical damage may not occur because urate is a radical scavenger [30]. It should be mentioned here that free radicals are not only generated by xanthine oxidase and leucocytes but also in the metabolic pathways of catecholamines and prostaglandins. It is, however, felt that because of the very low concentrations of these precursors the contribution to damage may be negligible. Free radicals that have been demonstrated with electron spin resonance (ESR) cannot be directly traced to place and system of origin. Several earlier reports using ESR may not have taken into consideration all sources of error arising from the preparation of tissue for ESR-analysis during which free radicals can be generated [31].

The most likely place for free radical generation in the myocyte is the mitochondrion where about 2% of the respired oxygen is present as free radical. Glutathione and glutathione peroxidase (present in mM-concentrations in heart) are used for the 'mopping-up' of free radicals under physiological conditions. Although it has been shown that the ischemic reperfused heart loses glutathione, the loss occurs over a period of one hour after reperfusion, whereas so-called 'reperfusion-injury' occurs immediately after the onset of reperfusion. It may be that the loss of glutathione is also an epi-phenomenon, i.e. it may occur after death.

There is no doubt that oxygen radicals, if artificially generated [32], produce myocardial injury. However, the presence of naturally generated oxygen radicals and their importance for ischemic and post-ischemic cell death remain inconclusive.

Experiments on the existence of reperfusion injury

We have designed and carried out different types of experiments to try to conclusively prove or disprove the existence of reperfusion injury.

Infarct size experiments

If reperfusion could add to the damage of ischemia then infarcts should be larger within a certain window of time *with* reperfusion. This hypothesis is very difficult to study because there is no method available that allows the detection of necrosis *and* the quantitative measurement of infarct size without reperfusion. All methods based on formatan production from tetrazolium salts have a practical time limit of infarct detection without reperfusion of at least 3 hours after coronary occlusion, a time after which most cells are dead as judged by other methods (i.e. electron microscopy).

We reported years ago [33] that the size of reperfused infarcts is not different from the size of unreperfused infarcts at t=3 hours after coronary occlusion. This was observed in the presence of tissue which could have become infarcted if ischemia and reperfusion (or no reperfusion) were prolonged. At 6 hours after occlusion the infarcts were larger than at 3 hours with or without reperfusion at 6 hours.

From our experiments, we concluded that rather than adding to the 3-hour ischemia, reperfusion actually salvaged ischemic myocardium which would have become necrotic had the occlusion lasted longer.

Experimental studies

In our laboratory, two different groups of experiments were carried out to evaluate the effects of reperfusion on ischemic myocardium. Since one of the main problems in the evaluation of reperfusion injury is the difficulty in differentiating the effects of ischemia alone versus the combined effects of ischemia plus reperfusion, we decided to apply the following experimental protocol: produce period of ischemia → take biopsy at end of ischemia → initiate reperfusion → take biopsies at different time intervals → terminate experiment. All biopsies underwent examination by electron microscopy using our own [34] semiquantitative evaluation system for the determination of the degree of ischemic injury (Table 1). Electron microscopy seems to be a very suitable tool for this kind of study because it allows a direct evaluation of all changes at different time intervals, and it also correlates well with metabolic and functional changes occurring during ischemia and reperfusion [34]. The hypothesis is that if reperfusion aggravates ischemic cell damage then the incidence of more severe degrees of injuries should increase in reperfusion.

Material and methods

1. In 9 anesthetized dogs, the left anterior descending artery was occluded for time intervals of 45, 90 and 180 minutes, respectively(3 dogs per subgroup). At the end of the ischemic time, a needle biopsy was taken from the center of the ischemic area. Reperfusion was allowed for 48 hours. Before sacrifice of the animal, a biopsy was taken from the same area.

2. A second group of experiments was designed to test the effects of early reperfusion on ischemic myocardium. In 7 anesthetized dogs the LAD was occluded for 90 minutes and reperfusion was reinstituted. Biopsies were taken at three time intervals: at the end of ischemia, 5 minutes after the onset of reperfusion and at 30 minutes, then the animals were sacrificed.

All tissues from the different experimental groups were separated in subendocardial and subepicardial samples, which were imediately fixed in cold 2% glutaraldehyde in 0.1 M cacodylate buffer and embedded in epon

Table 1. Scoring of the most typical ultrastructural symptoms leading to the classification of different degrees of ischemic injury versus normal myocardial cells. Irreversible injury is indicated by the presence of flocculent densities in the mitochondrial matrix.

State of the myo-cardium:	Ultrastructure							
	Mitochondria				Grading of nuclei		Myofilaments	
Normal or degree of ischemic injury	Normal granules + or –	Flocculent densities + or –	Grading of matrix and cristae light	broken	Light	Pycnotic	Con-tracted or relaxed	Con-tracture bands + or –
Normal	+	–	–	–	–	–	contracted	+/–
Slight	–	–	+	+	–	–	contracted	+/–
Moderate	–	–	++	++	+	+	contracted	+
Severe	–	–	+++	+++	+	+	contracted	+
Irreversible	–	+	+++	+++	++	++	relaxed	++

using routine procedures. All samples were then studied and photographed in the electron microscope and subsequently evaluated using the scoring system shown in Table 1. The ultrastructural evaluation was carried out by two trained observers who remained unaware of whether the tissue was taken from ischemic or ischemic-reperfused tissue until all the biopsies were diagnosed.

Effects of 48 hours of reperfusion on ischemic myocardium

Ischemia of differing durations produced injury to the myocardium of varying degrees as can be seen from Table 2. 45 minutes of coronary artery occlusion caused reversible injury varying from slight to severe, with the subendocardium exhibiting more progressed injury than the subepicardium. Longer periods of ischemia in most animals resulted in irreversible injury of the subendocardium, in two animals also in the subepicardium, i.e. transmural myocardial infarction. It clearly becomes evident from the data presented in Table 2 that the subendocardium is more susceptible than the subepicardium to the effects of ischemia. Duration of ischemia, therefore, seems to be only one of several factors influencing the speed of development of irreversible injury as has been pointed out in the first part of this chapter.

Reperfusion either caused recovery of ischemically injured myocardium or the degree of injury remained the same. In the case of reversible ischemic injury as seen in the subendocardium of dogs #3 and #4, this was interpreted

Table 2. Ultrastructural results of coronary occlusion and reperfusion in nine dogs.

Dog	Ischemia			Reperfusion		
	min	epi	endo	h	epi	endo
1	45	+	+++	48	n	+
2	45	++	+++	48	+	++
3	45	++	++	48	+	++
4	0	++	++	48	n	++
5	90	+	irre	48	++	irre
6	90	++	irre	48	+	irre
7	180	irre	irre	48	irre	irre
8	180	++	++	48	n	+
9	180	irre	irre	48	irre	irre

endo = endocardial layer; epi = epicardial layer; h = hours; min = minutes;

n	= normal
+	= slight
++	= moderate
+++	= severe
irre	= irreversible

as a delay of recovery similar to the delayed recovery of adenine nucleotide content of reperfused ischemic canine myocardium as described by Reimer and Jennings [35]. Irreversible injury was not observed in myocardium which was only reversibly injured at the end of ischemia, indicating that reperfusion did not have any deleterious effects on ischemic myocardium. Tissue which was irreversibly injured by ischemia showed further progression of cellular destruction.

It may be concluded from these experiments that ischemia causes injury of differing degrees of severity in the canine heart and that reperfusion of longer duration did not have any additional harmful effects but led to structural recovery of the formerly ischemic myocardium.

Effects of early reperfusion in ischemic myocardium

In 6 dogs which underwent coronary artery occlusion for 90 minutes, three biopsies were taken for ultrastructural evaluation as described above. Table 3 lists the severity of ischemic injury as determined for each tissue sample. Ischemia caused a wide range of injury varying from slight to irreversible, and the subendocardium was more severely afflicted than the subepicardium. One animal showed transmural infarction at the end of ischemia and irreversible injury persisted during reperfusion. Neutrophilic leucocytes were found to be present in irreversibly injured tissue, both in capillaries and venoles as well as extravascularly, closely attached to irreversibly injured cells. Neutrophils were also found in the subendocardial tissue exhibiting irreversible injury

Table 3. Effects of early reperfusion on ischemic myocardium.

Dog	Ischemia 90 min		Rep 5 min		Rep 30 min	
	epi	endo	epi	endo	epi	endo
1	+++	irre	++	irre	+	irre
2	+	++	+	++	n	++
3	irre	irre	irre	irre	irre	irre
4	++	++	++	++	+	++
5	+++	irre	++	irre	++	irre
6	+	+	+	+	n	n

Scores indicate severity of ischemic injury.
n   = normal
+   = slight
++   = moderate
+++ = severe
irre   = irreversible

when the subepicardium was only reversibly injured, i.e. when subendocardial infarction was present. In all other animals, only reversible injury was found at the end of ischemia, and that was usually less severe at 30 minutes but remained unchanged at 5 minutes of reperfusion. Neutrophils were sometimes observed in blood vessels from reversibly injured tissue, but they were absent from the extravascular space.

This series of experiments failed to show any harmful effects of reperfusion of ischemic myocardium and it confirmed the data of our first study described here, that reversible injury caused by ischemia either persists for a longer period of time or becomes less severe during the course of reperfusion. Neutrophils were found to closely attach to irreversibly injured myocardial cells, probably destroying them further, but they were never found to be in close proximity to reversibly injured cells.

These experiments allow the conclusion that at the intervals studied, reperfusion salvaged rather than damaged ischemic myocardium.

References

1. Frommer PL (1968) The myocardial infarction research programm of the National Heart Institute. Am J Cardiol 22: 108–110
2. Reimer KA, Jennings RB (1979) The 'wavefront phenomenon' of myocardial ischemic cell death. II. Transmural progression of necrosis within the framework of ischemic bed size (myocardium at risk) and collateral flow. Lab Invest 40: 633–644
3. Schaper W, Frenzel H, Hort W (1979) Experimental coronary artery occlusion. I. Measurement of infarct size. Basic Res Cardiol 74: 46–53
4. Schaper W, Hofmann M, Mueller KD, Genth K, Carl M (1979) Experimental occlusion of two small coronary arteries in the same heart. A new validation method for infarct size manipulation. Basic Res Cardiol 74: 224–229

5. Reimer KA, Jennings RB, Cobb FR (1985) Animal models for protecting ischemic myocardium: results of the NIHBL cooperative study: comparison of unconscious and conscious dog models. Circ Res 56: 651–665

6. Schaper W, Binz K, Sass S, Winkler B (1987) Influence of collateral blood flow and of variations in MVO_2 on tissue-ATP content in ischemic and infarcted myocardium. J Mol Cell Cardiol 19: 19–37

7. Schaper J, Schaper W (1983) Reperfusion of ischemic myocardium: ultrastructural and histochemical aspects. J Am Coll Cardiol 1: 1037–1046

8. Schaper W (1984) Experimental infarcts and the microcirculation. In: DJ Hearse and DM Yellon (eds) Therapeutic Approaches to Myocardial Infarct Size Limitation. Raven Press, New York, pp 79–90

9. Gotsman MS, Lotan C, Weiss AT, Appelbaum D, Sapoznikov D, Hasin Y, Mosseri M (1989) Early and prehospital thrombolytic therapy in acute myocardial infaction. In: Schmutzler H, Rutsch W, Dougherty FC (eds) Limitation of Infarct Size. Springer Verlag, Berlin, Heidelberg, pp 107–130

10. Reimer KA, Jennings RB (1988) Reperfusion injury. In: Schettler G, Jennings RB, Rapaport E, Wenger NK, Bernhardt R (eds) Reperfusion and Revascularization in Acute Myocardial Infarction. Springer , pp 52–55

11. Schaper W (1987) Heart rate reduction, a new and old therapeutic principle? Eur Heart J 8 (Suppl L): 1–4

12. Smith GL, Allen DG (1988) Effects of metabolic blockade on intracellular calcium concentration in isolated ferret ventricular muscle. Circ Res 62: 1233–1236

13. Jennings RB, Schaper J, Hill ML, Steenbergen C Jr, Reimer KA (1985) Effect of reperfusion late in the phase of reversible ischemic injury. Changes in cell volume, electrolytes, metabolites, and ultrastructure. Circ Res 56: 262–278

14. Schaper J (1979) Ultrastructure of the myocardium in acute ischemia. In: Schaper W (ed) The Pathophysiology of Myocardial Perfusion. Elsevier, Amsterdam, New York, Oxford, pp 581–673

15. Uraizee A, Reimer KA, Murry CE, Jennings RB (1987) Failure of superoxide dismutase to limit size of myocardial infarction after 40 minutes of ischemia and 4 days of reperfusion in dogs. Circulation 75: 1237–1248

16. Lucchesi BR, Mullane KM (1986) Leukocytes and ischemia-induced myocardial injury. Ann Rev Pharmacol Toxicol 26: 201–224

17. Lucchesi BR, Romson JL, Jolly SR (1984) Do leucocytes influence infarct size? In: Hearse DJ, Yellon DM (eds) Therapeutic Approaches to Myocardial Infarct Size Limitation. Raven Press, New York, pp 219–248

18. Schott RJ, Nao BS, McClanahan, Simpson PJ, Todd RF, Stirling MC, Gallagher KP (1988) Anti-Mol monoclonal antibody does not alter myocardial stunning. Circulation 78,II–78: 310 (abstr)

19. Klein HH (1987) Thesis, Universität Göttingen

20. Hearse DJ, Humphrey SM, Chain EB (1973) Abrupt reoxygenation of the anoxic potassium-arrested perfused rat heart – A study of myocardial enzyme release. J Mol Cell Cardiol 5: 395

21. Hearse DJ, Manning AS, Downey JM, Yellon DM (1986) Xanthine oxidase: a critical mediator of myocardial injury during ischemia and reperfusion? Acta Physiol Scand 548 (Suppl): 65–78

22. Akizuki S, Yoshida S, Chambers D, Eddy L, Parmley L, Yellon D, Downey J (1984) Blockage of the O2-radical producing enzyme, xanthine-oxidase, reduces infarct size in the dog. Fed Proc 43: 540 (abstr)

23. Akizuki S, Yoshida S, Chambers DE, Eddy LJ, Parmley LF, Yellon DM, Downey JM (1985) Infarct size limitation by the xanthine oxidase inhibitor allopurinol, in closed-chest dogs with small infarcts. Cardiovasc Res 19: 686–692

24. Simpson PJ, Mickelson J, Fantone JC, Gallagher KP, Lucchesi BR (1987) Iloprost inhibits neutrophil function *in vitro* and *in vivo* and limits experimental infarct size in canine heart. Circ Res 60: 666–673

25. Ambrosio G, Weisfeldt ML, Jacobus WE, Flaherty JT (1987) Evidence for a reversible oxygen radical-mediated component of reperfusion injury: reduction by recombinant superoxide dismutase administered at the time of reflow. Circulation 75: 282–291

26. Reimer KA, Murray CE, Jennings RB (1986) Failure of superoxide dismutase to limit myocardial infarct size in a canine ischemia/reperfusion model. Circulation 74 (Suppl II): 484 (abstr)

27. Eddy LJ, Stewart JR, Jones HP, Engerson TD, McCord JM, Downey JH (1987) Free radical-producing enzyme, xanthine oxidase, is undetectable in human hearts. Am J Physiol 253: H709–H711

28. Podzuweit T, Beck H, Müller A, Görlach G, Scheld HH (1988) Absence of xanthine oxidase activity in the human myocardium. J Mol Cell Cardiol 20 (Suppl V): 131 (abstr)

29. Muxfeldt M, Schaper W (1987) The activity of xanthine oxidase in heart of pigs, guinea pigs, rabbits, rats and humans. Basic Res Cardiol 82: 486–492

30. Ames BN, Cather R, Schiers E, Hochstein P (1981) Uric acid provides an antioxidant defense in humans against oxidant and radical caused aging and cancer: a hypothesis. Proc Natl Acad Sci USA 78: 6858–6862

31. Garlick PB, Shuter SL, Davies MJ, Hearse DJ, Slater TF (1988) ESR spectroscopy: preparative techniques may cause artefactual generation of radicals. J Mol Cell Cardiol 20 (Suppl V): 180 (abstr)

32. McCord JM (1984) Are free radicals a major culprit? In: Hearse DJ, Yellon DM (eds) Therapeutic Approaches to Myocardial Infarct Size Limitation. Raven Press, New York, pp 209–218

33. Hofmann M, Hofmann M, Genth K, Schaper W (1980) The influence of reperfusion on infarct size after experimental coronary artery occlusion. Basic Res Cardiol 75: 572–582

34. Schaper J, Mulch J, Winkler B, Schaper W (1979) Ultrastructural, functional, and biochemical criteria for estimation of reversibility of ischemic injury: A study on the effects of global ischemia on the isolated dog heart. J Mol Cell Cardiol 11: 521–541

35. Reimer KA, Hill ML, Jennings RB (1981) Prolonged depletion of ATP and of the adenine nucleotide pool due to delayed resynthesis of adenine nucleotides following reversible myocardial ischemic injury in dogs. J Mol Cell Cardiol 13: 229–239

PART VI

The role of calcium

Subcellular calcium shifts in ischemia and reperfusion

HERBERT K. HAGLER and L. MAXIMILIAN BUJA

Department of Pathology, The University of Texas Southwestern Medical Center at Dallas, 53235 Harry Hines Blvd., Dallas, Texas 75235-9072, USA

Abstract

Subcellular calcium shifts and pathological calcification are observed under conditions of myocardial ischemia and/or reperfusion cell injury and represent the more severe manifestations of abnormal calcium (Ca^{2+}) homeostasis. The use of specialized techniques for measurement of intracellular electrolytes such as electron probe x-ray microanalysis and the use of the fluorescent Ca^{2+} indicator, fura 2, are providing new insights into regulation of intracellular Ca^{2+} and the role of altered Ca^{2+} homeostasis in the pathogenesis of myocardial cell injury. During the progression of myocardial cell injury, investigations indicate that increased intracellular Ca^{2+} develops in association with other manifestations of membrane injury, including other electrolyte alterations, altered cell volume regulation, and altered membrane phospholipids.

Introduction

The accumulation of calcium during myocardial ischemic injury is well recognized [1–5]. In the peripheral regions of myocardial infarcts produced by a permanent coronary occlusion and infarcts produced by temporary coronary occlusion followed by reperfusion, pathological calcification is routinely observed by transmission electron microscopy. The severest calcification occurs in the peripheral regions of infarcts produced by permanent coronary occlusions and in subendocardial infarcts produced by temporary coronary occlusion with reperfusion, as illustrated in Fig. 1. The pathological calcification is an indicator of severe cellular and membrane damage and has been associated with the uptake of diagnostic indicators of myocardial infarction such as technetium-99m stannous pyrophosphate. These observations have served to stimulate investigations into the potential role of perturbed calcium homeostasis in the pathogenic manifestations of myocardial ischemic injury, including arrhythmogenesis, contractile dysfunction, and cell death.

H.M. Piper (ed.) Pathophysiology of severe ischemic myocardial injury, 283–296.
© 1990 Kluwer Academic Publishers, Dordrecht –

284

PROLONGED ISCHEMIA

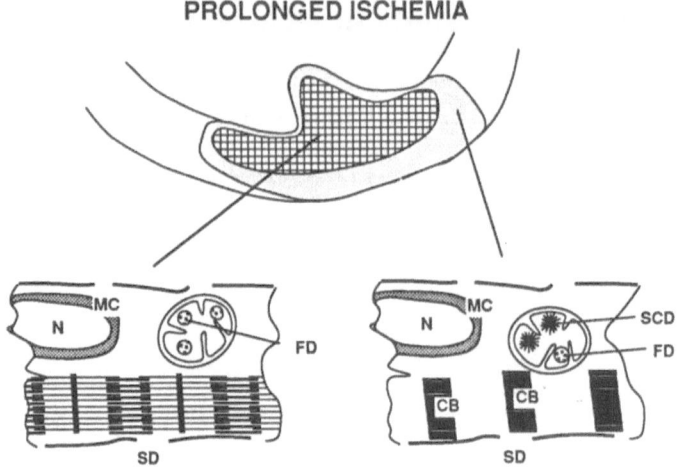

TEMPORARY ISCHEMIA WITH REPERFUSION

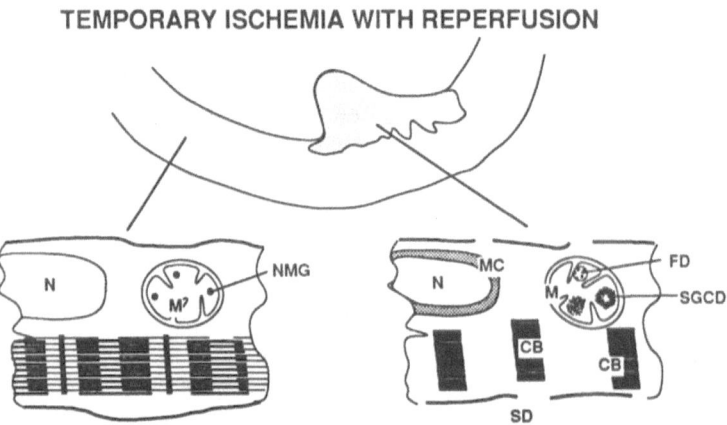

Fig. 1. Summary of morphological features of myocardial cell injury present in different regions of prolonged transmural infarcts (upper panel) and temporary ischemia followed by reperfusion (lower panel). With prolonged ischemia, the myofibrils in the central region are hyperrelaxed as compared to the normal tissue depicted in the lower panel, and the mitochondria contain flocculent densities composed of denatured lipid and protein, whereas the myofibrils in the periperal region are formed into contraction bands and the mitochondria show calcium deposits as well as flocculent densities. With temporary ischemia and reperfusion, injury is limited to the subendocardium and is characterized by myofibrillar contraction bands and early mitochondrial calcification. N, nucleus; MC, marginated chromatin; SD, sarcolemmal defect; FD, flocculent (amorphous) density; NMG, normal matrix granule; CB, contraction band; LCD large (spicular) calcium deposit; SCD, small (granular) calcium deposit.

Total calcium changes during myocardial infarction

After a coronary occlusion, necrosis progresses from the subendocardium to the subepicardium [1]. Reperfusion after 40–60 minutes of occlusion will limit necrosis to the papillary muscle and the adjacent subendocardium (Fig. 1). At 3 to 6 hours of occlusion the necrotic region will extend from the subendocardium to the subepicardium. In most cases necrosis within the myocardial bed-at-risk is complete and the area of necrosis cannot be limited by reperfusion. In general, the ultimate infarct size is determined by the duration and severity of the ischemia, the collateral blood flow after occlusion, and the size of the bed-at-risk. Necrosis tends to proceed faster in the subendocardium than the subepicardium. This is probably related to a poorer oxygen supply-demand ratio in the subendocardium and possibly to intrinsic metabolic differences in the populations of myocytes from the two regions.

The morphological differences reflect differences in the progression of injury within the subendocardium and subepicardial regions. The central zone of the infarct contains predominantly necrotic fibers with relaxed myofibrils (Fig. 1). The mitochondria do not contain calcium deposits but predominantly exhibit amorphous (flocculent) densities of denatured protein and lipid. In more peripheral regions the necrotic fibers are associated with hypercontracted, disrupted myofibrils (contraction bands) and the mitochondria contain both amorphous densities and calcium deposits. Non-necrotic cells in this peripheral region contain lipid droplets which indicate alteration of metabolism, but do not exhibit other signs associated with irreversible injury.

The morphological changes also correlate with studies of ^{45}Ca accumulation during evolving myocardial infarction. ^{45}Ca accumulation occurs to a greater degree, and earlier, in the course of myocardial infarction following permanent coronary occlusion in the subepicardium than in the subendocardium [4]. If reperfusion is provided after 1 to 3 hours of coronary occlusion, ^{45}Ca accumulation is greatly increased across the myocardial wall [5]. Although calcium accumulation is less prominent in the central ischemic zone, this does not exclude shifts of Ca^{2+} from extracellular to intracellular space and from organelles into the cytoplasm, thereby leading to activation of Ca^{2+} mediated degradative processes.

Potential mechanisms of membrane injury

There is quite a bit of evidence supporting the concept that changes in membrane phospholipids contribute to the functional changes of membrane transport systems and structural alterations found in ischemic and hypoxic myocardium. Chien *et al.* reported small (10%) decreases in total phospholipids and certain phospholipid species, i.e., phosphotidylethanolamine and phosphotidylcholine in the ischemic canine subendocardium after 1 to 3 hours of permanent occlusions [6]. Increases in free fatty acids, including arachidonic acid, were measured in the ischemic myocardium after 40 to 60 minutes of coronary occlusion in the dog model [7]. Since membrane phospholipids normally contain arachidonic acid, a marker of increased phospholipid degradation would be the accumulation of free arachidonate. Similar phospholipid changes have been found with global ischemia in an isolated rat heart model [8]. Others have reported progressive changes in free fatty acids and other amphiphatic lipids and transient increases in lysophospholipids in ischemic myocardium [9, 10]. The phospholipid and fatty acid changes in ischemic myocardium are large enough to induce Ca^{2+} permeability defects in isolated cardiac membranes [6].

Membrane stability is dependent on a balance between degradation, including deacylation (removal of fatty acids), and synthesis, including *de novo* synthesis and reacylation. Data indicate that an increase in $[Ca^{2+}]_i$ leads to an accelerated phospholipid degradation. The exact mechanism of action, whether it is activation of phospholipases, a direct effect of $[Ca^{2+}]_i$ on phospholipids or a free radical-mediated effect is unknown. There is evidence of accelerated phospholipid degradation in *in vivo* and *in vitro* models of ischemia. The resynthesis of phospholipids does involve ATP-dependent processes [7]. It is conceivable that if ATP levels are sufficiently preserved, reacylation of phospholipids could occur and preserve membrane integrity. Conversely, it is postulated that when myocytes are energy depleted in the presence of an increase in $[Ca^{2+}]_i$, then accelerated phospholipid degradation develops in association with an impaired ability to reacylate membrane phospholipids. In addition Ca^{2+}-mediated activation of proteases may contribute to the cytoskeletal damage observed in ischemic myocardium [11, 12]. There also may be a role for Ca^{2+} in free radical-mediated membrane damage [10].

In order to investigate the relationship between phospholipid degradation and calcium homeostasis, experiments were performed using mepacrine, an alkyl acridine, and U26,384 (Upjohn Pharmaceutical Company), a steroidal diamine. Mepacrine has been reported to inhibit phospholipase A_2, and U26,384 inhibits phospholipase activities from human neutrophils, platelets, and hog pancreas *in vitro* [13]. Cultured cardiac myocytes that were treated with these compounds were protected against phospholipid degradation and electrolyte changes as measured by x-ray microanalysis, including calcium accumulation [13]. The treated cells maintained normal morphological structure including protection against hypercontraction and blebbing. In another study the protective effect of chlorpromazine pretreatment in an isolated perfused myocardium subjected to ischemia was observed [14]. A protective effect of mepacrine in a pig model of temporary myocardial ischemia and reperfusion has been reported by Das *et al.* [15]. The specificity and mechanism of action of these compounds has not been determined. However, in the setting of impaired energy metabolism, these compounds prevent the progressive release of fatty acids from membrane phospholipids and are associated with prevention of calcium overloading and preservation of cellular integrity.

Altered calcium homeostasis and other electrolyte alterations

The postulated sequence of events leading to the membrane damage and gross calcium overloading discussed above is as follows. Ischemia and its underlying component, hypoxia, produce alterations of energy metabolism which result in progressive loss of ATP, acidosis, and lactate accumulation [1–3]. In general it is thought that the altered metabolic status can cause discrete changes in membrane function which lead to disturbances in electrolyte homeostasis and receptor function [1–3, 16]. Myocardial ischemia initially causes excitation-contraction uncoupling with a result efflux of K^+ from the myocytes [17] followed by cell swelling, increases in cell water and Na^+, and further efflux of K^+ [1, 18, 19]. An increase in free cytosolic calcium $[Ca^{2+}]_i$ is postulated to develop at this stage of injury [1–3]. Net $[Ca^{2+}]_i$ influx into the cell could be attributed to changes in the Na^+-K^+ ATPase, the Na^+-Ca^{2+} exchanger, receptor and voltage dependent Ca^{2+} channels, and the Ca^{2+}-ATPase efflux system. There may also be an intracellular redistribution of Ca^{2+} from the sarcoplasmic reticulum and possibly the mitochondria. This initial change probably involves free Ca^{2+} without an increase in total calcium. Increased $[Ca^{2+}]_i$ may stimulate a number of intracellular events, including increased ATP degradation due to activation of Ca^{2+}-dependent ATPases, impairment of ATP synthesis due to Ca^{2+} loading of the mitochondria, activation of Ca^{2+} dependent lipases and proteases, and, possibly, enhancement of various free radical mediated reactions. These alterations could lead to progressive ATP depletion and membrane damage with the potential for marked calcium overloading and cell death. The onset of irreversible injury correlates with the development of a membrane permeability defect to multivalent ions and associated severe contractile depression as judged by findings from lanthanum tracer experiments in isolated hypoxic and ischemic myocardial preparations [14, 20].

Intracellular calcium alterations

The assessment and measurement of intracellular calcium is integral with the investigation of the above hypotheses. Many approaches have been used [21, 22] including, a) the measurement of total calcium using atomic absorption measurements combined with intracellular and extracellular markers, b) ^{45}Ca measurements of Ca^{2+} content and flux, c) probes of membrane permeability defects such as ionic lanthanum, d) measurement of subcellular electrolytes including total calcium using electron probe x-ray microanalysis (EPMA), e) use of ion selective electrodes to measure Ca^{2+} activity, and f) the use of dyes such as aequorin and the carboxylate indicators to measure free Ca^{2+} levels. Since all these methods have strengths and weaknesses, our laboratory has used several of them to measure altered calcium homeostasis. We have developed methods using EPMA to measure total (free plus bound) subcellular electrolytes, including calcium, and the carboxylate indicator, fura-2, to measure $[Ca^{2+}]_i$. These methods have been applied to investigate several of the issues in cardiac pathophysiology [23–26, 5, 27–28].

A number of studies have implicated calcium accumulation in the pathogenesis of myocardial ischemic injury, yet have not provided direct evidence for cellular increases in calcium. These deficiencies have been due to inadequate methods for measuring calcium changes in intact myocardial preparations. In efforts to measure directly cellular changes in total and free calcium we have employed a cultured neonatal rat cardiac myocyte model. This model is compatible with analytical techniques including electron probe x-ray microanalysis for the measurement of intracellular total electrolyte concentrations, including total calcium, and the recently developed technique of introducing an intracellular Ca^{2+} sensitive fluorescent dye, fura-2, to measure quantitative dynamic Ca^{2+} changes. The combination of the isolated myocyte model with the above techniques has allowed a number of studies relating calcium overloading, adenosine triphosphate (ATP) depletion, and membrane phospholipid degradation to be performed [25, 29, 30]. Release of tritiated arachidonic acid into the culture medium was used as an indicator of phospholipid degradation in this model. Myocytes were prelabeled for 24 hours with tritiated arachadonic acid prior to the experiments. High pressure chromatography was used for measurements of ATP.

A number of metabolic inhibitors of high energy phosphate metabolism were used including deoxyglucose (DOG), cyanide (CN), oligomycin (OG) and iodoacetic acid (IAA) (see Fig. 2). In cells treated with IAA (30 μM), a glycolytic inhibitor and alkylating agent, ATP was mildly reduced after one hour followed by marked decreases following two hours treatment. Arachidonate release was at control levels after one hour and increased after longer exposures. In general, the release of arachidonate did not occur until a 50% reduction of ATP occurred. As ATP was reduced to very low levels, there was an accelerated arachidonate release [25, 29, 30]. In static fura-2 measurements of cells on coverslips in a standard spectrofluorometer, there was no change in $[Ca^{2+}]_i$ from control values of 80 ± 6.6 nM (n=5) after one hour, and after two hours $[Ca^{2+}]_i$ increased five-fold to 496 ± 116 nM (n=5). Dynamic measurements of $[CA^{2+}]_i$ performed on groups of cells by microspectrofluorometry indicated an initial reduction associated with loss of contractile activity. There was a precipitous increase in $[Ca^{2+}]_i$ to the micromolar range at the point of development of hypercontrature and cell blebbing [5, 27]. Normal levels of electrolytes in the cytoplasm (Fig. 3) and mitochondria (Fig. 4) were found using electron probe x-ray microanalysis after one

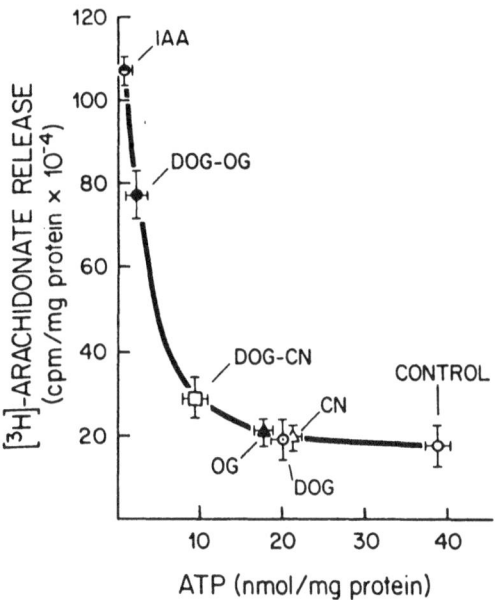

Fig. 2. Arachidonate release plotted versus ATP concentration for various metabolic inhibitors of ATP synthesis. IAA, iodoacetic acid; DOG-CN deoxyglucose in combination with cyanide; DOG-OG, deoxyglucose in combination with oligomycin; DOG, deoxyglucose alone; CN, cyanide alone; OG, oligomycin alone. Reprinted with permission from Gunn *et al.* [30].

hour exposure to iodoacetate, but after 1.5 to 2 hours of exposure, elemental changes occurred including increased sodium, chlorine and calcium with decreases in potassium and magnesium [8]. Morphological changes included hypercontracture and bleb formation. X-ray microanalysis showed densities in the mitochondria consistent with an uptake of calcium by these organelles. The metabolic inhibitors 20 mM deoxyglucose and 1 mM cyanide showed generally similar dynamic calcium changes to that shown with iodoacetic acid, however, with DOG and CN, the $[Ca^{2+}]_i$ increase was more rapid but with less total increase [5, 27].

A series of studies using Na^+-K^+ pump inhibition in 0 mM K^+ medium or $10^{-3}M$ ouabain were performed for comparison with the metabolic studies. After 30–45 minutes of sodium pump inhibition with ouabain there was an increase in $[Ca^{2+}]_i$ by fura-2 measurements (Fig. 5), and an increase in Na, decrease in K, and an increase in Ca by EPMA [5, 26, 27]. The electrolyte alterations occurred much more rapidly than with metabolic inhibition. The mechanism appears to involve Na^+ accumulation followed by activation of Na^+-Ca^{2+} exchange. Cultures subjected to Na^+-K^+ pump inhibition were characterized by a significant increase in arachidonic acid release after 60 minutes, and a continuing release at later time points. There was only a moderate decrease in ATP at 1 to 3 hours. The cultures returned to normal

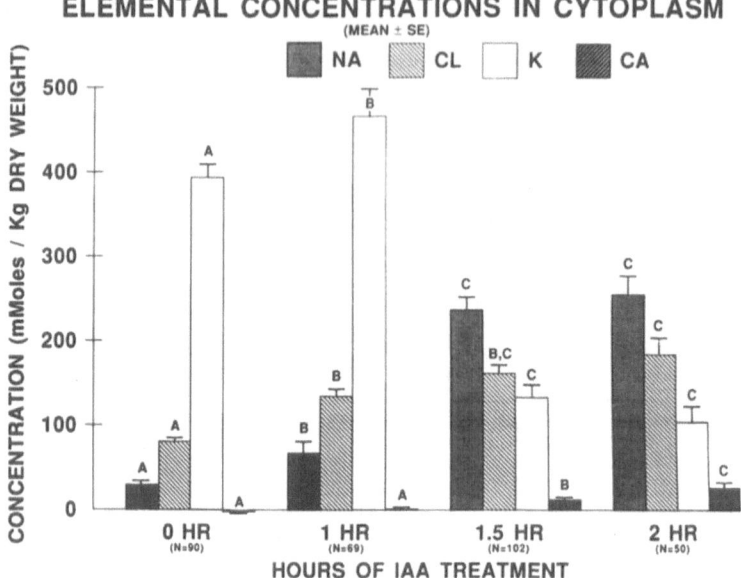

Fig. 3. Elemental concentrations in cytoplasm as measured by electron probe x-ray microanalysis versus time of exposure to IAA (iodoacetic acid) in cultured neonatal rat ventricular myocytes. Data presented with analysis of variance and Duncans multiple range test. Groups with different letter designations are significantly different at the p<0.05 level. Data summarized from Buja *et al.* [25].

medium after one hour of Na$^+$-K$^+$ pump inhibition, showed complete recovery of ATP at 24 hours and exhibited normal ultrastructure by electron microscopy. The cultures treated for two to three hours of N$^+$-K$^+$ pump inhibition gave incomplete recovery of ATP levels after 24 hours. Electron microscopy documented a mixed population of myocytes showing relatively normal ultrastructure and another population with features of irreversible injury.

The response of myocytes to metabolic and Na$^+$-K$^+$ pump inhibition are quite distinct. The metabolic inhibitors cause a progressive decline in ATP levels. Once the ATP reaches a critical level, the myocytes develop calcium loading, release arachidonate, and progress through contracture to cell death. With Na$^+$-K$^+$ pump inhibition there is a rapid rise in intracellular calcium and a progressive increase in arachidonate release. There was a moderate decrease in ATP and the development of contracture. Even though there was calcium accumulation and arachidonate release, the injury was mostly reversible after one hour of Na$^+$-K$^+$ pump inhibition. This is consistent with an initial resistance to Ca^{2+} accumulation produced by this mechanism as observed by others [31]. However, after 3 hours inhibition there was a significant number of myocytes which were irreversibly injured. These results are in agreement with observations in isolated adult rat papillary muscle prepara-

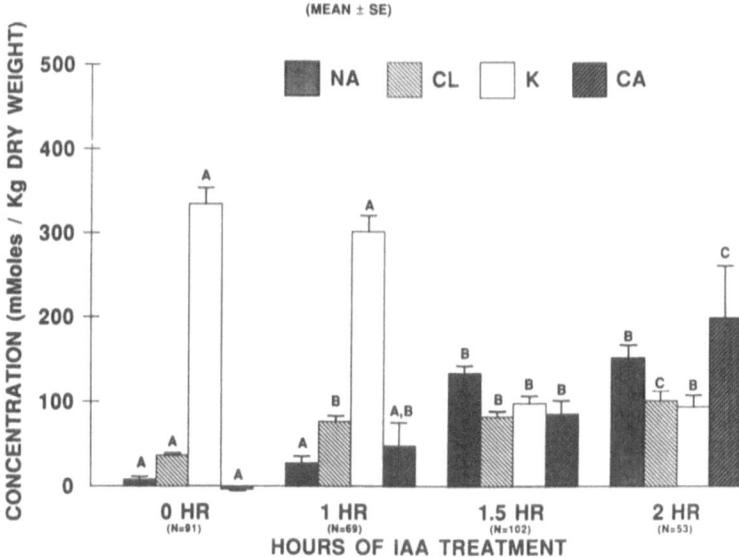

Fig. 4. Elemental concentrations in mitochondria as measured by electron beam x-ray microanalysis versus time of exposure to IAA (iodoacetic acid) in cultured neonatal rat ventricular myocytes. Data presented with analysis of variance and Duncans multiple range test. Groups with different letter designations are significantly different at the p<0.05 level. Data summarized from Buja *et al.* [25].

tions exposed to Na⁺-K⁺ pump inhibition. After exposure to potassium free buffer for 3 hours and then a return to normal buffer for one hour, the muscles exhibited persistent electrolyte alterations (measured by x-ray microanalysis) and contractile depression. In significant numbers of myocytes there was increased cytoplasmic and mitochondrial Ca accumulation [32].

There are several conclusions which may be drawn from these observations: a) recovery following a calcium loading of the myocytes is influenced by the mechanism, magnitude and duration of the loading conditions; b) an increase in intracellular calcium, such as occurs with Na⁺-K⁺ pump inhibition, leads directly to phospholipid degradation and release of arachidonic acid; c) the ATP levels at the time of calcium loading influence the severity of injury; d) the extent of energy impairment and the cell's ability to produce ATP has an influence on the potential for recovery following calcium loading conditions. Thus, there appears to be an important link between calcium accumulation and impaired energy metabolism on the progression of membrane and cellular injury. In spite of different experimental and animal models, this link between ATP levels and calcium accumulation is supported by work reported from other laboratories [33–37].

Early studies looking for early increases in calcium with hypoxia or metabolic inhibition produced inconclusive results [38]. Recently Barry *et al.*,

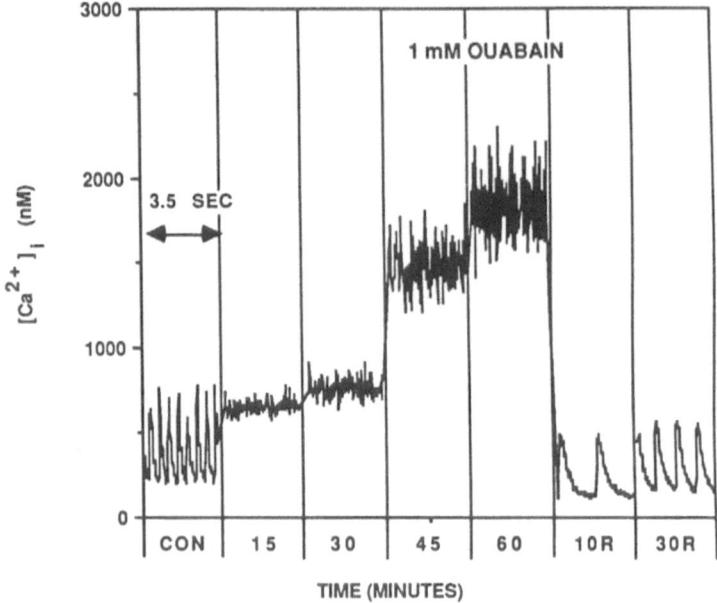

Fig. 5. Cultured neonatal rat cardiac myocytes incubated with fura-2 for measurement of dynamic changes in $[Ca^{2+}]_i$ under control conditions and after treatment with 1 mM ouabain for 15, 30, 45, and 60 minutes followed by recovery in ouabain free media for 10 and 30 minutes. The 340/380 ratios were calibrated according to the methods of Grynkiewicz *et al.* [22] and shown as calcium concentration. Rmax and Rmin were determine using 20 μM bromo-A23187 and 5 mM EGTA, respectively. Most groups of myocytes recovered spontaneous beating activity after 30 minutes of recovery.

using indo-1 to measure $[Ca^{2+}]_i$, have shown increases associated with contracture in metabolically inhibited cultured neonatal chick heart cells [33]. Recent studies using isolated perfused heart preparations loaded with the fluorescent indicator indo-1 [39] and hearts loaded with the nuclear magnetic resonance indicator F-BAPTA [40, 41] indicate an increase in cell $[Ca^{2+}]_i$ during the first 30 minutes of ischemia. Thus, there is now strong evidence that, during metabolic inhibition, hypoxia, and ischemia, there is an early increase in $[CA^{2+}]_i$. Future work has to be directed towards the mechanisms by which increased $[Ca^{2+}]_i$ leads to membrane and electrolyte alterations.

Reperfusion injury

Reperfusion injury implies additional damage to injured myocytes caused by reperfusion after a previous episode of ischemia [1, 42]. This injury may involve further impairment of function, induction of arrhythmias and progression to cell death. Free radical generation, calcium overloading and impaired energy metabolism are mechanisms which have been postulated to explain reperfusion injury. After brief periods of coronary occlusion of as little as 15 minutes, a persistent contractile depression has been observed up to 24 hours. This phenomenon, referred to as myocardial stunning [1, 42], has been insufficient to cause myocardial necrosis. Coronary occlusion for 2 to 4 hours in which necrosis is limited to the subendocardium are responsible for even longer intervals of persistent coronary depression. In studies after 2 hours of coronary occlusion, recovery of contractile function was found to require 1–4 weeks of reperfusion, but after 4 hours of occlusion there was no functional recovery after 4 weeks of reperfusion [43].

Interventions designed to stimulate the rate of ATP synthesis have not appeared to change the recovery rate of the stunned myocardium [1, 42]. In spite of depressed ATP levels, the contractile reserve of myocardium can be stimulated with inotropic interventions [1, 42]. Free radical bursts with reperfusion have been observed in isolated heart models and the use of free radical scavengers has been beneficial in some models, but appear to be time and model dependent [1, 42].

Some evidence supports calcium accumulation as having a role in reperfusion injury. Calcium loading can involve several possible mechanisms, including Na^+ activation of Na^+-Ca^+ exchange, Ca^{2+} channels, and impaired Ca^{2+} regulation by the sarcoplasmic reticulum [1, 42–44]. Electron probe x-ray microanalysis data presented by Walsh and Tormey [45] is consistent with a release of Ca^{2+} from the sarcoplasmic reticulum into the cytoplasm after reperfusion of ischemic myocardium. Reperfusion causes massive calcium accumulation in a population of injured cells, and there is some evidence that mildly injured cells also develop transient calcium loading. Although calcium accumulation is greatest in the necrotic subendocardium with reperfusion, ^{45}Ca studies indicate a transmural increase in calcium accumulation after 1–3 hours of coronary occlusion followed by reperfusion, suggesting that calcium loading also involves injured but salvageable myocardium [4]. Some observations from studies using technetium-99m stannous pyrophosphate (^{99m}Tc-PYP) provide some insight into this phenomenon [46]. It was found that when ^{99m}Tc-PYP was injected at the onset of reperfusion following a 3-hour occlusion, the uptake of ^{99m}Tc-PYP overestimated the myocardial infarction. If the administration was delayed for 90 minutes following reperfusion, the ^{99m}Tc-TYP infarct size correlated closely with the infarct size as measured using the triphenyl tetrazolium chloride staining technique. Thus there may be a population of injured myocytes which initially develop ^{99m}Tc-PYP uptake and calcium load which are later able to recover normal function. There have been beneficial effects of treatment with diltiazem, a calcium channel antagonist, on temporarily ischemic, reperfused myocardium. Earlier work indicated that diltiazem and propranolol, a beta adrenergic antagonist, permitted improved functional recovery and a smaller infarct size one month after a 4-hour coronary occlusion followed by reperfusion [43]. It was also found that diltiazem treatment increased the rate of function recovery in stunned myocardium over the first 24 hours of recovery following 15 minutes of coronary occlusion [47].

The role of Ca^{2+} loading in myocardial dysfunction and cell injury following coronary occlusion and reperfusion seems to be very important. The above observations are consistent with observations in the cultured cell model that suggest the ultimate fate of cells in terms of recovery and irreversible injury depends on a very complex interrelation between the severity of metabolic injury and the duration and amount of calcium accumulation.

Acknowledgements

Work from our institution was supported in part by NIH Ischemic Heart Disease SCOR Grant HL17669 and the Moss Heart Fund, Dallas, Texas.

References

1. Reimer KA, Jennings RB (1986) Myocardial ischemia, hypoxia, and infarction. In: HA Fozzard, E Haber, RB Jennings, AM Katz, HE Morgan (eds) The Heart and Cardiovascular System. Raven Press, New York, pp 1133–1201
2. Buja LM (1984) Basic pathologic processes of the heart: relationship to cardiomyopathies. In: N Sperelaiks (ed) Physiology and Pathophysiology of the Heart. Martinus Nijhoff Publishing, Boston, pp 43–57
3. Hagler HK, Burton KP, Buja LM (1981) Electron probe x-ray microanalysis of normal and injured myocardium: methods and results. In: TE Hutchinson, AP Somlyo (eds) Microprobe Analysis of Biological Systems. Academic Press, New York, pp 127–155
4. Buja LM, Burton KP, Hagler HK, Roan P, Willerson JT (1980) Calcium and lipid accumulation during evolution of experimental myocardial infarction. Circulation 62 (Suppl III): III–144
5. Morris AC, Hagler HK, Willerson JT, Buja LM (1989) Relationship between calcium loading and impaired energy metabolism during Na^+, K^+ pump inhibition and metabolic inhibition in cultured neonatal Ra^+ cardiac mydyotes. J Clin Invest 83: 1876–1887
6. Chien KR, Reeves JP, Buja LM, Bonte FJ, Parkey RW, Willerson JT (1981) Phospholipid alterations in canine ischemic myocardium. Temporal and topographical correlations with Tc-99m-PPi accumulation and an *in vitro* sarcolemmal Ca^{2+} permeability defect. Cir Res 48: 711–719
7. Chien KR, Han A, Sen A, Buja LM, Willerson JT (1984) Accumulation of unesterified arachidonic acid in ischemic canine myocardium: relationship to a phosphatidylcholine deacylation-reacylation cycle and depletion of membrane phospholipids. Cir Res 54: 313–322
8. Burton KP, Buja LM, Sen A, Willerson JT, Chien KR (1986) Accumulation of arachidonate in triacylglycerols and unesterified fatty acids during ischemia and reflow in the isolated rat heart: correlation with the loss of contractile function and the development of calcium overload. Am J Pathol 124: 238–245
9. Corr PB, Gross RW, Sobel BE (1984) Amphiphatic metabolites and membrane dysfunction in ischemic myocardium. Circ Res 55: 135–154
10. Burton KP (1988) Evidence of direct toxic effects of free radicals on the myocardium. Free Radical Biology and Medicine 4: 15–24
11. Steenbergen C, Hill ML, Jennings RB (1987) Cytoskeletal damage during myocardial

ischemia: changes in vinculin immunofluorescence staining during total *in vitro* ischemia in canine heart. Circ Res 60: 478–486

12. Ganote CE, Vander Heide RS (1987) Cytoskeletal lesions in anoxic myocardial injury: a conventional and high-voltage electron-microscopic and immunofluorescence study. Am J Pathol 129: 327–344

13. Sen A, Miller JC, Reynolds RC, Willerson JT, Buja LM, Chien KR (1988) Inhibition of the release of arachidonic acid prevents the development of sarcolemmal membrane defects in cultured rat myocardial cells during ATP depletion. J Clin Invest 82: 1333–1338

14. Burton KP, Hagler HK, Willerson JT, Buja LM (1981) Relationship of abnormal intracellular lanthanum accumulation to progression of ischemic injury in isolated perfused myocardium: effects of chlorpromazine. Am J Physiol 241: H714–H723

15. Das KD, Engleman RM, Rousou JA, Breyer RH, Otani H, Lemeshow S (1986) Role of membrane phospholipids in myocardial injury induced by ischemia and reperfusion. Am J Physiol 251: H71–H79

16. Buja LM, Muntz HK, Rosenbaum T, Haghani Z, Buja DK, Sen A, Chien KR, Willerson JT (1985) Characterization of a potentially reversible increase in beta adrenergic receptors in isolated, neonatal rat cardiac myocytes with impaired energy metabolism. Circ Res 57: 640–645

17. Shine KI (1981) Ionic events in ischemia and anoxia. Am J Pathol 102: 256–261

18. Willerson JT, Scales F, Mukherjee A, Platt MR, Templeton GH, Fink GC, Buja LM (1977) Abnormal myocardial fluid retention as an early manifestation of ischemic injury. Am J Pathol 87: 159–188

19. Buja LM, Willerson JT. (1981) Abnormalities of volume regulation and membrane integrity: in myocardial tissue slices after early ischemic injury in the dog: Effects of mannitol, polyethylene glycol and propranolol. Am J Pathol 103: 79–95

20. Burton KP, Hagler HK, Templeton GH, Willerson JT, Buja LM (1977) Lanthanum probe studies of cellular pathophysiology induced by hypoxia in isolated cardiac muscle. J Clin Invest 60: 1289–1302

21. Blinks JR (1986) Intracellular [Ca^{2+}] measurements. In: HA Fozzard, E Haber, RB Jennings, AM Katz, HE Morgan (eds) The Heart and Cardiovascular System: Scientific Foundations. Raven Press, New York, pp 671–701

22. Grynkiewicz G, Poenie M, Tsien RY (1985) A new generation of Ca^{2+} indicators with greatly improved flourescence properties. J Biol Chem 260: 3440–3450

23. Hagler HK, Lopez LE, Flores JS, Lundswick RJ, Buja LM (1983) Standards for quantitative energy dispersive x-ray microanalysis of biological cryosections: validation and application to studies of myocardium. J Microsc 131: 221–234

24. Hagler HK, Buja LM (1986) Effect of specimen preparation and section transfer techniques on the preservation of ultrastructure, lipids and elements in cryosections. J Microsc (Oxford) 141: 311–317

25. Buja LM, Hagler HK, Parsons D, Chien K, Reynolds RC, Willerson JT (1985) Alterations of ultrastructure and elemental composition in cultured neonatal rat cardiac myocytes after metabolic inhibition with iodoacetic acid. Lab Invest 53: 397–412

26. Buja LM, Williams PK, Buja DK, Chien KR, Willerson JT (1986) Comparative effects of cardiac myocyte injury induced by inhibition of the Na^+-K^+ pump and intermediary metabolism. Clin Res 34: 627A

27. Morris AC, Hagler HK, Buja LM (1988) Alterations in ionic calcium homeostasis in neonatal rat ventricular myocytes with metabolic inhibition. FASEB J 2: A1157

28. Jones RL, Miller JC, Williams PK, Chien KR, Willerson JT, Buja LM (1987) The relationship between arachidonate release and calcium overloading during ATP depletion in cultured neonatal rat cardiac myocytes. Fed Proc 46: 1152

29. Chien KR, Sen A, Reynolds RC, Chang A, Kim Y, Gunn MD, Buja LM, Willerson JT (1985) Release of arachidonate from membrane phospholipids in cultured neonatal rat myocardial cells during adenosine triphosphate depletion. J Clin Invest 75: 1770–1780

30. Gunn MD, Sen A, Chang A, Willerson JT, Buja LM, Chien KR (1985) Mechanisms of accumulation of arachidonic acid in cultured myocardial cells during ATP depletion. Am J Physiol 249: H1188–H1194

31. Murphy E, Jacob R, Lieberman M (1985) Cytosolic free calcium in thick heart cells: its role in cell injury. J Mol Cell Cardiol 17: 221–231

32. Parsons D, Burton KP, Hagler HK, Buja LM (1987) Contractile and elemental changes induced by calcium overload in papillary muscles. Fed Proc 46: 1404

33. Barry WH, Peeters GA, Rasmussen CAF Jr, Cunningham MJ (1987) Role of changes in $[Ca^{2+}]_i$ in energy deprivation contracture. Circ Res 61: 726–734

34. Ishida H, Kohmoto O, Bridge JHB, Barry WH (1988) Alterations in cation homeostasis in cultured chick ventricular cells during and after recovery from adenosine triphosphate depletion. J Clin Invest 81: 1173–1181

35. Kim D, Cragoe EJ Jr, Smith TW (1987) Relations among sodium pump inhibition, Na-Ca and Na-H exchange activities, and Ca-H interaction in cultured chick heart cells. Circ Res 60: 185–193

36. Kim D, Okada A, Smith TW (1987) Control of cytosolic calcium activity during low sodium exposure in cultured chick heart cells. Circ Res 61: 29–41

37. Haworth RA, Goknur AB, Hunter DR, Hegge JO, Berkoff HA (1987) Inhibition of calcium influx in isolated adult rat heart cells by ATP depletion. Circ Res 60: 586–594

38. Cheung JY, Bonventre JV, Malis CD, Leaf A (1986) Calcium and ischemic injury. New Engl J Med 314: 1670–1676

39. Lee H-C, Smith N, Mohabir R, Clusin WT (1987) Cytosolic calcium transients from the beating mammalian heart. Proc Natl Acad Sci USA 84: 7793–7797

40. Steenbergen C, Murphy E, Levy L, London RE (1987) Elevation in cytosolic free calcium concentration early in myocardial ischemia in perfused rat heart. Circ Res 60: 700–707

41. Marban E, Kitakaze M, Kusuoka H, Porterfield JK, Yue DT, Chacko VP (1987) Intracellular free calcium concentration measured with 19F NMR spectroscopy in intact ferret hearts. Proc Natl Acad Sci USA 84: 6005–6009

42. Weisfeld ML (1987) Reperfusion and reperfusion injury. Clin Res 35: 13–20

43. Bush LR, Buja LM, Tilton G, Wathen M, Apprill P, Ashton J, Willerson JT (1985) Effects of propranolol and diltiazen alone and in combination on the recovery of left ventricular segmental function after long-term reperfusion following temporary coronary occlusion in conscious dogs. Circulation 72: 413–430

44. Kusuoka H, Porterfield JK, Weisman HF, Weisfeldt ML, Marban E (1987) Pathophysiology and pathogenesis of stunned myocardium: depressed Ca^{2+} activation of contraction as a consequence of reperfusion-induced cellular calcium overload in ferret hearts. J Clin Invest 79: 950–961

45. Walsh LG, Tormey J McD (1988) Subcellular shifts of electrolytes during myocardial ischemia and reperfusion. Am J Physiol 255: H917–H928

46. Jansen DE, Corbett JR, Buja LM, Hansen C, Ugolini V, Parkey RW, Willerson JT (1987) Quantification of myocardial injury produced by temporary coronary artery occlusion and reflow with technetium-99m pyrophosphate. Circulation 75: 611–617

47. Taylor AL, Golino P, Buja LM, Eckels RM (1987) Is post ischemic systolic dysfunction principally caused by reperfusion? Circulation 76 (Suppl IV): IV–228

Causes and effects of changes in cytosolic free calcium in the hypoxic myocardial cell

ASHLEY P. ALLSHIRE and PETER H. COBBOLD

Department of Human Anatomy and Cell Biology, The University of Liverpool, P.O. Box 147, Liverpool L69 3BX, UK

Key words: Ca_i, contracture, rigor, Na-Ca exchange, Na_i

Abstract

We review cytosolic free calcium (Ca_i) measurements in hypoxic single cardiomyocytes, isolated heart tissue and intact myocardium. In single cells the seminal event may be a shortening which is (largely) Ca_i-independent and probably corresponds to hypoxic contracture of intact tissue. This shortening is soon followed by a Ca_i rise and net Ca^{2+} ingress across the sarcolemma which is sensitive to the Na^+ electrochemical gradient, suggesting that Na-Ca exchange occurs, and that a Na_i imbalance precedes the Ca_i rise. Reoxygenation of single cells triggers spontaneous mechanical activity (and oscillation of Ca^{2+} between cytosol and sarcoplasmic reticulum) analogous to reoxygenation arrhythmias in intact myocardium, and provided that Ca_i has not risen above several micromolar it is returned to resting levels. We interpret the Ca_i-independent shortening as a rigor which activates the myosin ATPase and thereby accelerates ATP depletion so that ATPase-linked ion pumps in the cell membranes become limited thermodynamically. An ensuing Na_i rise leads through depressed Na-Ca exchange to a Ca_i rise. Such a model highlights rigor-compex mediated activation of myosin S1-ATPase as the fundamental target for interventions to ameliorate ischemic damage to the myocardium.

Introduction

Calcium overload has for many years been proposed as a fundamental mechanism in the ischemic injury of the myocardium [1]. At some point during deterioration of cellular metabolism the cytosolic concentration of free calcium ions (Ca_i) must rise. The electrochemical gradient for Ca^{2+} across the sarcolemma is of the order of 10^6 and must be maintained by active processes which are susceptible to metabolic blockade. In this chapter, we relate measured changes in Ca_i to other pathophysiological processes such as changes in the cell's mechanical properties, ATP status, rigor activation of

H.M. Piper (ed.) Pathophysiology of severe ischemic myocardial injury, 297–314.
© *1990 Kluwer Academic Publishers, Dordrecht*

actomyosin, and other intracellular ions, especially Na^+. Having established temporal relationships, we propose a sequence of events in which Ca_i rises relatively late, and propose a causal interrelation between falling ATP, rigor activation of myosin ATPase, further rapid depletion of ATP leading to alteration of Na^+ gradients and ending in perturbation of calcium homeostasis through impaired Na-Ca exchange. Since most myocardial injury occurs during readmission of oxygen to metabolically inhibited cells ('oxygen paradox') we also consider the role of Ca_i here, notably the large-amplitude Ca_i oscillations that have been measured in reoxygenated myocytes.

The pathophysiological phenomena that we attempt to explain are summarised by the simultaneous recordings made by Allen and Smith [2] of Ca_i and tension in ferret papillary muscle depleted of glycogen and poisoned with cyanide (Fig. 1). This article concentrates solely upon the adult myocardial cell whether in isolation, within a multicellular preparation (usually papillary muscle) or *in situ* in the whole heart.

Effects of metabolic blockade on sarcosolic free Ca^{2+} concentration

The past decade has seen enormous improvements in techniques for measuring Ca_i in cells, from the use of fluorescent and bioluminescent probes in single isolated cells or multicellular preparations, to fluorescent and NMR probes in whole hearts. Here we relate Ca_i measurements to the mechanical properties of the myocytes in the preparation (e.g. cell shape, papillary muscle tension, intra-ventricular pressure) and draw together information from poisoned single cells through to the whole hypoxic heart.

Ca_i in single isolated cardiomyocytes

In the absence of manageable procedures for monitoring the tension developed by a single isolated cardiomyocyte, workers in this field have had to resort to recording the shape of the cell, normally a rod-shaped structure of about $100 \times 20 \times 6-10$ µm. Glucose-free anoxia eventually leads to a shortening of the cell and loss of distinct sarcomeres, but retention of the polygonal outline. Reoxygenation then leads, essentially, to either retention of the rod-shaped form (with or without some relengthening) or to a rounding-up of the cell and blebbing of the cell surface. Stern *et al.* [3] have shown that the time elapsed since the cell shortens determines its response to reoxygenation: the longer the time the greater the probability of rounding-up and blebbing, which they term hypercontracture. If a cell is still unshortened, reoxygenation does not trigger this hypercontraction [3]. Thus shortening of the myocyte represents a turning point in its response to reoxygenation. It is a significant event in the deterioration of the cell and needs to be understood. In several studies Ca_i was monitored in myocytes undergoing the transition

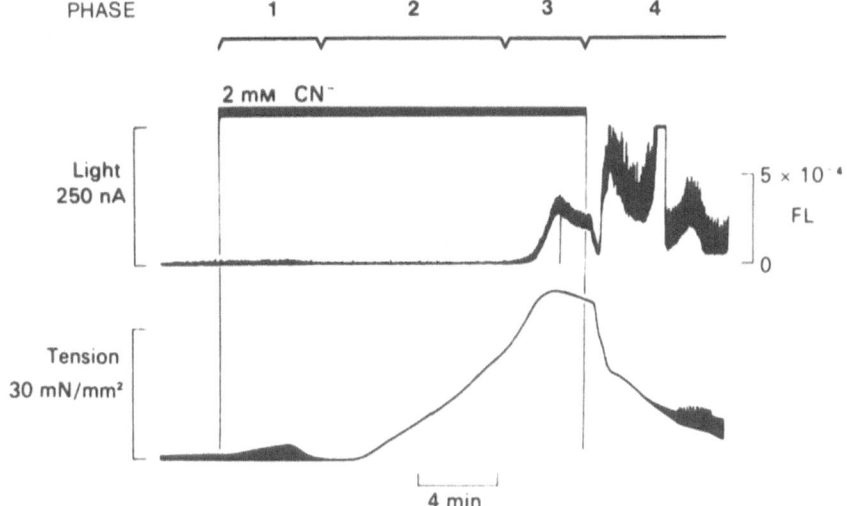

Fig. 1. Cyanide effect on Ca$_i$-dependent aequorin light (upper panel; FL, fractional luminescence) and tension (lower panel) in a paced ferret papillary muscle. The muscle had been depleted of glycogen by prolonged stimulation before cyanide was added to inhibit oxidative phosphorylation. Temperature, 30°C. [Reprinted in adapted form by permission from J. Physiol. (London) *369*, 92P. © 1985 The Physiological Society.]

Phase (1), contractile failure; (2), contracture develops while Ca$_i$ remains at the control 'diastolic' level; (3), Ca$_i$ begins to rise during the later stage of contracture; (4), removal of cyanide leads to a gradual reverse of contracture and recovery of contractility; Ca$_i$ falls transiently, rises again, then gradually and erratically returns toward control levels.

from rod-shaped (healthy controls) to shortened and thence to rounded-up; Fig. 2 summarises the data.

A broad view of the data presented in Fig. 2 suggests that isolated cardiomyocytes shorten while Ca$_i$ remains low, or if a small rise has occurred Ca$_i$ is still too low to explain shortening on the basis of Ca-troponin C-mediated activation of actomoysin. The shortening event itself usually occurs over a relatively short period, about half a minute, but no accompanying transient rise in Ca$_i$ is apparent. Rather, Ca$_i$ increases once shortening is complete. In those cases where a small rise prior to shortening has been reported [4], Ca$_i$ still rises markedly after shortening. Whether Ca$_i$ starts to rise slightly prior to shortening, or not, may depend upon the protocol used for attaching the cell to the substrate. In Fig. 2, cells in panels a and b were cocooned in agarose gel and free to contract, in panel c they had been allowed to settle and attach to a glass coverslip. In a recent study, anoxic cardiomyocytes attached to a silicone substratum did not shorten although Ca$_i$ as measured with Fura-2 rose to micromolar; however, less firmly attached cells shortened before the Ca$_i$ rise began [5]. Other differences may be attributable to the intensity of metabolic blockade; the more intense the blockade the more rapid the onset of pathophysiological decay and the less chance of

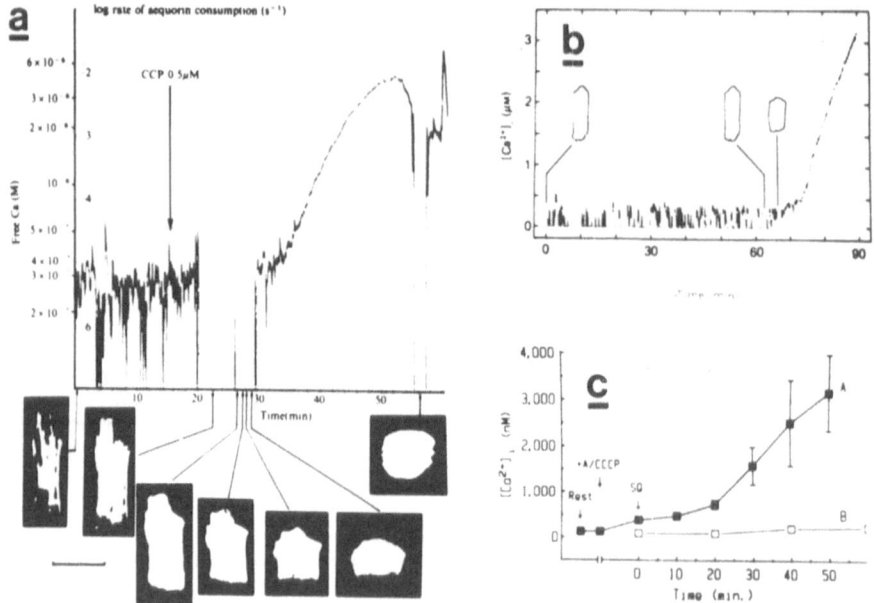

Fig. 2. Ca$_i$ and shape changes in individual rat cardiomyocytes during anoxia/'chemical' hypoxia. Temperature, 37°C.

a: Shortening of a cell before Ca$_i$ begins to rise, following exposure to the mitochondrial uncoupler carbonyl cyanide *m*-chlorophenylhydrazone (CCP). Scale bar, 50 μm. [Reprinted by permission from Nature *312*, 444–446, © 1984 Macmillan Magazines Ltd.]

b: Anoxia. In this cell Ca$_i$ was not significantly different before and after shortening (means 183 nM over 1000 sec, and 258 nM over 60 sec, respectively; p>0.05). Ca$_i$ remained below 350 nM for 78 sec and below 400 nM for 109 sec after shortening was first detected (p < 0.05). [Reprinted by permission from Biochem. J. *244*, 381–385; © 1987 The Biochemical Society, London.]

c: ATP depletion with amytal and CCP (A); control, (B). Cell shortening complete at SQ. [Reprinted by permission from Am. J. Physiol. *255*, C162–C168, © 1988 The American Physiological Society.]

resolving subtle temporal differences in the time-course of the decay processes. If, as we propose later, shortening itself leads to accelerated ATP consumption, then in experimental protocols in which rapid ATP depletion is induced by the experimental intervention *per se* the effect of the endogenous ATP depletion may be masked. We therefore place more emphasis on those experiments in which metabolic inhibition takes a relatively long time to develop (e.g. panel b).

Studies on populations of isolated myocytes by Haworth *et al.* support the conclusion that shortening can occur without a rise in Ca$_i$. The time-course of the onset of shortening of cells in a population is independent of extracellular calcium [9] and indo-1 measurements show that Ca$_i$ rises very little in cells in contracture despite depletion of 96% of their ATP content[10,11].Buffering of Ca$_i$ to about 10 nM with quin2 at high intracellular concentrations had no effect on either the time-course of onset, or the extent of myocyte shortening. While these experiments involve extreme metabolic blockade to deplete ATP levels rapidly and synchronously within the population, they do illustrate that myocyte shortening can occur independently of any rise in Ca_i.

Ca_i in multicellular preparations

In papillary muscle preparations tension and Ca_i can be monitored simultaneously in either small populations or even single cells. The pioneering work of Allen and colleagues (as in Fig. 1) showed clearly a rise in diastolic tension prior to any rise in Ca_i above the detection limit of about 400 nM [2]. Later work from this group, using either hypoxia or metabolic poisons, also demonstrated a contracture tension while Ca_i was not raised by more than a factor of 1.4 above resting levels [12]. Indeed Ca_i begins to rise only about 10 minutes later, by which time tension has reached two or three times the developed tension in the healthy muscle [13]. Studies using the mitochondrial uncoupler FCCP in conjunction with either aequorin [14] or Ca-selective microelectrodes [15] also revealed tension rises without an accompanying rise in Ca_i. Thus data from papillary muscle indicate that considerable Ca_i-independent tension can be generated during metabolic inhibition.

Ca_i in the whole heart

Indo-1 has been used to follow contraction transient failure in ischemia by monitoring surface fluorescence of the whole heart [16] but has not yet, to our knowledge, been used to study prolonged ischemic contracture. Measurements with the NMR probe 5F-BAPTA showed that global ischemia induces no immediate change in Ca_i despite a rapid decline in the NMR signals from creatine phosphate and ATP [17]. However, these data lack adequate resolution to resolve the time course of Ca_i changes in relation to contracture (monitored as intraventricular pressure). Resting tension rose markedly after 7–8 minutes; Ca_i was normal over 5–6 minutes but was raised after 9–10 minutes.

Thus the effects of ischemia on Ca_i and tension in intact heart have yet to be shown to differ dramatically from the sequence in isolated cells or papillary muscle.

Rigor complexes activate actomyosin in metabolically inhibited cardiomyocytes

We have shown above that metabolic blockade can induce mechanical activity (shortening, tension development) while Ca_i remains at, or very close to, resting levels. The most likely mechanism by which this Ca_i-independent tension is generated is through the formation of rigor complexes between myosin and actin. A rigor complex is formed between a nucleotide-free myosin S1-ATPase and an adjacent actin. A rigor complex can activate adjacent S1-ATPases in the absence of a rise in Ca_i. This process could thereby induce tension development and provide another route for ATP hydrolysis. Here we summarise evidence for the involvement of rigor complexes in contracture of the hypoxic myocardial cell.

Rigor complexes in vitro

If a muscle is first cooled and then permeabilised and washed free of ATP it forms an inelastic structure in which all the myosin head groups are attached by ATP-free rigor complexes to adjacent actins. A sarcomere spacing representative of the relaxed state is retained, and such material has long been popular for biophysical and crystallographic studies. If, however, the muscle is not cooled, despite rigorous chelation of calcium it will contract during permeabilisation. It seems that levels of ATP intermediate between those needed for full dissociation of myosin from actin (about 0.1 mM) and zero can activate actomyosin. This is thought to occur by a rigor complex impeding relaxation of tropomyosin within the groove along the actin filament, thereby allowing adjacent myosins along the 7-actin grouping controlled by that tropomyosin molecule to become actin-activated. Providing some ATP is present, a Ca-independent activation of actomyosin can thus occur. The rigor complexes essentially mimic the tropomyosin configuration normally endowed by Ca-troponin C. Rigor complex activation of myosin S1-ATPase was first described *in vitro* by Bremel and Weber [8] and further characterised by Murray *et al.* [19]. As ATP was reduced below 0.1 mM the Ca-independent activity of the S1-ATPase rose. Bremel and Weber concluded that 'rigor complexes elicit a co-operative response from actin filaments which causes all actin molecules of the filament to be "turned on" in the absence of calcium [18].'

A second effect of low ATP levels (about 0.1 mM) is to enhance the affinity of troponin C for calcium, possibly through rigor complex formation [20]. This effect can only generate 10% or so of the maximal Ca-activated tension, whereas rigor complex-activation can easily exceed Ca-mediated tension development.

Evidence for rigor complex formation in the myocardial cell

Here we offer an explanation for the data summarized above which show that myocardial contracture can occur without any rise in Ca_i. The evidence supporting rigor-mediated contracture comes from studies on papillary muscle and whole heart.

Analysis of the response of hypoxic papillary muscle to perturbations in length [21] showed that contracture involved a stiffness independent of active force development (however, reoxygenation contracture could be explained in terms of Ca_i-dependent active force development). Ventura-Clapier and Vassort observed that cyanide or hypoxia progressively impaired tension recovery following quick releases of papillary muscle [22]. They concluded that the rise in resting tension following metabolic inhibition is mediated by the formation of rigor bridges rather than by activation of the contractile proteins by calcium. Holubarsch [23] used a similar protocol and reached the same conclusion. Previously Holubarsch et al. [24] had monitored heat production of papillary muscle and concluded, again, that hypoxic contracture results from rigor-like cross-bridges with no, or very little, heat production, consistent with slowly cycling cross-bridges.

ATP levels promoting rigor complexes

In vitro studies of myosin S1-ATPase in the presence of tropomyosin-decorated F actin indicate that rigor complex activation requires 10–100 μM ATP [19]. However, these data were obtained at low ionic strength and in dilute solution and may not be applicable to thick and thin filaments in situ. Fabiato and Fabiato [20] detected rigor activation in permeabilised cells at about 50 μM MgATP. These studies used pure MgATP, whereas inorganic phosphate (Pi) is likely to increase during metabolic blockade in vivo to as much as 30 mM [25] and has been shown to weaken rigor complexes in skinned fibres [26]. So, the rise in Pi in vivo might be expected to impair rigor tension developing at a given MgATP concentration (rigor tension would be approximately halved in the presence of 20 mM Pi). Permeabilised isolated cardiomyocytes undergo Ca_i-independent shortening when the concentration of MgATP in the bathing medium is reduced. Altschuld et al. [27] observed shortening at 1–10 μM MgATP, and Haworth et al. [9] at 50–100 μM MgATP (corresponding to 0.15 nmol ATP mg-1 wet weight).

ATP levels in isolated myocytes and whole hearts

The first measurements of ATP in suspensions of isolated cells were complicated by asynchrony between the myocytes' shortening [9]. Recently Haworth et al. have used a synchronous ATP-depletion protocol [11] to deplete ATP very rapidly indeed, and found that cells shorten only when about 95% of their ATP content is lost (Ca_i remains below 100 nM – ref. [10]). Unfortunately such whole cell measurements cannot resolve cytosolic and mitochondrial ATP pools, so a direct comparison with permeabilised cells is difficult.

Measurements of ATP in the whole heart are complicated by regional differences, differences in cell types, extracellular volume, speed of contractile failure, perfusion and so forth, as well as the above-mentioned sub-compartmentation. Allen and Orchard [25] provide a recent overview. In our view the complexity of these whole organ studies make it unlikely that a clear-cut relationship between ATP and mechanical properties could be expected.

We conclude that rigor complexes forming at MgATP levels in the cytosol of around 10–100 µM (or lower when Pi is elevated) are the most likely cause of the observed Ca_i-independent mechanical changes, including shortening of isolated myocytes, increased diastolic tension in papillary muscle and the rise in intraventricular pressure of the ischemic heart.

Why and how does Ca_i rise?

Ca_i begins to rise after rigor complexes have activated actomyosin in a Ca-independent fashion (see Figs. 1, 2). Why should Ca_i rise, and which fluxes into and out of the cytosolic compartment predominate? The most detailed understanding has come from direct measurement of Ca_i in single cells or small populations.

The Ca_i rise depends upon an influx of Ca^{2+}

Here we summarise recent data from our laboratory, in which aequorin was used to monitor Ca_i in single isolated rat cardiomyocytes.

a) Metabolic poisoning or glucose-free anoxia in nominally Ca-free media causes myocytes to shorten without a subsequent rise in Ca_i (Fig. 3a).

b) Ca_i rises can be reversed by a period in Ca-free medium (Fig. 3b). However, when Ca is returned a few minutes later, Ca_i jumps to approximately the level it would have reached had the level of extracellular Ca been maintained throughout. Similar observations have been made in papillary muscle [13, Fig. 10], and in single cardiomyocytes loaded with Fura-2 [8, Fig. 2]. Thus a progressive resetting of the equilibrium between the fluxes moving calcium into and out of the cytosol, leading to increasing Ca_i, appears to occur rather than a 'filling-up' of the cytosol with calcium.

c) Net Ca ingress is blocked by Ni (Fig. 3c) Co, Mn and La but is apparently insensitive to either verapamil (Fig. 3d) or lidoflazine. Thus instead of leaking through gross 'holes' in the sarcolemma, we envisage Ca entering cells via a channel(s) probably distinct from the voltage-gated Ca channel (i_{si}). This pharmacological profile strongly resembles that described by Poole-Wilson *et al.* for ^{45}Ca influx into hypoxic interventricular septum [1].

d) The flux of ^{45}Ca into shortened myocytes is actually *slower* than in healthy cells [10]. ATP depletion also impairs both ^{45}Ca influx and the rate

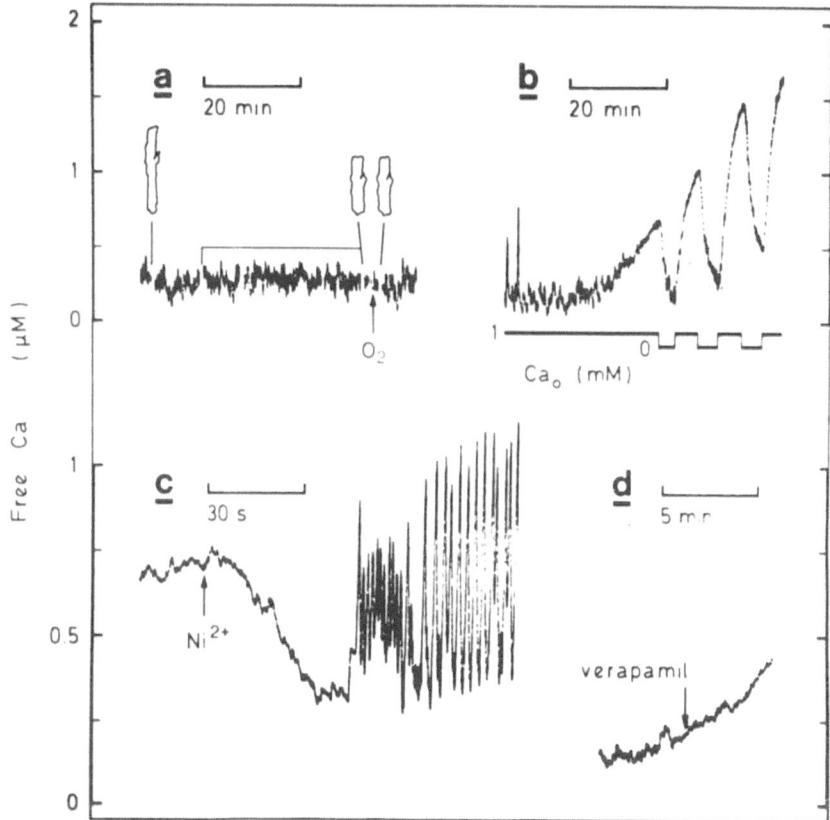

Fig. 3. Aequorin measurements of Ca$_i$ in single cardiomyocytes under anoxia (a) or 'chemical' hypoxia, i.e. 2 mM cyanide and 5 mM 2-deoxyglucose (b-d). The aequorin signal was calibrated at 1 mM free Mg^{2+}; temperature, 37°C; other conditions as in 7, 28.

Effects of (a) nominally Ca^{2+}-free superfusion medium on Ca$_i$ and cell shape, and effects on the Ca$_i$ rise of (b) changes in the extracellular Ca^{2+} concentration (data exponentially smoothed with time constant of 5 sec), (c) 1 mM NiCl$_2$ (time constant 0.5 sec; reprinted in adapted form by permission from Biochem. Soc. Trans. *15*, 960, © 1987 The Biochemical Society, London), and (d) 5 µM verapamil.

of Ca$_i$ rise [8]. The Ca$_i$ rise which takes place must therefore reflect a more than commensurate reduction of Ca efflux from the cytosol. Finally, the measured rise in Ca$_i$ will underestimate the amount of Ca entering the cell if part is sequestered by the sarcoplasmic reticulum.

Causes of raised Ca$_i$

A rise in Ca$_i$ that depends on extracellular calcium but involves a reduction in ^{45}Ca influx requires a still greater reduction of Ca efflux from the cytosol. Since the Ca$_i$ rise follows myocyte shortening, which we have shown to result from rigor complexes forming as a result of severe ATP depletion, an

306

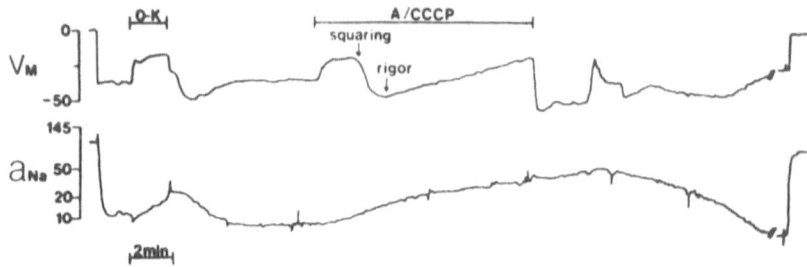

Fig. 4. Membrane potential (Vm) and Na$^+$ activity (a_{Na}) measured by microelectrode in a single isolated cardiomyocyte during and after an episode of ATP depletion. A/CCCP, amytal (3 mM) + CCP (2 μM). [Reprinted by permission of the publisher from Li *et al.*, *in* Biology of isolated adult cardiac myocytes (W.A. Clark *et al.*, eds.) pp. 342–345, copyright 1988 by Elsevier Science Publishing Co., Inc.]

impairment of ATP-dependent ion pumps could underlie the reduced efflux. Although the sarcolemmal Ca,Mg-ATPase could begin to reverse at low ATP concentrations, this is unlikely to be important because it would enhance rather than curtail Ca influx. A diminution of ATPase-linked Ca efflux may indeed occur, but the low capacity of this route suggests that effects on Na-Ca exchange may be more important.

The effectiveness of the Na-Ca exchanger in removing Ca^{2+} from the cytosol depends upon the Na$^+$ electrochemical gradient across the sarcolemma, and hence upon the Na,K-ATPase. This pump may become thermodynamically limited by the declining free energy of ATP hydrolysis at around the time the cell shortens. Impaired Na pumping would cause the concentration of Na$^+$ in the cytosol, Na$_i$, to rise. Electrode measurements have shown that Na$_i$ increases steadily in both papillary muscle during glucose-free hypoxia [29] and in metabolically poisoned single cardiomyocytes [30]. Li *et al.* [30] found that Na$_i$ begins to rise (from less than 10 mM) a minute or so before the cell shortens, and reaches 50 mM some 13 minutes later (Fig. 4). Elevated Na$_i$ may depress Ca^{2+} extrusion via Na-Ca exchange, so that a Ca$_i$ rise follows the Na$_i$ rise. However, simultaneous measurements of Ca$_i$, Na$_i$ and membrane voltage in the same cell will be needed to test this linkage. Ultimately a progressive rise in Na$_i$ would deplete the Na$^+$ electrochemical gradient to the extent that it can no longer drive Ca^{2+} extrusion, whereupon the exchange reverses and Na$^+$ extrusion is coupled to Ca^{2+} ingress and dissipation of the Ca^{2+} gradient. However, in the early stages of the Ca$_i$ rise Na-Ca exchange is likely to run in the 'forward' mode since depletion of cell ATP reduces Ca^{2+} influx [10]. Instead, the still further reduced efflux which must pertain (if Ca$_i$ is to rise) probably represents a depressed Na-Ca exchange due to elevated Na$_i$ and perhaps an as yet undefined role for ATP in modulating the activity of the exchanger (discussed by Haworth *et al.*, ref [10]) In aequorin-injected cardiomyocytes the Ca$_i$ rise is accelerated and retarded, respectively, by small (10 mM) decreases or increases in extracellular Na [31, and unpublished results]. Hence the exchanger is still functional, although its contribution to Ca^{2+} efflux and/or influx has not yet been established. Nevertheless, it is possible that the rise in Ca_i does reflect a resetting of the Na-Ca exchange flux as Na_i rises because of a curtailed extrusion of Na^+ on the ATPase-linked pump.

With the introduction of new fluorescent probes of Na_i more direct tests of the contribution of sodium perturbation to the Ca_i rise should be feasible. At present we favour this route for the net Ca^{2+} ingress over earlier speculation that ATP depletion leads to partial reversal of the sarcolemmal Ca^{2+} pump [31].

Importance of the rise in Ca_i

Since cardiomyocytes have already lost their primary function, contractility, by the time Ca_i begins to rise we may ask whether it is particularly important to study it. Indeed, if the cell does not have its ATP supply restored Ca_i presumably rises to levels sufficiently high to activate Ca-dependent proteases and phospholipases, thereby inducing irreparable damage to cell structure and compartmentalisation. The extent of the rise in Ca_i is, however, of key importance when we consider the effects of reoxygenation.

Reoxygenation

The oxygen paradox is central to understanding reperfusion injury in the ischemic heart. It is during the few minutes of reoxygenation that most myocardial injury occurs. Here we survey measurements of Ca_i under these conditions and discuss the large amplitude Ca_i oscillations which follow reoxygenation or removal of metabolic blockade, and attempt to account for their generation.

Ca_i in single isolated myocytes

Aequorin-injected rat cardiomyocytes subjected to glucose-free anoxia first shorten, then Ca_i starts to rise. If reoxygenation is carried out when Ca_i has reached 1–3 µM we observe a response like that shown in Fig. 5a [7, 32]: Ca_i first falls toward resting levels over 20–30 s, then begins to oscillate. The largest transient in this train (not shown) had a duration of about 2 seconds and reached a Ca_i of 4 µM from a 'diastolic' level of approximately 500 nM. Finally, after 5–15 min the transients cease and Ca_i returns to resting levels. During this period the cell either retains its truncated shape or rounds up (probably very promptly, within seconds of readmitting O_2), and twitches in concert with the Ca_i spikes. In other experiments, we have reoxygenated

308

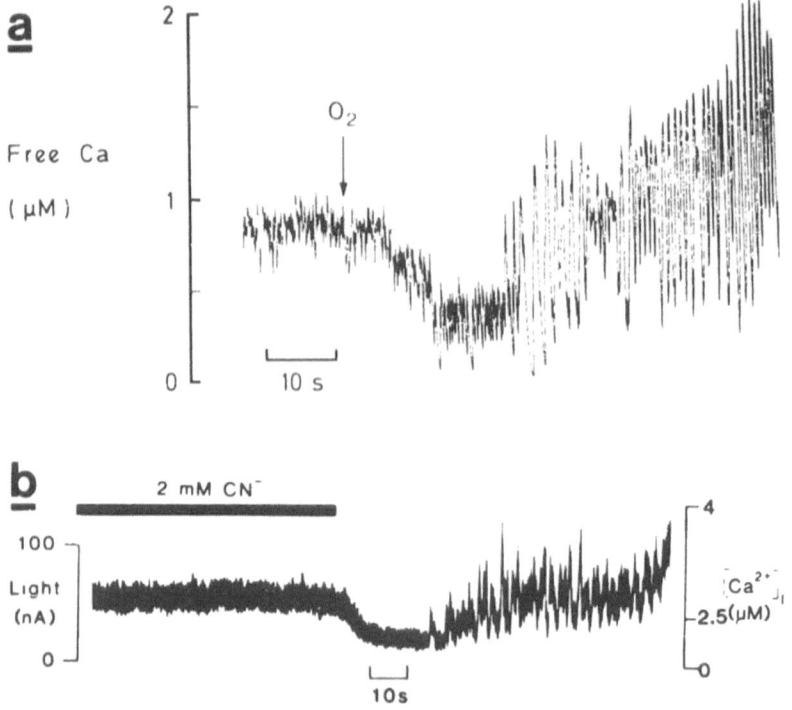

Fig. 5. The Ca$_i$ oscillations which follow removal of metabolic blockade, measured with aequorin.

a: Reoxygenation of an isolated anoxic rat cardiomyocyte. Temperature, 37°C (other conditions given in 7); time constant 0.1 sec. [Reprinted in adapted form by permission from *Phil. Trans. R. Soc. Lond. B 320*, 325–343, © 1988 The Royal Society, London.]

b: Removal of cyanide from a glycogen-depleted ferret papillary muscle. [Reprinted by permission of The American Heart Association, Inc., from Smith, G.L., Allen, D.G. (1988) Effects of metabolic blockade on intracellular calcium concentration in isolated ferret ventricular muscle. *Circ Res 62*, 1223–1236.]

shortened cells while Ca$_i$ was still less than 1 μM; in this case the cells remained rod-shaped, but an episode of Ca$_i$ oscillations and mechanical activity lasting several minutes occurred before the cells restored Ca$_i$ to resting levels and became quiescent again. These different effects of reoxygenation upon cell shape have been emphasised by Stern *et al.* [3]; the responses of both cell shape and Ca$_i$ are markedly dependent on the time elapsed since shortening. The underlying cause appears to be the Ca$_i$ rise which develops during this period. If Ca$_i$ is allowed to exceed about 3 μM before oxygen is reintroduced, there is at most only a partial fall in Ca$_i$ before it goes on to still higher levels and exhausts remaining aequorin. These cells quickly and invariably round up and bleb; it is unlikely that Ca$_i$ is returned to resting levels after the aequorin has been fully discharged, so by this criterion such cells could be regarded as non-viable.

Ca$_i$ in papillary muscle

Allen and colleagues have described the fall in Ca$_i$ and subsequent oscillations in aequorin-injected cells *in situ* in ferret papillary muscle. Figure 1 shows that wash-out of cyanide leads to just such a response of free Ca, although the oscillations in individual cells were not resolved within the preparation which included several hundred cells injected with aequorin. Presumably, the oscillations are not synchronised between cells (as suggested too by the lack of oscillations in the tension recording). After about 5 minutes, the aequorin signal and tension return toward control levels. Smith and Allen [13] obtained similar recordings from both glycogen-depleted papillary muscle and from single cells *in situ* on removing cyanide. Figure 5b is reproduced from ref. [13] – the resemblance to the record from single isolated cardiomyocytes during reoxygenation (Fig. 5a) is striking. Smith and Allen refer to these Ca$_i$ oscillations after the removal of metabolic blockade as arrhythmias, which are a characteristic feature of the oxygen paradox. Such oscillatory behaviour of Ca$_i$ could underlie much of the unco-ordinated mechanical activity and tissue injury that occurs upon reoxygenation. A further parallel with isolated cells is the failure of papillary muscle to recover low Ca$_i$ levels if metabolic blockade was not removed until Ca$_i$ exceeded about 2.5 μM [13].

Mechanism of the reoxygenation-induced Ca$_i$ oscillations

Smith and Allen [13] argue that the Ca$_i$ oscillations result from a Ca overload within the sarcoplasmic reticulum, the Ca^{2+} being cyclically released and resequestered only when ATP is resupplied. However, the experiment shown in Fig. 3c demonstrates that net ATP resupply is not necessary to the production of either the fall in Ca$_i$ or the subsequent oscillations. Superfusing a cyanide/2-deoxyglucose-poisoned cardiomyocyte with 1 mM Ni causes Ca$_i$ to fall then oscillate, much as we see upon reoxygenation (Fig. 5a). Similar responses can be induced with Mn and Co but, interestingly, not with La (which induces the fall in Ca$_i$ but no subsequent oscillations). That the Ca$_i$ responses correspond so closely is remarkable, bearing in mind that the reoxygenated cell will have rapidly regenerated ATP to about 25% of control levels [33] whereas the Ni-treated cell will remain depleted of ATP. The Ni-induced oscillations reveal that a cell severely deficient in ATP retains an ability to generate rapid Ca^{2+} fluxes into and out of the cytosol; clearly Ca$_i$ cannot be described as being 'out of control' under these conditions.

What is the role of the putative calcium overload in the SR? Smith and Allen [13] note similarities in the Ca$_i$ oscillations in muscle with oscillations induced in Ca-loaded cardiac cells. We have shown that caffeine, which blocks Ca^{2+} uptake and induces Ca^{2+} release from the SR, also blocks the Ca$_i$ fall and oscillations induced by reoxygenation [7, 32], and prevents the oscillations (but only slows the initial fall) in Ni-treated cells [28]. Why the SR should release Ca^{2+} cyclically is not known. Smith and Allen [13] suggest that spontaneous Ca^{2+} release from the SR triggers (Ca^{2+}-activated) transient inward Ca currents which in turn induce the next episode of Ca^{2+} release from the SR. However, since Ni blocks Ca channels, experiments like that in Fig. 3c argue against the involvement of an inward Ca current: under these conditions, and perhaps on reoxygenation, a cyclical uptake and release of Ca^{2+} from the SR can proceed independently of specific sarcolemmal Ca channels. (On the other hand, Smith and Allen report Ni as depressing the Ca_i oscillations provoked by cyanide removal (Fig. 11 of ref. [13])). Fabiato has described calcium-induced release of calcium by SR in the absence of sarcolemma [34], but this is probably distinct from Ca^{2+} release from over-loaded SR, or from caffeine-induced release.

Removal of extracellular Ca or addition of La do not induce oscillations despite inducing an initial fall in Ca_i to 500 nM or less, which suggests that the oscillations may require an entry of Ca^{2+} across the sarcolemma. It is conceivable in view of the ability of La or low extracellular Ca, but not Ni, Mn, Co or verapamil, to abolish these oscillations that the trigger calcium crosses the sarcolemma by a route that is insensitive to classical divalent channel antagonists. Phasic contractions which propagate spontaneously from either end of non-excited cardiomyocytes also suggest the existence of a Ca^{2+} influx which is unaffected by Ca channel antagonists. The route might consist of remnants of gap junctions in the intercalated disc region of the cell, and permit Ca^{2+} entry in the presence of competing ions. The effect of La could be explained in these terms if it too entered the cell and blocked initiation of Ca^{2+} release from the SR. However, the mechanism of reoxygenation-induced Ca_i oscillations clearly requires further study, particularly in view of the ability of caffeine, ryanodine and transient low-Ca perfusion to lessen perfusion-induced arrhythmias in the ischemic heart [35, 36].

Hypothesis for mechanisms of hypoxia-reoxygenation injury

The hypothesis we propose here is in broad agreement with that of Smith and Allen [13], but we place greater emphasis on the time-course of events, which is more readily discerned and resolved in single cells. Figure 6 summarises the sequence we envisage. Its main features include:

a) Shortening of the myocyte represents a significant turning point in deterioration of the cell, as noted by Stern et al. [3]. We think that shortening may be accompanied by a sudden depletion of the remaining cellular ATP through activation of myosin ATPase by rigor complexes, so that ATP-dependent Na^+ pumping is impaired and Na_i rises. This concept is consistent with the 'asynchronous ATP depletion' model of Haworth et al. [11]. Unfortunately, direct measurements of ATP in single cells are not yet feasible, but such a hypothesis would explain why both Na_i and Ca_i start to rise significantly above resting levels once cells have shortened. Presum-

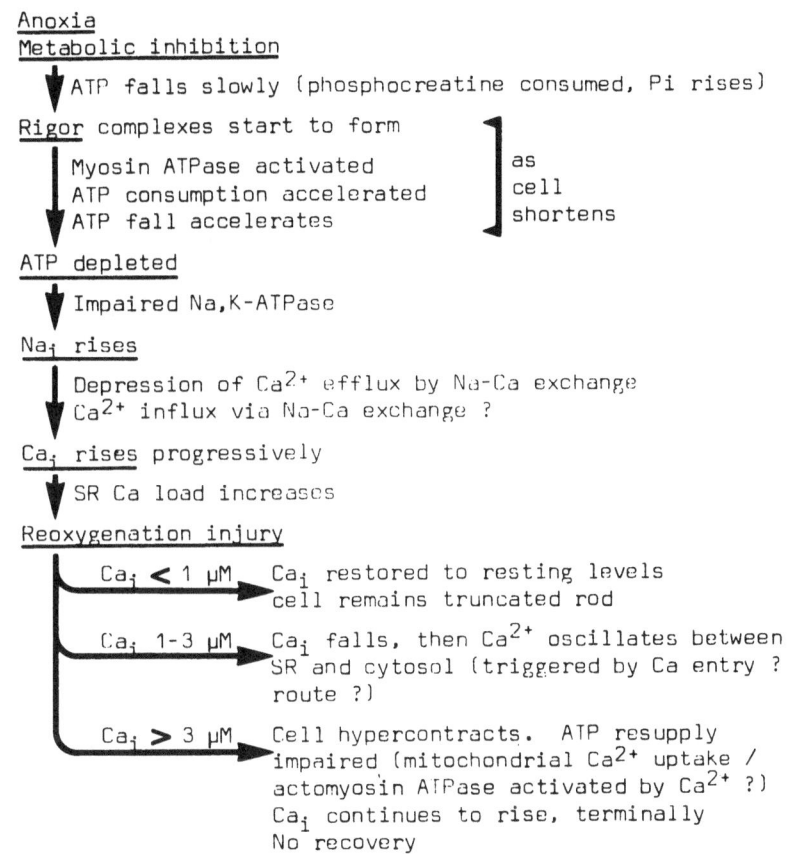

Anoxia
Metabolic inhibition

▼ ATP falls slowly (phosphocreatine consumed, Pi rises)

Rigor complexes start to form

| Myosin ATPase activated
| ATP consumption accelerated   } as cell shortens
▼ ATP fall accelerates

ATP depleted

▼ Impaired Na,K-ATPase

Na_i rises

| Depression of Ca^{2+} efflux by Na-Ca exchange
▼ Ca^{2+} influx via Na-Ca exchange ?

Ca_i rises progressively

▼ SR Ca load increases

Reoxygenation injury

Ca_i < 1 µM → Ca_i restored to resting levels cell remains truncated rod

Ca_i 1-3 µM → Ca_i falls, then Ca^{2+} oscillates between SR and cytosol (triggered by Ca entry ? route ?)

Ca_i > 3 µM → Cell hypercontracts. ATP resupply impaired (mitochondrial Ca^{2+} uptake / actomyosin ATPase activated by Ca^{2+} ?) Ca_i continues to rise, terminally No recovery

Fig. 6. Cardiomyocyte deterioration during anoxia or metabolic blockade: proposed sequence of events.

ably, as the overlap between thick and thin filaments increases during cell shortening, rigor complex-activated myosin ATPase activity will increase; ATP depletion could be stretch sensitive therefore.

b) The rise in Ca_i (which is not reflected in any appreciable acceleration of Ca^{2+} influx and may even occur while Ca^{2+} influx is reduced) is sensitive to extracellular Ni, Co, Mn and removal of external Ca, but is unaffected by calcium channel antagonists such as verapamil. The Ca_i rise probably reflects a curtailed Ca^{2+} efflux, leading to a net gain of Ca by the cell. Reduction of Ca^2 efflux on the Na-Ca exchanger may be the most important process.

c) The extent to which Ca_i has risen determines the fate of the cell at reoxygenation. If Ca_i already exceeds 3 µM then readmission of oxygen triggers sudden rounding, blebbing and terminal injury to the cell, possibly as a result of Ca^{2+}-activated actomyosin activity and mitochondrial Ca^{2+} uptake both attenuating the restoration of adequate ATP levels.

d) Reoxygenation before Ca_i has reached 3 μM causes a drop in Ca_i to 300–500 nM, followed by dramatic Ca_i oscillations and synchronous 'twitching' of the cell.

e) The Ca_i oscillations are blocked by caffeine and thus involve cyclical uptake and release from the SR, perhaps because of Ca^{2+} overload. They depend on the entry of Ca^{2+} across the sarcolemma by an undefined route distinct from the classical Ca channel.

f) Most curiously, extracellular Ni (or Co or Mn) can substitute for reoxygenation to induce a temporary fall and oscillations in Ca_i. In this situation ATP resynthesis will not have occurred, demonstrating the capability of metabolically impaired myocytes to generate relatively rapid Ca fluxes between the cytosol and the SR lumen.

g) Conceivably, an influx of calcium through remnant gap junctions in intercalated discs may trigger regenerative release of Ca^{2+} from the overloaded SR.

Future directions

Do these insights into the deterioration of the hypoxic myocardial cell suggest how the ischemic myocardium might be protected? The hypothesis highlights several potential targets for manipulations aimed at delaying the onset of ionic imbalance, for instance blockade of Na-Ca exchange or of the routes for Na^+ influx. However, these interventions would be largely *post hoc* in character, aimed at treating those symptoms we recognize (ionic changes) while leaving other aspects of the deterioration to progress. We believe that prevention of the putative ATP depletion by the rigor-complex activated myosin ATPase would be a useful target. If an acceleration of ATP depletion via the Sl-ATPase is found to coincide with the shortening of the cardiomyocyte, then not only ionic imbalances but a whole spectrum of deleterious events triggered by falling ATP levels could be attenuated by delaying rigor. Clearly such an agent would need to inhibit rigor complex formation between myosin and actin without impairing the activation of actomyosin mediated by Ca-tropomyosin at normal ATP levels.

Acknowledgement

We are grateful to the British Heart Foundation for project grant funding.

References

1. Poole-Wilson PA, Harding DP, Bourdillon PDV, Tones MA (1984) Calcium out of control. J Mol Cell Cardiol 16: 175–187
2. Allen DG, Smith GL (1985) Intracellular calcium in metabolically depleted ferret ventricular muscle during exposure to cyanide and its removal. J Physiol (Lond.) 369: 92P
3. Stern MD, Chien AM, Capogrossi MC, Pelto DJ, Lakatta EG (1985) Direct observation of the 'oxygen paradox' in single rat ventricular myocytes. Circ Res 56: 899–903
4. Eisner DA, Nichols CG, O'Neill SC, Smith GL, Valdeolmillos M (1989) The effects of metabolic inhibition on intracellular calcium and pH in isolated rat ventricular cells. J Physiol (Lond.) 411: 393–418
5. Piper HM, Jacobson SL, Schwartz JL, Mealing GAR, Whitfield JF (1988) Disturbance of Ca^{2+} homeostasis in restrained cardiomyocytes under anoxia and reoxygenation. J Mol Cell Cardiol 20 (Suppl V): abstract 51
6. Cobbold PH, Bourne PK (1984) Aequorin measurements of free calcium in single heart cells. Nature 312: 444–446
7. Allshire A, Piper HM, Cuthbertson KSR, Cobbold PH (1987) Cytosolic free Ca^{2+} in single rat heart cells during anoxia and reoxygenation. Biochem J 244: 381–385
8. Li Q, Altschuld RA, Stokes BT (1988) Myocyte deenergization and intracellular free calcium dynamics. Am J Physiol 255: C162–C168
9. Haworth RA, Hunter DR, Berkoff HA (1981) Contracture in isolated adult rat heart cells. Role of Ca^{2+}, ATP, and compartmentation. Circ Res 49: 1119–1128
10. Haworth RA, Goknur AB, Hunter DR, Hegge JO, Berkoff HA (1987) Inhibition of calcium influx in isolated adult rat heart cells by ATP depletion. Circ Res 60: 586–594
11. Haworth RA, Nicolaus A, Goknur AB, Berkoff HA (1988) Synchronous depletion of ATP in isolated adult rat heart cells. J Mol Cell Cardiol 20: 837–846
12. Allen DG, Orchard CH (1983) Intracellular calcium concentration during hypoxia and metabolic inhibition in mammalian ventricular muscle. J Physiol (Lond.) 339: 107–122
13. Smith GL, Allen DG (1988) Effects of metabolic blockade on intracellular calcium concentration in isolated ferret ventricular muscle. Circ Res 62: 1223–1236
14. Eisner DA, Orchard CH, Allen DG (1984) Control of intracellular ionized calcium concentration by sarcolemmal and intracellular mechanisms. J Mol Cell Cardiol 16: 137–146
15. Chapman RA (1986) Sodium/calcium exchange and intracellular calcium buffering in ferret myocardium: an ion-sensitive micro-electrode study. J Physiol (Lond.) 373: 163–179
16. Lee HC, Mohabir R, Smith N, Franz MR, Clusin WT (1988) Effect of ischemia on calcium-dependent fluorescence transients in rabbit hearts containing indo 1. Circulation 78: 1047–1059
17. Steenbergen C, Murphy E, Levy L, London RE (1987) Elevation in cytosolic free calcium concentration early in myocardial ischemia in perfused rat heart. Circ Res 60: 700–707
18. Bremel RD, Weber A (1972) Cooperation within actin filament in vertebrate skeletal muscle. Nature New Biol 238: 97–101
19. Murray JM, Knox MK, Trueblood CE, Weber A (1982) Potentiated state of the tropomyosin actin filament and nucleotide-containing myosin subfragment 1. Biochemistry 21: 906–915
20. Fabiato A, Fabiato F (1975) Effects of magnesium on contractile activation of skinned cardiac cells. J Physiol (Lond.) 249: 497–517
21. Lewis MJ, Housmans PR, Claes VA, Brutsaert DL, Henderson AH (1980) Myocardial stiffness during hypoxic and reoxygenation contracture. Cardiovasc Res 14: 339–344
22. Ventura-Clapier R, Vassort G (1981) Rigor tension during metabolic and ionic rises in resting tension in rat heart. J Mol Cell Cardiol 13: 551–561
23. Holubarsch Ch (1983) Force generation in experimental tetanus, KCl contracture, and oxygen and glucose deficiency contracture in mammalian myocardium. Pflügers Arch 396: 277–284

24. Holubarsch Ch., Alpert NR, Goulette R, Mulieri LA (1982) Heat production during hypoxic contracture of rat myocardium. Circ Res 51: 777–786

25. Allen DG, Orchard CH (1987) Myocardial contractile function during ischemia and hypoxia. Circ Res 60: 153–168

26. Mekhfi H, Ventura-Clapier R (1988) Dependence upon high-energy phosphates of the effects of inorganic phosphate on contractile properties in chemically skinned rat cardiac fibres. Pflügers Arch 411: 378–385

27. Altschuld RA, Wenger WC, Lamka KG, Kindig OR, Capen CC, Mizuhira V, Vander Heide RS, Brierley GP (1985) Structural and functional properties of adult rat heart myocytes lysed with digitonin. J Biol Chem 260: 14325–14334

28. Allshire A, Cobbold PH (1987) Ca^{2+} flux into metabolically deprived cardiomyocytes. Biochem Soc Trans 15: 960

29. Guarnieri T (1987) Intracellular sodium-calcium dissociation in early contractile failure in hypoxic ferret papillary muscles. J Physiol (Lond.) 388: 449–465

30. Li Q, Altschuld RA, Biagi BA, Stokes BT (1988) Cation and membrane potential alterations in energy depleted cardiac myocytes. In: Biology of isolated adult cardiac myocytes. Clark WA, Decker RS, Borg TK (eds) Elsevier, New York, pp 342–345

31. Allshire AP, Cobbold PH (1989) Cytosolic Ca^{2+} in hypoxic cariomyocytes. In: Isolated adult cariomyocytes. Piper HM, Isenberg G (eds) CRC Press, Boca Raton, Florida. Vol 1, pp 287–308

32. Berridge MJ, Cobbold PH, Cuthbertson KSR (1988) Spatial and temporal aspects of cell signalling. Phil Trans R Soc Lond B 320: 325–343

33. Hohl C, Ansel A, Altschuld R, Brierley GP (1982) Contracture of isolated rat heart cells on anaerobic to aerobic transition. Am J Physiol 242: H1022–H1030

34. Fabiato A (1985) Time and calcium dependence of activation and inactivation of calcium-induced release of calcium from the sarcoplasmic reticulum of a skinned canine cardiac Purkinje cell. J Gen Physiol 85: 247–289

35. Thandroyen FT, McCarthy J, Burton KP, Opie LH (1988) Ryanodine and caffeine prevent ventricular arrhythmias during acute myocardial ischemia and reperfusion in rat heart. Circ Res 62: 306–314

36. Tosaki A, Hearse DJ (1987) Protective effect of transient calcium reduction against reperfusion-induced arrhythmias in rat hearts. Am J Physiol 253: H225–H233

PART VII

Mechanical factors: rigor and contracture

Rigor and contracture: the role of phosphorus compounds and cytosolic Ca^{2+}

G.J.M. STIENEN and G. ELZINGA
The Laboratory for Physiology, Free University, van der Boechorststraat 7, 1081 BT Amsterdam, The Netherlands

Abstract

Since in the intact myocardium the effects of ischemia lead to changes in the composition of the sarcoplasm, the sarcoplasmic factors which affect mechanical performance in ischemia cannot effectively be studied at the level of complexity found in the intact cell. Much has been learned in this respect from skinned muscle preparations, i.e. preparations where the cellular membrane is made permeable so that the 'intracellular' composition can be controlled by the composition of the bathing solution. These studies show that the contractile apparatus is not only sensitive to calcium, which is essential for contraction, but also to pH, inorganic phosphate, ATP, and ADP amongst others.

Phosphate and acidification have a depressive effect on force production, which is more pronounced at the calcium levels, normally found in the beating heart, which do not cause maximum force production. ADP has a potentiating effect on force but it depresses shortening velocity, probably by acting as a competitive inhibitor of ATP induced crossbridge detachment. A decrease of ATP, in the presence of calcium, increases force until a concentration of about 100 μM is reached. When ATP drops even below this level, force decreases but never disappears as rigor develops at these low levels. Shortening velocity decreases when ATP falls. The ATPase activity related to contraction varies with Ca^{2+} concentration in proportion to force production. It is depressed by ADP at larger concentrations, and by ATP at low concentrations.

Introduction

Under normal conditions, cardiac muscle excels in long term stability and reliability of its mechanical performance. These properties, essential for proper functioning of the ventricular pump, result from the intimate coupling between metabolism and performance, and powerful cellular control me-

H.M. Piper (ed.) Pathophysiology of severe ischemic myocardial injury, 317–336.
© *1990 Kluwer Academic Publishers, Dordrecht*

chanisms. It is difficult therefore, to single out the determining factors of cardiac failure during hypoxia or ischemia when studying the whole heart and it can be expected that insight can be gained from studies on isolated cardiac tissue in which the action of cellular control mechanisms is prevented.

In this chapter, a summary will be given of properties of the contractile system. Much of this knowledge is directly obtained from isolated preparations and is essential to understand the changes in myocardial performance during ischemia, which are often associated with rigor and contracture.

Rigor and contracture can be described as follows:

RIGOR is a state in which the tissue is virtually depleted of ATP. In this state, the tissue is inexcitable and a low level of permanent force and high stiffness is maintained. The distance over which (isotonic) shortening is possible is quite small. The general opinion is that permanent links are formed between the contractile proteins, and that no ATP is split.

CONTRACTURE is a certain state of contraction in which force development takes place during a prolonged period. The contractile system not only generates force, but also induces shortening and can split ATP. A contracture occurs, for instance, when the extracellular medium contains a high potassium concentration. It is also found when the integrity of the cell membrane is lost, resulting somehow in a high calcium ion concentration.

In this overview, attention will be focused in particular on the physiological and biochemical effects of phosphorus compounds and cytosolic Ca^{2+} concentrations on the mechanical and energetic properties of so-called skinned muscle tissue. Such preparations are particularly useful in studying the mechanisms involved in rigor and contracture. In these preparations, the cell membrane is either removed by microdissection [1, 2] or made permeable by means of a detergent (Triton X-100, saponin or digitonin). In both cases, the composition of the 'intracellular' milieu can be manipulated. An overview of the methods involved and a description of the functional properties of skinned preparations has been given by Stephenson [3].

A number of different intracellular components affect the force produced during contraction. It is difficult, therefore, to give a complete description of the whole spectrum of contractile performance which ranges from physiological to severe pathophysiological behaviour. However, from an account of the effects of Ca^{2+}, ATP, ADP, P_i, creatine phosphate, and pH on mechanical performance, the relative importance of the various components in this respect may be judged. Several high quality review articles have been published in related areas of research [4–7].

Muscle contraction, a result of molecular interaction

In order to understand the effects of the various compounds affecting muscle contraction, it is necessary to gain insight into the nature of the molecular interaction. In striated muscle, the actin (thin) and myosin (thick) filaments

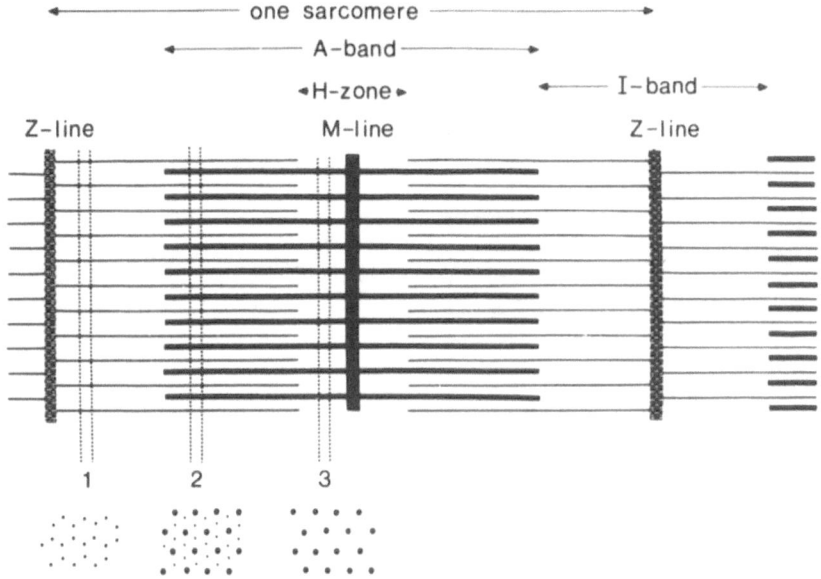

Fig. 1. Diagram of the sarcomere containing myosin (thick) filaments and actin (thin) filaments with definitions of the different parts and cross-sectional views at three locations (Reproduced with permission and modified from [81]).

within each sarcomere are ordered into a regular lattice (Fig. 1). The thick filaments are arranged in a hexagonal array and the thin filaments are positioned in the centre of a triangle formed by three neighbouring thick filaments. Force development is generally thought to result from chemical bonding between the myosin head and the actin filament: crossbridge formation. Crossbridge formation is, even when the contraction is isometric, part of a cyclic process in which myosin heads attach to and detach from actin. During shortening of the muscle, the crossbridges detach and reattach further along the thin filament, thereby sliding the actin and myosin filaments past each other. During the crossbridge cycle, chemical energy available from the hydrolysis of ATP is converted into mechanical work and heat. The crossbridge cycle and its relation to the actomyosin ATPase, based on the scheme of Lymn and Taylor (1971) [8] are schematically depicted in Fig. 2.

The scheme valid for the elementary steps of actomyosin ATPase activity derived from biochemical measurements is shown in Fig. 3. In the absence of actin, or calcium ions, myosin ATPase takes place at a very low rate (bottom row in Fig. 3) as compared to the actin activated actomyosin ATPase (upper row). ATP binds tightly to myosin ($K_1 = 10^{11}$ M^{-1}; K_i is the equilibrium constant of the ith reaction) and is split rapidly ($k_{3d} > 150$ s^{-1}, $k_{-3d} \cong 15$ s^{-1}; k_{+i} and k_{-i} denote the forward and backward rate constants, respectively). P_i dissociates very slowly ($k_{5d} \cong 0.06$ s^{-1}), then ADP dissociates and ATP binds again.

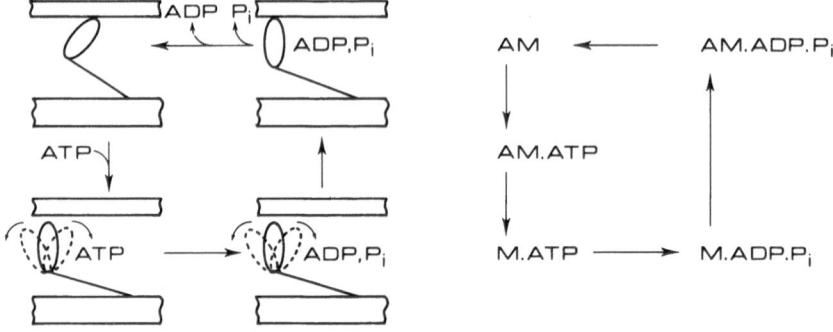

Fig. 2. Simplified scheme for the crossbridge cycle and its relation to the actomyosin ATPase [8]. The myosin head, the globular part of the myosin molecule which sticks out of the myosin filament, is able to bind to the actin filament. The attached states are characterized by two preferred orientations (angles) of the AM and AM.ADP.P$_i$ bonds. The dissociated heads have some degree of rotational freedom. (Reproduced, with the permission from the Annual Review of Biophys Biophys Chem, Volume 15, © 1986 by Annual Reviews Inc. [6]).

Actin activates the myosin ATPase by binding to M.ADP.P$_i$ (step 4), thereby accelerating P$_i$ release (step 5a). ADP release (step 9a) and ATP binding (step 1a) then follow rapidly. ATP binding results in breaking of the actomyosin complex. The hydrolysis step occurs both with myosin attached to actin (step 3a) and with dissociated myosin (step 3d). The state AM'.ADP, which is capable of binding P$_i$, is different from AM.ADP. It is not clear whether AM.ADP is an intermediate of the hydrolysis reactive sequence. AM'.ADP might, for example, dissociate directly to AM.

This scheme (Fig. 3) and the values presented were derived from biochemical studies on fast skeletal actin and myosin. It is likely that the scheme is also valid for slow skeletal and cardiac muscle [9]. The numerical values for cardiac muscle, however, are in many cases lower than the values presented above. It has been found, for instance, that the overall rate of the *in vitro* AM.ATPase of cardiac muscle is at least a factor of 5 smaller than that of fast skeletal muscle. The rate constant of ADP dissociation from actomyosin is also at least a factor of 5 slower in cardiac muscle than in fast skeletal muscle. The association constant for ADP binding is about 200 times smaller in cardiac than in fast skeletal muscle. However, the following rate and equilibrium constants are approximately the same in cardiac and fast skeletal muscle: the second-order rate constant for the dissociation of actomyosin by MgATP, the second-order rate constant of myosin and myosin-ADP binding to actin, and the association constant of myosin to actin [10–13].

Understanding of the correspondence between the mechanically distinct states for the crossbridge and the biochemical states is still limited. The reason for this is twofold. Firstly, the experimental conditions for the bio-

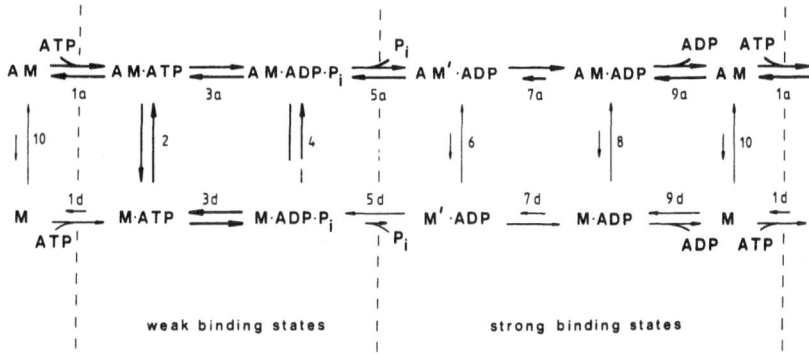

Fig. 3. A kinetic scheme of the elementary steps of the actomyosin ATPase. 'A' represents actin, 'M' is myosin subfragment 1. The heavy solid arrows indicate the predominant cyclic reaction pathway in the presence of actin. The relative lengths of the forward and reverse arrows qualitatively indicate the change in free energy across the corresponding step [82]. (Reproduced, with permission, from the Annual Review of Physiology, Volume 49, © 1987 by Annual Reviews Inc.).

chemical measurements are necessarily different from the *in vivo* situation. Secondly, *in vivo*, there exists a mechanical influence on the transition rates as is evidenced by the Fenn effect [14], which is necessarily absent in studies on isolated proteins.

However, some further progress may be expected here from recent developments in experimental techniques which allow simultaneous measurements of mechanical and biochemical properties on skinned preparations. It is, for instance, possible to monitor simultaneously the mechanical performance and the ATPase activity in solutions which mimic different intracellular environments. New insight may also be gained from studies on fragments of myosin molecules and actin filaments, whose motion can be determined by means of fluorescent labelling [15]. A further development is that a photochemical technique has become available which allows the study of the fast rate constants (c.f. Fig. 3) in skinned fibres. The diffusion limitations which make these preparations unsuitable for the study of rapid biochemical transients are overcome by the use of caged compounds. Caged ATP, for instance, is an inert photolabile precursor of ATP. Upon illumination by means of an intense pulse from a UV-laser, ATP is liberated (leaving its cage) and capable of reacting with the contractile proteins [16]. Some of the results obtained with caged compounds will be described below. So far, the general finding is that the kinetic scheme for the actomyosin ATPase, as derived from biochemical studies (Fig. 3), does indeed apply to skinned muscle as well. However, the way in which some of the crossbridge transitions are influenced by mechanical action is still unclear. In order to fully understand the interrelation between physiological and biochemical properties, more study is required.

Chemical composition of the sarcoplasm

The chemical composition of the sarcoplasm in the millimolar range is already accurately known. Part of our knowledge originates from biochemical analysis of extracts from rapidly frozen muscles, but more recently ^{31}P-*Nuclear Magnetic Resonance* (NMR) has proved to be a powerful tool in revealing part of the chemical composition of the sarcoplasm and changes thereof during active contraction. The resolution of NMR is still limited in most cases to the whole heart. In some studies, however, new methods have been used which give local, time-resolved information [17–19]. Here we will limit ourselves to a description of the steady state metabolic levels and will not be covering the NMR-field too extensively.

Under normal aerobic conditions, the following values are regularly reported in the literature [20–22].

MgATP concentration	= 4–8 mM
MgADP concentration	= 10–50 μM
Free Mg^{2+} concentration	= 1 mM
Creatine phosphate (PCr) concentration	= 30 mM
Inorganic phosphate (P_i) concentration	= 1–5 mM
K^+ concentration	= 120 mM
Na^+ concentration	= 10 mM

Several other components are present in the sub-millimolar range such as NAD, NADH.

It is well known that during ischemia, changes in phosphorus-containing metabolites occur due to inhibition of ATP synthesis by oxidative phosphorylation. A simulation of the changes which occur during ischemia or anoxia as a function of the amounts of P_i formed (or time) is shown in Fig. 4 [4]. It is clear that the ATP, PCr, P_i and AMP concentrations change when ATP synthesis is not sufficient. Apart from these changes, it has been shown that cystosolic free calcium concentration increases within 9–15 minutes of myocardial ischemia from a time-averaged level of 0.61 μM to at least 3 μM [23].

The effects of cytosolic Ca^{2+}, phosphorus compounds, and pH on force development, shortening velocity, and ATPase activity in cardiac muscle

Effects of Ca^{2+}

Force development of cardiac muscle is a function of the internal Ca^{2+} concentration (Fig. 5) and this function again depends upon the MgATP concentration, the free Mg^{2+} concentration, phosphate concentration, pH, temperature, ionic strength of the solution, and sarcomere length [1, 2, 24–31]. It is generally thought that the calcium sensitivity of force development

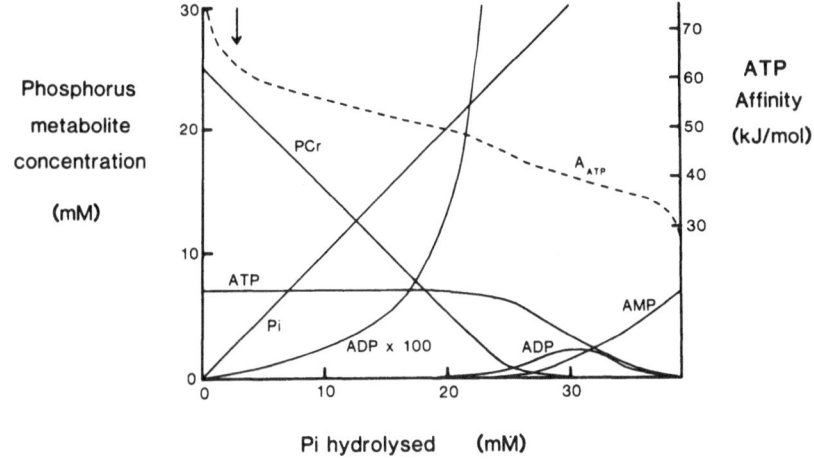

Fig. 4. Model of concentrations of PCr, ATP, ADP, AMP, and P_i in the presence of creatine kinase and myokinase as ATP is hydrolysed. The thermodynamic affinity (free energy change) of ATP (A_{ATP}) hydrolysis is also shown. A_{ATP} was calculated using the equation $A_{ATP} = -\Delta G_o + RT\ln\{[ATP]/[ADP]\cdot[P_i]\}$, with $-\Delta G_o = 30$ kJ/mol. The arrow represents the approximate concentration of P metabolites in aerobic perfused hearts at low or moderate workloads. Note that, as plotted, the abscissa has units of moles of P_i hydrolysed. However, during a period when there is net consumption of ATP in excess of production, the figure can be used to indicate the way in which P metabolites will change as a function of time [4].

reflects the affinity of calcium binding to the multiple Ca^{2+} binding sites of troponin C (TnC). However, the force-pCa curves are too steep for TnC to be the sole determinant. Evidence has been accumulated that neighbouring binding sites along the thin filament show some degree of co-operative interaction [32]. Studies by Babu *et al.* [33] [34] and Moss *et al.* [35] have shown that extracting cardiac troponin C and substituting it with fast skeletal troponin C affects the force-pCa curve. The dependence of the force-pCa curves on the free Mg^{2+} concentration is probably due to the competitive action of Ca^{2+} and Mg^{2+}. The way in which MgATP (Fig. 5) and P_i (Fig. 8) affect the force-pCa relationships is not yet fully understood. Qualitatively, it appears that the binding of crossbridges plays a modulatory role. It has been shown, for instance, that several factors which influence maximum force development also modulate its calcium sensitivity [36].

The shortening velocity at zero external load (V_{max}) is probably limited by the maximum rate at which crossbridges are able to detach in a contracting muscle. If Ca^{2+} indeed only plays a modulatory role in crossbridge attachment, it is to be expected that the maximum velocity of shortening would be very insensitive to the Ca^{2+} concentration. A long-standing controversy exists in the literature on this point. Julian [37] found that the force-velocity relationship at low Ca^{2+} concentrations was different from the relationship found at saturating calcium concentrations. Podolsky and Teichholz [38], on

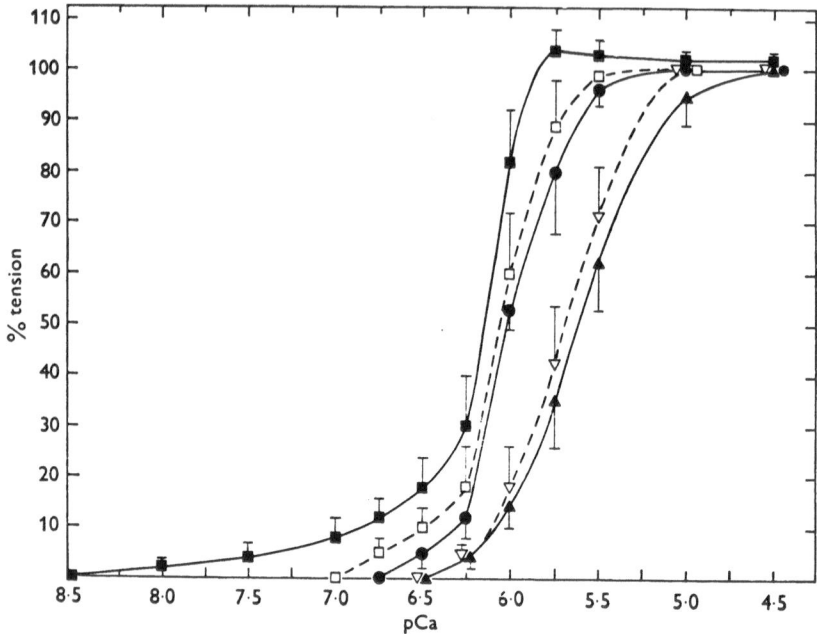

Fig. 5. Curves of the tension developed by skinned cardiac cells of 9–13 μm width and 35–60 μm length as a function of pCa for various pMg and pMgATP (▲ – ▲ pMg 2.50, pMgATP 1.80; ▽ – ▽ pMg 2.50, pMgATP 2.50; ● – ● pMg 3.50, pMgATP 2.50; □ – □ pMg 4.50, pMg ATP; 2.50; ■ – ■ pMg 4.50, pMgATP 3.50).For each medium applied to a given cell, the tension is expressed by the percentage of the tension developed by the same cell at pCa 5.0, pMg 3.50 and pMgATP 2.50. The zero percent of tension is defined by the tension developed at pCa 9.0, pMg 3.50 and pMgATP 2.50.

the other hand, claimed that there was no such effect. The discussion is still by no means closed as can be seen from recent publications [35]. Biochemical evidence also indicates that the role of Ca^{2+} is more complex than that of merely switching the actin filament on or off [39].

Most estimates of the ATPase rate under isometric conditions in cardiac muscle are obtained from heat, oxygen consumption, or NMR measurements. Gibbs and Loiselle [40] reported a stable maintenance heat production of tetanized papillary muscle of the rat at 27 °C of 30.4 mW/g, which corresponds to an overall ATPase rate of about 0.5 mM/s. Assuming that 40% of this is associated with the ATPase activity of the sarcoplasmic reticulum, a value of 0.3 mM/s is obtained for the actomyosin ATPase. Similar values can be derived from oxygen consumption measurements on cat papillary muscle [41] or from NMR studies in rat heart [42]. More direct information is obtained from *in vitro* measurements [43] and from glycerinated muscle [44, 45]. These results indicate that the ATPase rate and force at different Ca^{2+} concentrations are proportional. Recent experiments carried out in our laboratory on skinned cardiac trabeculae [46] confirm this notion.

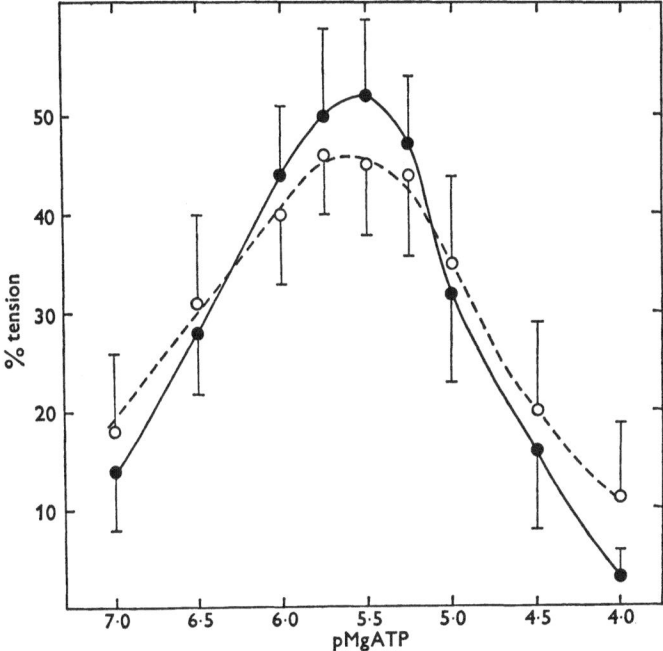

Fig. 6. Curve of tension developed by skinned cardiac cells of 9–13 μM width and 35–60 μm length (● – ●) and by segments of skinned fibres of frog semi-tendinosus of 8–12 μm width and 30–60 μm length (○ -- ○) as a function of pMgATP at pCa 9.50. For each medium applied to a given cell the tension is expressed by the percentage of the tension developed by the same cell at pCa 5.0 (cardiac cell) or 4.50 (skeletal muscle fibre), with pMg 3.50 and pMgATP 2.50. The zero percent of tension is defined by the tension developed at pCa 9.0 pMg and pMgATP 2.50 [1, 2].

In addition, it can be noted that by means of caged ATP, Barsotti and Ferenczi [47] determined a rate of ATP hydrolysis in chemically skinned trabeculae at 12°C of 63 μM/s. This value corresponds well with the values derived from oxygen and heat measurements, when adjusted to account for the large effect of temperature on the ATPase activity (a four-fold increase with a rise in temperature of 10°C).

Effects of MgATP

The relationship between force and the cytosolic MgATP concentration is rather complicated. It has been found that in the absence of MgATP force can be generated. The extent to which shortening can occur, however, is in that case very limited (less than 1%). In Fig. 6, isometric force in the absence of Ca^{2+} is shown as a function of the MgATP concentration. Force at zero or very low MgATP concentrations is about 15% of maximum active force under

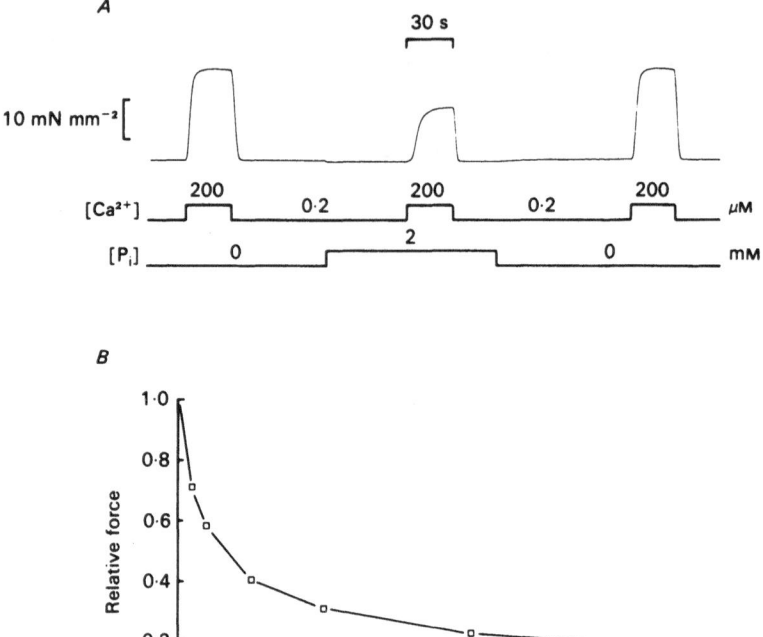

Fig. 7. A. Chart record of force in a skinned trabecula in the presence of 0.2 µM Ca^{2+} or 200 µM Ca^{2+}. For the middle period 2 mM P$_i$ (K salt) was added to the relaxing and activating solutions and the ionic strength was kept constant by reduction of K propionate concentration. Experimental conditions: pH 7.0, 22°C, 5 mM ATP, 10 mM PCr, mean muscle diameter = 100 µm.
B. Relationship between the maximum Ca^{2+} regulated force (obtained at 200 µM Ca^{2+}) and P$_i$ concentration in the activating solution. Force is expressed relative to the maximum force obtained in P$_i$ free solution [30].

physiological conditions; it reaches an optimum between 1 and 10 µM MgATP and decreases at higher MgATP concentrations. In order to explain the optimum in force, it has to be assumed that attached crossbridges can exist in a low force producing rigor state, i.e. the AM complex in Fig. 3 [48], in which crossbridges accumulate in the absence of ATP and a high force producing state which is part of the crossbridge cycle. The increase of ATP at low concentrations causes a shift of the occupancy from the low to the high force producing state. A further increase in MgATP concentration causes an increase in the rate of crossbridge dissociation via step 1a (Fig. 3) which results in a net decrease in the number of attached crossbridges and, eventually, causes force relaxation.

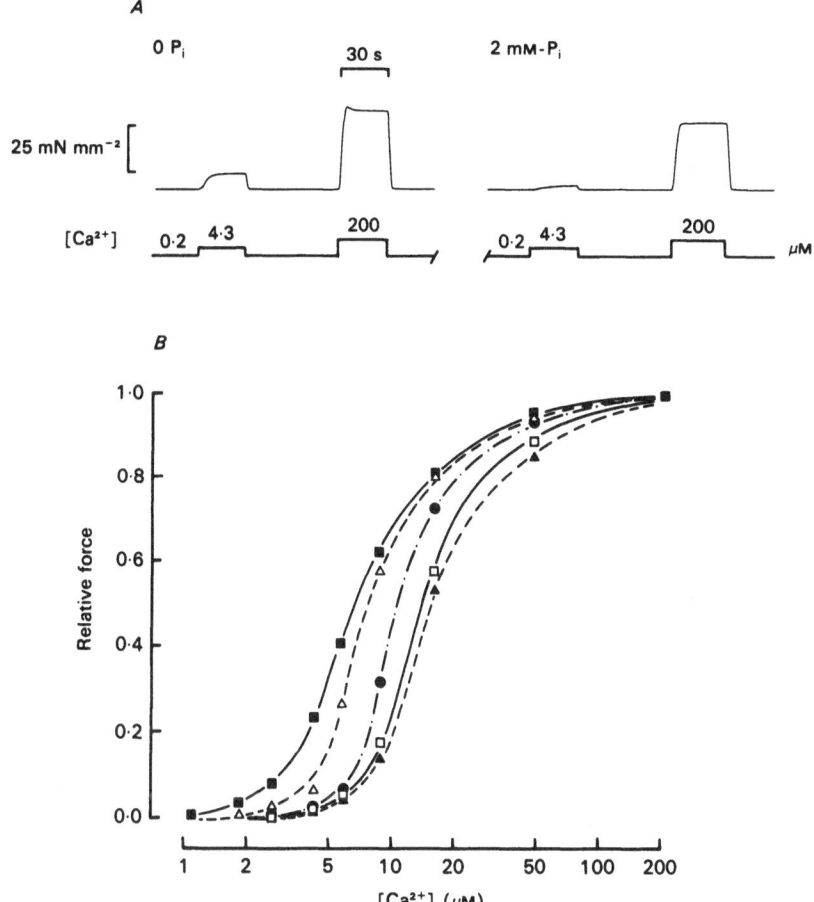

Fig. 8. A. Chart record of force at two Ca^{2+} concentrations (4.3 µM and 200 µM) in the absence and presence of P_i. Muscle diameter 140 µM.
B. Force–$[Ca^{2+}]$ relationships at various concentrations of P_i (mM):
0 (■) , 2(△) , 5(●) , 10(□) , 20(▲). Force at each P_i concentration is expressed relative to the maximum force at the same P_i [30].

The active force production in the presence of a saturating Ca^{2+} concentration also depends on the MgATP concentration [2]. The active component of force, appearing on an increase in Ca^{2+} concentration, is small at very low ATP concentrations, and reaches a maximum around 100 µM MgATP of about 140% of the force at 5 mM MgATP. An example of this relationship, obtained on fast skeletal muscle, is shown in Fig. 9. At low ATP concentrations up to 100 µM this relationship is also determined by the presence of rigor complexes. The decrease of force at higher ATP concentration is probably due to the dissociating effect of MgATP [49, 50].

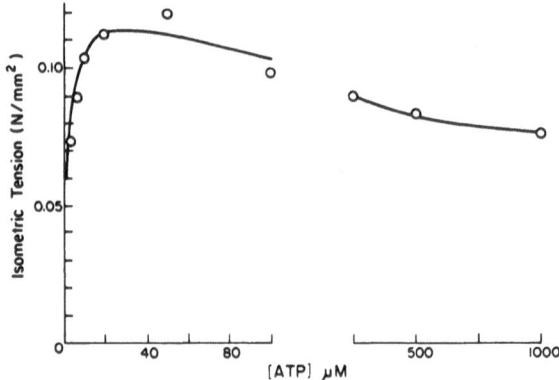

Fig. 9. The isometric tension is plotted as a function of the ATP concentration at 10°C. The isometric tension at 5 mM ATP (not shown) was 85% of that at 1 mM ATP, and at 10 mM ATP it was 81% of that at 1 mM ATP. Reproduced by permission from [51].

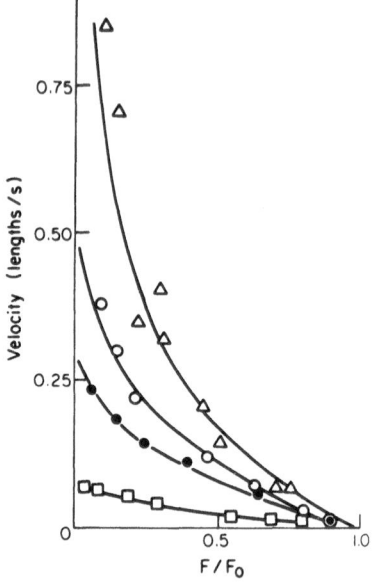

Fig. 10. Force-velocity curves for different ATP concentrations: 10 μM (□), 50 μM (●), 100 μM (○), and 500 μM (△) [51]. Reproduced by permission from [51].

The relationship between the velocity of shortening and the MgATP concentration (Fig. 10) has also been studied extensively [51, 52], because it is regarded as an important measure of muscle performance. The curvature of the force-velocity relationship has been found to increase with a decrease in MgATP concentration. The maximum velocity of shortening decreases in a hyperbolic fashion with the MgATP concentration being half the maximum at about 0.5 mM in fast muscles [50, 53] and at about 0.15 mM in slow muscle fibres [53]. These measurements are not performed in cardiac muscle tissue at 37°C, and therefore, it is by no means certain that the decrease in the cytosolic MgATP concentration seen during ischemia has no effect on short-ening velocity in heart muscle.

As mentioned above, the maximum turnover rate of ATP in intact cardiac tissue can be estimated from heat, oxygen consumption and NMR measure-ments. The values obtained have to be used with care, because they are obtained via indirect approaches, and because they are species and highly temperature dependent and age related. A typical value in intact mammalian muscle at body temperature is probably around 1 mM/s. Assumpting that the concentration of myosin heads is about 0.2 Mm, and that all heads participate, this implies a maximum turnover rate for each crossbridge of about 5 s^{-1}. In view of the results in fast rabbit psoas muscle [54], this rate, in cardiac muscle, will also probably depend on the MgATP concentration in hyperbolic fashion with a rather low K_m (the concentration at which the rate is half the maximum) of about 20 µM.

Effects of P_i

Inorganic phosphate in the millimolar range depresses force development [e.g. 55–57]. This finding has considerable impact on the behavior of cardiac and skeletal muscle during ischemia or fatigue. It is clear that the depression of force by phosphate (Figs. 7 and 8) is more pronounced in cardiac than in skeletal muscle [28]. There is some uncertainty about the mechanism under-lying the phosphate effect. Nosek *et al.* [56], in following a suggestion from Dawson *et al.* [58], found that in fast skeletal rabbit muscle at different pH that it is the diprotonated form of inorganic phosphate which affects force, while Kentish [31] showed that in cardiac muscle it is the total concentration which matters. The mechanism involved is probably related to the reversal of step 5 in Fig. 3 [59].

As far as we know, the relationship between shortening velocity and P_i has not been investigated in cardiac muscle. The results in skeletal muscle indicate, however, that there is no effect of P_i on V_{max} [60]. Recent experi-ments carried out in our laboratory [61] on skinned rabbit psoas fibres indicate that the velocity of isotonic lengthening is considerably depressed in the presence of 15 mM P_i.

The dependency of the rate of ATP hydrolysis on P_i has been investigated in skeletal and smooth muscle [62, 63], and also in cardiac muscle [64]. These results indicate that there is only a small decrease in the rate of ATP hydrolysis at higher P_i concentrations. This finding is rather surprising be-cause the current kinetic scheme (Fig. 3) implies that force and AM.ATPase are equally affected by phosphate. It might well be that more complicated schemes are required to account for this discrepancy [62] or that the correlation between force generation and ATPase activity is less direct than envisaged at present, i.e. by co-operative interaction between the two heads of the myosin molecule [65].

Effects of MgADP

To study the effects of ADP by changing the ADP concentration in the bathing solution of skinned preparations is quite difficult. The reason for this is that in order to vary the ADP concentration, the ATP regenerating system needed for the resynthesis of ATP from ADP has to be omitted from the solutions. This results in gradients of ADP and ATP in the preparations which have to be taken into account in the analysis of the results [60] or have to be dealt with otherwise [66]. Cooke and Pate [60] and Hoar et al. [67] found a potentiating effect on force development.

The effect of ADP on rigor force (in the absence of ATP and Ca^{2+}) is probably minor or absent altogether [68]. The mechanism proposed to account for the increase in active force [60] is that an increase of the ADP concentration inhibits ATP binding and the subsequent dissociation of the crossbridge, so that the number of attached crossbridges is increased.

It has been shown [10, 11] that the dissociation of ADP from the actomyosin complex is sufficiently slow to limit the maximum shortening velocity. For bovine ventricular muscle at 30°C, for instance, a rate constant of 700 s^{-1} has been estimated which is, under certain assumptions, compatible with the maximum shortening velocity in this type of muscle, which is measured to be about 4 L_0/s. Release of ADP is required before ATP binding can occur. It was observed in fast skeletal muscle that the maximum shortening velocity decreases when the ADP concentration is raised. This indicates that ADP may act as a competitive inhibitor of ATP induced detachment. Several studies indicate that inhibition might be half the maximum at about 200–300 μM [54, 60, 69].

A similar inhibitory mechanism has been proposed for the effect of ADP on the rate of ATP hydrolysis. The results of Cooke and Pate indicate that the value for the inhibition constant for the rate of ATP hydrolysis might be the same as that of the maximum shortening velocity. However, in cardiac muscle, ADP dissociation is too fast to really limit the steady state of ATP hydrolysis (about 5 s^{-1}).

Effects of creatine phosphate

There are several reports in the literature which show that creatine phosphate at high concentrations depresses force production [30, 70]. It has been shown by Kentish [30], however, that these effects might in part be due to contami-

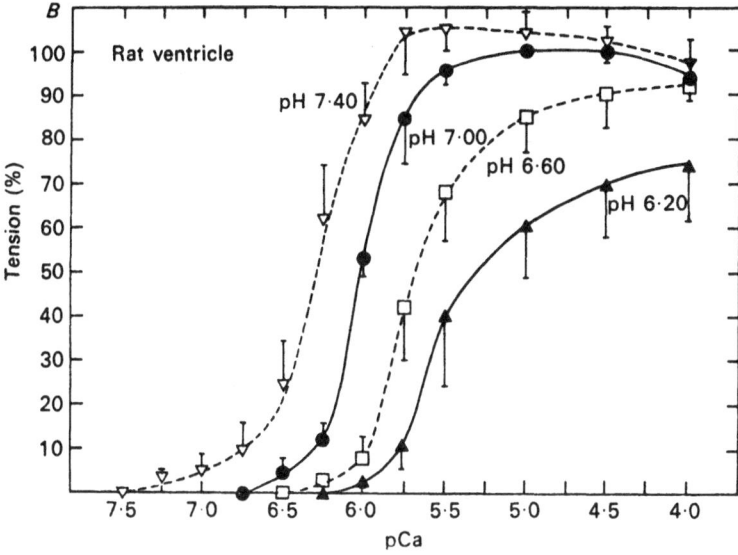

Fig. 11. Effects of varying pCa and pH on the tension developed by segments of skinned cardiac muscle cells at pMg 3.50 and pMgATP 2.50. The tension developed by each segment at a given pCa and a given pH was expressed as a percentage of the tension developed by the same segment at pCa 5.00 and pH 7.00. Reproduced by permission from [24].

nant phosphate present in the creatine phosphate. Moreover, force in the absence of creatine phosphate might be elevated because of depletion of ATP and build-up of ADP, leading to an over-estimation of the effects at high creatine phosphate concentrations. It has also been shown that the shortening velocity decreases with increasing creatine phosphate concentrations. However, it seems likely that this is also caused by depletion of ATP as a result of inadequate resynthesis of ATP.

Effects of pH

Within the pH range found in intact muscle cells, isometric force development of skinned muscle increases with pH [24, 71]. This suggests that the steady state isometric force level decreases during ischemia or fatigue. However, the impact of this effect is not very great. At submaximal Ca^{2+} concentrations, as found during contraction in intact cardiac muscle, these effects are enhanced by a decrease in Ca^{2+} sensitivity and a change in threshold for activation (Fig. 11). The force at saturation of Ca^{2+} is more depressed on a decrease in pH in the acidic rather than in the alkaline range. The origin of these effects is not yet clear. The data do not correspond with a simple competition between H^+ and Ca^{2+} for a single class of binding sites on troponin [24]. In addition, it can be noted that several of the biochemical reactions of the kinetic scheme are possibly pH dependent [72]. Maximum shortening velocity is also reduced at low pH [66], but the effect is less in slow muscle than in fast muscle [73].

The free energy of ATP hydrolysis

In the previous section the effects of the isolated separate compounds were discussed. Since muscle contraction is a process requiring energy, it must ultimately depend on the free energy change associated with ATP hydrolysis. The free energy available from ATP hydrolysis is:

$$dG/d\xi = \Delta G°_{obs} + RTln\{[ADP].[P_i]/[ATP]\} = -60 \text{ kJ/mol},$$

in which [ATP], [ADP], [P_i] denote free cytosolic concentrations, $\Delta G°_{obs} =$ –30 kJ/mol and R and T are the usual thermodynamic constants.

When the concentration of phosphorus compounds in the cell changes, the free energy of ATP hydrolysis will also change. As is shown in Fig. 4, it might even become –30 kJ/mol, when the creatine phosphate reservoir is exhausted. It has been pointed out by several authors [4, 74, 76] that the energy requirement of ionic transport processes is around 40 kJ/mol. This indicates that a lack of free energy may lead to impairment of the function of the SR Ca-pump, the Na-K pump and the surface membrane Ca pump. The free energy change associated with crossbridge cycling is also about 40 kJ/mol, indicating that the mechanical performance and the rate of ATP splitting are also affected. In this respect, it can be noted that Dawson et al. [77] found that the rate of ATP splitting during fatigue decreases when the creatine phosphate concentration is close to zero.

The fact that ADP and [P_i] appear in the nominator and ATP in the denominator of the free energy expression, suggests an antagonistic action by these substances during muscle contraction. A process in which ADP and ATP compete for the same binding site corresponds with this idea. If [P_i] release is required for ADP release, this would also be valid. The overall picture would then be that ADP and [P_i] promote crossbridge formation, while ATP promotes crossbridge dissociation. However, the results described in the previous section show that the changes in mechanical performance and in the ATPase activity do not follow this general rule. This indicates that other transitions are involved or that the mechanism of energy transduction is more complex [78].

Mechanical changes during ischemia; rigor or contracture

When coronary blood flow is reduced or stopped, mechanical activity declines within a few minutes (acute ischemic failure), and after about 15 minutes a gradual rise in diastolic pressure occurs (ischemic contracture).

The factors involved in acute ischemic failure were summarized recently by Allen and Orchard [4]. They distinguish: activation factors, i.e. shortening of the action potential duration, probably resulting in a reduction of calcium release from the sarcoplasmic reticulum, and metabolic factors such as a rise in phosphate concentration and a fall in pH, which both diminish force production directly, and indirectly via a change in the calcium sensitivity (section about effects of cytosolic Ca^{2+} and phosphorus compounds).

The gradual rise in diastolic pressure, after about 15 minutes of ischemia, might be related to a decrease in ATP concentration, since it is accompanied by a reduction of the heat-tension ratio [79]. It is unclear, however, whether the ATP level falls below the level required for a significant decrease in the AM.ATPase rate (about 50μM). If this is indeed the case, it would imply that occupancy of the AM (rigor) state would increase and the mechanical behaviour of the tissue would be intermediate between a rigor and an actively contracting muscle. It remains to be established whether or not the rise in Ca^{2+} concentration occurring during prolonged ischemia is an important factor in the development of the ischemic contracture [80].

Acknowledgement

We thank Mr. J. de Zeeuw for expert secretarial assistance.

References

1. Fabiato A, Fabiato F (1975a) Contractions induced by a calcium-triggered release of calcium from the sarcoplasmic reticulum of single skinned cardiac cells. J Physiol 249: 469–495
2. Fabiato A, Fabiato F (1975b) Effects of magnesium on contractile activation of skinned cardiac cells. J Physiol 249: 497–517
3. Stephenson EW (1981) Activation of fast skeletal muscle: contributions of studies on skinned fibers. Am J Physiol 240: C1–C19
4. Allen DG, Orchard CH (1987) Myocardial contractile function during ischemia and hypoxia. Circ Res 60: 153–168
5. Gibbs CL (1978) Cardiac energetics. Physiol Rev 58: 174–254
6. Hibberd MG, Trentham DR (1986) Relationships between chemical and mechanical events during muscular contraction. Ann Rev Biophys Biophys Chem 15: 119–161
7. Woledge RC, Curtin NA, Homsher E (1985) Energetic aspects of muscle contraction. Monographs of the Physiological Society. London: Academic Press
8. Lymn RW, Taylor EW (1971) Mechanism of adenosine triphosphate hydrolysis by actomyosin. Biochemistry 10: 4617-4624
9. Taylor EW (1979) Mechanism of actomyosin ATPase and the problem of muscle contraction. CRC Crit Rev Biochem 6: 103–164
10. Siemankowski RF, White HD (1984) Kinetics of the interaction between actin, ADP, and cardiac myosin-S1. J Biol Chem 259: 5045–5053
11. Siemankowski RF, Wisemann MO, White HD (1985) ADP dissociation from actomyosin subfragment 1 is sufficiently slow to limit the unload shortening velocity in vertebrate muscle. Proc Natl Acad Sc 82: 658–662

12. Smith SJ, White HD (1985)   Kinetic mechanisms of 1-N6-etheno-2-aza-ATP and 1-N6-ethano-2-aza-ADP binding to bovine ventricular actomyosin-S1 and myofibrils. J Biol Chem 260: 15156–15162

13. Marston SB, Taylor EW (1980)   Comparison of the myosin and actomyosin ATPase mechanisms of four types of vertebrate muscles. Biochim Biophys Acta 1: 573–600

14. Fenn WO (1923)   A quantitative comparison between the energy liberated and the work performed by the isolated sartorius of the frog. J Physiol 58: 175–203

15. Yanagida T, Arata T, Oosawa F (1985)   Sliding distance of actin filament induced by a myosin crossbridge during one ATP hydrolysis cycle. Nature 316: 366–369

16. Goldman YE, Hibberd MG, McCray JA, Trentham DR (1982)   Relaxation of muscle fibres by photolysis of caged ATP. Nature 300: 701–705

17. Balaban RS, Kantor HL, Katz LA, Briggs RW (1986)   Relation between work and phosphate metabolite in the *in vivo* paced mammalian heart. Science 232: 1121–1123

18. Bittl JA, Balschi JA, Ingwall JS (1987)   Contractile failure and high-energy phosphate turnover during hypoxia: 31P–NMR surface coil studies in living rat. Circ Res 60: 871–878

19. Blackledge MJ, Rajagopalan B, Oberhaensli RD, Bolas NM, Styles P, Radda GK (1987)   Quantitative studies of human cardiac metabolism by ^{31}P rotating-frame NMR. Proc Natl Acad Sc 84: 4283–4387

20. Mattews PM, Bland JL, Gadian DG, Radda GK (1982)   A ^{31}P-NMR saturation transfer study of the regulation of creatine kinase in the rat heart. Biochim Biophys Acta 721: 312–320

21. Clarke K, O'Connor AJ, Willis RJ (1987)   Temporal relation between energy metabolism and myocardial function during ischemia and reperfusion. Am J Physiol 253: H412–H421

22. Katz LA, Swain JA, Portman MA, Balaban RS (1988)   Intracellular pH and inorganic phosphate content of heart *in vivo*: a ^{31}P-NMR study. Am J Physiol 255: H189–H196

23. Steenbergen C, Murphy E, Levy L, London RE (1987)   Elevation in cytosolic free calcium concentration early in myocardial ischemia in perfused rat heart. Circ Res 60: 700–707

24. Fabiato A, Fabiato F (1978)   Effects of pH on the myofilaments and the sarcoplasmic reticulum of skinned cells from cardiac and skeletal muscles. J Physiol 276: 233–255

25. Kentish JC, Jewell BR (1984)   Some characteristics of Ca^{2+}-regulated force production in EGTA-treated muscles from rat heart. J Gen Physiol 84: 83–99

26. Godt RE, Lindley BD (1982)   Influence of temperature upon contractile and isometric force production in mechanically skinned muscle fibers of the frog. J Gen Physiol 80: 279–297

27. Fink RHA, Stephenson DG, Williams DA (1986)   Potassium and ionic strength effects on isometric force of skinned twitch muscle fibres of rat and toad. J Physiol 370: 317–337

28. Kentish JC, ter Keurs HEDJ, Ricciardi L, Bucx JJJ, Noble MIM (1986)   Comparison between the sarcomere length-force relations of intact and skinned trabeculae from rat right ventricle. Circ Res 58: 755–768

29. Kentish JC (1984)   The inhibitory effects of monovalent ions on force development in detergent-skinned ventricular muscle from the guinea pig. J Physiol 352: 353–374

30. Kentish JC (1986)   The effects of inorganic phosphate and creatine phosphate on force production in skinned muscles from rat ventricle. J Physiol 370: 585–604

31. Kentish JC (1987)   The inhibitory action of acidosis and inorganic phosphate on the Ca^{2+}-regulated force production of rat cardiac myofibrils. J Physiol 390: 59P

32. Brandt PW (1984)   The thin filament of vertebrate skeletal muscle cooperatively activates as a unit. J Mol Biol 180: 379–384

33. Babu A, Scordilis SP, Sonneblick EH, Gulati J (1989) The control of myocardial contraction with skeletal fast muscle troponin C. J Biol Chem 262, 12: 5815–5822

34. Babu A, Sonnenblick E, Gulati J (1988)   Molecular basis for the influence of muscle length on myocardial performance. Science 240: 74–76

35. Moss RL (1986)   Effects on shortening velocity of rabbit skeletal muscle due to variations in the level of thin-filament activation. J Physiol 377: 487–505

36. Brandt PW, Cox RN, Kawai M, Robinson T (1982)   Regulation of tension in skinned muscle fibers. Effect of cross-bridge kinetics on apparent Ca^{2+} sensitivity. J Gen Physiol 79: 997–1016

37. Julian FJ (1971) The effect of calcium on the force-velocity relation of briefly glycerinated frog muscle fibres. J Physiol 218: 117–145
38. Podolsky RJ, Teichholtz LE (1970) The relation between calcium and contraction kinetics in skinned muscle fibres. J Physiol 211: 19–35
39. Chalovich JM, Eisenberg E (1986) The effect of troponin-tropomyosin on the binding of heavy meromyosin to actin in the presence of ATP. J Biol Chem 261: 5088–5093
40. Gibbs CL, Loiselle D (1978) Energy output of tetanized cardiac muscle: species differences. Pflügers Arch 373: 31–38
41. Cooper G (1976) The myocardial energetic active state. I. Oxygen consumption during tetanus of cat papillary muscle. Circ Res 39: 695–704
42. Spencer RGS, Balschi JA, Leigh Jr JS, Ingwall JS (1988) ATP synthesis and degradation rates in the perfused heart. Biophys J 54: 921–929
43. Bhatnagar GM, Walford GD, Beard ES, Humphreys S, Lakatta EG (1984) ATPase activity and force production in myofibrils and twitch characteristics in intact muscle from neonatal, adult, and senescent rat myocardium. J Mol Cell Cardiol 16: 203–218
44. Portzehl H, Zaolarek P, Gaudin J (1969) The activation by Ca^{2+} of the ATPase of extracted muscle fibrils with variation of ionic strength, pH and concentration of MgATP. Biochim Biophys Acta 189: 440–448
45. Saeki Y, Kato C, Totsuka T, Yanagisawa K (1987) Mechanical properties and ATPase activity in glycerinated cardiac muscle of hyperthyroid rabbit. Pflügers Arch 408: 578–583
46. van den Berg C, Elzinga G, Stienen GJM (1989) Relation between ATPase activity and force development in chemically skinned cardiac trabeculae of rat. J Physiol 415: 114P
47. Barsotti RJ, Ferenczi MA (1988) Kinetics of ATP hydrolysis and tension production in skinned cardiac muscle of the guinea pig. J Biol Chem 263, 32: 16750–16756
48. Bremel RD, Weber A (1972) Cooperation within actin filament in vertebrate skeletal muscle. Nature (Lond) New Biol 238: 91–101
49. Ferenczi MA, Simmons RM, Sleep JA (1982) General considerations of cross-bridge models in relation to the dependence on MgATP concentration of mechanical parameters of skinned fibers from frog muscle. In: Twarog BM, Levine RJC, Dewey MM (eds) Basic Research of Muscles: A Comparative Approach. New York: Raven Press, pp 91–107
50. Ferenczi MA, Goldman YE, Simmons RM (1984) The dependence of force and shortening velocity on substrate concentration in skinned muscle fibres from Rana temporaria. J Physiol 350: 519–543
51. Cooke R, Bialek W (1979) Contraction of glycerinated muscle fibers as a function of the ATP concentration. Biophys J 28: 241–258
52. Chaen S, Kometani K, Yamada T, Shimizu H (1981) Substate-concentration dependence of tension, shortening velocity and ATPase activity of glycerinated single muscle fibers. J Biochem 90: 1611–1621
53. Stienen GJM, van der Laarse WJ, Elzinga G (1988) Dependency of the force velocity relationships on MgATP in different types of muscle fibers from Xenopus laevis. Biophys J 53: 849–855
54. Glyn H, Sleep JA (1985) Dependence of adenosine triphosphatase activity of rabbit psoas muscle fibres and myofibrils on substrate concentration. J Physiol 365: 259–276
55. Rüegg JCM, Schadler GJ, Steiger, Muller G (1971) Effects of inorganic phosphate on the contractile mechanism. Pflügers Arch 325: 359–364
56. Nosek TM, Fender KY, Godt RE (1987) It is the dipronated inorganic phosphate that depresses force in skinned skeletal muscle fibers. Science 236: 77–97
57. Cooke R, Franks K, Luciani GB, Pate E (1988) The inhibition of rabbit skeletal muscle contraction by hydrogen ions and phosphate. J Physiol 395: 77–97
58. Dawson MJ, Smith S, Wilkie DR (1986) The $[H_2PO_4^{-1}]$ may determine cross-bridge cycling rate and force reduction in fatiguing muscle. Biophys J 49: 268a
59. Hibberd MG, Dantzig JA, Trentham DR, Goldman YE (1985) Phosphate release and force generation in skeletal muscle fibers. Science 228: 1317–1319

336

60. Cooke R, Pate E (1985) The effects of ADP and phosphate on the contraction of muscle fibers. Biophys J 48: 789–798
61. Elzinga G, Stienen GJM, Versteeg PGA (1989) Effect of inorganic phosphate on length responses to changes in load in skinned rabbit psoas fibres. J Physiol 415: 132P
62. Kawai M, Güth K, Winnekes K, Haist C, Rüegg JC (1987) The effect of inorganic phosphate on the ATP hydrolysis rate and tension development in chemically skinned rabbit psoas fibres. Pflügers Arch 408: 1–9
63. Gagelman M, Güth K (1987) Effects of inorganic phosphate and Ca^{2+} sensitivity in skinned taenia coli smooth muscle fibers. Biophys J 51: 457–463
64. Herzig JW, Peterson JW, Rüegg JC, Solaro RJ (1981) Vanadate and phosphate ions reduce tension and increase cross-bridge kinetics in chemically skinned heart muscle. Biochim Biophys Acta 672: 191–196
65. Chaen S, Shimada M, Sugi H (1986) Evidence for cooperative interactions of myosin heads with thin filament in the force generation of vertebrate skeletal muscle fibers. J Biol Chem 261: 13632–16636
66. Chase PB, Kushmerick MJ (1988) Effects of pH on contraction of rabbit fast and slow skeletal muscle fibers. Biophys J 53: 935–946
67. Hoar PE, Mahoney CW, Kerrick WGL (1987) MgADP increases maximum tension and Ca^{2+} sensitivity in skinned rabbit soleus fibers. Pflügers Arch 410: 30–36
68. Schoenberg M, Eisenberg E (1987) ADP binding to myosin cross-bridges and its effect on the cross-bridge detachment rate constants. J Gen Physiol 89: 905–920
69. Johnson RE, Adams PH (1984) ADP binds similarly to rigor muscle myofibrils and to actomyosin-subfragment one. FEBS Letters 174: 11–14
70. Ventura-Clapier R, Mekhfi H, Vassort G (1987) Role of creatine kinase in force development in chemically skinned rat cardiac muscle. J Gen Physiol 89: 815–837
71. Robertson SP, Kerrick WGL: The effects of pH on Ca^{2+}-activated force in frog skeletal muscle fibers. Pflügers Arch 380: 41–45
72. Metzger JM, Moss RL (1988) Depression of Ca^{2+} insensitive tension due to reduced pH in partially troponin-extracted skinned skeletal muscle fibers. Biophys J 54: 1169–1173
73. Metzger JM, Moss RL (1987) Greater hydrogen ion-induced depression of tension and velocity in skinned single fibres of rat fast than slow muscles. J Physiol 393: 727–742
74. Kammermeier H, Schmidt P, Jungling E (1982) Free energy change at ATP-hydrolysis: a causal factor of early hypoxic failure of the myocardium? J Mol and Cell Cardiol 14: 267–277
75. Kammermeier H (1987) High energy phosphate of the myocardium: concentration versus free energy change. In: Jacob RHJ, Just, and Holubarsch CH (eds) Cardiac energetics. Darmstadt, Steinkopff Verlag, pp 31–36
76. Kushmerick MJ (1987) Energetics studies of muscles of different types. In: Jacob RHJ, Just, Holubarsch CH (eds) Cardiac energetics Darmstadt, Steinkopff Verlag pp 17–30
77. Dawson MJ, Gadian DG, Wilkie DR (1980) Mechanical relaxation rate and metabolism studied in fatiguing muscle by phosphorus nuclear magnetic resonance. J Physiol 299: 465–484
78. Eisenberg E, Hill TL, Chen Y (1980) Cross-bridge model of muscle contraction. Biophys J 29: 195–227
79. Holubarsch C, Alpert NA, Goulette R, Mulieri LA (1982) Heat production during hypoxic contracture of rat myocardium. Circ Res 51: 777–786
80. Smith GL, Allen DG (1988) Effects of metabolic blockade on intracellular calcium concentration in isolated ferret ventricular muscle. Circ Res 62: 1223–1236
81. Jung DWG (1988) Dynamic properties of cross-bridges in frog skeletal muscle fibres. Thesis, Amsterdam
82. Goldman YE (1987) Special topic: molecular mechanism of muscle contraction. Ann Rev Physio 49: 629–654

Importance of mechanical factors in ischemic and reperfusion injury

CHARLES E. GANOTE and RICHARD S. VANDER HEIDE

Department of Pathology, Northwestern University Medical School, 303 East Chicago Avenue, Chicago, Illinois 60611, USA

Introduction

Acute myocardial cell death is associated with complex biochemical and morphological changes which depend upon the type of cell injury sustained by the myocardium. Of the many changes associated with acute ischemic or anoxic myocardial cell death, intracellular calcium overload is a prominent feature of ischemia-reperfusion injury as has been shown in many experimental models. Consequently, early hypotheses and investigative research regarding acute myocardial death centered around calcium overload and determining the events and/or series of events which lead to cellular calcium overload. During our investigations of the mechanism(s) of cell damage associated with cellular injury, evidence appeared that cellular contracture and/or physical stress may be involved with acute cellular death in some experimental systems. Recently there is a growing body of evidence to suggest that cells irreversibly injured by hypoxia or ischemia may become fragile and therefore not able to withstand physical stresses associated with reperfusion or reoxygenation. This suggests that calcium overload may not be the primary cause of cell death. This chapter will evolve a discussion of the role of mechanical factors in the development of irreversible myocardial cellular injury and cell death.

$$\text{CELL} \xleftrightarrow{} \underset{\text{reflow}}{\overset{\text{ischemia}}{\text{REVERSIBLE}}} \dashrightarrow \overset{\text{ischemia}}{\text{IRREVERSIBLE}} \underset{\text{reflow}}{\longrightarrow} \text{DEATH} \longrightarrow \text{NECROSIS}$$

CONCEPT OF IRREVERSIBLE INJURY

Concepts of reversible and irreversible injury

Myocardial cells can withstand brief temporary episodes of ischemia or hypoxia. Although metabolically altered, the cells are capable of regaining normal structure and function if blood flow or oxygen is restored before a critical period of anoxia/ischemia has elapsed. However, full functional

H.M. Piper (ed.) Pathophysiology of severe ischemic myocardial injury, 337–355.
© 1990 Kluwer Academic Publishers, Dordrecht

recovery may be delayed. Such cells are considered to have sustained *reversible injury*. If the period of ischemia or hypoxia is prolonged, the cells become more severely damaged such that upon reperfusion or reoxygenation the cells do not recover, but continue to degenerate and die. These cells are considered to be *irreversibly injured*. It is important to recognize that irreversibly injured cells are not dead. It is true that such cells would die if returned to a normal environment, but if the cells are kept under special conditions they theoretically may be able to survive indefinitely. Thus irreversibly injured cells may be capable of relatively normal metabolic activities including ATP-production, electrolyte pump activity, and perhaps even synthetic activities that would allow repair of the damage. Such events cannot occur in nature but are possible under laboratory conditions or with therapeutic interventions. Irreversible injury, then, is a relative rather than an absolute term.

Cell death is an absolute term. When a cell dies it cannot carry out normal cellular functions under *any* conditions. However, a practical definition is needed to provide a basis for experimental studies of cellular reactions to injury. Cell death is defined as occurring at the time that the plasma membrane of the cell is no longer capable of maintaining a barrier between the intracellular and the extracellular space. The term 'loss of membrane integrity' is commonly used to designate this condition. Loss of the semipermeable properties of the membrane allows release of metabolites and necessary enzymatic proteins out of the cell and influxes of calcium and extracellular markers into the cell. *Necrosis* refers to the degenerative changes occurring after cell death.

The canine *in vivo* regional infarct model in dogs

The canine open-chested posterior papillary muscle infarct model was developed by Jennings *et al.* [1]. This model remains the most widely used for study of regional infarction. In this model the circumflex coronary artery was temporarily ligated for varying periods of time followed by reflow. Infarct size was determined by microscopic examination 1–7 days later. They found that irreversible injury of the papillary muscle occurred after as little as 20 minutes of total ischemia.

Following permanent ischemia, the dead cells in the infarct regions exhibited features of coagulation necrosis. The cells are elongated due to bunching of the myofibrils in the regional area of the ischemic infarct, creating the characteristic I-bands in the sarcomeres. Although I-bands are normally seen in relaxation, these stretched sarcomeres are actually in rigor contracture. The cell is massively swollen and as a result the sarcolemma is raised away from the surface of the sarcomeres forming subsarcolemmal blebs. The mitochondria are swollen and contain amorphous or flocculant densities, which are classically considered a hallmark of irreversible injury. Close examination of the sarcolemma overlying the blebs by electron microscopy usually reveals defects in the plasma membrane.

Following temporary ischemia, the reflow of blood into regions of irreversibly injured myocardium causes severe cellular contracture characterized by irregular zones of hypercontracted and greatly overstretched sarcomeres which have torn away from the intercalated disc. These alternating zones produce a banding pattern which has been termed *contraction band necrosis*. In addition, the cells undergo explosive and massive swelling with formation of large subsarcolemmal blebs. There is a massive and sudden release of cytosolic proteins from the cells accompanied by a large influx of calcium into the cell. The excess calcium is accumulated in the mitochondria and form annular, granular, dense bodies also called calcium accumulation granules. Finally, large defects in the plasma membrane are easily demonstrable by electron microscopy [2].

Perfused heart models

The oxygen paradox

Our use of the isolated perfused rat heart for the study of mechanisms of irreversible injury began in the laboratories of Dr. Winifred Nayler, then at the Cardiothoracic Institute in London. David Hearse's laboratory had been studying the phenomenon of oxygen-induced enzyme release in perfused rat hearts. These workers [3] had reported that following a period of hypoxic perfusion, the reintroduction of oxygen produced a rapid release of enzymes from the heart. This was considered to be a parodoxical response of the cells to oxygen and thus the term *oxygen paradox* was coined to describe the phenomenon. Since enzyme release is a commonly used marker for irreversible myocardial injury, we conducted a morphologic study of the effects of permanent and temporary hypoxic perfusions on isolated perfused rat hearts. The results showed that during permanent hypoxia, enzyme release first began after about 60 minutes of hypoxic perfusion. At the times during which enzyme release occurred, the cells appeared similar to those that had undergone coagulation necrosis after ischemic injury. The hypoxic cells contained swollen mitochondria (with flocculent densities), subsarcolemmal blebs (with associated plasma membrane defects), and there was a generalized swelling and vacuolization of cytoplasmic components [4].

The events caused by reoxygenation of hypoxic rat myocardium were similar to those seen with reperfusion of ischemic myocardium in the canine model. In contrast to the delayed enzyme release with permanent hypoxia, reoxygenation of hearts after 20–30 minutes of hypoxia produced a sudden peak of enzyme release. The longer the hypoxic interval prior to reperfusion the greater was the magnitude of enzyme release and the extent of irreversible injury. Enzyme release began within seconds of reoxygenation and

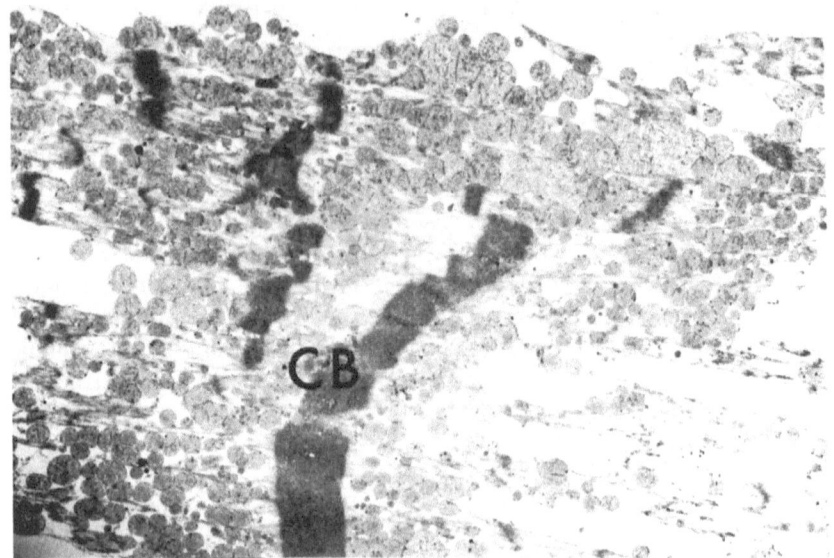

Fig. 1. Electron micrograph of an irreversibly injured cell after the oxygen paradox showing a prominent contraction band and cellular and mitochondrial swelling. The sarcolemmal membrane would show focal defects and loss of costamere attachments to the sarcolemma.

peaked by 2–3 minutes. Morphological examination of hearts at early times following reoxygenation showed that the cells rapidly hyper-contracted with contraction band formation beginning within 30–60 seconds. Later, by 2–5 minutes, the cells showed massive swelling. The ultrastructural lesions found were essentially identical to those seen in reperfused myocardium with contraction band necrosis (Fig. 1).

A variety of mitochondrial uncouplers and inhibitors administered at the time of reoxygenation completely prevented *both contraction banding and oxygen-induced enzyme release.* Since inhibitors and uncouplers of oxidative phosphorylation would presumably prevent the cell from resuming production of ATP following the resupply of oxygen, we reasoned that the resupply of ATP to the irreversibly injured cells could initiate cellular contraction and thereby cause the contraction band formation and enzyme release observed during the oxygen paradox.

In any case, the evidence indicated that cells had undergone irreversible injury after 20–30 minutes of hypoxic perfusion, yet cells retained intact plasma membranes for a considerable time thereafter. Thus, loss of membrane permeability *per se* was not a cause of irreversible injury. It follows, then, that irreversible injury must occur earlier than the loss of membrane permeability and furthermore that reoxygenation either causes additional injury, i.e. free radical generation, or exposes latent cell injury. We have subsequently found that free-radical active agents, such as dimethylthiourea and catalase, do not influence the oxygen paradox [5]. Since we had found that contraction banding occurred temporally co-incident with enzyme release, we hypothesized from these observations that mechanical stresses caused by contraction banding might in turn cause rupture of plasma membranes and enzyme release [6].

The calcium paradox

The *calcium paradox* originally described by Zimmerman and Hulsmann [7] refers to the phenomenon which occurs when a heart perfused for a brief (usually 3–5 minute) period with calcium-free perfusate is re-exposed to calcium-containing perfusate. Following re-exposure to calcium, hearts develop irreversible contracture, release cytoplasmic enzymes and develop severe contraction band necrosis. Coincident to reperfusion, the heart also accumulates massive amounts of calcium from the perfusate. Initial studies hypothesized that acute calcium overload was the major cause of cellular injury and the calcium paradox was considered a model of calcium overload injury similar to that caused during ischemia-reperfusion [8]. Our studies suggest another pathogenesis that better explains the observed experimental results.

Muir provided the first ultrastructural study of the calcium paradox [see 13]. He showed that calcium depletion and repletion caused separations of myocardial cells at the intercalated disc regions and the formation of contraction bands. A variety of methods have been shown to provide partial or complete protection from the calcium paradox. Studies that documented complete protection usually also documented unique morphological characteristics different from those observed in unprotected hearts. Interventions which provided protection from cellular damage reduced the extent of separation at the intercalated discs and also prevented the additional lesion of lifting of the outer lamina of the sarcolemma (basement membrane) from the plasma membrane [9]. It has subsequently been found that manganese, when used to replace calcium, will prevent the intercalated disc separations but not the lifting of the basement membrane from the sarcolemmal plasma membrane. However, hearts treated in this manner do not develop a calcium paradox, showing that the basement membrane lesion is not the critical lesion leading to the paradox.

Our studies of the calcium paradox were begun during attempts to study the role of calcium in hypoxic injury. When hearts that were irreversibly injured by 40–60 minutes of hypoxia were reperfused with *calcium-free*, oxygenated media total cell injury was increased, an unanticipated result. Similarly, hearts perfused with hypoxic calcium-free media showed a sustained enzyme release much earlier than was ever seen with hypoxia alone. These unexpected results led to a study of the morphology of calcium-free anoxic hearts which revealed that the principal lesions observed were contracture of the myocytes, wide separations of cells at the intercalated discs junctions and rupture of the plasma membranes adjacent to nexus (tight) junctions. The cells had separated at fascia adherens junctions but the nexus junctions had remained virtually intact. These lesions were nearly identical to those of the calcium paradox.

Contracture and the calcium paradox

Structure of the intercalated disc
The fascia adherens junction serves as the internal attachment site of sarcomere chains and therefore are the major structures responsible for mechanical force transduction between myocardial cells. The internal face of the disc membrane is a modified Z-band containing alpha-actinin which cross links the f-actin thin filaments. The actin filaments are also attached to the plasma membrane by a complex of proteins containing vinculin as a principal component. Some proteins of the complex are thought to span the membrane and to connect to a 135-kD adherens junction-specific cell adhesion molecule (A-CAM) [10]. This is a calcium-dependent glycoprotein which serves as the 'glue' which binds adjacent cells. In the absence of extracellular calcium the adhesive properties of the A-CAM molecules are lost and cells separate from one another and from substrate attachments.

Nexus junctions provide a low resistance coupling between myocardial cells [11]. They are formed from barrel-shaped complexes of nexin molecules which span the membranes of adjacent cells forming open channels between two cells. Crystalloid arrays of nexus complexes form membrane patches which are focal points of cellular contact. These 'tight junctions' are not calcium dependent and therefore remain intact in calcium-free environments.

Desmocalin is the extracellular calcium-dependent glycoprotein in macula adherens junctions. These junctions contain desmoplakins and serve as attachment points of intermediate (desmin) filaments of the myocardial cytoskeleton. The forces resisted by these junctions may be those of passive stretching rather than active contraction.

In calcium-free medium, the calcium-dependent fascia and macula adherens junctions separate leaving only the nexus junctions as points of cell attachment (Fig. 2). If contraction were to occur when cells were attached in this tenuous manner all mechanical forces of contraction would be transmitted to the plasma membrane at the inherently weaker nexus junctions, instead of along the stronger pathways involving fascia adherens junctions.

Physical stresses and cell injury
To determine if the induction of physical or mechanical stress in myocardial cells previously weakened by calcium-free perfusion could produce membrane injury, we induced contracture in calcium deprived hearts. In the first experiments, a rapid contracture was induced in calcium-free hearts by the

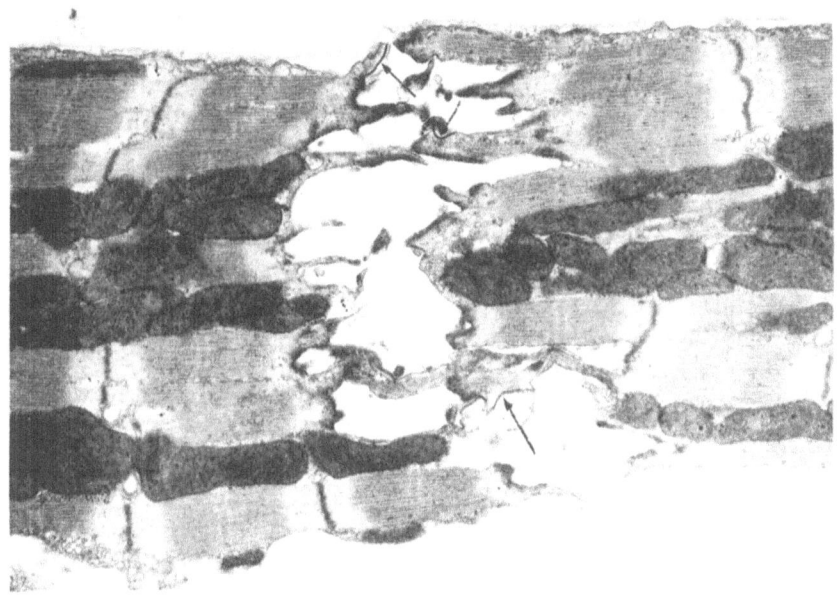

Fig. 2. Electron micrograph of the intercalated disc junction between two myocytes after calcium-free perfusion. The fascia adherens junctions are widely separated but the nexus junctions remain intact. With calcium repletion and contracture of the cells the membranes rupture at the nexus junctions as the cells separate. Figure 12B from Vander Heide RS, Ganote CE (1985). Caffeine-induced injury in calcium-free perfused rat hearts. Am J Pathol 118: 55–65.

administration of the mitochondrial uncoupling agent dinitrophenol (DNP) [12]. DNP leads to a rapid contracture, because in addition to uncoupling electron transport from oxidative phosphorylation, DNP also activates mito- chondrial ATPases which consume any remaining intracellular ATP. DNP- induced contracture caused the release of myoglobin from calcium-free hearts. In a second series of experiments, the effects of balloon-induced expansion of the ventricular cavity was determined to see if physical stress alone could cause myoglobin release and intercalated disc separations in calcium-free hearts. However, since calcium-free hearts are relaxed, they could be easily distended by the balloon without offering significant resistance and therefore consequently sustained little damage. To cause the hearts to stiffen and thereby provide resistance against physical distension, we induced hypoxic contracture prior to calcium deprivation. Distension of calcium-free (but not control) hearts caused a large myoglobin release that corresponded to the degree of distension induced by the intraventricular balloon. These results indicated that mechanical stress, in the presence of previously weakened intercalated discs, was able to cause significant membrane damage and cell death [13].

The results were clear, but in the above experiments the expression of physical stress-induced injury required the combination of hypoxia and calcium depletion. The definitive experiments showing a correlation between contracture (without hypoxia) and cell injury in calcium-free hearts were performed in our laboratory using caffeine [14]. Caffeine releases only that calcium stored in the sarcoplasmic reticulum (SR) and thus enough calcium to produce a maximum contracture, but not enough to produce 'calcium overload'. Caffeine-induced contracture caused cellular injury in calcium-free hearts similar in nearly all respects to that seen after the calcium paradox. The only difference, as expected, was that the mitochondria of caffeine-treated hearts did not show marked swelling or calcium accumulation granules, since no calcium was available to them from the perfusate.

Additional support for the hypothesis that mechanical stresses resulting from contracture can cause the membrane lesions in the calcium paradox comes from experiments showing that agents that inhibit contracture, but which do not prevent membrane electrolyte fluxes or interfere with mitochondrial function, also prevent calcium-induced injury. Dimethylsulfoxide (DMSO), an agent which prevents contracture and enzyme release in the oxygen paradox, was found also to protect hearts from calcium paradox injury. The argument that the effects of DMSO could be derived from its ability to scavenge free radicals is not tenable since another agent, beta-diacylmonoxamine (BDM or DAM), which inhibits contraction but which is not a free radical scavenger, also protects hearts from the calcium paradox [14].

Pathogenesis of the calcium paradox
The experiments discussed above strongly support the hypothesis that the calcium paradox is the result of the weakening of the intercalated disc adherens junctions during calcium-free perfusion. These lesions remain latent until the discs are exposed to a physical stress that causes separation of cells and tearing of the plasma membranes near the nexus junctions [13].

$$\text{CELL} \underset{\text{Ca}^{2+}}{\overset{\text{Ca}^{2+}\text{-free}}{\longleftrightarrow}} \text{REVERSIBLE} \overset{\text{Ca}^{2+}\text{-free}}{-\:-\:-\:\to} \text{disc} \overset{\text{(fragility)}}{\underset{\text{separations Ca}^{2+}}{\longrightarrow}} \text{DEATH} \overset{\text{(Contracture)}}{\longrightarrow} \text{NECROSIS}$$

PATHOGENESIS OF CALCIUM PARADOX

Contracture and the oxygen paradox

Observations of cell fragility

The observations that agents which prevent contraction banding during reoxygenation, whether by preventing ATP repletion (cyanide, amytal,

DNP) or by direct inhibition of interaction of contractile proteins (DMSO, BDM) [15], also protect hearts from membrane damage and enzyme release associated with reoxygenation, suggested that mechanical forces could be the cause of membrane injury in the oxygen paradox.

To test our hypothesis that mechanical stress was responsible for membrane rupture and enzyme release, perfused rat hearts were subjected to periods of anoxic perfusion that resulted in graded degrees of irreversible injury. The degree of injury (as tested by the amount of oxygen-induced enzyme release in a parallel series of control hearts), ranged from none to nearly total injury. We utilized two separate experimental protocols, each designed to produce varying amounts of physical stress in anoxic rat hearts. Hearts were either (1) subjected to varying amounts of physical distension with an intraventricular balloon or (2) were subjected to varying degrees of osmotic swelling. Damage was assessed by monitoring enzyme release and cellular morphology. In the first group, inflation of the intraventricular balloon in control hearts (which were in anoxic contracture but which were not yet irreversibly injured), caused little or no enzyme release. In contrast, hearts subjected to irreversible periods of anoxia prior to distension released intracellular enzymes, the amount of which correlated with both the volume of balloon inflation and the duration of the anoxic interval prior to balloon inflation. These results demonstrated that physical stress alone could cause membrane rupture of irreversibly injured but not reversibly injured cells.

The effects of osmotic swelling on perfused hearts were then determined [16]. Control hearts perfused with control medium of 295–300 mOsm could be subjected to sudden severe osmotic swelling by switching the perfusate to a 150 mOsm medium, with no apparent damage and no enzyme release. Anoxic hearts, however, sustained cellular damage and released intracellular enzymes, the amount of which was dependent on both the degree of preceding injury to the hearts (anoxic interval) and the osmolality of the perfusate (Fig. 3). The gradation of injury clearly showed that as injury progressed, the cells in the heart became progressively more osmotically fragile. As these experiments were conducted entirely under hypoxic conditions it can also be concluded that oxygen played no role in initiating or exposing the injury.

The morphological studies showed that the major cellular lesions seen following the oxygen paradox were reproduced in the absence of oxygen by mechanical stresses. These included the separation of sarcomere attachments to the internal face of the fascia adherens junctions and the shredding and lysis of Z-bands. The swelling produced large subsarcolemmal blebs and rupture of the plasma membranes (Fig. 4). The observations that both mechanical stretching and osmotic swelling of myocytes would injure hypoxic but not control cells allows the conclusion that *irreversibly injured myocardium is fragile and this fragility can be exposed by either mechanical or osmotic stresses.*

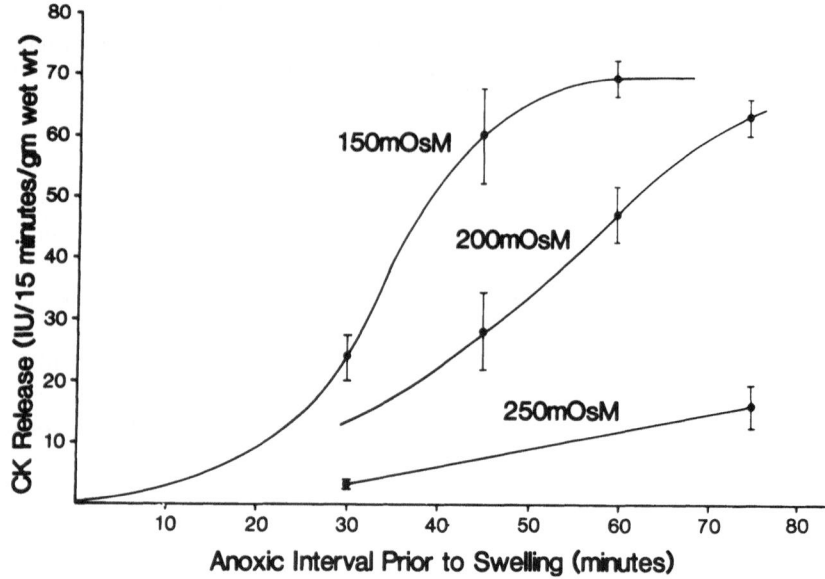

Fig. 3. Graph of the effects of cellular swelling with solutions of various osmolalities on enzyme release from anoxic perfused rat hearts. Both the duration of anoxic perfusion and the osmolality of the perfusate influence enzyme release. These results demonstrate that as anoxic injury becomes more severe the cells become increasingly osmotically fragile. Figure 5 from Vander Heide RS, Ganote CE (1987). Increased myocyte fragility following anoxic injury. J Mol Cell Cardiol 19: 1085–1103.

Cytoskeletal structure

The myocyte cytoskeleton is basically similar to that of other cells but is more highly specialized. Stress fibers present in more primitive cell types have been reorganized into the sarcomeres in myocardial cells and the attachment plaques usually seen at the periphery of cells are concentrated at the interca- lated disc. The barbed ends of the actin thin filaments (6–8nm) are cross linked in the Z-band regions and the intercalated discs by alpha-actinin, a cytoskeletal protein which composes much of the dense material present in these structures. Intermediate filaments (IF) (8–14nm) are made up of poly- mers of desmin subunits. They form a well organized network of longitudinal and transverse filaments that interconnect most of the cytoplasmic organelles and make connections to the sarcolemma and the nuclear membranes. The longitudinal fibers also make connections to the macula adherens junctions of the intercalated discs. The IF system in myocardial cells is believed to maintain the register of the Z-bands in both longitudinal and transverse directions and to determine the resting length of the cell.

The sarcolemma or cell membrane is composed of the lipid bilayer, an outer lamina or basement membrane, and a subcortical lattice. The tensile

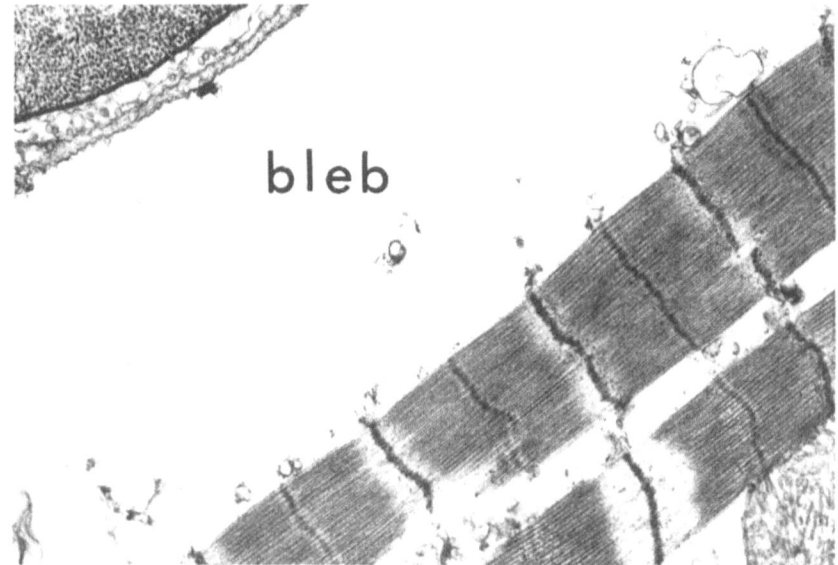

Fig. 4. Electron micrograph of a large subsarcolemmal bleb on an anoxically injured and osmotically swollen myocardial cell. There is lysis of the lateral costamere junctions between the sarcolemma and the Z-line attachments to the plasma membrane. Distortion of Z-lines can also be seen. It is proposed that lesions in the attachment sites of the cytoskeleton account for the increased osmotic fragility of irreversibly injured myocardial cells.

strength of the sarcolemma is thought to be derived from the subcortical layer. Similar to red blood cells, the sarcolemma contains spectrin molecules which may serve as attachment sites for intermediate filaments. A subcortical lattice surrounds each myocardial cell at the Z-band region. The lattice is composed principally of vinculin, a protein that connects the sarcolemma of the myocardial cell to the periphery of the sarcomeres at the Z-bank [18]. This sarcolemmal-sarcomere attachment complex produces the characteristic scalloped pattern of the sarcolemma seen with electron microscopy. These junctions are called costamere junctions. Costameres are thought to also interact with membrane-spanning proteins to form attachments to the extracellular matrix. A layer of dense material can be seen on the inner surface of the sarcolemma arranged in periodic plaques which may correspond to leptomeres. The function of leptomeres is not known but they may serve as cytoskeletal attachment sites.

Microtubules are especially numerous near the nucleus. They course through the cytoplasm at varying angles and connect to cellular organelles and the sarcolemma. They are dynamic structures composed of tubulin polymeres and are sensitive to both ATP and calcium levels. Microtubules are believed to provide a motive force for particle transport, to help organize the golgi apparatus and to play a role in myofibrillogenesis.

Cytoskeletal lesions in irreversible injury

Steenbergen, Hill, and Jennings [19] were the first to suggest that lesions involving the attachment of cytoskeletal proteins to the sarcolemma were responsible for the occurrence of subsarcolemmal blebs and membrane ruptures in irreversibly injured ischemic myocardium and ischemia-reperfusion injury. Reperfusion of hypertonic ischemic cells with isotonic fluid caused swelling of the cells and consequent rupture of cell membranes [20, 21]. These authors were able to demonstrate that irreversibly injured ischemic dog myocardium had diminished immunofluorescense staining for the cytoskeletal protein vinculin and suggested that alterations in the sub-sarcolemmal cytoskeletal lattice was a possible contributing cause to membrane damage following irreversible periods of ischemia [19].

To test our hypothesis that lesions in the cytoskeletal support system are responsible for the formation of subsarcolemmal blebs and the observed increased cellular fragility following irreversible anoxic injury, we conducted a study of the cytoskeleton of injured myocardial cells using high voltage electron microscopic (HVEM) and immunofluorescence techniques [22]. These studies demonstrated that an intact cytoskeletal network could be well visualized in osmotically swollen control cells. In contrast, this same cyto-skeletal network was severely disrupted in osmotically swollen anoxic cells. There was loss of desmin connections to both nuclear and sarcolemmal attachments and the extensive microtubular system had disappeared. The cells that contained subsarcolemmal blebs had loss of the dense layer of protein (leptomeres) normally present immediately subjacent to the lipid bilayer. Immunofluorescence studies demonstrated a loss of vinculin staining both at the intercalated discs and at the lateral costamere junctions. In addition, alpha-actinin staining was significantly decreased in irreversibly injured anoxic cells.

In summary, the demonstration of cytoskeletal lesions by conventional and high voltage EM and the loss of immunofluorescent staining of two cyto-skeletal proteins in irreversibly injured anoxic cells provides a plausible explanation for our observation that irreversibly injured cells are mechani-cally fragile when compared to control cells. Furthermore, the major lesions appeared to reside in the cytoskeleton and the development of increased cell fragility coincident with irreversible injury could explain the cell damage seen in the oxygen paradox.

Isolated adult myocyte models

Characteristics of isolated myocytes

The healthy isolated myocyte is calcium tolerant and remains elongated as a rod-shaped form and is quiescent in physiologic concentrations of extracellu-lar calcium [21]. Trypan blue, a non-toxic viable dye, has been extensively

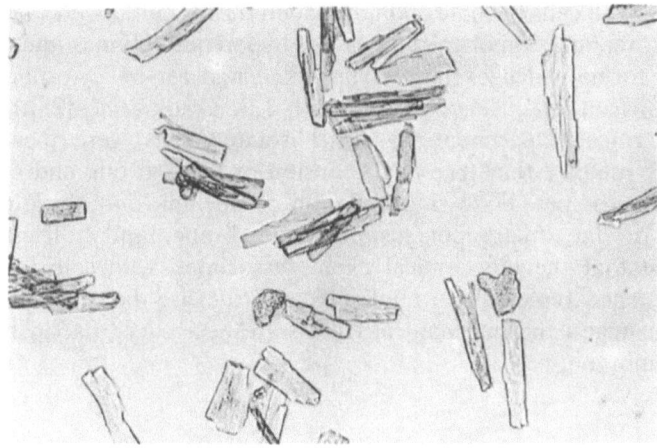

Fig. 5. Light micrograph of a control suspension of isolated myocytes. The cells are mainly elongated rod-shaped cells which exclude the extracellular marker dye trypan blue.

used in isolated myocyte studies to assess cell viability. Cells that exclude trypan blue from the intracellular space are viable in that they are capable of carrying out homeostatic metabolic functions (Fig. 5). A variety of conditions can cause the elongated rod-shaped cells to contract into rounded forms [23, 24].

Round cells that exclude trypan blue have been shown to carry out normal metabolic function and maintain normal ionic gradients [23]. However, round cells are more fragile than rod cells and become easily damaged by minor trauma such as vigorous stirring of cell suspensions. The cell damage that occurs is reflected by both biochemical alterations in the cells and the loss of cytosolic enzymes as well as the admission of trypan blue to the cell interior [25].

When isolated cells are made anoxic without prior inhibition of anaerobic glycolysis, they slowly round up. However, when the cells are subjected to rapid complete metabolic inhibition by the additional blockade of anaerobic metabolism using iodoacetate, the cells retain their rod shape until the available supply of ATP is exhausted and then rapidly contract into a square shape [26]. This square-form is the *in vitro* equivalent of rigor contracture [27]. Square cells are stable in form for the duration of an extended incubation period. In the discussion below, cells excluding trypan blue are considered to be viable cells regardless of cell shape while those unable to exclude trypan blue are considered non-viable.

The calcium paradox

The calcium paradox does not occur in isolated myocytes if the cells are in suspension. Calcium can be repeatedly depleted and repleted without causing cell injury. If the cells become sodium-loaded during prolonged calcium-free incubations, readmission of calcium causes hypercontraction of the myocytes into round forms which exclude trypan blue and retain cytosolic proteins indicating no cell death has occurred [27]. J.S. Frank *et al.* [28] have performed a critical experiment in which isolated cells were incubated in calcium-free media either free in suspension or fixed at one end by attachment to a micropipet. Following repletion of calcium, only those cells that were fixed to the micropipet sustained membrane injury. These results demonstrate that the biochemical events associated with calcium influxes across an intact sarcolemma are not sufficient to cause the calcium paradox, but instead suggest that mechanical factors are necessary to actually disrupt the cell membrane.

The oxygen paradox

Early studies of the oxygen paradox in isolated myocytes by Altschuld *et al.* [24] demonstrated that following a prolonged period of hypoxia, most of the cells assumed a square configuration, indicating that they were in 'rigor contracture'. Reoxygenation caused one population of cells to contract further and become round cells while a separate population of cells relaxed and assumed the rod-shaped configuration. There was, however, no loss of cell viability or release of enzymes from either group of cells. Piper *et al.* [29] have confirmed that a classical oxygen paradox does not occur in briefly cultured isolated myocytes. Stern *et al.* [30] have shown that while the time to contracture of rod cells into square forms (a measure of the rate of ATP-depletion) is highly variable, the interval from contracture to the point where reoxygenation of square cells results in cell rounding and not relaxation is relatively constant. The heterogeneity of cell squaring may relate to variable energy demands of the individual cells. The energy demand of the cells may vary according to the rate of sodium leakage into cells and the rates of ATP consumption of the various electrolyte pumps of the cell. Viable isolated myocytes do not spontaneously contract and therefore the sodium/potassium pump and the calcium pump become the principal consumers of available energy. Normally these processes comprise only 10–20% of the energy demands of a contracting myocyte. Once ATP has become severely depleted the sarcomeres undergo rigor contracture and cells become square shaped.

Round cells which result from reoxygenation of hypoxic square cells are actually disc-shaped, resulting from hypercontraction of the sarcomeres into a single central contraction band. The ability of cells in suspension to contract without physical restraint, such that the mechanical stresses of contraction are not focally transmitted to the sarcolemma, probably accounts for the maintenance of an intact plasma membrane during reoxygenation contracture [31].

Fragility of isolated myocytes

Since the occurrence of the oxygen paradox upon reoxygenation of intact ischemic or anoxic hearts had been the only way to unequivocally test for irreversible injury, the study of injury in isolated myocytes which do not show an oxygen paradox has had no firm basis on which to determine when irreversible injury occurs. The close correlation between the onset of osmotic fragility and irreversible injury in both ischemic dog hearts [32] and ischemic and anoxic perfused rat hearts suggested that the onset of osmotic fragility could be a useful marker of irreversible injury in isolated myocytes.

Myocardial cells are relatively resistant to osmotic swelling and do not show ideal behavior when exposed to hypotonic solutions [33]. It has been shown that the resistance to swelling resides within the cell itself. It is thought that the cytoskeleton of the cell restricts the ability of the cell to deform during swelling. Tissue slices from control hearts can be exposed to solutions as low as 60mOsm without sustaining membrane damage [20].

Increased osmotic fragility during the metabolic inhibition of isolated myocytes has been documented in our laboratory [32]. Control myocytes isolated and incubated in 320–340 mOsm media (the increased osmolality is due to supplemental substrates and amino acids) were exposed to hypotonic media prepared by dilution of the control media with an equal volume of deionized water. During a 60-minute incubation aliquots were removed and mixed with trypan blue-containing fixative and cell counts were performed. There was no difference in the number of viable rod cells between the two preparations. The only difference was that, as expected, the round cells in the hypotonic preparation stained blue at a more rapid rate than round cells during isotonic incubation. Metabolic inhibition of similar preparations of cells resulted in squaring of the rods as ATP-depletion occurred. The rates of squaring were similar in isotonic and hypotonic media. In both media, squaring was complete by 10–15 minutes, indicating that the rates of energy consumption were similar in both preparations. There was a striking difference in the rates at which myocytes developed trypan blue permeability. By 60 minutes of incubation about 20% of isotonic square cells had stained while nearly 50% of hypotonic cells stained with trypan blue.

To test the effect of acute cell swelling on cell viability, metabolically inhibited myocytes were incubated for 25 minutes in isotonic media and then tranferred to either isotonic or hypotonic media. The transfer of cells to isotonic media resulted in a negligibly small increase of non-viable (trypan blue-staining) square cells. The transfer of cells to hypotonic media (acute cell swelling) caused nearly twice as many cells to stain with trypan blue. A majority of cells that had turned blue in hypotonic media developed multiple dome-shaped blebs of the sarcolemmal membranes. Blebs were rarely seen on viable cells. The blebs occurred both on the lateral surfaces of cells and on the ends of cells and were similar to those seen in injured cells in intact tissues

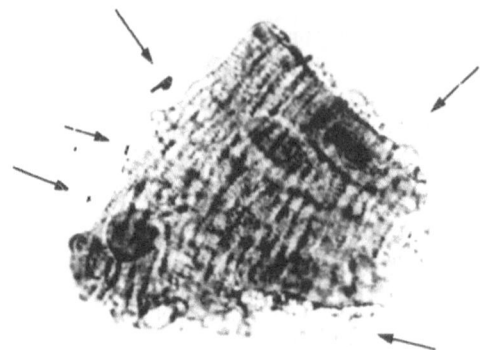

Fig. 6. Light micrograph of an isolated myocyte following metabolic inhibition with sodium amytal and iodacetic acid. The cell has contracted into a square-shape as a result of ATP-depletion rigor contracture. This cell has been suspended in hypotonic medium and the resultant swelling has produced large blebs on the cell surface.

(Fig. 6). Thus an early onset of osmotic fragility occurs as a result of metabolic inhibition of isolated myocytes.

Preliminary experiments to determine the effect of ischemia on isolated myocyte fragility were carried out by incubation of a concentrated slurry of cells under a layer of oil at 37°C (C.E. Ganote, R.S. Vander Heide, unpublished). The cells under these conditions rapidly consume all available oxygen so that the cells become nearly totally anoxic and most of the cells squared-up. The cells were then diluted into hypertonic, isotonic and hypotonic media to assess their osmotic fragility. Similar to the metabolically inhibited cells it was found that after 25 minutes of ischemia resuspension of cells in hypertonic (460 mOsm) or isotonic (320 mOsm) media resulted in a small increase in the number of non-viable square cells, while suspension in hypotonic (160 mOsm) buffer which presumably caused acute cell swelling resulted in a much larger proportion of non-viable square cells (34.2%, vs. 21.3%, vs. 6.2% viable cells in the hyper-, iso-, and hypotonic buffers, respectively). The non-viable, swollen, blue cells showed numerous blebs on the sarcolemmal membranes. These results demonstrate that osmotic fragility may also be a prominent feature of ischemic injury to isolated myocytes.

Hypothesis: Cytoskeletal lesions, cell fragility, mechanical factors, and irreversible injury

The results of the studies described in this chapter provide support for the hypothesis that irreversible ischemic and anoxic injury occurs when yet undefined lesions in the cytoskeletal support system of the myocardial cell occur. Cytoskeletal lesions can explain the increased myocyte fragility which can be demonstrated at the same time cells become irreversibly injured. Recent studies have shown that similar events may also occur in other cell systems. Buja *et al.* [35] have described blebs on cultured neonatal myocytes following metabolic inhibition with iodoacetate. Schwartz *et al.* [36] describe numerous microblebs forming on the surface of anoxic cultured adult myocytes. Herman *et al.* [37], in studies of cultured hepatocytes, found that numerous small membrane blebs form on the surface of the cells following anoxic incubation. With reoxygenation, early bleb formation was reversible and the cells recovered normal morphology. After longer anoxic incubation periods the smaller blebs coalesced into larger ones and cell death occurred as a result of sudden swelling and rupture of the large blebs. The osmotic fragility of cells with blebs was not determined. A reversible reorganization of actin stress fibers and vinculin- and alpha-actinin-containing attachments has been observed during ATP depletion and repletion in cultured PtK$_2$ cells, suggesting that dynamic changes in the cytoskeleton may occur during anoxia.

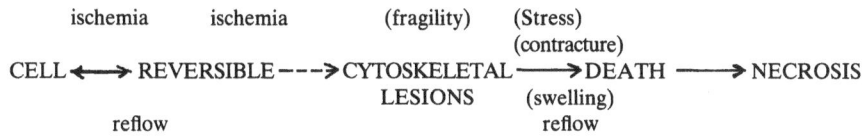

Pathogenesis of ischemic/anoxic injury

Although future studies will be required to determine the precise mechanism(s) by which anoxic and ischemic injury cause cytoskeletal lesions and increased cell fragility, it is clear that the induction of a mechanical stress (such as contracture or acute cell swelling), in myocytes previously rendered fragile by irreversible injury, can account for the membrane rupture and acute cell death which occurs during reoxygenation of hypoxic myocardium or reperfusion of ischemic myocardium.

References

1. Jennings RB, Wartman WB, Zudyk ZE (1957) Production of a homogeneous myocardial infarction in the dog. Arch Pathol 63: 580–585
2. Kloner RA, Ganote CE, Whalen DA, Jennings RB (1974) Effects of a transient period of ischemia on myocardial cells. II. Fine structure during the first few minutes of reflow. Am J Pathol 74: 399–422
3. Hearse DJ, Humphrey SM, Chain EB (1973) Abrupt reoxygenation of the anoxic potassium-arrested perfused rat heart: A study of myocardial enzyme release. J Mol Cell Cardiol 5: 395–407
4. Ganote CE, Seabra-Gomes R, Nayler WG, Jennings RB (1975) Irreversible injury in anoxic perfused rat hearts. Am J Pathol 81: 179–198
5. Vander Heide RS, Sobotka PA, Ganote CE (1987) Effects of the free radical scavenger DMTU and mannitol on the oxygen paradox in perfused rat hearts. J Mol Cell Cardiol 19: 615–625

6. Ganote CE (1983) Contraction band necrosis and irreversible myocardial injury. J Mol Cell Cardiol 15: 67–73

7. Zimmerman ANE, Hulsmann WC (1966) A paradoxical influence of calcium ions on the permeability of the cell membrane of the isolated rat heart. Nature 211: 646–647

8. Yates JC, Dhalla NS (1975) Structural and functional changes associated with failure and recovery of hearts after perfusion with Ca^{2+}-free medium. J Mol Cell Cardiol 7: 91–103

9. Crevey BJ, Langer GA, Frank JS (1978) Role of Ca^{2+} in maintenance of rabbit myocardial cell membrane structural and functional integrity. J Mol Cell Cardiol 10: 1081–1100

10. Volk T, Geiger B (1986) A-CAM: A 135-kD receptor of intercellular adherens junctions. II. Antibody-mediated modulation of junction formation. J Cell Biol 103: 1451–1454

11. De Mello WC (1982) Intercellular communication in cardiac muscle. Circ Res 51: 1–9

12. Ganote CE, Grinwald PM, Nayler WG (1984) 2,4-Dinitrophenol (DNP)-induced injury in calcium-free hearts. J Mol Cell Cardiol 16: 547–557

13. Ganote CE, Nayler WG (1985) Contracture and the calcium paradox. J Mol Cell Cardiol 17: 733–745

14. Vander Heide RS, Ganote CE (1985) Caffeine-induced injury in calcium-free perfused rat hearts. Am J Pathol 118: 55–65

15. Elz JS, Nayler WG (1988) Contractile activity and reperfusion-induced calcium gain after ischemia in the isolated rat heart. Lab Invest 58: 653–659

16. Vander Heide RS, Ganote CE (1987) Increased myocyte fragility following anoxic injury. J Mol Cell Cardiol 19: 1085–1103

17. Tokuyasu KT, Dutton AH, Singer SJ (1983) Immunoelectron microscopic studies of desmin (skeletin) localization and intermediate filament organization in chicken cardiac muscle. J Cell Biol 96: 1736–1742

18. Geiger B, Avnur Z, Kreis TE, Schlessinger J (1984) The dynamics of cytoskeletal organization in areas of cell contact. In: Cell and Muscle Motility. Vol 5. Plenum Press: JW Shay (ed), New York and London

19. Steenbergen C Jr, Hill ML, Jennings RB (1987) Cytoskeletal damage during myocardial ischemia: Changes in vinculin immunofluorescence staining during total *in vitro* ischemia in canine heart. Circ Res 60: 478–486

20. Steenbergen C Jr, Hill ML, Jennings RB (1985) Volume regulation and plasma membrane injury in aerobic, anaerobic and ischemic myocardium *in vitro*: Effect of osmotic swelling on plasma membrane integrity. Circ Res 57: 864–875

21. Jennings RB, Reimer KA, Steenbergen C (1986) Myocardial ischemia revisited. The osmolar load, membrane damage and reperfusion. Editorial. J Mol Cell Cardiol 18: 769–680

22. Ganote CE, Vander Heide RS (1988) Irreversible injury of isolated adult rat myocytes: Osmotic fragility during metabolic inhibition. Am J Path 132: 212–222

23. Haworth RA, Hunter DR, Berkoff HA (1981) Contracture of isolated rat heart cells: Role of Ca^{2+}, ATP and compartmentation. Circ Res 49: 1119–1128

24. Altschuld RA, Gibb L, Ansel A, Hohl C, Kruger FA, Brierley GP (1980) Calcium tolerance of isolated rat heart cells. J Mol Cell Cardiol 12: 1383–1395

25. Lambert MR, Johnson JD, Lamka KG, Brierley GP, Altschuld RA (1986) Intracellular free calcium and the hypercontracture of adult rat heart myocytes. Arch Biochem Biophys 245: 426–435

26. Hohl C, Ansel A, Altschuld R, Brierley GP (1982) Contracture of isolated rat heart cells on anaerobic to aerobic transition. Am J Physiol 242: H1022–H1030

27. Altschuld RA, Hostelter JR, Brierley GP (1981) Response of isolated rat heart cells to hypoxia, reoxygenation and acidosis. Circ Res 49: 307–316

28. Frank JS, Brady AJ, Farnsworth S, Mottino JG (1986) Ultrastructure and function of isolated myocytes after calcium depletion and repletion. Am J Physiol 250: H265–H275

29. Piper HM, Spahr R, Huttner JF, Spieckermann PG (1985) The calcium and the oxygen paradox: Non-existent on the cellular level. Basic Res Cardiol 80: 159–163

30. Stern MD, Chien AM, Capogrossi C, Pelto DJ, Lakatta EG (1985) Direct observation of the 'oxygen paradox' in single rat ventricular myocytes. Circ Res 56: 899–903

31. Piper HM (1988) Evaluation of anoxic injury in isolated adult cardiomyocytes. In: WA Clark, RS Decker, TK Borg (eds) Biology of Isolated Adult Cardiac Myocytes. Elsevier Sci Publ Co, Inc, New York, pp 68–81

32. Sage MD, Jennings RB (1988) Cytoskeletal injury and subsarcolemmal bleb formation in dog heart during *in vitro* total ischemia. Am J Pathol 133: 327–337

33. Roos KP (1986) Length, width, and volume changes in osmotically stressed myocytes. Am J Physiol 151: H1373–H1378

34. Ganote CE, Vander Heide RS (1987) Cytoskeletal lesions in anoxic myocardial injury: A conventional and high voltage electron microscopic and immunofluorescence study. Am J Path 129: 327–344

35. Buja LM, Hagler HK, Parsons D, Chien K, Reynolds RC, Willerson JT (1985) Alterations of ultrastructure and elemental composition in cultured neonatal rat myocytes after metabolic inhibition with iodoacetic acid. Lab Invest 53: 397–411

36. Schwartz P, Piper HM, Spahr R, Spieckermann PG (1984) Ultrastructure of cultured adult myocardial cells during anoxia and reoxygenation. Am J Pathol 115: 349–361

37. Herman B, Nieminen A-L, Gores GJ, Lemasters JJ (1988) Irreversible injury in anoxic hepatocytes precipitated by an abrupt increase in plasma membrane permeability. FASEB J 2: 146–151

PART VIII

The role of endothelial cells and neurons

Sensitivity of the endothelium to hypoxia and reoxygenation

H.M. PIPER, S. BUDERUS, A. KRÜTZFELDT, T. NOLL, S. MERTENS
and R. SPAHR
Institut für Physiologie I, Universität Düsseldorf, Moorenstr. 5, D-4000 Düsseldorf, FRG

Introduction

The endothelium of the coronary system performs a great number of specific physiological and metabolic functions, such as the regulation of vascular tone, transport of nutrients, blood coagulation, and it also acts as a selective permeability barrier. Endothelial injury has severe consequences for the pump function of the heart and, ultimately, for metabolic and structural integrity of the whole organ. Endothelial performance depends on a sufficient supply of metabolic energy. Current knowledge of substrate and energy metabolism of endothelial cells in general, and of those in the coronary vasculature in particular, is very limited. In the heart, in which 90% of the organ mass consists of cardiomyocytes [1] with a large energy demand, the relative contribution of endothelial cells, which comprise only 2–3% of the organ mass [2], to the energy metabolism of the whole organ is very difficult to identify. For this reason, culture models have come into use to study specifically the metabolic properties of coronary endothelial cells.

When the oxygen supply of myocardial tissue falls short, the endothelium may contribute to the development of tissue injury in a positive or a negative manner, depending on the degree of its own alteration. It has been discussed whether the role of the endothelium may be that of reducing the impending tissue injury during the early phase of oxygen deficiency. This is because hypoxic endothelial cells can release increased amounts of vasodilatory auta-coids, i.e. endothelium-derived relaxing factor (EDRF) and prostacyclin [3] that increase the flow of blood into the undersupplied region if these media-tors gain access to the arterioles. When the metabolic function of endothelial cells becomes seriously altered, their malfunction may exacerbate tissue injury. A decisive deleterious role has been attributed to endothelial cells in the 'oxygen paradox' since they might be the source of oxygen radicals generated by xanthine oxidase [4], an enzyme localized only in the endothe-lial cell compartment [5].

This chapter deals primarily with three questions about coronary endothe-lial cell function: (1) What are the physiological substrates for the energy

H.M. Piper (ed.) Pathophysiology of severe ischemic myocardial injury, 359–379.
© *1990 Kluwer Academic Publishers, Dordrecht*

metabolism of coronary endothelial cells? (2) What does 'hypoxia' mean to their respiratory function? (3) Does endothelial cell integrity deteriorate before or after cardiomyocyte integrity in the ischemic/hypoxic-reoxygenated heart? To answer these questions, the use of cultures of coronary endothelial cells has been essential. Some caution is required, however, in extrapolating absolute quantities of data from cultures to the endothelium *in vivo*, even though current knowledge indicates great similarity between the coronary endothelial cells in culture and those in heart tissue. For the isolation and culture of coronary endothelium several protocols have been described [6–9]. By these procedures a certain average fraction of all coronary endothelial cells is isolated. Since more than 90% of the endothelial cells contained in the heart are localized in the microvascular bed [2], these preparations are understood to represent coronary microvascular endothelial cells. The protocol used in our laboratory comprises two major steps: first, the heart is perfused with collagenase to dissociate all the cells contained within, and second, endothelial cells are purified from the resulting suspension of cells and grown in culture to confluent monolayers.

Aerobic substrate metabolism of coronary endothelial cells

Adenine nucleotide contents

Coronary endothelial cells, in confluent monolayers of two-week old cultures, contain high levels of adenine nucleotides: 21.4 nmol ATP/mg protein, 1.8 nmol ADP/mg protein, and 0.5 nmol AMP/mg protein [9]. Calculated from these values, the adenylate energy charge [10] EC = (ATP + 0.5 ADP) / (ATP + ADP + AMP) amounts to 0.94. This energy charge indicates a well - energized metabolic state [10]. Half the protein from the cultured cells can be removed by brief treatment with trypsin, so that the adenine nucleotide contents per mg of the remaining cell protein are twice as high as the values given above. On a cell protein base, therefore, the endothelial adenine nucleotide contents exceed those of the myocardial tissue. This finding is consistent with the results previously reported by Nees *et al.* [11].

Glycolytic and oxidative energy production

Among the metabolic substrates tested, glucose is of predominant importance for coronary endothelial cells in confluent monolayer cultures. But almost all energy obtained by catabolizing glucose is generated glycolytically. This is not due to a lack of oxygen, as demonstrated by the finding that increased oxygen supply, by incubation of cultures under 100% O_2 instead of 21% O_2 (air), did not alter this metabolic behavior [9].

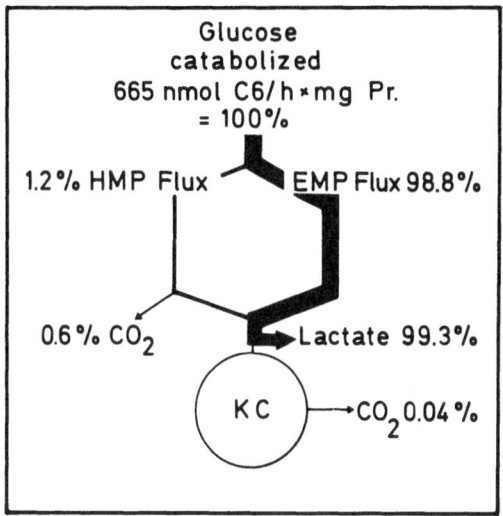

Glucose, 5 mM

Fig. 1. Scheme of glucose catabolism of rat coronary endothelial cells in 2-week-old confluent cultures, incubated in Tyrode solution with 5 mM glucose. Rates are given as percentages of total glucose breakdown. HMP, hexose monophosphate pathway; EMP, Embden Meyerhof pathway; KC, Krebs cycle. (Reproduced with permission from ref. [17].)

At concentrations of glucose above 1 mM, the catabolic rates for glucose are constant. At the physiological concentration of 5 mM the catabolism of glucose to CO_2 and lactate was not influenced by palmitate, lactate or glutamine [9]. Findings on glucose uptake in macrovascular endothelial cells suggest that the uptake of glucose through the plasma membrane represents the rate limiting step for endothelial glucose utilization [12]. Coronary endothelial cells are responsive to insulin [7], but its effect on steady state degradation rates of 5 mM glucose is only small. With 10^{-7}M insulin, glycolytic flux could be stimulated only by 20% [9].

In the presence of 5 mM exogenous glucose alone, the portion of glucose diverted to the hexose monophosphate shunt is small, but it accounts for almost all CO_2 produced from glucose (Fig. 1). Interestingly, at concentrations of glucose below 1 mM, the amount of glucose oxidized in the Krebs cycle is greater than at higher concentrations, and lactate production is conversely decreased (Fig. 2). Thus, oxidative metabolism is inhibited at physiological glucose concentrations. The inhibitory effect of glucose on mitochondrial oxidation also affects other substrates degraded in the Krebs cycle, i.e. palmitate, lactate and amino acids. The oxidation of these substrates (300 μM palmitate, 1mM lactate, 0.5 mM glutamine) is reduced by 50% or more in the presence of 5 mM glucose (Fig. 3). The inhibitory effect of glucose on mitochondrial respiration has been termed the 'Crabtree effect' [13, 14].

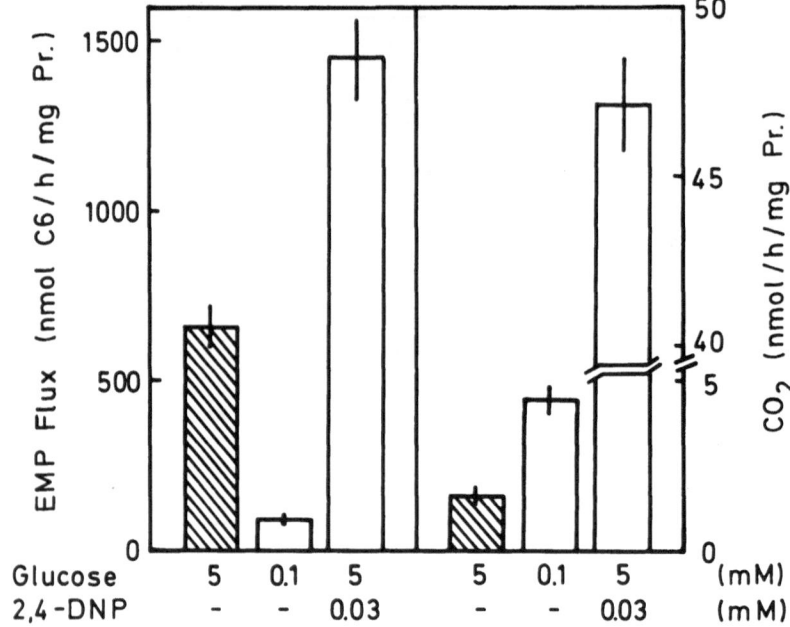

Fig. 2. Rat coronary endothelial cells in 2-week-old confluent cultures, incubated in Tyrode solution: Catabolism of exogenous glucose through the Emden Meyerhof pathway (EMP) and to CO_2 within the mitochondria. The methods are described in ref. [9]. 2,4-DNP, 2,4-dinitrophenol. ($\bar{x} \pm$ S.E.M.; n = 5 cultures).

Expression of the Crabtree effect by these cells demonstrates a loose coupling between glycolytic flux and Krebs cycle activity. In cells exhibiting the Crabtree effect, the allosteric control of phosphofructokinase and/or pyruvate kinase by a high cytosolic phosphorylation potential seems to be weak or absent [14, 15]. In this metabolic state glycolytic flux, and thereby the production of NADH, can be stimulated irrespective of the capacity of the mitochondrial respiratory chain to re-oxidize the surplus in reducing equivalents. Consequently, the cytosol becomes more reduced and, according to the mass action ratio of the near-equilibrium reaction catalyzed by the lactate dehydrogenase, pyruvate is predominantly turned into lactate. It is thought that the increase in glycolytic intermediates and cytosolic ATP production causes a shortage of ADP and P_i at the mitochondrial site and thus leads to inhibition of oxidative energy production [14, 15]. Consistent with this hypothesis is the finding that in experiments in which mitochondrial respiration was uncoupled from ATP synthesis by 2,4-dinitrophenol, oxidation of 5 mM glucose in the Krebs cycle was indeed stimulated thirty times (Fig. 2).

The capacity of the hexose monophosphate pathway greatly exceeds its activity under control conditions. When cellular NADPH is oxidized by the presence of methylene blue (0.4 mM), the flux through the hexose monophosphate pathway becomes greatly stimulated, comprising 81% of total glucose

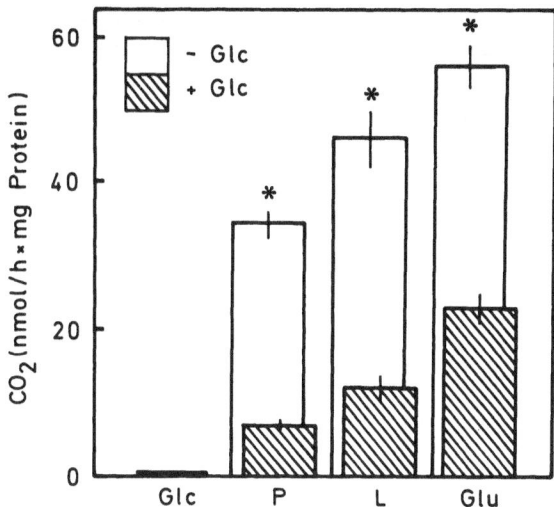

Fig. 3. Rat coronary endothelial cells in 2-week-old confluent cultures, incubated in Tyrode solution: Production of labelled CO_2 in the Krebs cycle from labelled exogenous substrates without and with presence of 5 mM glucose (Glc). P, 300 µM palmitate complexed to 60 µM albumin; L, 1 mM lactate; Glu, 0.5 mM glutamine. ($\bar{x} \pm$ S.E.M.; n = 5 cultures.) Asterisks symbolize statistical differences, $p < 0.05$, according to Student's paired t-test. (Reproduced with permission from ref. [17].)

catabolism [9]. This demonstrates that coronary endothelial cells possess a large potential capacity of the hexose monophosphate pathway. A similar observation has been made before on microvascular endothelial cells of other origin [16].

Cultured coronary endothelial cells contain endogenous stores of glycogen (170 nmol C6/mg culture protein), sufficient to replace exogenous glucose for many hours [9]. But glycogen is degraded only at low rates, indicating low glycogen phosphorylase activity. To maintain their energy balance in the absence of glucose, endothelial cells increase the oxidative use of other substrates, exogenous or endogenous, and thereby augment their oxygen demand (Fig. 4). In the heart, fatty acids and lactate are the most important energetic substrates under aerobic conditions. Coronary endothelial cells are also able to utilize lactate and palmitate as fuels for oxidative phosphorylation; but they are even better suited to oxidize amino acids [9, 17].

The oxygen uptake of coronary endothelial cells is low in comparison with that of the whole heart. In stirred suspensions of two-week-old cultures, oxygen is taken up at a rate of 8 nmol/min/mg cell protein, when 0.2 mM palmitate is the only exogenous substrate. Under the same supply conditions, the beating myocardium requires 50 to 100 nmol O_2/min/mg protein at a low to moderate work load. Oxygen consumption by coronary endothelial cells in fact comes close to the demand of the arrested myocardium. When the ATP/O ratio is taken as 2.8, the oxygen consumption mentioned above is equivalent to 45 nmol ATP/min/mg protein. When glucose is added to the

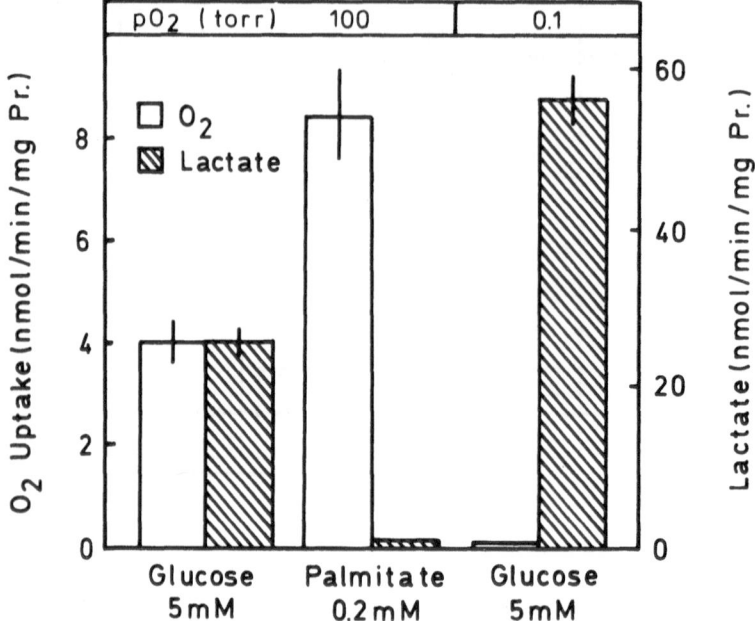

Fig. 4. Rat coronary endothelial cells from 2 week-old confluent cultures, suspended in Tyrode solution with 5 mM glucose or 100 μM palmitate, complexed to 20 μM albumin: Oxygen uptake and production of lactate, at high and low oxygen tension. The methods are described in ref. [30]. ($\bar{x} \pm$ S.E.M.; n = 5 cultures).

cells, oxygen consumption drops by 50%, equivalent to 22 nmol ATP/min/mg protein. But then lactate is produced at a rate of 25 nmol/min/mg protein corresponding to 25 nmol ATP/min/mg protein (1 mol ATP/mol lactate), so that the calculated total energy production amounts to 47 nmol ATP/min/mg, i.e. the same as in the presence of palmitate.

Substrate metabolism of endothelial cells of other origin

The described results on glucose metabolism in cultures of coronary endothelial cells resemble in several respects those obtained on cultures of microvascular endothelium from penis corpus cavernosum [16] and on isolated brain microvessels [18, 19]. High activity of glutamine metabolizing enzymes has also been reported for pulmonary microvascular cells [20]. This suggests great similarity of microvascular endothelium of different sources in the investigated aspects of energy metabolism.

It may be of significance for the heart as a whole that coronary microvascular endothelial cells only break down glucose to lactate. This is because lactate is a much better oxidative substrate for the cardiomyocyte than glucose. In producing lactate, they are supported by the cellular contents of the vascular space. Leucocytes [21] and lymphocytes [22] can also express a pronounced Crabtree effect and erythrocytes produce lactate by necessity, since they lack oxidative metabolism.

Hypoxic energy metabolism of coronary endothelial cells

Oxygen sensitivity of the whole heart

The whole heart responds to the gradual reduction of oxygen supply with a gradual reduction of oxygen uptake and a steady increase in lactate production. The respiratory function of individual cardiomyocytes is unaltered unless the ambient oxygen tension drops below a few torr. It has been concluded, therefore, that the gradual changes in the perfused heart can be explained as a statistical phenomenon: the lower the total amount of oxygen supplied to the heart per unit of time, the fewer cells along the perfusion path can satisfy their oxygen demand. The oxygen sensitivity of the respiratory function of endothelial cells has been determined in our laboratory.

Specific precautions are needed to determine accurately the oxygen sensitivity of individual cells. This is because oxygen gradients in unstirred layers at the cell surface have to be avoided, and defined medium pO_2 values must be maintained for some length of time. An experimental system ('oxystat') meeting these requirements has been developed by Noll et al.[23] (Fig. 5). The results reported in the following have been obtained by use of this system.

Oxygen sensitivity of the respiratory function of coronary endothelial cells

At oxygen tensions above 3 torr, the uptake of oxygen by coronary endothelial cells is constant; below 3 torr oxygen consumption gradually declines (Fig. 6). The rate of oxygen consumption is half the maximum at a pO_2 of 0.8 torr. The relationship between the rate of oxygen uptake and oxygen tension apparently obeys Michaelis-Menten kinetics (Fig. 6, inset). The sensitivity of oxygen uptake to oxygen tension was found to be the same when exogenous glucose, palmitate, or glutamine were supplied, and when only endogenous substrates could be oxidized. In the presence of glucose, however, oxygen uptake rates above 3 torr O_2 are 50% lower than in its absence, due to the contribution of glycolysis to energy metabolism.

In isolated mitochondria, 0.2 torr represents the K_m of oxygen consumption by the cytochrome c oxidase [24, 25]. Whole cells generally have a reduced apparent affinity to oxygen, due to intra- and extracellular gradients of oxygen. In the oxystat system, the formation of an extracellular oxygen gradient is prevented by rapid mixing of the medium. Therefore, the pO_2 of the half-maximal oxygen consumption by coronary endothelial cells, i.e. 0.8 torr, indicates that within the endothelial cell there is a gradient of 0.6 torr

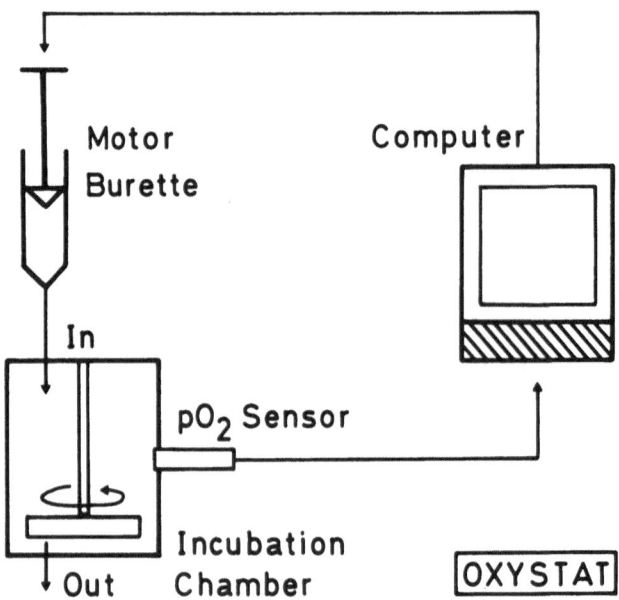

Fig. 5. Oxystat system. The cells are suspended in the incubation chamber, in which the oxygen tension is maintained at a selected value by injecting appropriate amounts of oxygen saturated medium using a feedback controlled motor burette. The oxygen consumption in the chamber is determined from the medium addition needed to keep a constant pO_2.

towards the inner mitochondrial membrane. This value accords closely with estimates of intracellular oxygen gradients in other cell types [26]. The sensitivity of individual endothelial cells to oxygen is comparable to that of cardiomyocytes [27]. Physiologically, oxygen tensions of 1 torr and below are extremely low, since they are two orders of magnitude below the normal arterial oxygen tension. They will occur locally, however, whenever the heart responds with signs of anaerobic metabolism to a mismatch between oxygen supply and demand [28].

The aerobic production of lactate in the presence of glucose, 5 mM, is unaffected by a reduction of medium pO_2 from 100 to 10 torr. At 1 and 0.1 torr, lactate production increased, inversely related to the decrease in oxygen consumption [30]. At a pO_2 of 0.1 torr, lactate production is increased 2.3 times as compared to well-oxygenated conditions (Fig. 4). This means that the Pasteur effect in coronary endothelial cells is small compared to its effect in the cardiac muscle cell. This finding is consistent with the pronounced Crabtree effect under aerobic conditions.

Energetic changes in hypoxic coronary endothelial cells

In anoxia ($pO_2 \leq 1$ torr) with exogenous supply of glucose, the adenine nucleotide contents of coronary endothelial cells remain unaltered for several

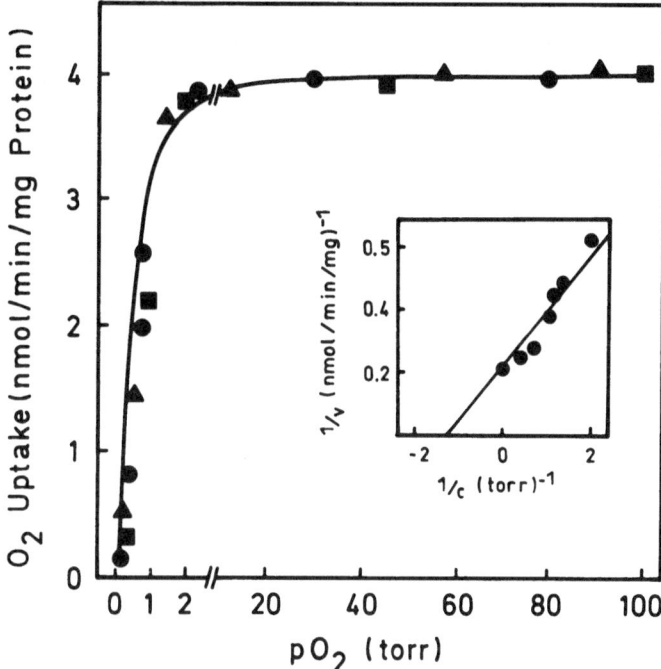

Fig. 6. Rat coronary endothelial cells from 2 week-old confluent cultures, suspended in Tyrode solution with 5 mM glucose: Relation of oxygen uptake to medium pO_2 (inset shows the Lineweaver-Burk plot). The methods are described in ref. [30]. Different symbols stand for different experiments.

hours (Fig. 7A). The increase in glycolytic energy production is sufficient to fully compensate for the lack of respiratory ATP supply. The calculated rates of ATP production under aerobic conditions (in the presence of 5 mM glucose: 47 nmol ATP/min/mg protein) and at 0.1 torr O_2 (55 nmol ATP/min/mg protein; see Fig. 4) are almost identical.

The importance of glucose for hypoxic energy production in coronary endothelial cells was tested in experiments in which glucose was omitted from the incubation medium and replaced by substrates that can only be used oxidatively (Fig. 7B). Under these conditions the production of lactate is very small and can be fully accounted for by the degradation of glycogen. In the absence of a supply of exogenous glucose, cellular contents of ATP decrease at oxygen tensions ≤ 2 torr. A decrease of ATP levels is accompanied by a transient increase of the AMP concentration. Greater reduction of pO_2 caused a greater reduction in cellular ATP levels. A return from 0.1 to 10 torr O_2 after 1 hour led to a rapid restoration of the initial oxygen uptake [30], indicating preservation of mitochondrial integrity. In 30 minutes of reoxygenation, cellular ATP contents recovered only incompletely (Fig. 7B), probably due to the purine loss from the cells.

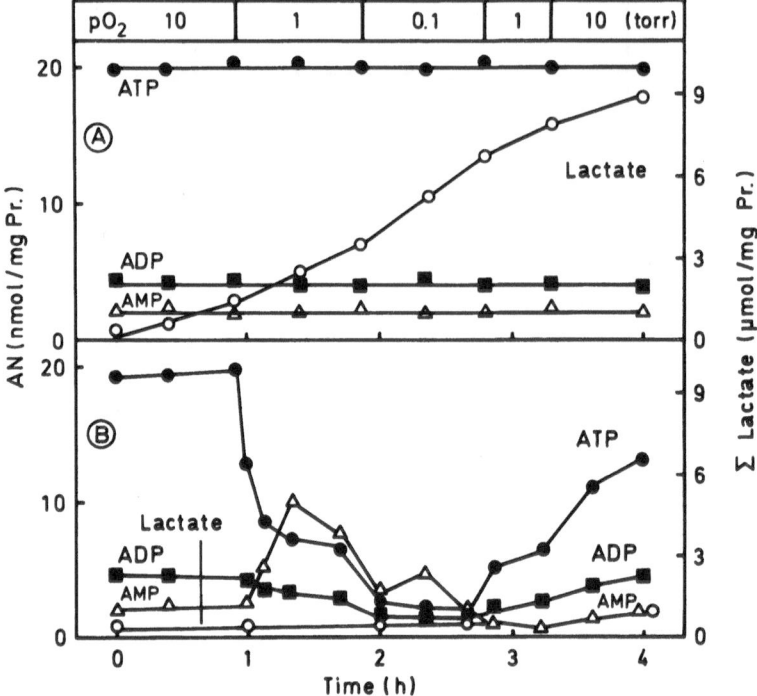

Fig. 7. Rat coronary endothelial cells from 2-week-old confluent cultures, suspended in Tyrode solution with (A) 5 mM glucose or (B) 100 μM palmitate, complexed to 20 μM albumin, plus 0.5 mM glutamine: Changes in adenine nucleotide contents and production of lactate at selected oxygen tensions. The methods are described in ref. [30]. Values from two single experiments.

Reaction to hypoxia by endothelial cells of other origin

As reported above for cultured microvascular endothelial cells, the energetic state of cultured macrovascular endothelial cells cannot be altered by inhibition of mitochondrial respiration alone; it needs the additional inhibition of glycolytic energy production to achieve energy depletion [29, 31, 32]. When glycolytic and oxidative energy production is inhibited, macrovascular endothelial cells become energy depleted at a rate comparable to that of coronary microvascular endothelial cells, i.e. slower than the heart muscle under identical conditions.

Trophic effects of hypoxia on cell proliferation and function have been studied in cultured macrovascular endothelial cells incubated for one or several days at reduced pO_2. In nominally oxygen free culture medium (containing glucose) bovine pulmonary artery cells were found to stop growing; but 20 torr O_2 were sufficient to obtain a growth rate equal to that at 140 torr [33]. In one study, proliferation of bovine aortic endothelial cells was found to be increased after 3 to 4 days under 14 torr O_2 as compared to 140 torr O_2, suggesting that hypoxia can stimulate the synthesis of growth factors [34]. Unfortunately, in none of these studies could the pO_2 at the surface of the cell layer be exactly defined; this makes it difficult to relate the results to a possible impairment of respiratory function.

Endothelial cells cultured at low oxygen tension exhibit signs of biochemical adaptation, apparently not related to changes in energy metabolism. Bovine aortic and pulmonary endothelial cells were cultured at 14 torr O_2. After 4 days, the activity of the glycolytic enzymes pyruvate kinase and phosphofructokinase was increased [35, 36]. These results suggest that endothelial cells, normally well-suited to survive episodes of oxygen deficiency, may become even better adapted to hypoxia by augmenting their glycolytic capacity.

Biochemical changes in endothelial cells induced by prolonged hypoxia can also be potentially disadvantageous from a therapeutic point of view. In bovine pulmonary artery and pulmonary microvascular endothelial cell cultures, incubated in nominally oxygen free medium, the plasminogen activator activity was found decreased and plasminogen activator inhibitor activity increased within a few hours [37]. Thus, the fibrinolytic potential of hypoxic endothelial cells decreases. If coronary endothelial cells reacted similarly *in vivo*, reduced fibrinolytic capacity of the coronary endothelium might contribute to re-occlusion of coronary arteries which were opened after a thrombotic blockade.

Low oxygen tension also has an effect on the endothelial metabolism of biogenic amines. Compared to normoxic conditions, serotonin uptake was increased in endothelial cells at 20 torr O_2 and even more in nominally oxygen free medium after 1 to 3 days [33]. Cell growth was reduced in nominally oxygen free medium, but not under 20 torr. This suggests that the oxygen sensing mechanism for induction/activation of the serotonin transport differs from the mechanism making cell growth hypoxia-sensitive.

Evidence for oxygen sensor mechanism(s) differing from the respiratory response of endothelial cells also comes from studies on endothelial autocoid release. In isolated segments of canine femoral and coronary arteries and in rat tail arteries, reduction of the luminal pO_2 to 40 torr in the glucose-containing perfusate was sufficient to cause a release of vasodilatory amounts of the prostaglandins PGI_2 and PGE_2 [38]. It has been suggested that the non-prostanoid endothelium-derived relaxing factor(s) (EDRF) also exhibit the same sensitivity to oxygen tension [3], since in many vessels the release of prostaglandins and EDRF occurs in parallel [39]. Considering the great affinity of endothelial cells to oxygen and their large capacity for glycolytic energy production, these results suggest that the oxygen sensor for release of vasodilatory autacoids is independent from the effects of hypoxia on respiratory function or the energetic state of the endothelium.

The synthesis of prostaglandins involves peroxidase reactions and therefore fails at extremely low oxygen concentrations [40]. EDRF seems to be almost identical to nitric oxide, synthesized from arginine in endothelial cells [41, 42] via an unknown reaction which apparently involves molecular oxygen. EDRF synthesis may therefore also cease in the absence of oxygen. Both the synthesis of vasodilatory amounts of prostaglandins [43] and of EDRF [44, 45] have been shown to depend on energy production. Conditions which lead to energy depletion of endothelial cells, therefore, abolish endothelium mediated vasodilation.

In summary, it may be possible that endothelial cells possess different oxygen sensor mechanisms for different metabolic functions, of which the respiratory response (cytochrome c oxidase) is the one with the highest affinity to oxygen. The present data, however, do not permit this conclusion with certainty, since unstirred layers with considerable oxygen gradients could account for the apparent metabolic response to oxygen tensions between 3 and 40 torr in the cited experiments.

Participation of coronary endothelium in severe myocardial injury

Alteration of structure and function of coronary endothelium in the ischemic-reperfused myocardium

Even though the ultrastructure of the endothelium in ischemic-reperfused myocardium has received less attention than the ultrastructure of the cardiomyocytes, several electron microscopic studies indicate that, in general, in ischemic myocardial tissue structural damage of the endothelium develops more slowly and is more easily reversed than that of the cardiomyocytes [46–48]. The spatial extent of severe endothelial injury never exceeds the extent of severe cardiomyocyte injury. Thus, in myocardium reperfused after prolonged regional ischemia, areas with persistent severe alterations of endothelial ultrastructure and with hemorrhage are always contained in larger areas of cardiomyocyte necrosis [49].

The most prominent effect of ischemia on endothelial structure is the swelling of the cells. The early studies by Poche et al. [46] demonstrated that endothelial swelling increases from anoxia, to ischemia, to anoxia plus hypercapnia, indicating that acidosis has a marked influence on endothelial cell swelling. Moderate endothelial cell swelling in the microvasculature is reversible [46, 47]. Extensive endothelial swelling occluding the capillary bed can be irreversible. But this is not because of the irreversibility of the changes within the endothelial cell itself. Extensive endothelial cell swelling prevents a restoration of normal supply conditions, a phenomenon termed 'no-reflow' [50]. Under such conditions, it cannot be truly determined whether the endothelial injury is inevitably deleterious.

Greater resistance of endothelial cells to ultimate cell injury does not exclude early onset of endothelial dysfunction. A function which can be tested in the ischemic-reperfused heart is the endothelial barrier function for water and solutes. Reperfused myocardium becomes edematous. Increased water flux across the endothelial lining can be due to altered transendothelial hydrostatic, oncotic and osmotic pressure gradients. To test permeability changes more specifically, the extravasation of colloidal particles [49] or macromolecules [51, 52] has been investigated. These studies show that the endothelial barrier function in the ischemic-reperfused heart is disturbed concomitantly with progressive myocardial injury.

The causes for the increase in endothelial permeability are not precisely known. The cited studies on ultrastructure and the results reported below demonstrate that early onset of increased permeability is not related to the necrosis of a substantial number of endothelial cells. Changes in microvascular permeability can be due to the opening of intercellular clefts. The barrier function of endothelial cells depends on the integrity of their cytoskeleton [53]. In cultured endothelial cells which were energy depleted, essential parts of the cytoskeleton, i.e. the actin microfilaments, became partly disassembled, and the cells retracted from one another [29, 32]. Changes in the actin microfilament structure occurred concomitantly to the decrease in cellular ATP levels. Interestingly, such cells became non-responsive to exogenous stimulators of cell retraction such as histamine [32].

After long periods of ischemia or hypoxia, the basement membrane and the surface coat of endothelial cells [54] may become altered. The extracellular matrix of the endothelial cells contributes to the selective permeability of the endothelial barrier [55]. The extracellular matrix may become altered for a number of reasons. It can be attacked by proteolytic enzymes released from leucocytes, and the resynthesis of new components may be impaired. Interestingly, the synthesis of matrix components can become reduced in hypoxia even without extensive energy depletion. This is concluded from experiments in which bovine pulmonary artery endothelial cells were exposed to 20 torr O_2 for 3 days in complete cell culture medium which included glucose [56]. These conditions did not change cell growth or cell morphology in light microscopy; nor did they cause trypan blue uptake. Marked energetic changes are not to be expected under such conditions (see above). Nevertheless, proteoglycan production by these cells was reduced. This finding also indicates an oxygen sensor mechanism not related to hypoxic energetic disturbance.

Absence of severe endothelial cell injury in the anoxic-reoxygenated heart

It has been hypothesized that dysfunction of the microvascular coronary endothelium contributes to the development of severe myocardial damage when hearts are reoxygenated after extended periods of ischemia or anoxia. The term "oxygen paradox" has been introduced for the abrupt exacerbation of tissue injury upon reoxygenation, which is characterized by development of contracture, cell disruption and a massive loss of enzymes [57, 58]. A particular role has been attributed to endothelial cells in the oxygen paradox since they might be the source of oxygen radicals generated by xanthine oxidase [4], an enzyme localized in the heart only in the microvascular endothelial cell compartment [5]. Since free oxygen radicals are very reactive, one would expect most damage to be at the site of their production, i.e. in the endothelium.

In the study described here [59] guinea pig hearts were anoxically perfused. The perfusate either contained or did not contain glucose, since the coronary endothelium possesses a large capacity for glycolytic energy production (see above) and, therefore, the extent of endothelial hypoxic injury could depend on glucose supply. In perfused guinea pig hearts, 60 minutes of anoxic perfusion caused a submaximal oxygen paradox with either perfusate. The severity of cell injury was evaluated by the loss of macromolecules. Loss of lactate dehydrogenase (LDH) and creatine kinase (CK) represents injury of the mass of myocardial cells. As indicator for the enzyme release from endothelial cells the marker enzyme purine nucleoside phosphorylase (PNP) was used. PNP has been demonstrated to be a specific marker enzyme for endothelial cells and pericytes in the heart [60]; cardiomyocyte preparations are devoid of this enzyme [61]. Absence of PNP release, therefore, indicates the absence of endothelial cell deterioration.

After 60 minutes of anoxia, hearts with and without glucose in the perfusate were depleted of ATP, but those in which glycolytic activity was higher ended up with slightly higher ATP contents (Fig. 8). Subsequent reoxygenation for 15 minutes restored ATP contents to half the control values. In hearts perfused anoxically without glucose, ATP levels after 60 minutes were even lower, i.e. 5%, and during 15 minutes reoxygenation no substantial recovery of ATP contents occurred. In anoxic hearts perfused with glucose, lactate efflux was 550 µmol/h/g dry weight, in those without 220 µmol/h/g dry weight. In hearts perfused with glucose during anoxia, contracture rose in one step within the first 5 minutes of reperfusion, whereas a gradual rise was observed in hearts perfused without glucose during anoxia [59]. Thus, the hearts with greater ATP resynthesis developed contracture more rapidly. Hearts perfused with glucose during anoxia also responded to reoxygenation with a faster and more extensive release of LDH and CK (Fig. 9).

A substantial increase in PNP loss remained absent during anoxia and subsequent reoxygenation, even though the release of LDH and CK indicated severe tissue injury. If endothelial damage is comparable to damage of the muscle cells, a loss of PNP synchronous to that of the other enzymes would be expected. The deviant behavior of PNP cannot be attributed to differences in molecular weight among the three investigated enzymes because they are all in the 100 kilodalton range (LDH 134 kD, CK 86 kD, PNP 90 kD). But the possibility exists that PNP activity is held back in endothelial cells even when they are already losing other macromolecules; this had to be ruled out in additional experiments.

Coronary microvascular endothelial cells contain all three enzymes. It was investigated , using a culture preparation of these cells, whether anoxic injury would result in any differences in the loss of LDH, CK and PNP. Endothelial

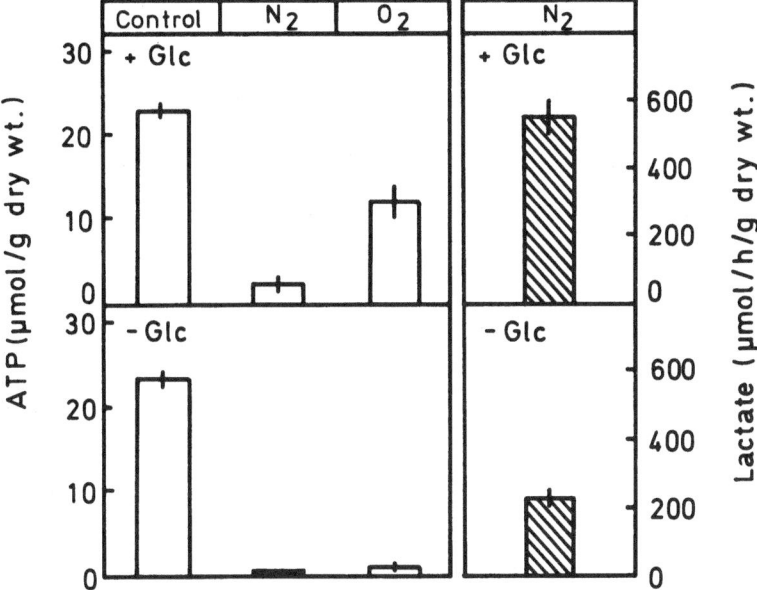

Fig. 8. Anoxic-reoxygenated guinea pig hearts, perfused with Tyrode solution. Left: Tissue contents of ATP under initial control conditions, after 60 min anoxia (N_2) and 15 min reoxygenation (O_2). Right: Amount of lactate produced in 60 min anoxia. ± Glc, anoxic perfusion ± 5 mM glucose. The methods are described in ref. [59]. ($\bar{x}$ ± S.D., n = 4 hearts.)

cells released only small amounts of these enzymes during 120 minutes of substrate free anoxic incubation. The relative losses of LDH, CK and PNP activities were not significantly different (Fig. 10). Digitonin treatment, used to selectively permeabilize the plasmalemma, caused an equal or much greater liberation of all three enzymes. These results demonstrate that PNP can be as easily released from injured endothelial cells as LDH and CK. The absence of greater PNP loss in the anoxic-reperfused heart, therefore, must be due to less severe injury of endothelial cells as compared to the injury of cardiomyocytes.

It appears as a paradox within the 'oxygen paradox' that those hearts which produce less energy and lose more high-energy phosphates in anoxia and, furthermore, fail to rapidly resynthesize ATP after resupply of oxygen and glucose, become less seriously injured immediately upon reoxygenation. These findings are, however, in accordance with the previous observation [58] that uncoupling or inhibition of mitochondrial respiration can reduce or prevent massive tissue disruptions upon reoxygenation. The fact that the lack of oxidative energy protects against the oxygen paradox has been explained by mechanical factors. According to this theory the critical step in eliciting the oxygen paradox is the development of Ca^{2+}–dependent contracture for which both elevated cytosolic Ca^{2+} levels and the presence of some ATP are required [62].

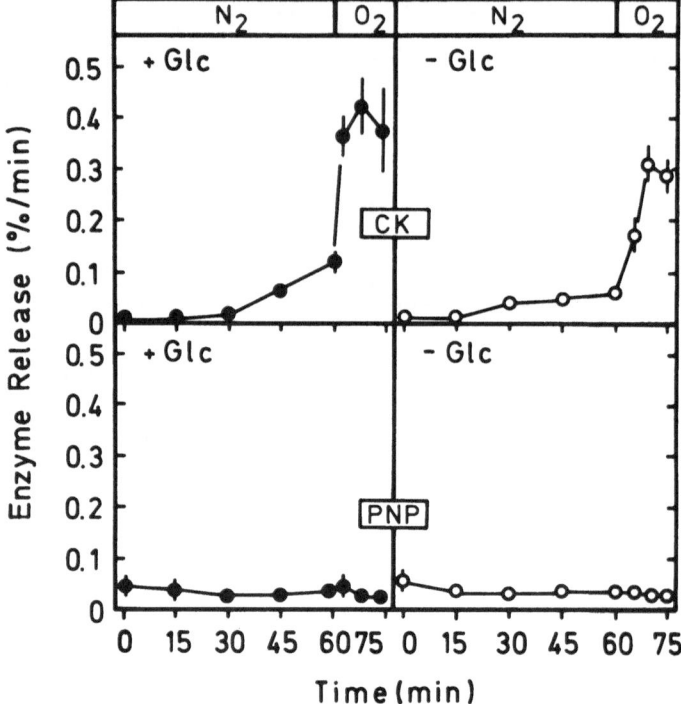

Fig. 9. Anoxic-reoxygenated guinea pig hearts, perfused with Tyrode solution. Release of CK and PNP during 60 min anoxic perfusion (N_2) and 15 min reoxygenation (O_2) as a percentage of the initial total tissue activity. ± Glc, anoxic perfusion ± 5 mM glucose. The methods are described in ref. [59]. ($\bar{x}$ ± S.E.M., n = 8 hearts.)

The absence of rapid endothelial cell deterioration upon reoxygenation can also be inferred from a study on endothelial macromolecule permeability in ischemic-reperfused rat hearts [51]. Ischemic periods of up to 30 minutes were tested which gradually increased the postischemic permeability. Free radical scavengers (superoxide dismutase, catalase, mannitol) and hypoxic reperfusion did not prevent increased postischemic permeability, suggesting that free radicals were not the cause.

The evidence for great tolerance of anoxia-reoxygenation and ischemia-reperfusion of coronary endothelium *in situ* is in apparent contrast to the conclusions drawn by Hülsmann and Dubelaar [63]. They suggested that the washout of enzymes from hearts after a period of ischemia indicated greater endothelial than cardiomyocyte injury. The evidence for preferential endothelial injury given in the cited study, however, seems questionable. This is mainly because the conclusion is based on a lower CK/LDH ratio in the effluent from reperfused tissue than in heart homogenates, assumed to be due to a preferential release of LDH from endothelial cells. But this assumption cannot be verified by the data given in the cited paper.

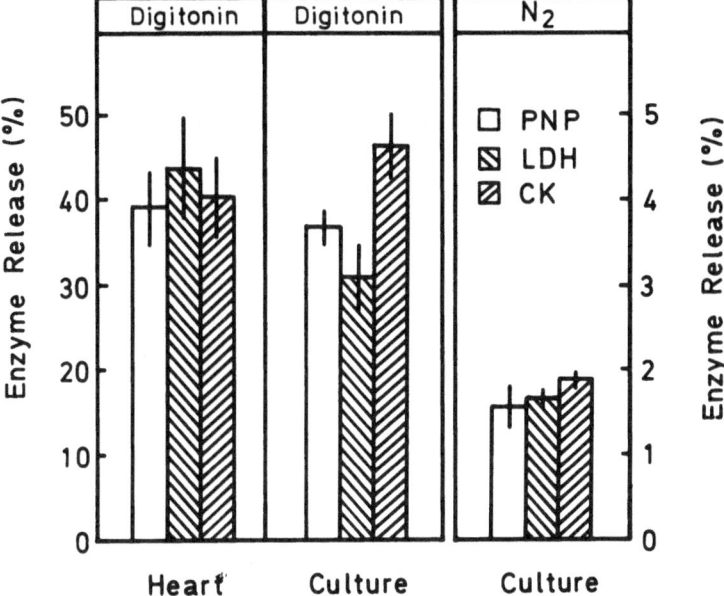

Fig. 10. Left: Comparison of the release of PNP, LDH und CK from guinea pig hearts perfused with 0.1 mg/ml digitonin for 10 min, and from rat coronary endothelial cell cultures incubated with 0.1 mg digitonin/ml far 1 min. Right: Comparison of enzyme release from endothelial cells within 120 min substrate free anoxia (N_2). Enzyme release is given as a percentage of the initial total tissue or culture activity. The methods are described in ref. [59]. ($\bar{x} \pm$ S.E.M., n = 4 hearts or 4 cultures.)

Conclusions

Coronary endothelial cells gain most of their metabolic energy by glycolytic ATP production. Since this happens in the physiological range of blood glucose concentrations, limited use of other substrates seems to characterize the physiological state of coronary endothelial cells.

Coronary endothelial cells have an energy demand similar to the arrested myocardium; this demand is low. This could be the main reason why in the anoxic perfused heart, both in the presence and absence of glucose, endothelial cell injury is less severe than that of the cardiomyocytes. In further contrast to cardiomyocytes, coronary endothelial cells tolerate reoxygenation better after an extended period of anoxia or ischemia. The reported data corroborate the hypothesis that the oxygen paradox is a genuine, energy-dependent phenomenon of the cardiomyocytes.

Even though endothelial cells seem better able to cope with oxygen deficiency than heart muscle cells, their malfunction may still jeopardize the survival of the whole ischemic area. It has been shown that in ischemic

376

myocardium the permeability of the endothelial barrier increases, which favours the development of interstitial edema upon reperfusion. Endothelial cells, even though far from disintegrating, may swell when they become depleted of energy; if this causes no-reflow, myocardial ischemia cannot be reversed. In this sense, endothelial dysfunction can limit the reversibility of ischemic myocardial injury.

Acknowledgement

This study was supported by the Ministerium für Wissenschaft und Forschung des Landes Nordrhein-Westfalen.

References

1. Dow JW, Harding NGL, Powell T (1981) Isolated cardiomyocytes. I. Preparation of adult myocytes and their homology with intact tissue. Cardiovasc Res 15: 483–548
2. Simionescu M, Simionescu N (1978) Isolation and characterization of endothelial cells from heart microvasculature. Microvasc Res 16: 426–452
3. Bassenge E, Busse R (1988) Endothelial modulation of coronary tone. Progr Cardiovasc Disease 30: 349–380
4. McCord JM (1985) Oxygen-derived free radicals in postischemic tissue injury. New Engl J Med 312: 159–163
5. Jarasch ED, Grund C, Bruder G, Heid HW, Keenan TW, Franke WW (1981) Localization of xanthine oxidase in mammary gland epithelium and capillary endothelium. Cell 25: 67–82
6. Nees S, Gerbes AL, Gerlach E (1981) Isolation, identification, and continuous culture of coronary endothelial cells from guinea pig hearts. Eur J Cell Biol 24: 287–297
7. Gerritsen ME, Burke TM (1985) Insulin binding and effects of insulin on glucose uptake and metabolism in cultured rabbit coronary microvessel endothelium. Proc Soc Exp Biol Med 180: 17–23
8. Mistry G, Drummond GI (1986) Adenosine metabolism in microvessels from heart and brain. J Mol Cell Cardiol 18: 13–22
9. Krützfeldt A, Spahr R, Mertens S, Siegmund B, Piper HM (1989) Metabolism of exogenous substrates by coronary microvascular endothelial cells in culture. J Mol Cell Cardiol, in press
10. Atkinson DE (1971) Adenine nucleotides as stoichiometric coupling agents in metabolism and as regulatory modifiers: the adenylate energy charge. In: Vogel HJ (ed) Metabolic Pathways, volume V, Metabolic Regulation. New York, Academic Press, pp 1–21
11. Nees S, Gerlach E (1983) Adenine nucleotides and adenosine metabolism in cultured coronary endothelial cells: formation and release of adenine compounds and possible functional implications. In: Berne RM, Rall TW, Rubio R (eds) Regulatory Function of Adenosine. The Hague, Martinus Nijhoff Publishers, pp 347–360
12. Olgemüller B, Schön J, Wieland OH (1985) Endothelial plasma membrane is a glucocorticoid-regulated barrier for the uptake of glucose into the cell. Mol Cell Endocrinol 43: 165–171
13. Crabtree HG (1929) Observation of the carbohydrate metabolism of tumors. Biochem J 23: 536–545
14. Wenner CE (1979) Pasteur and Crabtree effects – assay in cells. Meth Enzymol 55: 289–297
15. Gonsalvez M, Garcia-Suarez S, Lopez-Alarcon L (1978) Metabolic control of glycolysis in normal and tumor permeabilized cells. Cancer Res 38: 142–148

16. Dobrina A, Rossi F (1983) Metabolic properties of freshly isolated bovine endothelial cells. Bioch Biophys Acta 762: 295–301

17. Spahr R, Krützfeldt A, Mertens S, Siegmund B, Piper HM (1989) Fatty acids are not an important fuel for coronary microvascular endothelial cells. Mol Cell Biochem, in press

18. Chan CT, Brecher P, Haudenschild C, Chobanian AV (1979) The effect of cholesterol feeding on the metabolism of rabbit cerebral microvessels. Microvasc Res 18: 353–369

19. Hingorani V, Brecher P (1987) Glucose and fatty acid metabolism in normal and diabetic rabbit cerebral microvessels. Am J Physiol 252: E648–E653

20. Leighton B, Curi R, Hussein A, Newsholme EA (1987) Maximum activities of some key enzymes of glycolysis, glutaminolysis, Krebs cycle and fatty acid utilization in bovine pulmonary endothelial cells. FEBS Lett 225: 93–96

21. Rossi F, Zatti M (1966) Effect of phagocytosis on the carbohydrate metabolism of polymorphonuclear leucocytes. Biochim Biophys Acta 121: 110–119

22. Hume DA, Radik JL, Ferber E, Weidemann MJ (1978) Aerobic glycolysis and lymphocyte transformation. Biochem J 174: 703–709

23. Noll T, DeGroot H, Wissemann P (1986) A computer-supported oxystat system maintaining steady-state O_2 partial pressures and simultaneously monitoring O_2 uptake in biological systems. Biochem J 236: 765–769

24. Chance B (1965) Reaction of oxygen with the respiratory chain in cells and tissue. J Gen Physiol 49: 163–188

25. DeGroot H, Noll T, Sies H (1985) Oxygen dependence and subcellular partitioning of hepatic menadione-mediated oxygen uptake. Arch Biochem Biophys 243: 556–562

26. Clark A, Clark PAA, Connett RJ, Gayeski TEJ, Honig CR (1987) How large is the drop in PO_2 between cystosol and mitochondrion? Am J Physiol 252: C583–C587

27. Wittenberg BA, Wittenberg JB (1985) Oxygen pressure gradient in isolated cardiac myocytes. J Biol Chem 260: 6548–6554

28. Lübbers DW: Intercapillärer O_2-Transport und intracelluläre Sauerstoffkonzentration. In: Hess B, Staudinger HJ (eds) Biochemie des Sauerstoffs. Berlin, Springer Verlag, pp 67–92

29. Hinshaw DB, Armstrong BC, Beals TF, Hyslop PA (1988) A cellular model of endothelial cell ischemia. J Surg Res 44: 527–537

30. Mertens S, Noll T, Spahr R, Krützfeldt A, Piper HM (1989) The energetic response of coronary endothelial cells to hypoxia. Am J Physiol: in press

31. Shryrock JC, Rubio R, Berne RM (1988) Release of adenosine from pig aortic endothelial cells during hypoxia and metabolic inhibition, Am J Physiol 254: H223–H229

32. Wysolmerski RB, Lagunoff D (1988) Inhibition of endothelial cell retraction by ATP depletion. Am J Pathol 132: 28–37

33. Lee SL, Fanburg BL (1987) Glycolytic activity and enhancement of serotonin uptake by endothelial cells exposed to hypoxia/anoxia. Circ Res 60: 653–658

34. Meininger CJ, Schelling ME, Granger HJ (1988) Adenosine and hypoxia stimulate proliferation and migration of endothelial cells. Am J Physiol 255: H554–H562

35. Hance AJ, Robin ED, Simon LM, Alexander S, Herzenberg LA, Theodore J (1980) Regulation of glycolytic enzyme activity during chronic hypoxia by changes in rate-limiting enzyme content. J Clin Invest 66: 1258–1264

36. Cumminskey JM, Simon LM, Theodore J, Ryan US, Robin ED (1981) Bioenergetic alterations in cultivated pulmonary artery and aortic endothelial cell exposed to normoxia and hypoxia. Exp Lung Res 2: 155–163

37. Wojta J, Jones RL, Binder BR, Hoover RL (1988) Reduction in PO_2 decreases the fibrinolytic potential of cultured bovine endothelial cells derived from pulmonary arteries and lung microvasculature. Blood 71: 1703–1706

38. Busse R, Förstermann U, Matsuda H, Pohl U (1984) The role of prostaglandins in the endothelium-mediated vasodilatory response to hypoxia. Pflügers Arch 401: 77–83

39. De Nucci G, Gryglewski RJ, Warner TD, Vane JR (1988) Receptor-mediated release of endothelium-derived relaxing factor and prostacyclin from bovine aortic endothelial cells is coupled. Proc Natl Acad Sci USA 85: 2334–2338

378

40. Needleman P, Turk J, Jakschik BA, Morrison AR, Lefkowith JB (1986) Arachidonic acid metabolism. Ann Rev Biochem 55: 69–102
41. Palmer RMJ, Ashton DS, Moncada S (1988) Vascular endothelial cells synthesize nitric oxide from L-arginine. Nature 333: 664–666
42. Schmidt HHHW, Klein MM, Niroomand F, Böhme E (1988) Is arginine a physiological precursor of endothelium-derived nitric oxide? Europ J Pharmacol 148: 293–295
43. Griffith TM, Edwards DH, Newby AC, Lewis MJ, Henderson AH (1986) Production of endothelium derived relaxant factor is dependent on oxidative phosphorylation and extracellular calcium. Cardiovasc Res 20: 7–12
44. DeMey JG, Vanhoutte PM (1981) Anoxia and endothelium-dependent reactivity of the canine femoral artery. J Physiol 335: 65–74
45. Ku DD (1982) Coronary vascular reactivity after acute myocardial ischemia. Science 218: 576–578
46. Poche R, Arnold G, Nier H (1969) Die Ultrastruktur der Muskelzellen und der Blutkapillaren des isolierten Rattenherzens nach diffuser Ischämie und Hyperkapnie. Virchows Arch Abt A Pathol Anat 346: 239–268
47. Schaper J, Hehrlein F, Schlepper M, Thiedemann KU (1977) Ultrastructural alterations during ischemia and reperfusion in human hearts during cardiac surgery. J Mol Cell Cardiol 9: 175–189
48. Kloner RA, Rude RE, Carlson N, Maroko PR, DeBoer LWV, Braunwald E (1980) Ultrastructural evidence of microvascular damage and myocardial injury after coronary artery occlusion: which comes first? Circulation 62: 945–952
49. Fishbein MC, Y-Rit J, Lando U, Kanmatsuse K, Mercier JC, Ganz W (1980) The relationship of vascular injury and myocardial hemorrhage to necrosis after reperfusion. Circulation 62: 1274–1279
50. Kloner RA, Ganote CE, Jennings RB (1974) The "no-reflow" phenomenon after temporary coronary occlusion in the dog. J Clin Invest 54: 1496–1508
51. Sunnergren KP, Rovetto MJ (1987) Myocyte and endothelial injury with ischemia reperfusion in isolated rat hearts. Am J Physiol 252: H1211–H1217
52. Tilton RG, Larsen KB, Udell JR, Sobel BE, Williamson JR (1983) External detection of early microvascular dysfunction after no-flow ischemia followed by reperfusion in isolated rabbit hearts. Circ Res 52: 201–225
53. Shasby DM, Shasby SS, Sullivan JM, Peach MJ (1982) Role of endothelial cell cytoskeleton in control of endothelial permeability. Circ Res 51: 657–661
54. Haack DW, Bush LR, Lucchesi BR (1981) Lanthanum staining of coronary microvascular endothelium: effects of ischemia reperfusion, propranolol, and atenolol. Microvasc Res 21: 362–376
55. Curry FE, Michel CC (1980) A fibre matrix model of capillary permeability. Microvasc Res 20: 96–99
56. Humphries DE, Lee SL, Fanburg BL, Silbert JE (1986) Effects of hypoxia and hyperoxia on proteoglycan production by bovine pulmonary artery endothelial cells. J Cell Physiol 126: 249–253
57. Hearse DJ, Humphrey SM, Chain EB (1973) Abrupt reoxygenation of the anoxic potassium-arrested perfused rat heart: A study of myocardial enzyme release. J Mol Cell Cardiol 5: 395–407
58. Ganote CE (1983) Contraction band necrosis and irreversible myocardial injury. J Mol Cell Cardiol 15: 67–73
59. Buderus S, Siegmund B, Spahr R, Krützfeldt A, Piper HM (1989) Resistance of coronary endothelial cells to anoxia-reoxygenation in isolated guinea pig hearts. Am J Physiol 257: H488–H493
60. Rubio VR, Weidemeier T, Berne R (1972) Nucleoside phosphorylase: localisation and role in the myocardial distribution of purines. Am J Physiol 222: 550–555
61. Bowditch J, Brown AK, Dow JW (1983) Accumulation and salvage of adenosine and inosine by isolated mature cardiac myocytes. Biochim Biophys Acta 844: 119–128

62. Piper HM (1989) Energy deficiency, calcium overload or oxidative stress: Possible causes of irreversible ischemic myocardial injury. Klin Wschr 67: 465–476
63. Hülsmann WC, Dubelaar ML (1987) Early damage of vascular endothelium during cardiac ischaemia. Cardiovasc Res 21: 674–677

Release and effects of catecholamines in myocardial ischemia

ALBERT SCHÖMIG, RUTH STRASSER and GERT RICHARDT

The Department of Cadiology, University of Heidelberg, Heidelberg, FRG

Summary

Clinical and experimental studies suggest that in myocardial ischemia the sympathetic activity of the heart is closely related to the progression of cell injury and the incidence of malignant arrhythmias. Adrenergic stimulation of the ischemic myocardium is caused by increased local noradrenaline concentrations in the heart, while the plasma catecholamine levels are of minor relevance. In early ischemia, efferent sympathetic nerves are activated due to pain, anxiety, and fall in cardiac output or arterial blood pressure. However, excessive accumulation of noradrenaline is prevented since adenosine, formed in the ischemic myocardium, effectively suppresses the exocytosis of noradrenaline, and because released noradrenaline is rapidly removed as long as catecholamine re-uptake is functional.

With progression of ischemia to more than 10 minutes, however, the myocardium is no longer protected against excess catecholamine accumulation in the interstitial space since local metabolic release mechanisms become increasingly important. This release, which is independent from central sympathetic activity and from extracellular calcium, occurs in two steps: first, noradrenaline escapes from its intracellular storage vesicles and cumulates in the cytoplasma of the neuron. In a second, rate-limiting step, noradrenaline is transported accross the plasma membrane into the interstitial space, using the neuronal uptake carrier in reverse of its normal transport direction. The latter step requires increased intraneuronal sodium concentrations since noradrenaline leaves the nerve cell by a co-transport with the sodium ion.

Despite excessive interstitial noradrenaline concentrations, capable of rapidly desensitizing the ß-adrenergic receptor under normoxic conditions, myocardial ischemia induces a persistent 30% increase of ß-adrenergic receptor number.

The increased ß-receptor number causes enhanced sensitivity of the heart to catecholamines in the early phase of ischemia. In addition, the effector enzyme adenylatecyclase becomes temporarily supersensitive, followed by a rapid inactivation of the enzyme and its coupling protein G_s. In the α-adrenergic system the receptor number at the cell surface is not consistently elevated and receptor-independent mechanisms lead to a self-potentiating sensitization of the post-receptor components of the α_1-adrenergic system.

H.M. Piper (ed.) Pathophysiology of severe ischemic myocardial injury, 381–412.

Evidence for the significance of adrenergic mechanisms in ischemia-induced myocardial injury is derived from studies with acute and chronic sympathetic denervation prior to ischemia and from interventions using antiadrenergic agents. It was concluded from these studies that local metabolic, rather than centrally induced noradrenaline release is critically involved in progressive ischemic cell damage and the occurrence of ventricullar fibrillation in early ischemia. As a consequence of local metabolic catecholamine release, extracellular noradrenaline reaches 100–1000 times the normal plasma concentration within 20 minutes of ischemia. The deleterious combination of these extremely high noradrenaline concentrations with at least a temporarily enhanced responsiveness of the tissue to catecholamines is thought to accelerate the propagation of the wavefront of irreversible cell damage in the ischemic myocardium. Moreover, the heterogeneous distribution of catecholamine excess within the heart is considered to promote malignant arrhythmias by unmasking and enhancing electrophysiological disturbances in early ischemia such as automaticity and inhomogeneities in conduction and refractoriness.

Introduction

The course of acute myocardial infarction is considered to be heavily influenced by cardiac sympathetic activity. Experimental and clinical studies suggest that catecholamines accelerate the progression of myocardial injury, and arrythmogenic effects of enhanced sympathetic activity or elevated cardiac catecholamine concentrations are well documented. By these detrimental effects, cardiac sympathetic activity is thought to be a major determinant of the patient's outcome in acute myocardial infarction.

The aim of this review is to outline the reasons for excess sympathetic stimulation of the ischemic myocardium and its effects. The main emphasis will be placed on the causes of sympathetic hyperactivity in the ischemic heart which involve the mechanisms of extracellular catecholamine accumulation within the ischemic myocardium and the supersensitivity of the myocytes to adrenergic stimuli. The effects of adrenergic overstimulation on myocyte injury, perfusion of the ischemic area, and early arrhythmias induced by ischemia will be discussed more briefly, since excellent reviews covering these areas are already available [1–6].

Increased catecholamine concentrations within the ischemic myocardium

Three different mechanisms may be involved in the increase of catecholamine concentrations within the extracellular space of the ischemic myocardium: (a) increased plasma concentrations of catecholamines; (b) reflex increase in cardiac sympathetic activity accompanied by local release of catecholamines from the sympathetic nerve endings of the myocardium; and (c) local metabolic release from sympathetic neurons in the ischemic myocardium irrespective of central sympathetic activity.

Increased concentrations of circulating catecholamines

There is agreement in the literature that plasma catecholamine concentrations are increased in early myocardial infarction [7–16]. However, in uncomplicated infarction, plasma noradrenaline and adrenaline concentrations hardly exceed five times the normal levels at rest. Similar plasma concentrations are found in healthy subjects during moderate physical excercise. Dramatically elevated plasma concentrations, which can be expected to have detrimental effects, have been observed in patients with pulmonary edema or cardiogenic shock [12].

Plasma catecholamine concentrations in early infarction have been shown to depend on the amount of damaged myocardium and the hemodynamic consequences of infarction. In experimental studies, Karlsberg *et al.* demonstrated a correlation between plasma catecholamine concentrations and the anatomic size of myocardial necrosis as well as the reduction of cardiac output following coronary occlusion [17]. In human infarction, a reasonable correlation was found between plasma concentrations of noradrenaline and adrenaline and the angiographically determined reduction of left ventricular ejection fraction [16].

Following reperfusion of the ischemic myocardium – induced by lysis of the coronary clot within the first 3 hours of infarction – the plasma catecholamine concentrations briskly returned to nearly normal values [16], in spite of a still compromised hemodynamic performance of the heart [18]. This effect of early reperfusion on plasma catecholamine concentrations may be due to a reduced activity of cardiosystemic reflexes directly activated by metabolic consequences of ischemia (see below) in the underperfused myocardium [19].

The effect of increased plasma catecholamines in further damaging the ischemic myocardium cannot be assumed to be of major importance since ischemic myocardial areas are cut off from systemic circulation and cannot easily be reached by circulating plasma catecholamines. Experimental and clinical evidence of a causal relationship between plasma catecholamines and both the progression of myocardial damage and the development of malignant arrhythmias in infarction [14, 15] is rather vague, and the sparse data supporting this hypothesis can easily be interpreted as parallel phenomena.

Plasma catecholamine concentrations are not helpful as indicators of increased local catecholamine concentrations in the ischemic myocardium, since the contribution of the heart to total net noradrenaline release of the organism is in the range of 2–3% [20]. Moreover, in myocardial ischemia, the noradrenaline washout from the underperfused areas is severely hampered. Increased plasma catecholamines in infarction reflect enhanced activity of the whole sympathetic system rather than local activity in the heart.

Local catecholamine release in the myocardium due to reflex stimulation of sympathetic activity

Pain, anxiety, and a reflex activation of the sympathetic system not only cause an increased peripheral catecholamine release but also enhance sympathetic nerve activity to the heart. Reflex increase in sympathetic activity is mainly determined by two different mechanisms: (a) cardiovascular reflexes, induced by activation of pressor and volume receptors following a decrease in blood pressure and cardiac output, and (b) reflexes which are activated by afferents from ischemic myocardial areas [19]. Local acidosis, accumulation of metabolites, and increased wall stretch [21] are important factors in activating these reflexes. These reflexes, which originate in the ischemic myocardium, are different in anterior and posterior wall infarctions and may well lead to both increase or even depression of cardiac sympathetic activity [22]. Therefore, in experimental coronary occlusion, often only a slight and short-term increase in the impulse rate of sympathetic cardiac nerves is observed.

In the normally perfused myocardium, an acceleration in the impulse rate of cardiac efferent nerves causes a higher noradrenaline release and consequently an increase in sympathetic stimulation of the myocardial cells. In contrast, poorly perfused myocardium is protected within the first few minutes of ischemia against high local concentrations of catecholamines by several mechanisms [23–25]. Excessive accumulation of the neurotransmitter is prevented by rapid elimination of released noradrenaline via neuronal uptake (uptake$_1$) [23]. This re-uptake mechanism depends, for its energy, on an intact sodium gradient across the cell membrane of the sympathetic neuron [26, 27]. In total ischemia or anoxia this is active at least up to the 10th minute of ischemia [28] or anoxia [29]. In early ischemia, the reduced perfusion results in an increased neuronal elimination of noradrenaline because of prolonged exposure of the catecholamines to the uptake process. Extraneuronal elimination of noradrenaline (uptake$_2$) is of minor importance in ischemia [30].

Richard *et al.* [24] have demonstrated that in ischemia stimulation-induced exocytotic release of noradrenaline is modulated by presynaptic receptors. While the most effective modulators under conditions of normal oxygen supply are adrenergic α_2-receptors [31, 32], in ischemia inhibition of release by adenosine is more important. In ischemia, adenosine concentrations are reached within 3 minutes in the extracellular space which inhibit stimulation-induced noradrenaline release by two-thirds [24]. This suppression of noradrenaline release is transmitted by A1-adenosine receptors and can be ceased by adequate antagonists of the receptor such as 8-phenyltheophylline

[24]. Myocardial energy metabolism in early ischemia therefore has a considerable effect, through the formation of adenosine, on exocytotic release of noradrenaline from the sympathetic neuron.

With increasing duration of ischemia (longer than 10 minutes) the sympathetic neurons become severely depleted of ATP. Under these circumstances, exocytotic noradrenaline release ceases, since this release mechanism requires high-energy phosphates [33, 34].

The above-mentioned mechanisms (efficient noradrenaline elimination from the extracellular space, presynaptic inhibition of release by adenosine, and ATP dependency of exocytosis) all effectively inhibit excess accumulation of noradrenaline in the myocardium within the first few minutes of ischemia.

This is in contrast to the previous publications of Wollenberger and Shahab, who described a massive release of catecholamines within the first 3 minutes of ischemia, both in isolated hearts [35] and following coronary ligation in the anesthetized dog [36]. However, these results could neither be reproduced in the isolated organ [28, 30, 37–39] nor in the intact animal [40–42] and no major extracellular catecholamine accumulation has been demonstrated in the ischemic myocardium of various species such as rat, guinea pig, rabbit, canine, and pig during the very first minutes of ischemia.

Correspondingly, in the human heart no enhanced net cardiac release of noradrenaline during short-term myocardial ischemia could be demonstrated [43]. During percutaneous transluminal angioplasty with total occlusion of the left anterior descending coronary artery for 30–150 seconds, no significant increase in noradrenaline concentration was found in the coronary sinus during occlusion, nor during the subsequent reperfusion period.

Local metabolic release of noradrenaline

With the progression of ischemia, the myocardium is no longer protected against excess adrenergic stimulation, since local metabolic release mechanisms become more and more important. This release is independent from the central activation of sympathetic nerves and does not become relevant before the 10th minute in total ischemia [30]. With longer periods of ischemia, increasing quantities of catecholamines are released (Fig. 1) and within 40 minutes of ischemia, more than 30% of the total noradrenaline content of the heart will have been released. Adrenaline and dopamine together account for less than 5% of the corresponding noradrenaline release [30]. This release from sympathetic terminals is histologically reflected by reduction or disappearance of neuronal catecholamine fluorescence due to redistribution of noradrenaline from nerve terminals to other tissue compartments [44–46].

Since ischemia-induced transmitter release from the heart can only be measured during reperfusion, it is not possible, without referring to release kinetics, to decide whether release from sympathetic neurons occurs during ischemia or in the reperfusion phase. The time course of release can, as a

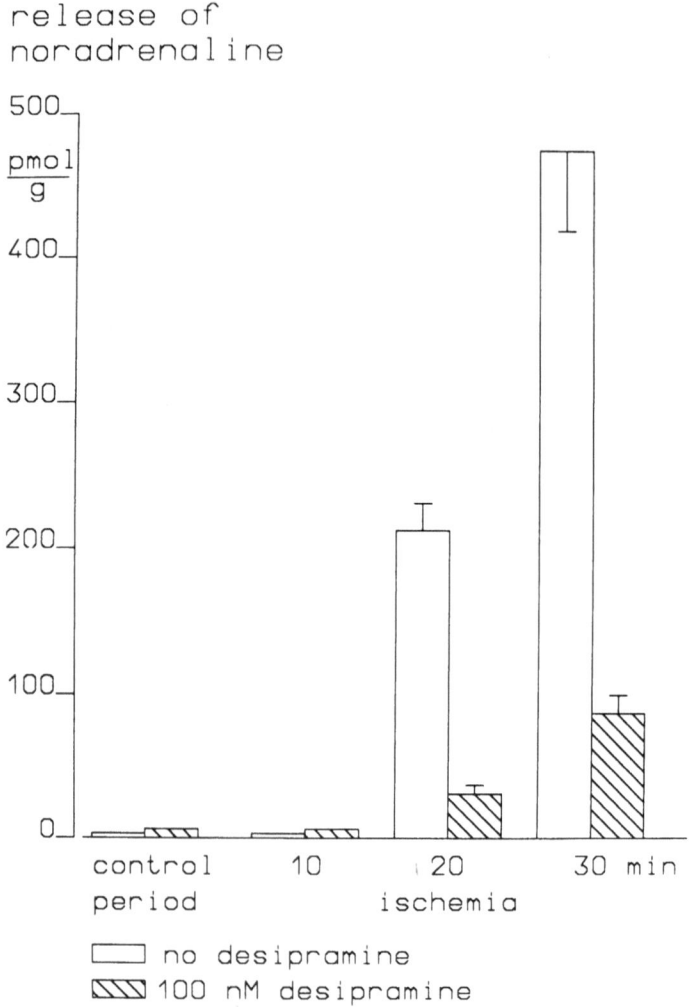

release of
noradrenaline

Fig. 1. Effect of global and total ischemia and desipramine on noradrenaline release from isolated perfused rat hearts.
Noradrenaline release was determined by an HPLC method from the reperfusate after various periods of isothermic perfusion stop. During normoxic control conditions and after ten minutes of ischemia only minor amounts of noradrenaline were collected in the perfusate, which slightly increased following application of desipramine. In contrast, during 20 and 30 minutes of ischemia noradrenaline release dramatically increased, rapidly reaching micromolar concentrations in the interstitial space (calculated from noradrenaline in reperfusate). During 20 and 30 minutes of ischemia, desipramine effectively suppressed the ischemia-induced local metabolic noradrenaline release.

good approximation, be described by means of a two-compartment model [47]. The first compartment corresponds to the washout kinetics from the extracellular space [48]. In 20 minutes of ischemia, this compartment comprises about 90% of total release. The remaining 10% are associated to a release induced by reperfusion. A further argument against major reperfusion-induced release and in favor of release during ischemia, is the fact that the blockade of energy metabolism combined with normal perfusion flow (e.g., anoxia or cyanide intoxication in combination with glucose depletion) also produces a noradrenaline release. It shows similar quantities and identical characteristics as ischemia-induced release. The amine release rapidly ceases after reoxygenation or after the addition of glucose. Likewise with low flow ischemia, noradrenaline release has been shown to occur during the ischemic phase [49]. In this experimental model, flow distribution is heterogeneous and noradrenaline is released into regions of particularly profound ischemia from which it is subsequently eluted during reperfusion.

Assuming uniform distribution of released noradrenaline in the extracellular space, during 20 to 40 minutes of ischemia, extracellular concentrations reach the micromolar range, which is 100 to 1,000 times the normal plasma concentration. Catecholamine concentrations of this order are capable of producing myocardial necrosis even in the non-ischemic heart [50].

Possible causes of extracellular catecholamine accumulation in ischemia

Several release mechanisms may play a role in this extracellular catecholamine accumulation during ischemia: (a) Exocytotic release is induced by depolarization of the nerve ending and requires calcium [33, 34, 51] and high-energy phosphates [33, 34]. It is combined with the release of peptides such as neuropeptide Y, which may therefore serve as a marker of exocytosis [52]. (b) Catecholamine diffusion through neuronal plasma membranes is of minor importance with intact membranes due to the low lipophilia of catecholamines [53, 54]. This mechanism gains significance during longer periods of ischemia when irreversible cell damage occurs and the neuronal membranes leak. (c) Noradrenaline efflux via specific transport systems in the neuronal plasma membrane was first suggested by Paton [55], and several authors have described pharmacological conditions for such carrier-mediated efflux of catecholamines from sympathetic nerve cells [56–58].

In contrast to other neurotransmitters which are enzymatically degraded in the extracellular spaces (such as acetylcholine and peptides), catecholamines are mainly inactivated by uptake into the sympathetic neuron (uptake$_1$) or uptake into extraneuronal cells (uptake$_2$). Both uptake$_1$ and uptake$_2$ are substrate specific, energy-consuming transmembrane transport processes [26] which can be inhibited by drugs such as tricyclic antidepressants (uptake$_1$) [59, 60] and steroids (uptake$_2$) [61]. Reduced activity and/or inhibition of these elimination processes results in extracellular accumulation of catecholamines, even if release remains unaltered.

Local metabolic noradrenaline release induced by ischemia and anoxia is nonexocytotic

Noradrenaline release in early ischemia shows characteristics assigning it to a transmembrane efflux via a specific transport system, identified as the uptake$_1$ carrier. During the ischemia it reverses transport direction and enables a carrier-mediated efflux of noradrenaline from the neuronal cytoplasm to the extracellular space.

This release is independent from extracellular calcium and not even the addition of EGTA to the calcium-free perfusate inhibits the release [30]. The inhibitory effect of high concentrations of organic calcium antagonists such as verapamil and diltiazem on ischemia-induced amine release described by Nayler and Sturrock [62, 63] is completely independent from extracellular calcium [64]. Therefore it cannot be attributed to the calcium channel blocking properties of the agents. The inhibition of release depends rather on an interference of the drugs with the carrier-mediated noradrenaline transport itself.

The release is not enhanced, as would be expected, by blockade of the neuronal uptake, but is markedly reduced. Release reduction by uptake blockade is more than 80% up to 30 minutes of ischemia [30]. The release can be suppressed by different inhibitors of neuronal uptake (for example, desipramine, cocaine, oxaprotiline, and nisoxetine). The concentrations necessary to suppress release are in the same range as those of uptake blockade [30].

Presynaptic receptors do not modulate the release, and consequently the α_2-antagonist yohimbine, which more than doubles exocytotic release, is without any effect in the case of ischemia-induced release [43].

While exocytotic noradrenaline release is accompanied by the liberation of neuropeptide Y from cardiac sympathetic nerve endings [52], total ischemia for 5 to 30 minutes or anoxia (up to 90 minutes) did not induce the release of neuropeptide Y like immunoreactivity from the guinea pig heart [65]. Identical release characteristics are found when catecholamine release is induced by anoxia or cyanide intoxication in the absence of glucose [66, 67], indicating a common release mechanism caused by energy depletion of the heart that cannot be explained by the concept of exocytosis.

Release of catecholamines from the heart by passive diffusion of the transmitter from the neuron can also be seen to have little importance in ischemia of up to 40 minutes. If release occurs by passive diffusion or efflux through leaky membranes, inhibition of neuronal re-uptake cannot result in reduced accumulation of catecholamines in the extracellular space. Only in ischemia of longer duration can release be explained by leak diffusion since, after 60 minutes, inhibition of neuronal re-uptake no longer causes a reduction in release [30].

Metabolic requirements of nonexocytotic noradrenaline release

Stop flow ischemia permits little variation of metabolic conditions whereas experimental models with depleted energy (such as anoxia and cyanide intoxication) and unchanged perfusion flow provide less complex experimental situations in which to study the metabolic requirements of nonexocytotic noradrenaline release. On the basis of those studies [66, 67], the energy state of the sympathetic nerve terminal appears to be the main determinant of nonexocytotic amine release. Both the interruption of oxidative phosphorylation (either by oxygen deficiency or by cyanide poisoning) and the inhibition or exhaustion of anaerobic glycolysis are necessary for a significant release of noradrenaline from the nerve terminals. Activity of either of the energy-providing processes is sufficient to strongly reduce the release. Thus, ongoing glycolysis completely prevents noradrenaline release even during complete anoxia or cyanide intoxication. Similar protective effects of glucose were found in incomplete (low flow) or regional ischemia [67, 68].

Energy depletion of the nerve terminal is both a necessary and sufficient cause for nonexocytotic noradrenaline release to occur during ischemia. Other factors implicated in ischemia, such as acidosis, increased interstitial potassium concentrations and accumulation of metabolites, are not likely to play a major role in this release because in experimental models with ongoing flow they are present to a much lower degree. The cumulative noradrenaline release, however, is even higher than during total ischemia.

Mechanism of local metabolic catecholamine release in ischemia (Fig. 2)

Under conditions of energy depletion, as is the case in myocardial ischemia, anoxia, or cyanide intoxication, catecholamine release has been demonstrated to be a two-step process [66, 69]. First, noradrenaline escapes from the storage vesicles resulting in enhanced axoplasmic amine concentrations. Second, noradrenaline is transported across the plasma membrane into the extracellular space using the uptake$_1$ carrier in reverse of its normal transport direction.

By accumulation of protons within the neuronal catecholamine storage vesicles the H$^+$-ATPase located in the vesicular membrane generates a transmembrane H$^+$ electrochemical potential of close to 200 mV which is composed of the vesicular membrane potential (inside positive) and a proton gradient (inside pH 5.5) [70–72]. The proton potential is the driving force of vesicular noradrenaline uptake, and amine inward transport is coupled with proton outward transport by a specific reserpine-sensitive carrier located

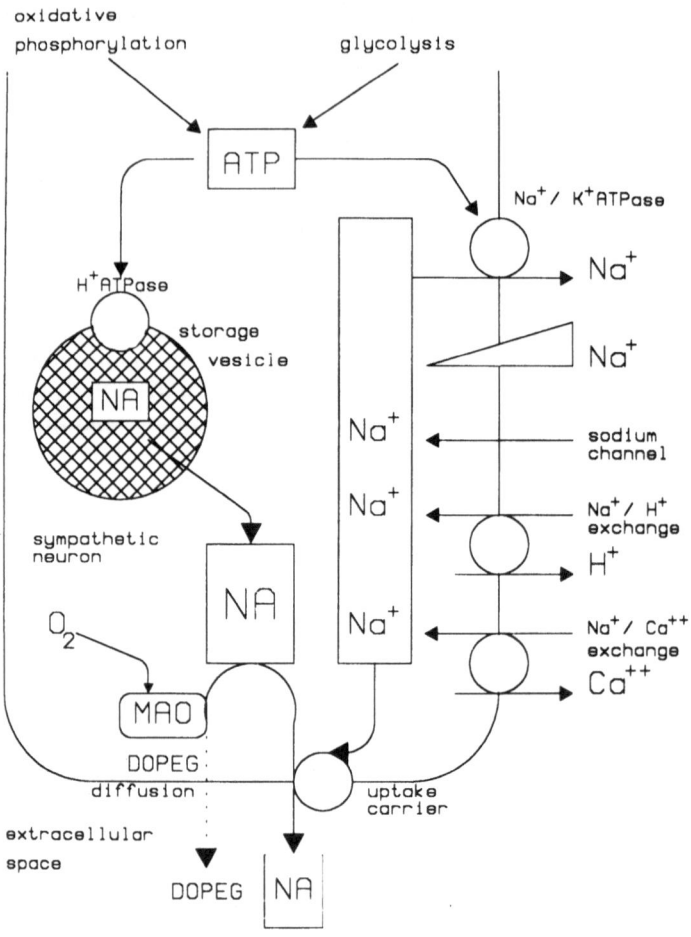

Fig. 2. Scheme of nonexocytotic, calcium independent noradrenaline (NA) release (left part) and its relation to neuronal sodium homeostasis (right part).

Energy depletion of the nerve terminal or blockade of vesicular H^+-ATPase disturb vesicular storage function and result in a loss of noradrenaline from storage vesicles into the axoplasma. Enhanced axoplasmic noradrenaline concentration can be detected by increased dihydroxyphenylethylenglycol (DOPEG) release. Enhanced axoplasmic noradrenaline concentrations do not cause relevant noradrenaline release from the nerve ending as long as neuronal sodium homoeostasis is undisturbed. The combined increase of noradrenaline and sodium within the cytoplasma results in major noradrenaline release via uptake$_1$ which reverses its normal transport direction under these conditions. Blockade of uptake$_1$ by desipramine-like agents inhibits nonexocytotic noradrenaline release but not DOPEG overflow.

Several mechanisms may interfere with neuronal sodium homeostasis (right part) and thereby modify nonexocytotic noradrenaline release. Inhibition of Na^+/K^+-ATPase by digitalis glycosides and/or increased sodium influx into the neuron cause noradrenaline release, if high cytoplasmic noradrenaline concentrations are present. A disturbed energy state, induced by ischemia or anoxia of the sympathetic nerve terminal interferes with both vesicular function and sodium homeostasis and therefore results in nonexocytotic noradrenaline release. Na^+/H^+-exchange has been identified to be a major route of neuronal sodium influx in early ischemia.

within the vesicular membrane [70–72]. A disturbed neuronal energy metabolism leads to dissipation of the proton potential and a loss of noradrenaline from the vesicles into the axoplasm [73, 74]. Ongoing glycolysis is sufficient to prevent this vesicular catecholamine loss even in the absence of functional oxidative phosphorylation [66].

In the presence of oxygen, axoplasmic noradrenaline is readily degraded by monoamine oxidase and the inactive metabolite DOPEG is formed [75]. Thus both exhaustion of glycolysis and hypoxia are required to cause major noradrenaline accumulation in the axoplasm of the sympathetic neuron.

Increased axoplasmic noradrenaline concentrations are not sufficient to induce outward transport of noradrenaline across the plasma membrane of the neuron because under normal conditions, catecholamine transport by the uptake carrier is directed from extracellular space to cytoplasm. Energetics and direction of this cotransport of catecholamines with sodium ions depend on the transmembrane sodium gradient [76–79]. Only an increase of intracellular sodium, which is assumed to occur during early ischemia [80, 81], enables a carrier-mediated efflux of noradrenaline into the extracellular space [76–79]. Blockade of the carrier by trycyclic antidepressants, such as desipramine, inhibits both inward and outward transport of catecholamines, and thus effectively suppresses nonexocytotic noradrenaline release.

In myocardial ischemia, the rise of intracellular sodium is caused by both a failure of Na^+/K^+-ATPase activity due to progressive energy depletion and an increased sodium influx across the plasma membrane. Sodium-proton-exchange has been identified as the predominant pathway of sodium entry into the sympathetic nerve endings in ischemia. This carrier-mediated transport system plays a critical role in the regulation of intracellular pH and is maximally activated by intracellular acidosis [82, 83]. The extrusion of protons is coupled with sodium entry which leads to intracellular sodium accumulation, especially when Na^+/K^+-ATPase activity is suppressed. Inhibition of Na^+/H^+-exchange by amiloride and more specifically by ethylisopropyl-amiloride [84] markedly reduces ischemia induced noradrenaline release [69].

Time course and localization of catecholamine release in ischemia

It is possible to characterize three subsequent phases of catecholamine release in myocardial ischemia [30].

Phase 1 (ischemia up to 10 minutes): During this phase, the release of catecholamines occurs by exocytosis and depends on the activity of the efferent cardiac sympathetic nerves. The extracellular accumulation of noradrenaline is limited by the rate of the neuronal re-uptake process. During the first minutes of ischemia, the effect of central sympathetic neural activity is reduced by presynaptic inhibitory effects of adenosine. At the end of phase 1, sympathetic neurotransmission progressively fails, presumably due to energy depletion of the nerve cells.

Phase 2 (10–40 minutes of ischemia): A massive accumulation of noradrenaline and, to a lesser extent, of adrenaline and dopamine occurs in the extracellular space of the ischemic myocardium. The release is determined by local energy exhaustion rather than by centrally originating factors. The release is independent from calcium and is inhibited by blockers of neuronal uptake. The mechanism is different from exocytotic release and demonstrates the characteristics of a carrier-mediated efflux using the neuronal uptake carrier in reverse of its normal transport direction.

Phase 3: When ischemia lasts longer than 40 minutes, the sympathetic neurons within the ischemic area progressively deplete from noradrenaline. The release occurs parallel to the development of structural membrane defects and can no longer be blocked by inhibitors of neuronal uptake.

This time course of catecholamine release is derived from studies in the isolated heart and therefore cannot be extrapolated directly to *in vivo* conditions. In situations of variable and incomplete ischemia that are present in myocardial infarction, it may be assumed that a temporarily dispersed release would occur. The principal mechanisms, that were thought to account for the release would be expected to apply also to myocardial infarction in humans. The situation is even more complex however, as different release mechanisms are active simultaneously in closely related myocardial regions with unequal residual perfusion [49]. In severely ischemic areas, nonexocytotic local metabolic release may be found, which is inhibited by desipramine-like drugs and is unaffected by classical sympatholytic drugs such as clonidine. At the same time, in the non-ischemic or mildly ischemic myocardium release predominantly occurs by exocytosis and agents like desipramine result in an aggravated catecholamine accumulation. The border zone of ischemia is unpredictably influenced by both mechanisms through catecholamine diffusion. Such chronological and local inhomogeneities in adrenergic activation of the myocardium may play an important role in the pathogenesis of ischemia-induced arrythmias [6].

Adrenergic receptors in acute myocardial ischemia

Acute myocardial ischemia induces the release of large quantities of endogenous norepinephrine activating both ß-adrenergic and α-adrenergic receptors. Various studies have shown that activation of adrenergic receptors by receptor-agonists results in their rapid desensitization [85–88]. The desensitization of adrenergic receptors involves phosphorylation [87, 89], functional uncoupling, and internalization of the receptors from the cell surface [85, 89]. Therefore, under physiological conditions an increased release of catecholamines leads to a rapid reduction of both ß-adrenergic and α-adrenergic receptor numbers at the cell surface [85].

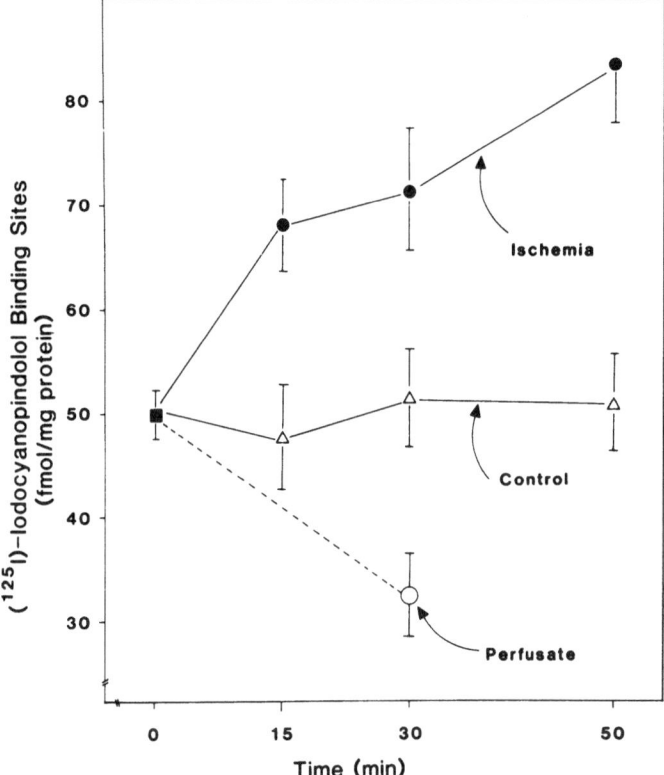

Fig. 3. β-adrenergic binding sites in isolated perfused rat hearts under normoxic conditions (*control* and *perfusate*) and during global and total ischemia.

Ischemia was induced by isothermic perfusion stop. The *perfusate* hearts were perfused for 10 minutes under normoxic conditions using the reperfusate from hearts which had been ischemic for 30 minutes.

In the isolated plasma membranes of the hearts the β-adrenergic receptors were determined using the radiolabelled β-antagonist (^{125}I) I-Iodocyanopindolol. Shown here are the specific β-adrenergic binding sites (± SEM, n=8) after various periods of perfusion or ischemia.

The perfusate derived from the ischemic hearts reduced the density of β-adrenergic receptors significantly. In contrast, total ischemia led to a rapid increase of the β-adrenergic receptors after 15 minutes with a further rise after 30 and 50 minutes of global ischemia.

β-adrenergic receptors

The amount of endogenous catecholamines released in ischemia would be quite sufficient both to activate and to regulate the ß-adrenergic receptors under normoxic conditions [90]. Likewise, the perfusion of isolated hearts with perfusate derived from globally ischemic hearts during the early reperfusion period led to a reduction of the ß-adrenergic receptors at the cell surface (Fig. 3). These data indicate that the ß-adrenergic receptors were activated by the catecholamines present in the perfusate. Moreover, this activation was closely linked to the inactivation of the ß-adrenergic system which involves receptor internalization [85]. However, despite the 100 to 1000 times increase in catecholamine concentrations in the ischemic myocardium, the density of ß-adrenergic receptors was increased by more than 30% in the cardiac plasma membranes of ischemic hearts. Similarly, in the dog heart, 5 hours after occlusion of the left anterior descending coronary artery the number of ß-adrenergic receptors present in isolated plasma membranes from the ischemic area was increased by about 30% [91]. The affinity of these receptors for antagonists was unchanged. Quite similar observations were described even after much shorter periods of ischemia in various *in vivo* models [92–96].

Predominantly local mechanisms have been identified to be responsible for this increase of ß-adrenergic receptors [90]. Thus in isolated perfused hearts global ischemia of 15 minutes induced an increased density of ß-adrenergic receptors at the cell surface (Fig. 3). The extent of the increase in this *in vitro* model system was similar to that observed in various *in vivo* systems using regional ischemia [97]. The increase of β-adrenergic receptors occurred very rapidly, persisted with prolonged ischemia, and was also rapidly reversible with reperfusion [98]. The fast time course indicates that new synthesis of ß-adrenergic receptors may not account for this increase of the receptor number at the cell surface. The number of receptors at the cell surface rather depends on a balance between receptor externalization and receptor internalization [99]. Under physiological conditions about 70% of the cellular ß-adrenergic receptors in the heart can be identified in the plasma membrane. The remaining 30% of the ß-adrenergic receptors are resident in a light membrane fraction [89, 90, 93]. This light membrane fraction represents an intracellular pool of membranes which lacks the classical plasma membrane markers [89]. Early myocardial ischemia leads to the increase of β-adrenergic receptors in the plasma membrane fraction at the expense of receptors in the light membrane fraction [93]. From these data, it was assumed that an increased externalization is responsible for the ischemia-induced rise of β-adrenergic receptors in the plasma membranes [93]. However, in isolated perfused hearts it has been demonstrated that with global ischemia and with the loss of high energy phosphates the agonist-promoted internalization was completely abolished [90, 98]. As a consequence of a reduced receptor internalization, the balance of receptor externalization and receptor internalization is shifted towards an increased density of receptors at the cell surface.

Little is known about structural alterations of the ß-adrenergic receptors in acute myocardial ischemia. Under physiological conditions, the occupancy of ß-adrenergic receptors by their agonists leads to receptor internalization and to receptor phosphorylation by a cAMP-independent beta-adrenergic receptor kinase [89, 100–102]. With ischemia, receptor internalization is abolished [90], but catecholamine-induced receptor phosphorylation might still occur.

Pharmacological data indicate that the binding site of the ß-adrenergic receptors are unaltered in acute myocardial ischemia [91, 103] and the affinities for their antagonists and their agonists remain unchanged [90]. Moreover, the coupling of the ß-adrenergic receptors to the postreceptor components of the adenylate cyclase system is not influenced by myocardial ischemia (see below). These data suggest that structurally and functionally the ß-adrenergic receptors remain intact in acute myocardial ischemia, and that the major ischemia-induced change is the enhanced density of ß-adrenergic receptors on the cell surface.

α-adrenergic receptors

Much less is known about the alterations and the role of the α-adrenergic receptors in acute myocardial ischemia. Using *in vivo* model systems for myocardial infarction in the dog [103–105] or in the cat [106–108] a significant increase of α_1-adrenergic receptors could be demonstrated in the plasma membranes derived from the ischemic zone. A similar increase was observed in guinea pigs *in vivo* [93, 109], whereas in an *in vitro* model using isolated perfused guinea pig heart, no change in the density of α_1-adrenergic receptors was found [110]. Similarly, in isolated rat hearts global ischemia failed to increase the α_1-adrenergic receptors in the plasma membranes [97, 111]. Therefore, at present it cannot be decided if these inconsistent data are due to the different species used or if the ischemia-induced increase of α_1-adrenergic receptors can be observed *in vivo* only. It may be speculated that in contrast to the ß-adrenergic receptor the modulation of α-receptors is rather due to systemic than to local mechanisms. The varying results on the density of α_1-adrenergic receptors in myocardial ischemia are reflected by controversial results concerning the role of α-adrenergic blockade in preventing ischemia induced arrhythmias [111–113].

The direct comparison of the ischemia-induced changes of ß-adrenergic and α-adrenergic receptor densities indicate that these two receptors are regulated by different mechanisms. In the isolated rat heart ischemia induces an increase of ß-receptors due to loss of receptor internalization, whereas the number of α_1-adrenergic receptors remains unchanged at the cell surface [97, 98, 111]. These data suggest that unspecific alterations like stiffness of the plasma membrane, which would influence all receptors in a similar way, are not responsible for receptor regulation in acute myocardial ischemia.

As with ß-adrenergic receptors, the pharmacological characteristics of α_1-adrenergic receptors remain unaltered in acute myocardial ischemia. Their affinities for agonists and antagonists remain constant [106, 107] and data indicate that the ligand binding site of the receptors remains intact. Under physiological conditions agonist occupancy of the α_1-adrenergic receptors induces receptor internalization and receptor phosphorylation [114–116].

The phosphorylation of the α_1-adrenergic receptors which is triggered by the protein kinase C [114–116] results in desensitization of the α_1-adrenergic system. However, it is still not known whether occupancy of the α_1-adrenergic receptor by endogenous noradrenaline induces receptor phosphorylation in acute myocardial ischemia.

Postreceptor components in myocardial ischemia

Both α_1- and ß-adrenergic receptors are activated by the endogenous catecholamines noradrenaline and adrenaline. However, they couple to and activate quite distinct signal transduction pathways. To evaluate the functional consequences of the ischemia-induced alterations at the receptor level, the accompanying modulation of the postreceptor components has to be considered.

Under physiological conditions of activation the α_1-adrenergic receptor couples to a guanine nucleotide binding regulatory protein (G_p or G_x). This activation of the G-protein leads to its dissociation in the α- and ßγ- subunit. The free α-subunit appears to activate the phospholipase C which in turn hydrolyses phosphatidylinositol 4.5-biphosphate to generate the two second messengers diacylglycerol and inositoltriphosphate (IP_3). IP_3 leads to the liberation of intracellular calcium whereas diacylglycerol activates the calcium and phosphatidylserine sensitive protein kinase C [116–120].

The postreceptor components of the ß-adrenergic system also involve a G-protein with its α-, ß- and γ-subunits. Again under physiological conditions, the activation of ß-adrenergic receptors leads to a dissociation of the α-subunit from the ßγ-subunit of this stimulatory G-protein of the adenylate cyclase system. It seems to be the free α-subunit which activates the adenylate cyclase to generate the second messenger cAMP [121].

There are only few data available on the ischemia-induced alterations of the α_1-adrenergic system. Thus the agonist-promoted high affinity state of the α_1-adrenergic receptor, indicating its ability to functionally couple to its G-protein, has not been evaluated in acute myocardial ischemia, and to date no biochemical data indicate whether α_1-adrenergic receptors are active or not in myocardial ischemia. Independent from α-receptors, the activity of the phospholipase C is enhanced in acute myocardial ischemia due to an increase of intracellular calcium [122]. Nonetheless, the pretreatment with prazosin and other α_1-adrenergic blockers has been shown to reduce the incidence of ventricular arrhythmias during coronary occlusion and reperfusion [122–125]. Part of this effect may be due to an attenuation of the ischemia-induced calcium overload [126].

Increased activity of protein kinase C indicates that independent from the alterations at the receptor level the α_1-adrenergic system is inadequately activated in acute ischemia [127]. Since protein kinase C becomes translocated from the cytosol to the plasma membranes with activation, this translocation was used as a parameter of enzyme activation [128–131]. In acute myocardial ischemia the ischemia-induced translocation could in fact demonstrate a rapid activation of protein kinase C [132]. It may be speculated that the enzyme is stimulated by the ischemia-induced release of phospholipids and fatty acids [124, 133] and/or by the calcium overload of the cardiomyocyte [127]. The activation of the protein kinase C may further promote the ischemia-induced calcium overload resulting in a vicious circle of enzyme activation and calcium accumulation.

Moreover, protein kinase C seems to be a link in a harmful interaction between the α_1- and the ß-adrenergic signal transduction system in acute myocardial ischemia. In acute myocardial ischemia the ß-adrenergic system becomes sensitized by two different mechanisms. One mechanism involves the ß-adrenergic receptors (see above) and the second mechanism is restricted to the enzyme itself. The previously described increase of ß-adrenergic receptors leads to an increased stimulation of the adenylate cyclase by ß-adrenergic agonists [90, 93, 134]. This observation corresponds well with the increased levels of cAMP in the ischemic zone [135, 153].

In early myocardial ischemia this increased ß-agonist effect is superimposed by an enzyme-specific activation of the adenylate cyclase [97, 98, 137] which is sensitive to direct stimulation by manganese or forskolin [138, 139]. The two sensitization processes have quite distinct time courses and are caused by different mechanisms.

The receptor-specific sensitization is based on the increased density of ß-adrenergic receptors at the cell surface and additionally on their increased ability to couple to their G-protein, the stimulatory G-protein (G_s). The increased coupling can be determined by the portion of receptors capable of forming an agonist-promoted ternary complex [140, 141]. Consequently, in early myocardial ischemia at any given concentration of the ß-agonist, more receptors couple more efficiently to the G_s-protein to activate the adenylate cylase [90]. These data also indicate that in the early period of ischemia the G_s-protein is intact and retains its ischemia-induced sensitization, indicating that this increased activity is due to a covalent modification of the enzyme [97, 98]. Protein kinase C, one of the secondary effector enzymes of the α-adrenergic pathway, seems to be involved in this early sensitization process [137]. This can be concluded from the finding that the protein kinase C inhibitor polymyxin B [142] prevents the ischemia-induced sensitization of the adenylate cyclase, whereas other protein kinase inhibitors like calcium/calmodulin inhibitors do not have this effect [137]. Phosphorylation of the enzyme which has previously been demonstrated in isolated cells *in vitro* [143] remains to be demonstrated in the ischemic heart. Activation of α_1-adrenergic receptors does not seem to be involved in the sensitization process of the adenylate cyclase. Consequently, the pretreatment with the α_1-blocker prazosin fails to prevent the ischemia-induced sensitization of the adenylate cyclase [137].

In contrast to the dual sensitization in early myocardial ischemia, the adenylate cyclase system becomes quite unresponsive on prolonged periods of ischemia, despite the persistent increase of functionally coupled receptors. Thus after one hour of global ischemia those receptors capable of forming the ternary complex remain persistently increased. However, both the GTPase activity and the total activity of the adenylate cyclase are greatly reduced after one hour of myocardial ischemia [144]. In addition, the response is reduced to direct stimulation of the adenylate cyclase is reduced by forskolin, indicating that the enzyme itself becomes inactivated after prolonged ischemia [137]. The persistent sensitization at the receptor level contrasts with an inactivation of the postreceptor components of the adenylate cyclase system. Thus different regulations of adrenergic receptors and postreceptor components may explain the variable reactions of the infarcted heart to adrenergic stimulation.

Contribution of catecholamines to ischemia-induced myocardial injury

Evidence for adrenergic effects in myocardial ischemia

Primarily, the assumption that catecholamines might be involved in mechanisms of myocardial ischemia and infarction came from observations of necroses in the hearts of patients with catecholamine producing pheochromozytoma [145, 146]. Similar cell damage could be produced by application of adrenaline to the heart with unchanged blood supply to the myocardium [4, 50].

In order to confirm the involvement of the sympathoadrenergic system in the progression of myocardial ischemia different surgical and pharmacological interventions have been studied. Leriche and Fontaine demonstrated that stellate gangliectomy reduced the extent of myocardial necrosis associated with coronary occlusion in the dog [148]. These early findings were strengthened by several other authors who found a significant reduction in infarct size when cardiac sympathectomy was combined with coronary ligation. In these studies, chronic denervation was much more effective than acute denervation [149–152]. Thus, after acute sympathectomy the size of infarction was reduced by about 25%, versus 90% after chronic denervation [151]. In accordance with the surgical intervention studies, various authors reported that ß-adrenergic blockade decreased the degree of ischemic damage [153–157].

Beta-adrenoceptor blockers have also been applied in human myocardial infarction. Cumulative data from controlled clinical trials indicate a 14% reduction of mortality within the first week following myocardial infarction [158–160]. Reduction of mortality by beta-blockers corresponded with a decrease of infarct size as assessed from cumulative enzyme release [159, 160].

From this protective effect of beta-adrenoceptor blockers in myocardial infarction, strong evidence can be derived that adrenergic overactivity enhances myocardial damage in ischemia. The dosage of the ß-blockers used and the negative results with isomeres which do not interact with the ß-adrenoceptor support the conclusion that these agents reduce myocardial ischemic injury through ß-adrenergic blockade rather than through unspecific actions [155, 160]. While the contribution of beta-adrenergic stimulation to the ischemic injury seems to be unequivocal, there is considerable controversy about the mechanisms involved in this effect.

In part, the injury of marginal, still contracting areas of ischemia may be explained by the augmented mechanical work caused by catecholamine release and ß-adrenergic overstimulation resulting in enhanced heart rate and contractility. However, changes in mechanical work cannot explain protection in the central zone of ischemia because the heart muscle in this zone is not contracting. Based on experimental findings, it may be assumed that ß-adrenergic stimulation further reduces high energy phosphates even in the non-contracting part of the ischemic zone, since ß-adrenergic stimulation is still capable of inducing formation of cyclic AMP under these conditions [135]. Formation of cyclic AMP is energy consuming itself and activates several intracellular processes which result in further degradation of high energy phosphates.

Among these energy consuming processes the activation of the sodium-potassium pump may be of major relevance. In different experimental settings the time course of extracellular potassium accumulation in the early phase of myocardial ischemia has been reported to be triphasic [40, 161, 162]. A rapid initial rise is followed by a plateau phase during which extracellular potassium may actually decrease. Subsequently, a second progressive increase takes place. It recently was demonstrated that catecholamines, by activating the sodium-potassium ATPase, are the precondition for the secondary decrease in extracellular potassium [163]. However, there are conflicting findings as to whether catecholamines stimulate the sodium-potassium pump directly, or through adenylate cyclase activation [164]. Calcium overload has been identified to play a crucial role in the pathogenesis of myocardial necrosis. In this context, the finding of an α-adrenergic mediated accumulation of calcium in reperfused myocardium [165] indicates involvement of α-receptor stimulation in ischemic cell damage , as well.

Receptor-independent cardiotoxic effects

Extremely high interstitial catecholamine levels (micromolar concentrations) during myocardial ischemia have raised the question about mechanisms of catechlamine-induced myocardial injury besides receptor stimulation. This assumption was supported by the finding that cardiotoxic effects of high catecholamine concentrations were not totally blocked by receptor antagonists and were not always accompanied by a parallel increase of cyclic AMP [166].

It was demonstrated that adenochromes, oxidation products of catecholamines, depress contractile activity and affect cardiac muscle cell membranes

[167]. Moreover, receptor-independent catecholamine-induced cardiotoxicity was connected to the formation of free radicals which may increase membrane permeability by promoting lipid peroxidation [4]. Although adenochrome formation may be an important factor for cardiac damage following exogenous administration of catecholamines its role in myocardial ischemia is challenged by the fact that oxygen tension rapidly decreases in the ischemic tissue and therefore major formation of these oxidation products is rather unlikely. For this reason, if they do at all, adenochromes are more likely to play a role in reperfusion injury.

Impeded blood flow to the ischemic area

Experiments with chronically sympathectomized dogs demonstrated that collateral perfusion to the central and peripheral ischemic zones of denervated hearts was two to four times higher in comparison to nonsympathectomized hearts [151]. It was concluded that impeded collateral flow is related to the sympathetic tone after coronary occlusion. Possible causes for impairment of coronary flow due to catecholamines can be divided into vascular, extravascular, and intravascular components. The coronary vasculature is influenced by both an α-adrenergic constrictor tone and an opposing ß-adrenergic vasodilator tone. Although under normal conditions the ß-adrenergic influence on the coronary vasculature predominates, α-adrenergic activity may increase under pathological conditions [168]. There is evidence that during experimental coronary occlusion α-adrenergic acitivity limits collateral flow to the ischemic myocardium [168, 169].

Catecholamines also increase extravascular compressive forces on the coronary vascular bed because they enhance intramyocardial pressure. Since coronary flow predominantly occurs in diastole, an accelerated heart rate, caused by adrenergic stimulation, will further diminish collateral flow.

In addition, there is evidence for an enhanced platelet aggregation induced by catecholamines in myocardial ischemia [170, 171]. These clinical results correspond with earlier *in vitro* findings of platelet aggregation caused by adrenaline and noradrenaline and transmitted by α-adrenoceptors [171, 173]. The hemostatic action of catecholamines may add an intravascular factor to the impairment of collateral flow in myocardial ischemia.

Adrenergic influences on arrhythmogenesis in myocardial ischemia

The relation of catecholamines to arrhythmias represents a similarly confusing and fascinating feature of adrenergic influences in acute myocardial ischemia. Evidence for a causal relationship came from experiments with both surgical and pharmacological interventions in adrenergic activity in myocardial infarction.

Chronic cardiac sympathetic denervation reduced the incidence of ventricular fibrillation, whereas acute sympathetic ablation failed to suppress ventricular fibrillation associated with ischemia [174, 175]. This apparent paradox might be solved by the finding that chronic denervation resulted in almost total depletion of myocardial catecholamines whereas acute denervation did not [175]. Thus, acute sympathetic denervation prevents catecholamine release evoked by central sympathetic activity, but not release induced by local metabolic processes. In contrast, the heart is protected from any kind of catecholamine release after chronic denervation.

It is remarkable that the same discrepancy was demonstrated for the effect of denervation in regard to infarct size (see above). Thus, it can be concluded that local metabolic catecholamine release in response to ischemia is critical for both the development of ventricular fibrillation and the degree of cell damage.

In accordance with the results obtained after surgical denervation, pharmacological depletion of myocardial catecholamines with 6-hydroxydopamine reduced the incidence of ventricular fibrillation following complete obstruction of the left anterior descendent coronary artery in dogs [176]. Comparable results were obtained in isolated heart preparations [177, 178]. Another approach to limit noradrenaline release during myocardial ischemia is the use of uptake$_1$-inhibitors which have been shown to suppress local metabolic noradrenaline release in ischemia (see above). As shown for catecholamine depletion, uptake$_1$-inhibitors such as desipramine and amitriptyline, dramatically reduce the incidence of ventricular fibrillation following coronary artery ligation in isolated perfused rat hearts [179, 180] and in dogs [181]. These data correspond with the hypothesis that local metabolic noradrenaline release in ischemia is critically involved in the inception of arrhythmias.

Matters become more complicated if one looks at the effects of unilateral and bilateral gangliectomy on ischemia-induced arrhythmias. Schwartz and colleagues have demonstrated that blockade of the left stellate ganglion was antiarrhythmic during ischemia, while blockade of the right stellate ganglion resulted in arrhythmogenic effect [182] and acute bilateral gangliectomy failed to influence arrhythmias [175]. It became apparent from these findings that the asymmetry in cardiac sympathetic innervation contributes to arrhythmogenesis during ischemia. The dominant effect of left stellate input is a shortening of ventricular refractory period, a phenomenon which is likely to enhance the propagation of ventricular arrhythmias due to re-entry mechanisms [183].

Several findings suggest that adrenergic effects on arrhythmogenesis in ischemia are mediated by the activation of beta-adrenergic receptors of the cardiomyocyte: On the one hand, adrenaline-induced vulnerability to ventricular fibrillation was accompanied by an increase in tissue cAMP [135, 184], on the other hand, beta-adrenergic blockade with propranolol, atenolol, and metoprolol attenuated ventricular arrhythmias in experimental myocardial infarction [176, 185–188].

Since in ischemia the antiarrhythmic effect of beta-adrenergic blockade was variable, whereas procedures depleting catecholamines or inhibiting their release appeared to be far more effective, the role of α-adrenergic stimulation was evaluated. In fact, α-receptor blockade by phentolamine and prazosin significantly reduced ventricular arrhythmias during coronary occlusion and especially during reperfusion in various species [190–192].

It has remained speculative which electrophysiological actions induced by adrenergic overactivity contribute significantly to the pathogenesis of ventricular arrhythmias during myocardial ischemia [1, 2, 5, 6]. On the cellular level, catecholamines interfere by stimulation of β-receptors with various components of the action potential, such as amplitude, duration, refractoriness, and conduction velocity, depending on the type of cardiac tissue [193]. Moreover, α-adrenergic mechanisms increase slow inward current and therefore may initiate delayed after depolarization and triggered activity [5, 194].

Experiments utilizing high catecholamine concentrations for coronary perfusion demonstrate that under normoxic conditions, in an electrically stable heart, these electrophysiological effects of catecholamines are not sufficient to induce malignant arrhythmias. In myocardial ischemia, however, heterogeneities of electrophysiological parameters such as resting potential, conduction velocity, and refractoriness are present as important preconditions for re-entry. These inhomogeneities correspond to metabolic and ionic gradients (cellular content of high energy phosphates and glycogen, extracellular potassium concentration, intra- and extracellular pH) between closely related areas with different ischemic injury [195, 196]. Superimposed are local and temporary inhomogeneities in noradrenaline release (see above) and catecholamine responsiveness of the myocytes (see above). This combination may be considered to aggravate variabilities of conduction and refractoriness and to promote ischemia-induced arrhythmias.

Apart from these direct electrophysiological effects, excess sympathetic stimulation facilitates arrhythmias by indirect actions [197]. These are enlargement of the ischemic area and increased heart rate which has been shown to unmask heterogeneities of conduction velocity in the ischemic zone [6, 198]. Thus, by direct and indirect interference with electrophysiological processes in the ischemic heart, excessive adrenergic stimulation promotes malignant arrhythmias and has a considerable effect on the outcome in acute myocardial infarction.

Acknowledgements

We are gratefully indebted to Karin Hornig for skilful preparation of the manuscript. The work was supported by a grant of the Deutsche Forschungsgemeinschaft (SFB 320 – Cardiac Function and its Regulation).

References

1. Corr PB, Gillis RA (1978) Autonomic neural influences on the dysrhythmias resulting from myocardial infarction. Circ Res 43: 1–9
2. Malliani A, Schwartz PJ, Zanchetti A (1980) Neural mechanisms in life-threatening arrhythmias. Am Heart J 100: 705–715
3. Ceremuzynski L (1981) Homoral and metabolic reactions evoked by acute myocardial infarction. Circ Res 48: 767–776
4. Rona G (1985) Catecholamine cardiotoxicity. J Mol Cell Cardiol 17: 291–306
5. Corr PB, Yamada KA, Witkowski FX (1986) Mechanisms controlling cardiac autonomic function and their relation to arrhythmogenesis. In: Fozzard HA, Jennings RB, Haber E, Katz AM, Morgan HE (eds) Heart and Cardiovascular Systems. Raven Press. NY 1343–1403
6. Janse MJ (1989) Why is increased adrenergic activity arrhythmogenic? In: Brachmann J, Schömig A (eds) Adrenergic System and Ventricular Arrhythmias in Myocardial Infarction. Springer Verlag, New York-Berlin-Heidelberg pp 353–363
7. Gazes PC, Richardson JA, Woods EF (1959) Plasma catecholamine concentrations in myocardial infarction and angina pectoris. Circulation 19: 657–661
8. Griffiths J, Leung F (1971) The sequential estimation of plasma catecholamines and whole blood histamine in myocardial infarction. Am Heart J 82: 171–179
9. Siggers DC, Salter C, Fluck DC (1971) Serial plasma adrenaline and noradrenaline levels in myocardial infarction using a new double isotope technique. Br Heart J 33: 878–883
10. Videbaek J, Christensen NJ, Sterndorff B (1972) Serial determination of plasma catecholamines in myocardial infarction. Circulation 46: 846–855
11. Strange RC, Rowe MJ, Oliver MF (1978) Lack of relation between venous plasma total catecholamine concentration and ventricular arrhythmias after acute myocardial infarction. Bri Med J 2: 921–922
12. Benedict CR, Graham-Smith DG (1979) Plasma adrenaline and noradrenaline concentrations and dopamine-ß-hydroxylase activity in myocardial infarction with and without cardiogenic shock. Br Heart J 42: 214–220
13. Nadeau RA, de Champlain J (1979) Plasma catecholamines in acute myocardial infarction. Am Heart J 98: 548–554
14. Karlsberg RP, Cryer PE, Roberts R (1981) Serial plasma catecholamine response early in the course of clinical acute myocardial infarction: Relationship to infarct extent and mortality. Am Heart J 102: 24–29
15. Bertel O, Bühler FR, Baitsch G, Ritz R, Burkart F (1982) Plasma adrenaline and noradrenaline in patients with acute myocardial infarction. Relationship to ventricular arrhythmias of varying severity. Chest 82: 64–68
16. Schömig A, Ness G, Mayer E, Katus H, Dietz R (1984) Sympathetic activity in patients with acute myocardial infarction before and after intracoronary thrombolytic therapy. Eur Heart J (Suppl 1) 5: 39 (abstract)
17. Karlsberg RP, Penkoske PA, Cryer PE, Corr PB, Roberts R (1979) Rapid activation of the sympathetic nervous system following coronary artery occlusion: Relationship to infarct size, site, and haemodynamic impact. Cardiovasc Res 13: 523–531
18. Ellis SG, Henschke CI, Sandor T, Wynne J, Braunwald E, Kloner RA (1983) Time course of functional and biochemical recovery of myocardium salvaged by reperfusion. J Am Coll Cardiol 1: 1047–1055
19. Malliani A, Schwartz PJ, Zanchetti A (1969) A sympathetic reflex elicited by experimental coronary occlusion. Am J Physiol 217: 703–709
20. Esler M, Jennings G, Korner P, Blombery P, Sacharias N, Leonard P (1984) Measurement of total and organ-specific norepinephrine kinetics in humans. Am J Physiol 247: E21–E28
21. Uchida Y, Murao S (1974) Excitation of afferent cardiac sympathetic nerve fibers during coronary occlusion. Am J Pharmacol 226: 1094–1099
22. Thames MD, Klopfenstein HS, Abboud FM, Mark AL, Walker JL (1978) Referential

distribution of inhibitory cardiac receptors with vagal afferents to the inferoposterior wall of the left ventricle activated during coronary occlusion in the dog. Circ Res 43: 512–519

23. Dart AM, Schömig A, Dietz R, Mayer E, Kübler W (1984) Release of endogenous catecholamines in the ischemic myocardium of the rat. Part B: Effect of sympathetic nerve stimulation. Circ Res 55: 702–706

24. Richardt G, Waas W, Kranzhöfer R, Mayer E, Schömig A (1987) Adenosine inhibits exocytotic release of endogenous noradrenaline in the rat heart: A protective mechanism in early myocardial ischemia. Circ Res 61: 117–123

25. Dart AM (1989) Influence of myocardial ischaemia on exocytotic noradrenaline release. In: Brachmann J, Schömig A (eds) Adrenergetic System and Ventricular Arrhythmias in Myocardial Infarction. Springer Verlag, New York-Berlin-Heidelberg pp 34–43

26. Iversen LL (1971) Role of transmitter uptake mechanisms in synaptic neurotransmission. Bri Pharmacol 41: 571–591

27. Sammet S, Graefe KH (1979) Kinetic analysis of the interaction between noradrenaline and Na$^+$ in neuronal uptake: Kinetik evidence for co-transport. Naunyn-Schmiedeberg's Arch Pharmacol 309: 99–107

28. Schömig A, Dietz R, Strasser R, Dart AM, Kübler W (1982) Noradrenaline release and inactivation in myocardial ischemia. In: Caldarera CM, Harris P (eds) Advances in Studies on Heart Metabolism CLUEB, Bologna, 239–244

29. Schömig A (1989) Increase of cardiac and systemic catecholamines in myocardial ischemia. In: Brachmann J, Schömig A (eds) Adrenergic System and Ventricular Arrhythmias in Myocardial Infarction. Springer Verlag, New York-Berlin-Heidelberg pp 61–77

30. Schömig A, Dart AM, Dietz R, Mayer E, Kübler W (1984) Release of endogenous catecholamines in the ischemic myocardium of the rat. Part A. Locally mediated release. Circ Res 55: 689–701

31. Starke K (1977) Regulation of noradrenaline release by presynaptic receptor systems. Rev Physiol Biochem Pharmacol 77: 1–124

32. Langer SZ (1981) Presynaptic regulation of the release of catecholamines. Pharmacol Rev 32: 337–362

33. Baker PF, Knight DE (1978) Calcium-dependent exocytosis in bovine adrenal medullary cells with leaky plasma membranes. Nature (Lond) 276: 620–622

34. Knight DE, von Grafenstein H, Maconochie DJ (1989) Intracellular requirements for exocytotic noradrenaline release. In: Brachmann J, Schömig A (eds) Adrenergic System and Ventricular Arrhythmias in Myocardial Infarction. Springer Verlag, New York-Berlin-Heidelberg pp 3–20

35. Wollenberger A, Shahab L (1965) Anoxia-induced release of noradrenaline from the isolated perfused heart. Nature 207: 88–89

36. Shahab L, Wollenberger A, Haase M, Schiller U (1969) Noradrenalinabgabe aus dem Hunderhezen nach vorübergehender Okklusion einer Koronararterie. Acta Biol Med Germ 22: 135–143

37. Rochette L, Didier J-P, Moreau D, Bralet J (1980) Effect of substrate on release of myocardial norepinephrine and ventricular arrhythmias following reperfusion of the ischemic isolated working rat heart. J Cardiovasc Pharmacol 2: 267–279

38. Abrahamsson T, Almgren O, Carlsson L (1983) Ischemia-induced noradrenaline release in the isolated rat heart: Influence of perfusion, substrate, and duration of ischemia. J Mol Cell Cardiol 15: 821–830

39. Carlsson L, Abrahamsson T, Almgren O (1985) Local release of myocardial norepinephrine during acute ischemia: An experimental study in the isolated perfused rat heart. J Cardiovasc Pharmacol 7: 791–798

40. Hirche HJ, Franz C, Bös L, Bissig R, Lang R, Schramm M (1980) Myocardial extracellular K$^+$ and H$^+$ increase and noradrenaline release as possible cause of early arrhythmias following acute coronary artery occlusion in pigs. J Mol Cell Cardiol 12: 579–593

41. McGrath BP, Lim SP, Leversha L, Shanahan A (1981) Myocardial and peripherial cate-

cholamine responses to acute coronary artery constriction before and after propranolol treatment in the anaesthetised dog. Cardiovasc Res 15: 28–34

42. Forfar JC, Riemersma RA, Oliver MF (1983) Alpha-adrenoceptor control of norepinephrine release from acutely ischemic myocardium: Effects of blood flow, arrhythmias, and regional conduction delay. J Cardiovasc Pharmacol 5: 752–759

43. Schömig A (1988) Adrenergic mechanisms in myocardial infarction: Cardiac and systemic catecholamine release. J Cardiovasc Pharmacol 12 (Suppl 1): 1–7

44. Holmgren S, Abrahamsson T, Almgren O, Eriksson BM (1981) Effect of ischaemia on the adrenergic neurons of the rat heart: A fluorescence histochemical and biochemical study. Cardiovasc Res 15: 680–689

45. Muntz KH, Hagler HK, Boulas HJ, Buja LM (1984) Redistribution of catecholamines in the ischemic zone of the dog heart. Am J Pathol 114: 64–78

46. Holmgren S, Abrahamsson T, Almgren O (1985) Adrenergic innervation of coronary arteries and ventricular myocardium in the pig: Fluorescence microscopic appearance in the normal state and after ischemia. Basic Res Cardiol 80: 18–26

47. Schömig A, Dart AM, Dietz R, Kübler W, Mayer E (1985) Paradoxical role of neuronal uptake for the locally mediated release of endogenous noradrenaline in the ischemic myocardium. J Cardiovasc Pharmacol 7 (Suppl 5): 40–44

48. Lindmar R, Löffelholz K (1974) Neuronal and extraneuronal uptake and efflux of catecholamines in the isolated rabbit heart. Naunyn-Schmiedeberg's Arch Pharmacol 284: 63–92

49. Dart AM, Riemersma RA (1988) Origins of endogenous noradrenaline overflow during reperfusion of the ischaemic rat heart. Clin Sci 74: 269–274

50. Waldenström AP, Hjalmarson AC, Thornell L (1978) A possible role of noradrenaline in the development of myocardial infarction. Am Heart J 95: 43–51

51. Rubin RP (1970) The role of calcium in the release of neurotransmitter substances and hormones. Pharmacol Rev 22: 389–428

52. Haass M, Cheng B, Richardt G, Lang RE, Schömig A (1989) Characterization and presynaptic modulation of stimulation-evoked exocytotic co-release of noradrenaline and neuropeptide Y in guinea pig heart. Naunyn-Schmiedeberg's Arch Pharmacol 339: 71–78

53. Mack F, Bönisch H (1979) Dissociation constants and lipophilicity of catecholamines and related compounds. Naunyn-Schmiedeberg's Arch Pharmacol 310: 1–9

54. Trendelenburg U, Bönisch H, Graefe KH, Henseling M (1980) The rate constants for the efflux of metabolites of catecholamines and phenethylamines. Pharmacol Rev 31: 179–203

55. Paton DM (1973) Mechanism of efflux of noradrenaline from adrenergic nerves in rabbit atria. Br J Pharmacol 49: 614–627

56. Raiteri M, del Carmine R, Bertollini A, Levi G (1977) Effect of desmethylimipramine on the release of ^{3}H-norepinephrine induced by various agents in hypothalamic synaptosomes. Mol Pharmacol 13: 746–758

57. Ross SB, Kelder D (1979) Release of ^{3}H-noradrenaline from the rat vas deferens under various in vitro conditions. Acta Physiol Scand 105: 338–349

58. Graefe KH, Fuchs G (1979) On the mechanism of neuronal efflux of axoplasmatic ^{3}H-(-)noradrenaline. In: Usdin E, Kopin IJ, Barchas J (eds) Basic and Clinical Frontiers, Vol 1. Pergamon Press, New York, Oxford, Toronto, Sydney, Frankfurt, Paris pp 268–270

59. Koe BK (1976) Molecular geometry of inhibitors of the uptake of catecholamines and serotonin in synaptosomal preparations of rat brain. J Pharmacol Exp Ther 199: 649–661

60. Dart AM, Dietz R, Kübler W, Schömig A, Strasser R (1983) Effects of cocaine and desipramine on the neurally evoked overflow of endogenous noradrenaline from the rat heart. Br J Pharmacol 79: 71–74

61. Iversen LL, Salt PJ (1970) Inhibition of catecholamine uptake$_2$ by steroids in the isolated rat heart. Br J Pharmacol 40: 528–530

62. Nayler WG, Sturrock WJ (1984) An inhibitory effect of verapamil and diltiazem on the release of noradrenaline from ischaemic and reperfused hearts. J Mol Cell Cardiol 16: 331–344

63. Nayler WG, Sturrock WJ (1985) Inhibitory effect of calcium antagonists on the depletion of cardiac norepinephrine during postischemic reperfusion. J Cardiovasc Pharmacol 7: 581–587

64. Richardt G, Schäfer H, Kanzler S, Haass M, Schömig A (1989) Einfluß von Kalzium-Antagonisten auf die kardiale Katecholaminfreisetzung bei Normoxie und Ischämie. Z Kardiol 78 (Suppl 1): 86 (abstract)

65. Franco-Cereceda A, Saria A, Lundberg JM (1989) Differential release of calcitonin gene-related peptide and neuropeptide Y from the isolated heart by capsaicin, ischaemia, nicotine, bradykinin and ouabain. Acta Physiol Scand 135: 173–187

66. Schömig A, Fischer S, Kurz Th, Richardt G, Schömig E (1987) Nonexocytotic release of endogenous noradrenaline in the ischemic and anoxic rat heart: Mechanism and metabolic requirements. Circ Res 60: 194–205

67. Dart AM, Riemersma RA, Schömig A, Ungar A (1987) Metabolic requirements for release of endogenous noradrenaline during myocardial ischaemia and anoxia. Br J Pharmacol 90: 43–50

68. Carlsson L (1988) A crucial role of ongoing anaerobic glycolysis in attenuating acute ischemia-induced release of myocardial noradrenaline. J Mol Cell Cardiol 20: 247–253

69. Schömig A, Kurz Th, Richardt G, Schömig E (1988) Neuronal sodium homoeostasis and axoplasmic amine concentration determine calcium-independent noradrenaline release in normoxic and ischemic rat heart. Circ Res 63: 214–226

70. Beers MF, Carty SE, Johnson RG, Scarpa A (1982) H^+-ATPase and catecholamine transport in chromaffin granules. Ann NY Acad Sci 402: 116–133

71. Phillips JH (1982) Dynamic aspects of chromaffin granule structure. Neurosci 7: 1595–1609

72. Winkler H, Apps DK, Fischer-Colbrie R (1986) The molecular function of adrenal chromaffin granules: Established facts and unresolved topics. Neuroscience 18: 261–290

73. von Euler US, Lishajko F (1963) Effect of adenine nucleotides on catecholamine release and uptake in isolated adrenergic nerve granules. Acta Physiol Scand 59: 454–461

74. Toll L, Howard BD (1978) Role of Mg^{2+}-ATPase and pH gradient in the storage of catecholamines in synaptic vesicles. Biochemistry 17: 2517–2523

75. Fowler CJ, Oreland L (1980) The nature of the substrate-selective interaction between rat liver mitochondrial monoamine oxidase and oxygen. Biochem Pharmacol 29: 2225–2233

76. Graefe KH, Zeitner CJ, Fuchs G, Keller B (1984) Role played by sodium in the membrane transport of ^{3}H-noradrenaline across the axonal membrane of noradrenergic neurones. In: Fleming WW (ed) Neuronal and extraneuronal Events in Autonomic Pharmacology. Raven Press, New York 51–62

77. Stute N, Trendelenburg U (1984) The outward transport of axoplasmic noradrenaline induced by a rise of the sodium concentration in the adrenergic nerve endings of the rat vas deferens. Naunyn-Schmiedeberg's Arch Pharmacol 327: 124–132

78. Trendelenburg U (1989) The dynamics of adrenergic nerve endings. In: Brachmann J, Schömig A (eds) Adrenergic System and Ventricular Arrhythmias in Myocardial Infarction. Springer Verlag, New York-Berlin-Heidelberg pp 53–60

79. Graefe KH (1989) On the mechanism of non-exocytotic release of noradrenaline from noradrenergic neurones. In: Brachmann J, Schömig A (eds) Adrenergic System and Ventricular Arrhythmias in Myocardial Infarction.Springer Verlag, New York-Berlin-Heidelberg pp 44–52

80. Fiolet JWT, Baartscheer A, Schumacher CA, Coronel R, Welle HF (1984) The change of the free energy of ATP hydrolysis during global ischemia and anoxia in the rat heart. Its possible role in the regulation of transsarcolemmal sodium and potassium gradients. J Mol Cell Cardiol 16: 1023–1036

81. Balschi JA, Frazer JC, Fetters JK, Clarke K, Springer CS, Smith TW, Ingwall JS (1985) Shift reagent and Na-23 nuclear magnetic resonance discriminates between extra and intracellular sodium pools in ischemic heart. Circulation 72 (Suppl III): 355 (abstract)

82. Lazdunski M, Frelin C, Vigne P (1985) The sodium/hydrogen exchange system in cardiac cells: Its biochemical and pharmacological properties and its role in regulating internal concentrations of sodium and internal pH. J Mol Cell Cardiol 17: 1029–1042

83. Aronson PS (1985)   Kinetic properties of the plasma membrane Na$^+$-H$^+$ exchanger. Ann Rev Physiol 47: 545–560
84. Vigne P, Frelin C, Cragoe Jr EJ, Lazdunski M (1983)   Ethylisopropylamiloride: A new and highly potent derivative of amiloride for the inhibition of the Na$^+$-H$^+$ exchange system in various cell types. Biochem Biophys Res Commun 116: 86–90
85. Harden TK (1983)   Agonist-induced desensitization of the beta-adrenergic receptor-linked adenylate cyclase. Pharmacol Rev 35: 5–32
86. Sibley DR, Lefkowitz RJ (1986) Molecular mechanisms of receptor desensitization using the beta-adrenergic receptor-coupled adenylate cyclase system as a model. Nature 317: 124–129
87. Strasser RH (1988) Phosphorylation of the beta-adrenergic receptor: Mechanisms of desensitization. In: Moudgil VK (ed) Receptor Phosphorylation. CRC Press, Boca Ration, FL p 199–226
88. Perkins JP (1983)   Desensitization of the response of adenylate cyclase to catecholamines. Curr Top Membr Transp 18: 85–108
89. Strasser RH, Stiles GL, Lefkowitz RJ (1984)   Translocation and uncoupling of the beta-adrenergic receptor in rat lung after catecholamine promoted desensitization *in vivo*. Endocrinology 115: 1392–1400
90. Strasser RH, Krimmer J, Marquetant R (1988)   Regulation of ß-adrenergic receptors: Impaired desensitization in myocardial ischemia. J Cardiovasc Pharmacol 12 (Suppl 1): 15–24
91. Mukherjee A, Wong TL, Buja M, Lefkowitz RJ (1979)   Beta adrenergic and muscarinic cholinergic receptors in canine myocardium. J Clin Invest 64: 1423–1428
92. Devos C, Robberecht P, Nokin P, Waelbroeck M, Clinet M, Camus JC, Beaufort P, Schoenfeld P, Christophe J (1985) Uncoupling between beta-adrenoceptors and adenylate cyclase in dog ischemic myocardium. Naunyn-Schmiedeberg's Arch Pharmacol 331: 71–75
93. Maisel AS, Motulsky HJ, Insel PA (1985)   Externalization of beta-adrenergic receptors promoted by myocardial ischemia. Science 230: 183–186
94. Vatner DE, Vatner SF, Fujii AM, Homcy C (1985)   Loss of high affinity cardiac beta adrenergic receptors in dogs with heart failure. J Clin Invest 76: 2259–2264
95. Vatner DE, Knight D, Shen YT, Thoma JXJ, Homcy CJ,   Vatner SF (1988) One hour of myocardial ischemia in conscious dogs increases beta-adrenergic receptors, but decreases adenylate cyclase activity. J Mol Cell Cardiol 20: 75–82
96. Insel PA, Maisel AS (1989)   Alpha$_1$- and beta-adrenergic receptors in myocardial ischemia and injury. In: Brachmann J, Schömig A (eds) Adrenergic System and Ventricular Arrhythmias in Myocardial Infarction. Springer Verlag, New York-Berlin-Heidelberg pp 81–90
97. Strasser RH, Dullaeus RB, Marquetant R (1989)   Dual sensitization of the adenylate cyclase system in acute myocardial ischemia. Circulation (in press)
98. Strasser RH, Dullaeus RB, Marquetant R, Kübler W (1988)   Dual sensitization of the ß-adrenergic system in early myocardial ischemia: Independent regulation of ß-receptors and adenylate cyclase. Circulation 78 (Suppl II): 482 1928 (abstract)
99. Lefkowitz RJ, Caron MG, Stiles GL (1984)   Mechanism of membrane-receptor regulation. Biochemical, physiological and clinical insights derived from studies of the adrenergic receptors. N Engl J Med 310: 1570–1579
100. Strasser RH, Sibley DR, Lefkowitz RJ (1986)   A novel catecholamine-activated cAMP-independent pathway for beta-adrenergic receptor phosphorylation in wild type and mutant S49 lymphoma cells: Mechanism of homologous desensitization of adenylate cyclase. Biochemistry 25: 1371–1377
101. Strasser RH, Benovic JL, Caron MG, Lefkowitz RJ (1986) Beta-agonist and prostaglandine E1-induced translocation of the beta-adrenergic receptor kinase: Evidence that the kinase may act on multiple adenylate cyclase coupled receptors. Proc Natl Acad Sci 83: 6363–6366
102. Benovic JL, Strasser RH, Caron MG. Lefkowitz RJ (1986)   Beta-adrenergic receptor kinase: Identification of a novel protein kinase which phosphorylates the agonist-occupied form of the receptor. Proc Natl Acad Sci 83: 2797–2801
103. Mukherjee A, McCoy KE, Duke RJ, Hogan M, Hagler H, Buja LM, Willerson JT (1982) Relationship between beta adrenergic receptor numbers and physiological responses during experimental canine myocardial ischemia. Circ Res 50: 735–741

104. Mukherjee A, Haghani Z, Brady J, Bush L, McBride W, Buja LM, Willerson JT (1983) Differences in myocardial α- and ß-adrenergic receptor numbers in different species. Am J Physiol 245: H957–H962

105. Mukherjee A, Hogan M, McCoy K, Buja LM, Willerson JT (1980) Influence of experimental myocardial ischemia on alpha$_1$-adrenergic receptors. Circulation 64 (Suppl III): 149 (abstract)

106. Corr PB, Shayman JA, Kramer JB, Kipnis RJ (1982) Increased α-adrenergic receptors in ischemic cat myocardium. J Clin Invest 67: 1232–1236

107. Corr PB, Witkowski FX, Sobel BE (1978) Mechanisms contributing to malignant dysrhythmias induced by ischemia in the cat. J Clin Invest 61: 109–119

108. Corr PB, Crafford WA (1981) Enhanced alpha-adrenergic responsiveness in the myocardium: Role of alpha adrenergic blockade. Am Heart J 102: 605–614

109. Maisel AS, Motulsky HJ, Zieglar MG, Insel PA (1987) Ischemia- and agonist-induced changes in ß-adrenergic receptor traffic in guinea pig hearts. Am J Physiol 253: H1159–H1166

110. Broadley KJ, Chess-Williams RG, Sheridan DF (1985) 3H-prazosin binding during ischemia and reperfusion in the guinea pig Langendorff heart. Br J Pharmacol 86: 759 (poster)

111. Dillon JS, Gu XH, Nayler WG (1988) Alpha$_1$-adrenoceptors in the ischemic and reperfused myocardium. J Mol Cell Cardiol 20: 725–735

112. Hamra M, Rosen MR (1988) Adrenergic receptor stimulation during simulated ischemia and reperfusion in canine cardiac purkinje fibers. Circulation 78: 1495–1502

113. Thandroyen FT, Worthington MG, Higginson LM, Opie LH (1983) The effect of alpha- and beta-adrenoceptor antagonist agents on reperfusion ventricular fibrillation and metabolic status in the isolated perfused rat heart. J Am Coll Cardiol 1: 1056–1066

114. Leeb-Lundberg LMF, Cotecchia S, DeBlasi A, Caron MG, Lefkowitz RJ (1987) Regulation of adrenergic receptor function by phosphorylation: Agonist-promoted desensitization and phosphorylation of α$_1$-adrenergic receptors coupled to inositol phospholipid metabolism in DDT1 MF2 smooth muscle cells. J Biol Chem 262: 3098–3105

115. Bouvier M, Leeb-Lundberg LMF, Benovic JL, Caron MG, Lefkowitz RJ (1987) Regulation of adrenergic receptor function by phosphorylation. Effects of agonist occupancy on phosphorylation of α$_1$- and ß$_2$-adrenergic receptors by protein kinase C and the cyclic AMP-dependent protein kinase. J Biol Chem 262: 3106–3113

116. Berridge MJ (1987) Inositol triphosphate and diacylglycerol: Two interacting second messengers. Ann Rev Biochem 56: 159–193

117. Berridge MJ (1984) Inositol triphosphate and diacylglycerol as second messengers. Biochem J 220: 345–360

118. Nishizuka Y (1986) Studies and perspectives of protein kinase C. Science 233: 305–312

119. Nishizuka Y (1984) The role of protein kinase C in cell surface signal transduction and tumor promotion. Nature 308: 693–698

120. Bell RM (1986) Protein kinase C activation by diacylglycerol second messengers. Cell 45: 631–632

121. Birnbaumer L, Codina J, Mattera R, Cerione RA, Hildebrandt D, Sunyer T, Rojas FJ, Caron M, Lefkowitz RJ, Iyenger R (1985) Structural basis of adenylate cyclase stimulation and inhibition by distinct guanine nucleotide regulatory proteins. In: Molecular mechanism of transmembranal signalling 4: 131–182

122. Hochachka PW (1986) Defense strategies against hypoxia and hypothermia. Science 231: 234–241

123. Wilber DJ, Lynch JJ, Montgomery DG, Lucchesi BR (1987) Adrenergic influences in canine ischemic sudden death: Effects of adrenoceptor blockade with prazosin. J Cardiovasc Pharmacol 10: 96–106

124. Suyatna FD, van Veldhoven PP, Borgers M, Mannaerts GP (1988) Phospholipid composition and amphiphile content of isolated sarcolemma from normal and autolytic rat myocardium. J Mol Cell Cardiol 20: 47–62

125. Benfey BG, Elfellah MS, Ogilvie RI, Varma DR (1984) Antiarrhythmic effects of prazosin

and propranolol during coronary artery occlusion and reperfusion in dogs and pigs. Br J Pharmacol 82: 717–725

126. Naylor WG, Gordon M, Stephens DJ, Sturrock WJ (1985) A protective effect of prazosin on the ischemic reperfused arrhythmium. J Mol Cell Cardiol 17: 685–699

127. Matthys E, Patel Y, Kreisberg J, Steward JH, Ventkatachalam M (1984) Lipid alterations induced by renal ischemia: Pathogenetic factor in membrane damage. Kidney 26: 153–161

128. Ebeling JG, Vandenbark GR, Kuhn LJ, Ganong BR, Bell RM, Niedel JE (1985) Diacyl-glycerols mimic phorbolester induction of leukemic cell differentiation. Proc Natl Acad Sci USA 82: 815–819

129. Kraft AS, Anderson WB (1983) Characterization of cytosolic calcium-activated phospholipid-dependent protein kinase activity in embryonal carcinoma cells. J Biol Chem 258: 9178–9183

130. Kreutter D, Caldwell AB, Moren MJ (1985) Dissociation of proteinkinase activation from phorbolester-induced maturation of HL-60 leukemia cells. J Biol Chem 260: 5979–5984

131. Yuan S, Sunahara FA, Sen AK (1987) Tumor-promoting phorbol esters inhibit cardiac functions and induce redistribution of protein kinase C in perfused beating rat heart. Circ Res 61: 372–378

132. Louis JC, Magal E, Yavin E (1988) Protein kinase C alterations in fetal rat brain after global ischemia. J Biol Chem 263: 19282–19285

133. Dobmeyer DJ, Kekec BK, Sobel BE, Corr PB (1988) Alpha$_1$-adrenergic mediated accumulation of lysophosphatidylcholine in isolated adult canine myocityes. Circulation 78 (Suppl II): 483 1925 (abstract)

134. Mori K (1976) Studies on adenyl cyclase system in myocardium (part II): Adenyl cyclase system in myocardial infarction of dogs. Nagoya J Med Sci 39: 9–14

135. Podzuweit T, Darby AJ, Cherry GW, Opie LH (1978) Cyclic AMP levels in ischemic and non-ischemic myocardium following coronary artery ligation: Relation to ventricular fibrillation. J Mol Cell Cardiol 10: 81–94

136. Krause EG, Wollenberger A (1980) Cyclic nucleotides in heart in acute myocardial ischemia and hypoxia. Adv Cyc Nucl Res 12: 49–61

137. Strasser RH, Dullaeus RB, Marquetant R, Kübler W (1989) ß-Rezeptorunabhängige Sensibilisierung der Adenylatzyklase in der akuten Myokardischämie. Z Kardiol 78 (Suppl 1): 88 303 (abstract)

138. Seamon KB, Daly JE (1981) Forskolin: A unique deterpene activator of cyclic AMP-generating systems. J Cyc Nucl Res 7: 201–224

139. Seamon KB, Padgett W, Daly JW (1981) Forskolin: Unique deterpene activator of adenylate cyclase in membranes and intact cells. Proc Natl Acad Sci 78: 3363–3367

140. Stadel JM, De Lean A, Lefkowitz RJ (1980) A high affinity agonist beta-adrenergic receptor complex is an intermediate for catecholamine stimulation of adenylate cyclase in turkey erythrocyte membranes. J Biol Chem 255: 1436–1441

141. Gilmann AG (1987) G proteins: Transducers of receptor-generated signals. Ann Rev Biochem 56: 615–649

142. Mazzei GJ, Katoh N, Kuo JF (1982) Polymyxin B is a more selective inhibitor for phospholipid-sensitive Ca^{2+}-dependent protein kinase than for calmodulin-sensitive Ca^{2+}-dependent protein kinase. Biochem Biophys Res Commun 109: 1129–1133

143. Bouvier M, Hausdorff WP, DeBlasi A, O'Dowd BF, Kobilka BK, Caron MG, Lefkowitz RJ (1988) Removal of phosphorylation sites from the ß$_2$-adrenergic receptors delays onset of agonist-promoted desensitization. Nature 333: 370–373

144. Susanni EE, Knight DR, Vatner DE, Vatner SF, Homcy CJ (1988) One hour of myocardial ischemia is associated with a decrease in the stimulatory guanyl nucleotide binding protein, Gs. Circulation 78 (Suppl II): 83 1926 (abstract)

145. Kline IK (1961) Myocardial alterations associated with pheochromocytomas. Am J Pathol 38: 539

146. van Vliet PD, Burchell HB, Titus JF (1966) Focal myocarditis associated with pheochro-

mocytoma. N Engl J Med 274: 1102

147. Raab W, Stark E, Macmillan WH, Gigee WR (1961) Sympathogenic origin and antiad-renergic prevention of stress-induced myocardial lesions. Am J Cardiol 8: 203–211

148. Leriche R, Fontaine R (1931) Les resultats actuels du traitment chirurgical de l'angine de poitrine. J Chir 38: 785

149. Cox WV, Robertson HF (1936) The effect of stellate ganglionectomy on the cardiac function of intact dogs and its effect on the extent of myocardial infarction and on cardiac function following coronary artery occlusion. Am Heart J 12: 285–300

150. Yodice A (1941) Sympathectomy and experimental occlusion of a coronary artery. Am Heart J 22: 545–548

151. Jones CE, Beck LY, DuPont E, Barnes GE (1978) Effect of coronary ligation on the chronically sympathectomized dog ventricle. Am J Physiol 235: H429–H434

152. Barber MJ, Thomas JX, Stephen JR, Jones B, Randall WC (1982) Effect of sympathetic nerve stimulation and cardiac denervation on MBF during LAD occlusion. Am J Physiol 12: H556–H574

153. Sommers HM, Jennings R (1972) Ventricular fibrillation and myocardial necrosis after transient ischemia. Effect of treatment with oxygen, procainamide, reserpine, and propranolol. Arch Intern Med 129: 780–789

154. Shatney CH, MacCarter DJ, Lillehei RC (1976) Effects of allopurinol, propranolol and methylprednisolone on infarct size in experimental myocardial infarction. Am J Cardiol 37: 572–580

155. Reimer KA, Rasmussen MM, Jennings RB (1976) On the nature of protection by propranolol against myocardial necrosis after temporary coronary occlusion in dogs. Am J Cardiol 37: 520–527

156. Abrahamsson T, Almgren O, Svensson L (1981) Local noradrenaline release in acute myocardial ischemia: Influence of catecholamine synthesis inhibition and ß-adrenoceptor blockade on ischemic injury. J Cardiovasc Pharmacol 3: 807–817

157. Bernauer W (1985) The effect of ß-adrenoceptor blocking agents on evolving myocardial necrosis in coronary ligated rats with and without reperfusion. Naunyn-Schmiedeberg's Arch Pharmacol 328: 288–294

158. Yusuf S, Peto R, Lewis J, Collins R, Sleight P (1985) Betablockade during and after myocardial infarction: An overview of the randomized trials. Prog Card Dis 27: 335–371

159. ISIS-I Collaborative Group (First International Study of Infarct Survival) (1986) Randomised trial of intravenous atenolol among 16027 cases of suspected acute myocardial infarction: ISIS-I. Lancet 2: 57–66

160. Cruickshank JM, Prichard BNC (1987) Beta-blockers in clinical practice. Chapter 5: Myocardial infarction. Churchill Livingstone, Edinburgh, London, Melbourne and New York, pp 435–504

161. Hill GC, Gettis CS (1980) Effect of acute coronary artery occlusion on local myocardial extracellular potassium concentration in K^+ activity in swine. Circulation 61: 768–778

162. Kleber AG (1983) Extracellular potassium accumulation in acute myocardial ischemia. J Mol Cell Cardiol 16: 389–394

163. Wilde AAM, Peters RJG, Janse MJ (1988) Catecholamine release and potassium accumulation in the isolated globally ischemic rabbit heart. J Mol Cell Cardiol 20: 887–896

164. Ellingsen O, Sejersted OM, Leraand S, Ilebekk A (1987) Catecholamine-induced myocardial potassium uptake mediated by $ß_1$-adrenoceptors and adenylate cyclase activation in the pig. Circ Res 60: 540–550

165. Sharma AD, Saffitz JE, Lee BI, Sobel BE, Corr PB (1983) Alpha adrenergic-mediated accumulation of calcium in reperfused myocardium. J Clin Invest 72: 802–818

166. Blaiklock RG, Hirsh EM, Lehr D (1978) Effect of cardiotoxic doses of adrenergic amines on myocardial cyclic AMP. J Mol Cell Cardiol 10: 499–509

167. Yates JC, Beamish RE, Dhalla NS (1981) Ventricular dysfunction and necrosis produced by adrenochrome metabolite of epinephrine: Relation to pathogenesis of catecholamine cardiomyopathy. Am Heart J 102: 210–221

411

168. Heusch G, Deussen A (1983)   The effects of cardiac sympathetic nerve stimulation on perfusion of stenotic coronary arteries in the dog. Circ Res 53: 8–15
169. Mudge GH, Grossman W, Mills RM, Lesch M, Braunwald E (1976)   Reflex increase in coronary vascular resistance in patients with ischemic heart disease. N Engl J Med 295: 1333–1337
170. Haft JI, Gershengorn K, Kranz P, Albert F, Oestreicher R, Fani K (1972)   The role of platelet aggregation in catecholamine-induced cardiac necrosis: Electron microscopic and drug studies. Am J Cardiol 29: 268
171. Haft JI, Fani K (1973)   Intravascular platelet aggregation in the heart induced by stress. Circulation 47: 353–358
172. O'Brian JR (1983)   Some effects of adrenaline and anti-adrenaline compounds on platelets in vitro and in vivo. Nature 200: 763–764
173. Mehta J, Mehta P, Ostrowski N (1985)   Increase in human platelet α-adrenergic receptor affinity for agonist in unstable angina. J Lab Clin Med 106: 661–666
174. Schaal SF, Wallace AG, Sealy WC (1969)   Protective influence of cardiac denervation against arrhythmias of myocardial infarction. Cardiovasc Res 3: 241–244
175. Ebert PA, Vanderbeek RB, Allgood RJ, Sabiston DC Jr (1970) Effect of chronic cardiac denervation on arrhythmias after coronary artery ligation. Cardiovasc Res 4: 141–147
176. Sethi V, Haider B, Ahmed SS, Oldewurtel HA, Regan TJ (1973) Influence of beta blockade and chemical sympathectomy on myocardial function and arrhythmias in acute ischaemia. Cardiovasc Res 7: 740–747
177. Penny WJ (1984)   The deleterious effects of myocardial catecholamines on cellular electrophysiology and arrhythmias during ischaemia and reperfusion. Eur Heart J 5: 960–973
178. Culling W, Penny WJ, Lewis MJ, Middleton K, Sheridan DJ (1984)   Effects of myocardial catecholamine depletion on cellular electrophysiology and arrhythmias during ischaemia and reperfusion. Cardiovasc Res 18: 675–682
179. Daugherty A, Frayn KN, Redfern WS, Woodward B (1986)   The role of catecholamines in the production of ischaemia-induced ventricular arrhythmias in the rat in vivo and in vitro. Br J Pharmacol 87: 265–277
180. Dietz R, Offner B, Dart AM, Schömig A (1989)   Ischaemia-induced noradrenaline release mediates ventricular arrhythmias. In: Brachmann J, Schömig A (eds) Adrenergic System and Ventricular Arrhythmias in Myocardial Infarction. Springer Verlag, Berlin-Heidelberg-New York pp 313–321
181. Wilkerson RD, Sanders PW (1978)   The antiarrhythmic action of amitriptyline on arrhythmias associated with myocardial infarction in dogs. Eur J Pharmacol 51: 193–198
182. Schwartz PJ, Snebold NG, Brown AM (1976)   Effects of unilateral cardiac sympathetic denervation on the ventricular fibrillation threshold. Am J Cardiol 37: 1034–1040
183. Schwartz PJ, Verrier RL, Lown B (1977) Effect of stellectomy and vagotomy on ventricular refractoriness in dogs. Circ Res 40 (Suppl 6): 536–540
184. Lubbe WF, Podzuweit Th, Daries PS, Opie LH (1978)   The role of cyclic adenosine monophosphate in adrenergic effects on ventricular vulnerability to fibrillation in the isolated perfused rat heart. J Clin Invest 63: 1260–1269
185. Pentecost BL, Austein WG (1966)   Beta-adrenergic blockade in experimental myocardial infarction. Am Heart J 72 (6): 790–796
186. Menken U, Wiegand V, Bucher P, Meesmann W (1979) Prophylaxis of ventricular fibrillation after acute experimental coronary occlusion by chronic beta-adrenoceptor blockade with atenolol. Cardiovasc Res 13: 588–594
187. Fearon RE (1967)   Propranolol in the prevention of ventricular fibrillation due to experimental coronary artery occlusion. Am J Cardiol 20: 222–228
188. Kupersmith J, Shiang H, Litwak RS, Herman MV (1976) Electrophysiological and antiarrhythmic effects of propranolol in canine acute myocardial ischemia. Circ Res 38: 302–307
189. Sheridan DJ, Penkoske PA, Sobel BE, Corr PB (1980) Alpha adrenergic contributions to dysrhythmia during myocardial ischemia and reperfusion in cats. J Clin Invest 65: 161–171

190. Stewart JR, Burmeister WE, Burmeister J, Lucchesi BR (1980) Electrophysiologic and antiarrhythmic effects of phentolamine in experimental coronary artery occlusion and reperfusion in the dog. J Cardiovasc Pharmacol 2: 77–91

191. Corr PB, Shayman JA, Kramer JB, Kipnis RJ (1981) Increased α-adrenergic receptors in ischemic cat myocardium. A potential mediator of electrophysiological derangements. J Clin Invest 67: 1232–1236

192. Williams LT, Guerrero JL, Leinbach RC, Gold HK (1982) Prevention of reperfusion dysrhythmias by selective coronary alpha adrenergic blockade. Am J Cardiol 49: 1046

193. Levy MN (1983) Neural control of cardiac rhythm and contraction. Chapter 4. In: Rosen MR, Hoffman BF (eds) Cardiac Therapy. Martinus Nijhoff Publishers, Boston, The Hague, Dodrecht, Lancaster pp 73–94

194. Lazzara R, Marchi S (1989) Electrophysiological mechanisms for the generation of arrhythmias with adrenergic stimulation. In: Brachmann J, Schömig A (eds) Adrenergic System and Ventricular Arrhythmias in Myocardial Infarction. Springer Verlag, New York-Berlin-Heidelberg pp 231–238

195. Coronel R, Fiolet JWT, Wilms-Schopman FJG, Schaapherder AFM, Johnson TA, Gettes IS, Janse MJ (1988) Distribution of extracellular potassium and its relation to electrophysiologic changes during acute myocardial ischemia in isolated perfused porcine heart. Circulation 77: 1125–1138

196. Janse MJ, Cinca J, Morena H, Fiolet JWT, Kleber AG, de Vries GP, Beckert AE, Durrer D (1979) The border zone in myocardial ischemia. An electrophysiological, metabolic and histological correlation in the pig heart. Circ Res 44: 576–588

197. Scherlag BJ, El-Sherif N, Hope RR, Lazzara R (1974) Characterization and localization of ventricular arrhythmias resulting from myocardial ischemia and infarction. Circ Res 35: 372–383

198. Verrier RL, Thompson PL, Lown B (1974) Ventricular vulnerability during sympathetic stimulation: Role of heart rate and blood pressure. Cardiovasc Res 8: 602–610

PART IX

Conclusions

Severe ischemic myocardial injury: Perspectives for therapy

HANS MICHAEL PIPER

Physiologisches Institut 1, Universität Düsseldorf, Moorenstr. 5, D-4000 Düsseldorf 1, FRG

Introduction

It is very much hoped that we might eventually be able to design specific strategies for saving myocardial tissue at different stages of progressive ischemic injury. At the point of irreversible injury, a causal therapeutic approach would have to intervene in the final process in which ischemic cell injury turns into irreversible damage. At present, the causal pathogenetic mechanisms of ischemia and reperfusion are only incompletely understood. Today's clinical therapeutic repertoire already contains a number of remedies applied to the ischemic and reperfused myocardium. For the development of future therapeutic concepts, however, the causal character of these approaches must be scrutinized (see Chapter 2).

It is a basic problem in evaluating 'cardioprotective' therapeutic approaches that most protocols used to test the therapeutic efficacy have only incomplete control of the biological variables. This often leads to an overestimate of the therapeutic value. The efficacy of a certain intervention is overestimated, for example, when the experimental control situation is one in which a crucial threshold in the development of injury has just passed, and a minor protective effect is sufficient to keep the treated sample in a particular state before this decisive threshold. If the degree of protection determined under such conditions is assumed to be generally valid, and the protective effects of different, causally unrelated therapeutic approaches are assessed, one can come to the absurd conclusion that protection of more than 100% is possible. Of course, such fallacies are unavoidable as long as the critical steps of the pathogenetic process remain unknown (Chapter 1).

Energy saving in ischemic myocardium

The development of cell injury in ischemic tissue starts from a deficit in energy production. The energy deficit leads to the slowing down or cessation of important metabolic functions, such as the control of the cellular cation

H.M. Piper (ed.) Pathophysiology of severe ischemic myocardial injury, 415–422.
© *1990 Kluwer Academic Publishers, Dordrecht –*

homeostasis. The key role of energy deprivation in the genesis of ischemic myocardial injury is clarified by the fact that myocardium under metabolic poisoning shows very similar characteristics of injury as ischemic myocardium.

When ischemic conditions persist, the degree of myocardial injury and the extent of energy loss increases. But neither this parallel nor the fact that energy depletion initiates the whole process implies that the final event of cell deterioration represents the immediate causal consequence of energy loss. The discussions in Chapters 3 and 4 show that the causal role of energy loss for the onset of irreversibility in ischemic injury is still unclear.

Most established therapeutic approaches to the ischemic myocardium are based on the principle of energy saving. They reduce myocardial energy demand and thereby prolong the time during which the tissue can be successfully reanimated. In open heart surgery, the most vigorous means of decreasing cardiac energy demand can be applied when the heart-lung machine is used to replace cardiac function. With complete cardioplegia, the main consumer of cardiac energy, i.e. contractile activity, can be omitted. In a patient with acute myocardial ischemia, the myocardial energy demand cannot be reduced quite so drastically, since his survival depends on the remaining hemodynamic function of the afflicted heart. Some savings in energy can be gained by the negative inotropic effect of, for example, β-blockers of calcium antagonists, and by an after-load reduction.

Unfortunately, therapeutic approaches based on energy saving rapidly lose their efficacy for the ischemic myocardium while the process of ischemic injury continues. This is because the myocardial energy demand is only high during the initial phase of ischemia, it decreases rapidly thereafter [1]. Consequently, measures to reduce energy expenditure affect the course of injury development only if they are applied before or very early on in ischemia [2–4]. Energy saving principles, therefore, cannot be used to rescue myocardium near to the pont of irreversible ischemic injury.

Improvement of the supply/demand ratio for the border zone

The amount of tissue jeopardized by ischemic injury after the occlusion of a coronary artery depends on the collateral blood flow to the area of risk. Collateral flow can reduce or completely prevent ischemic injury in the periphery of the affected area. When the oxygen demand in the periphery is low, more tissue can be kept alive by a given amount of collateral oxygen supply and the eventual size of a resulting infarct will be much smaller than the size of the area set at risk by coronary artery occlusion.

Since the oxygen demand of the heart muscle depends on the substrates utilized, the width of the border zone sufficiently supplied by collateral flow may depend on the substrates supplied. The oxidation of fatty acids by the heart muscle is disadvantageous under conditions of limited oxygen availability because it needs up to 30% more oxygen to produce ATP than the oxidation of glucose would need ('oxygen waste') [5]. Therefore, it has been attempted to 'stretch' oxygen supply in the periphery of ischemic tissue by a metabolic change from fatty acid to glucose oxidation [6].

In general, all steps to increase the supply/demand ratio in the periphery of the area at risk will help to reduce the size of the central severely ischemic area. This can be achieved by a reduction in the tissue's energy demand and by augmenting collateral flow. The energy demand can be reduced by negative inotropy. In addition, antiarrhythmic therapy will help to avoid unnecessary energy waste. When catecholamines released from the central ischemic area (Chapter 19) are prevented from stimulating energy metabolism by ß-blockade and from vasoconstriction by α-blockade [7], the supply/demand ratio in the border zone can be improved. Prostacyclin and its stable analogs seem to have a direct inhibitory effect on catecholamine release from ischemic nerve endings (Chapter 10). β-blockade may redistribute part of the coronary blood flow in favor of the collateral connections towards the ischemic area by an increase of vascular tone in the normal myocardium [8]. The use of vasodilators is not advisable unless they act specifically on the collateral vessels supplying the ischemic region, because general vasodilation can cause a diversion of flow away from the area at risk.

Cytoprotection of the ischemic myocardium

The term 'cytoprotective' may be used to characterize means which directly interfere with the causal chain of events leading to irreversible injury within individual myocardial cells. In this book, a number of metabolic mechanisms have been discussed which are suspected to represent key determinants of the development of severe ischemic injury.

The loss of cellular Ca^{2+} homeostasis is a sign of severe cell injury. As outlined in Chapters 14 and 15, the routes by which Ca^{2+} enters the cell are not yet known. Classical calcium antagonists have proved to be ineffective in preventing Ca^{2+} accumulation in the energy depleted myocardial cell (Chapter 15). A group of agents, unrelated to classical calcium antagonists, have been found to diminish or delay Ca^{2+} uptake in hypoxic or ischemic myocardial cells ('calcium entry blockers', Chapter 5). It is not yet known whether their effect is due to direct interference with the mechanism of Ca^{2+} uptake.

An interesting therapeutic approach for the future could be directed towards mitochondrial Ca^{2+} uptake (Chapter 6). At elevated cytosolic Ca^{2+} levels, reoxygenated respiring mitochondria must use part of their respiratory energy for the accumulation of Ca^{2+}. If this unnecessary energy expenditure could be prevented, respiratory energy could all be used for oxidative phosphorylation and mitochondria would also be protected from a massive Ca^{2+} overload. To date, any agents which could diffuse into myocardial cells and specifically block mitochondrial Ca^{2+} uptake have not been identified.

Table 1. Therapeutic interventions that save ischemic-reperfused myocardial tissue

---

1. Interventions which act 'protective' if given long before the manifestation of severe injury (energy savers)
   (a) Cardioplegia (high potassium, low calcium, cooling, Ca-antagonists, local anaesthetics)
   (b) Ca-antagonists
   (c) ß-blockers
      Common principle: Deceleration of energy turnover in the ischemic area.

2. Interventions that reduce infarct size by saving myocardium in the border zone (supply/demand modulators)
   (a) Flow redistribution (α-blockers, Ca-antagonists, ß-blockers)
   (b) Reduction of oxygen demand (reduction of energy demand, reduction of 'oxygen waste', antiarrhythmic drugs)
      Common principle: Improving the supply/demand ratio in the border zone with residual flow.

3. Interventions directed against key events in the pathogenesis of severe ischemia-reperfusion injury (cytoprotectives)
   (a) Blockers of calcium entry (sarcolemma, mitochondria)
   (b) Blockers of cross-bridge cycling
   (c) Phospholipase inhibitors
   (d) Anti-free radical interventions (scavengers, inhibitors of production)
   (e) Prevention of fatty acid accumulation
   (f) Lysosome stabilization
      Common principle: Direct interference with the pathogenesis of severe injury on the level of the myocardial cell.

4. Interventions which secure the effect of successful reperfusion (post-ischemic stabilizers)
   (a) Antihemostatic therapy
   (b) Vasodilators
   (c) Anti-inflammatory therapy
   (d) Antiarrhythmic drugs
      Common principle: Prevention of secondary reactions which can jeopardize a primarily successful reperfusion

---

Resumption of oxidative phosphorylation at the onset of reperfusion creates a dangerous situation in those myocardial cells which have accumulated high cytosolic levels of Ca^{2+} during ischemia. This is because the myofibrils develop contracture under these conditions (Chapters 16 and 17), with the consequence of massive disruption of cell structures. Drugs which could reduce myofibrillar cross-bridge cycling for the time needed to re-establish a normal cytosolic Ca^{2+} level could be a useful means of preventing severe reperfusion injury [9].

In ischemia, the cardiomyocyte becomes seemingly more fragile (Chapter 17) and this may be partly due to the hydrolysis of phospholipids in the sarcolemma (Chapter 9). A 'weakening' of the sarcolemmal structure, together with changes in the cytoskeletal connections between the sarcolemma and underlying cell structures, may facilitate cell deterioration.

Whether a loss of phospholipids from the sarcolemma during the reversible phase of cell injury is in itself so extensive that it is the immediate cause of sarcolemmal disruption, can be questioned from studies on hypoxic isolated cells [9]. It has been shown that phospholipase inhibitors exert a 'protective' effect on energy-depleted heart muscle cells, but the evidence that this effect is causally related to phospholipid stabilization is inconclusive (Chapter 9).

The importance of free radicals in the genesis of ischemic and reperfusion injury has been extensively discussed in recent years. As outlined in Chapters 6, 11, 12, 13 and 18, it is still a matter of debate whether oxygen radicals play a decisive role in the primary pathogenetic process of ischemia-reperfusion. If they do, they may exert part of their effect through the peroxidation of fatty acids in the phospholipid pool, which then become more easily attacked by phospholipases [10]. Therefore, both anti-free radical interventions (scavengers, inhibitors of production) and phospholipase inhibitors may act together to reduce the threat from oxygen radicals.

These pathogenetic mechanisms are by no means the only factor in the genesis of severe injury in ischemia-reperfusion. The accumulation of free fatty acids or fatty acyl carnitine or coenzyme A esters could also contribute to the development of cell injury. *In vitro*, amphiphilic long-chain acyl compounds in high concentrations can destabilize cell membranes by a detergent-like action (Chapter 8). It is not clear, though, whether they reach comparable intracellular free concentrations in the myocardial cell during the reversible phase of ischemia, as a large amount of these lipids can be bound to intracellular proteins, particularly the fatty acid binding protein.

The instability of lysosomes in the ischemic myocardial cell leads to the release of lysosomal enzymes which can attack cell structures thereby increasing cell injury. A cardioprotective effect of stabilization of lysosomes in the ischemic myocardial cell has been reported (Chapter 7). But the crucial role in the basic causal mechanism of cell injury in ischemia-reperfusion. has not yet been established.

Our knowledge is at present insufficient to state definitely which aspects of the complex process of changes in the ischemia-reoxygenated myocardial cell are of primary importance in the development of irreversible injury. This has the corollary that the primary targets of causal therapy are not clearly identified. It has recently been argued [9] that low energy levels and high cytosolic Ca^{2+} concentrations are common to all models of the ischemic/hypoxic myocardial cell at the point of impending irreversible injury. When the cell is reoxygenated under these conditions, contracture develops. In tissue, this leads to a mutual disruption of the cells, possibly facilitated by an increased fragility of the cells. In this context, the roles of phospholipid degradation, detergent effects of amphiphilic lipids, and free radical attack of cell structures are of only secondary importance. Accordingly, therapeutic efforts should be primarily directed towards the search for effective means of preventing Ca^{2+} uptake during ischemia/hypoxia and blocking Ca^{2+}-induced myofibrillar contracture during reperfusion.

Post-ischemic stabilization of the reperfused myocardium

Since the thrombotic occlusion of a coronary artery is the most common natural cause of myocardial ischemia, antihemostatic therapy is a basic element of all post-ischemic treatment. When a thrombotic occlusion was removed by physical force (such as balloon dilatation, laser abrasion), this site of the vessel wall is largely denuded from a functional endothelium and, therefore, also from its antithrombogenic potency. Lesions of the vessel wall further increase the probability of new thrombus formation. For these reasons, antihemostatic therapy is considered to be essential for the reperfused myocardium.

A re-occlusion of a successfully re-opened coronary artery may be due to a vasospasm. This may occur for a number of reasons; a deficit in the endothelium-dependent mechanism of vascular relaxation was recently discovered as such a possibility. Such a deficit is probably not confined to the acute phase of endothelial cell damage at the site of intervention, but seems to persist in the regenerating endothelium. It has been shown [11] that regenerating endothelium has a reduced capacity to produce the endothelium-derived relaxing factor.

Cell injury in the ischemic myocardium leads to the attraction and activation of leukocytes in the reperfused tissue. The release of hydrogen peroxide and proteolytic enzymes from these cells can damage the myocardial tissue at a time when it would otherwise have the best conditions to recover, since blood supply is re-established. As discussed in Chapter 12, therapeutic approaches are currently being investigated which may reduce the harmful potency of leukocytes to the reperfused myocardium.

Conclusions

Most currently used therapeutic approaches to ischemic and reperfused myocardium do not directly interfere, in all probability, with the crucial causal events in the development of myocardial cell injury in ischemia/reperfusion. Part of the therapy in the clinical emergency situation is not directed to the ischemic tissue itself, but is designed to avoid or lessen the consequences of cardiac failure (e.g. antiarrhythmic therapy). All therapeutic approaches to the ischemic tissue depend on the residual flow of blood into the ischemic area. Under favorable circumstances the flow can be augmented, thereby improving access to the injured tissue.

Measures designed to reduce energy expenditure of the tissue in the center of the ischemic area, where the blood supply is negligible, are only effective if given before or at the onset of ischemia. Later on, they can still improve the condition of the tissue in the periphery of this area by improving its supply/demand ratio. This ratio can also be enlarged by increasing the residual blood supply to the ischemic area. But vasodilators will only increase the blood supply to the ischemic area if the connecting vessels to the ischemic area are exclusively or at least predominantly dilated, general vasodilation may even lead to a diversion of the residual blood flow away from the collateral network.

Therapeutic approaches interfering directly with the causal key events in the process of ischemic cell deterioration are by no means completely established, mainly because of the lack of basic knowledge of the pathophysiology of severe ischemic/reoxygenation injury. Therapeutic principles of this kind, however, are much needed in the face of today's widespread use of techniques for the acute re-opening of coronary occlusions. In reperfused myocardium, attempts to improve the supply/demand ratio of the injured myocardial tissue are not really necessary since supply is re-established by the re-opening and demand is low due to the progressed stage of cell injury. It is a challenge for future research to find ways of interrupting the causal process of progressive injury and to prevent the immediate dangers of reperfusion (oxygen paradox injury). The next concern after the initial phase of successful reperfusion is to maintain the achieved state in order to allow the myocardial cells to recover.

Acknowledgements

This study was supported by the Deutsche Forschungsgemeinschaft, grants Pi 162/2–1 and A6 of SFB 242.

References

1. Kübler W, Spieckermann PG (1970) Regulation of glycolysis in the ischemic and the anoxic myocardium. J Mol Cell Cardiol 1: 351–377
2. Hearse DH, Yellon DM, Downey JM (1986) Can beta-blockers limit myocardial infarct size? Eur Heart J 11: 925–930
3. Cheung JY, Bonventre JV, Malis CD, Leaf A (1986) Calcium and ischemic injury. New Engl J Med 314: 1670–1676
4. Reimer KA, Jennings RB, Cobb FR, Murdock RH, Greenfield JC, Becker LC, Bulkley BH, Hutchins GM, Schwartz RP, Bailey KR, Passamani ER (1985) Animal models for protecting ischaemic myocardium: results of the NHLBI cooperative study. Comparison of conscious and unconscious dog models. Circ Res 56: 651–665
5. Hütter JF, Piper HM, Spieckermann PG (1985) Effects of fatty acid oxidation on efficiency of energy production in rat heart. Am J Physiol 249: H723–H728
6. Kjekshus JK, Mjos OD (1973) Effect of lipolysis on infarct size after experimental coronary artery occlusion. J Clin Invest 52: 1770–1778
7. Heusch G, Deussen A (1983) The effects of cardiac sympathetic nerve stimulation on the perfusion of stenotic coronary arteries in the dog. Circ Res 53: 8–15
8. Buck JD, Hardman HF, Warltier DC, Gross GJ (1981) Changes in ischemic blood flow distribution and dynamic severity of a coronary stenosis induced by beta blockade in the canine heart. Circulation 64: 708–715
9. Piper HM (1989) Energy deficiency, calcium overload or oxidative stress: possible causes of irreversible ischemic myocardial injury. Klin Wschr 67: 465–476

10. Weglicki BW, Dickens BF, Mak IT (1984) Enhanced lysosomal phospholipid degradation and lysophospholipid production due to free radicals. Biochem Biophys Res Commun 124: 229–235
11. Shimokawa H, Aarhus LL, Vanhoutte PM (1987) Porcine coronary arteries with regenerated endothelium have a reduced endothelium-dependent responsiveness to aggregating platelets and serotonin. Circ Res 61: 256–270

Index

426

Developments in Cardiovascular Medicine

Developments in Cardiovascular Medicine

100. J. Morganroth and E.N. Moore (eds.): *Risk/Benefit Analysis for the Use and Approval of Thrombolytic, Antiarrhythmic, and Hypolipidemic Agents.* Proceedings of the 9th Annual Symposium on New Drugs and Devices (1988). (forthcoming)
ISBN 0–7923–0294–X

101. P.W. Serruys, R. Simon and K.J. Beatt (eds.): *PCTA – An Investigational Tool and a Non-operative Treatment of Acute Ischemia.* 1990   ISBN 0–7923–0346–6

102. I.S. Anand, P.I. Wahi and N.S. Dhalla (eds.): *Pathophysiology and Pharmacology of Heart Disease.* 1990 (forthcoming)   ISBN 0–7923–0367–9

103. G.S. Abela (ed.): *Lasers in Cardiovascular Medicine and Surgery.* Fundamentals and Technique. 1990 (forthcoming)   ISBN 0–7923–0440–3

104. H.M. Piper (ed.): *Pathophysiology of Severe Ischemic Myocardial Injury.* 1990
ISBN 0–7923–0459–4

105. S.M. Teague (ed.): *Stress Doppler Echocardiography.* 1990   ISBN 0–7923–0499–3

106. P.R. Saxena, D.I. Wallis, W. Wouters and P. Bevan (eds.): *Cardiovascular Pharmacology of 5-Hydroxytryptamine.* Prospective Therapeutic Applications. 1990
ISBN 0–7923–0502–7

107. A.P. Shepherd and P.A. Öberg (eds.): *Laser-Doppler Blood Flowmetry.* 1990 (forthcoming)   ISBN 0–7923–0508–6

108. J. Soler-Soler, G. Permanyer-Miralda and J. Sagristà-Sauleda (eds.): *Pericardial Disease.* New Insights and Old Dilemmas. 1990   ISBN 0–7923–0510–8

109. J.P.M. Hamer: *Practical Echocardiography in the Adult.* With Doppler and Color Doppler Flow Imaging. 1990 (forthcoming).   ISBN 0–7923–0670–8

110. A. Bayés de Luna, P. Brugada, J. Cosin Aguilar and F. Navarro Lopez (eds.): *Sudden Cardiac Death.* 1990 (forthcoming)   ISBN 0–7923–0716–X

111. E. Andries and R. Stroobandt (eds.): *Hemodynamics in Daily Practice.* 1990 (forthcoming)   ISBN 0–7923–0725–9